RADIOLOGY SECRETS

DOUGLAS S. KATZ, MD
Assistant Professor of Radiology
State University of New York at Stony Brook
Stony Brook, New York
Associate Attending Radiologist
Winthrop-University Hospital
Mineola, New York

KEVIN R. MATH, MD
Assistant Professor of Radiology
Albert Einstein College of Medicine
Attending Radiologist
Physician-in-Charge of Musculoskeletal Imaging
Beth Israel Medical Center
New York, New York

STUART A. GROSKIN, MD
Associate Professor of Radiology and Medicine
State University of New York Health Science Center at Syracuse
Attending Radiologist
Chief, Section of Thoracic Imaging
University Hospital
Syracuse, New York

HANLEY & BELFUS, INC./ Philadelphia

Publisher: HANLEY & BELFUS, INC.
Medical Publishers
210 South 13th Street
Philadelphia, PA 19107
(215) 546-7293; 800-962-1892
FAX (215) 790-9330

United States sales and distribution:

Mosby
11830 Westline Industrial Drive
St. Louis, MO 63146

Note to the reader: Although the information in this book has been carefully reviewed for correctness of dosage and indications, neither the authors nor the editors nor the publisher can accept any legal responsibility for any errors or omissions that may be made. Neither the publisher nor the editors make any warranty, expressed or implied, with respect to the material contained herein. Experimental compounds and off-label uses of approved products are discussed. Before prescribing any drug, the reader must review the manufacturer's current product information (package inserts) for accepted indications, absolute dosage recommendations, and other information pertinent to the safe and effective use of the product described.

Library of Congress Cataloging-in-Publication Data

Katz, Douglas S., 1964–
    Radiology secrets / Douglas S. Katz, Kevin R. Math, Stuart A. Groskin.
        p.   cm. — (The Secrets Series)
    Includes bibliographical references and index.
    ISBN 1-56053-158-4 (alk. paper)
    1. Radiography, Medical—Examinations, questions, etc. I. Math,
Kevin R., 1962–   . II. Groskin, Stuart A., 1949–   . III. Title.
IV. Series.
    [DNLM: 1. Radiology—examination questions. WN 18.2 K19r 1997]
RC78.15.K38   1997
616.07'54'076—dc21
DNLM/DLC
for Library of Congress   97-31327
                                                                CIP

RADIOLOGY SECRETS   ISBN 1-56053-158-4

Last digit is the print number: 9 8 7 6 5 4 3 2

CONTENTS

CONTRIBUTORS

Michael M. Abiri, M.D.
Chairman and Associate Professor, Department of Radiology, Albert Einstein College of Medicine; Chairman, Department of Radiology, Beth Israel Medical Center, New York, New York

Ralf R. Barckhausen, M.D.
Chief Resident, Department of Diagnostic Radiology, Long Island College Hospital, Brooklyn, New York

Julie Barudin, M.D.
Department of Radiology and Breast Imaging, Hackensack University Medical Center, Hackensack, New Jersey

Richard D. Bellah, M.D.
Associate Professor of Radiology and Pediatrics, University of Pennsylvania School of Medicine; Department of Radiology, Children's Hospital of Philadelphia, Philadelphia, Pennsylvania

Robert J. Botash, M.D.
Assistant Professor, Department of Radiology, State University of New York Health Science Center at Syracuse, Syracuse, New York

Fred D. Cushner, M.D.
Director, Insall-Scott-Kelly Institute for Orthopaedics and Sports Medicine, New York, New York

Douglas R. DeCorato, M.D.
Assistant Professor of Radiology, Albert Einstein College of Medicine; Attending Radiologist, Beth Israel Medical Center, New York, New York

Corey D. Eber, M.D.
Assistant Professor, Department of Radiology, Albert Einstein College of Medicine, Beth Israel Medical Center, New York, New York

Ali M. Gharagozloo, M.D.
Clinical Instructor, Department of Radiology, State University of New York Health Science Center at Syracuse, Syracuse, New York

Bernard Ghelman, M.D.
Associate Professor of Radiology, Cornell University Medical College; Attending Radiologist, Hospital for Special Surgery, New York, New York

Eric L. Gingold, Ph.D.
Diagnostic Imaging Physicist, Department of Radiology, Hospital of the University of Pennsylvania, Philadelphia, Pennsylvania

Louise B. Godine, M.D.
Assistant Professor of Radiology, Albert Einstein College of Medicine; Attending Pediatric Radiologist, Beth Israel Medical Center, New York, New York

Burton M. Gold, M.D.
Associate Professor of Clinical Radiology, State University of New York at Stony Brook, Stony Brook, New York; Associate Chairman and Attending Radiologist, Department of Radiology, Winthrop-University Hospital, Mineola, New York

Stuart A. Groskin, M.D.
Associate Professor of Radiology and Medicine, State University of New York Health Science Center at Syracuse; Attending Radiologist and Chief, Section of Thoracic Imaging, University Hospital, Syracuse, New York

Zachary D. Grossman, M.D., FACR
Professor of Radiology, State University of New York at Buffalo; Chairman, Department of Radiology, The Roswell Park Cancer Institute, Buffalo, New York

Jonathan Hartman, M.D.
Chief Resident, Department of Radiology, Beth Israel Medical Center, New York, New York

M. Patricia Harty, M.D.
Assistant Professor, Department of Radiology, University of Pennsylvania School of Medicine; Staff Radiologist, Children's Hospital of Philadelphia, Philadelphia, Pennsylvania

Leo Hochhauser, M.D., FRCPC
Associate Professor of Radiology, Division of Neuroradiology, State University of New York Health Science Center at Syracuse; University Hospital, Syracuse, New York

Sunah A. Kang Feng, M.D.
House Officer, Department of Radiology, Beth Israel Medical Center, New York, New York

Douglas S. Katz, M.D.
Assistant Professor of Radiology, State University of New York at Stony Brook, Stony Brook, New York; Associate Attending Radiologist, Winthrop-University Hospital, Mineola, New York

Kim Kramer, M.D.
Instructor in Pediatrics, Cornell University Medical College; Attending Pediatrician, Memorial Sloan-Kettering Cancer Center, New York, New York

Terry L. Levin, M.D.
Clinical Associate Professor of Radiology, New York Medical College, Valhalla, New York; Attending Radiologist, St. Agnes Hospital, White Plains, New York

David P. C. Liu, M.D.
Assistant Professor of Radiology, Albert Einstein College of Medicine; Department of Radiology, Beth Israel Medical Center, New York, New York

William Kennedy Main, M.D.
Spine Surgeon, Department of Orthopaedic Surgery, Hospital for Special Surgery, New York, New York

Edward Math, M.D.
Radiology Resident, Duke University Medical Center, Durham, North Carolina

Kevin R. Math, M.D.
Assistant Professor of Radiology, Albert Einstein College of Medicine; Attending Radiologist and Physician-in-Charge of Musculoskeletal Imaging, Beth Israel Medical Center, New York, New York

Kenneth D. Murphy, M.D.
Assistant Professor and Interventional Radiology Fellowship Program Director, Department of Radiology, State University of New York Health Science Center at Syracuse, Syracuse, New York

Elmer Nahum, M.D.
Department of Radiology, State University of New York Health Science Center at Syracuse, University Hospital, Syracuse, New York

Susan Orel, M.D.
Assistant Professor, Department of Radiology, University of Pennsylvania School of Medicine; Presbyterian Hospital, Hospital of the University of Pennsylvania, Philadelphia, Pennsylvania

Rhonda P. Osborne, M.D.
Assistant Professor, Department of Radiology, Ultrasound Division, Long Island College Hospital, Brooklyn, New York

Steven Perlmutter, M.D.
Clinical Assistant Professor, Department of Radiology, State University of New York at Stony Brook, Stony Brook, New York; Chief, Genitourinary Section of Radiology, Winthrop-University Hospital, Mineola, New York

Robert B. Poster, M.D.
Associate Professor, Department of Radiology, State University of New York Health Science Center at Syracuse; University Hospital, Syracuse, New York

Carolyn L. Raia, M.D.
Attending Radiologist, Staten Island University Hospital, Staten Island, New York

Ernest M. Scalzetti, M.D.
Associate Professor of Radiology, State University of New York Health Science Center at Syracuse; University Hospital, Syracuse, New York

Giles R. Scuderi, M.D.
Associate Chief, Adult Knee Reconstruction, Beth Israel Medical Center; Director, Insall-Scott-Kelly Institute for Orthopaedics and Sports Medicine, New York, New York

Natalie Strutynsky, M.D.
Assistant Professor, Department of Radiology, Albert Einstein College of Medicine, Beth Israel Medical Center, New York, New York

John J. Wasenko, M.D.
Associate Professor, Department of Radiology, State University of New York Health Science Center at Syracuse, Syracuse, New York

Mark A. Westcott, M.D.
Department of Radiology, Beth Israel Medical Center, New York, New York

Barbara Zeifer, M.D.
Assistant Clinical Professor of Radiology, Albert Einstein College of Medicine; Section Director, Head and Neck Imaging, Beth Israel Medical Center; Director of Radiology, New York Eye and Ear Infirmary, New York, New York

DEDICATIONS

To the "Four Musketeers," Mark F, Dave "Sammy" F, Lon M, and Johnny "the Hawk" Z

To Evan M and Allison M for their friendship

To the Smiths for their continued mentorship in both medicine and life

Douglas S. Katz, MD

To the memory of my grandparents, Max, Tillie, Ben, and Etta

To my wonderful wife, Kim, and my parents, Ann and Philip

Kevin R. Math, MD

To my mother, Thelma, and my father, Morris, whose courage, love, and integrity have been and will always be a source of inspiration for me

To Jonathan and Margo, the two other most courageous and loving people I know

To Bryan, who, in going his own way, is becoming a fine young man

Stuart A. Groskin, MD

PREFACE

Radiology has undergone enormous technologic advancements and ever-broadening clinical applications since Roentgen discovered the x-ray in 1895. The progressive refinement of conventional radiography and the development of more sophisticated imaging modalities such as ultrasound, CT, and MRI have allowed radiology to emerge as one of the most exciting and challenging fields in medicine. A working knowledge of the principles of radiology is a powerful diagnostic tool, allowing one to translate the information on an image into a specific differential diagnosis, which can then be used to treat a patient. Radiology is a unique field in that it has applications in every specialty and subspecialty in medicine, and imaging studies are encountered by all health care deliverers, including physicians, medical students, physicians' assistants, and nurses. The specialty is ubiquitous, with radiology studies encountered on rounds, in conferences, in medical offices, and on examinations.

In *Radiology Secrets*, we have distilled an enormous amount of information in diagnostic and clinical radiology into 84 chapters, each written by a physician who subspecializes in that particular topic. Many of the most useful and practical facts and principles in radiology are passed down from one radiologist to the next in a manner that is difficult to duplicate in standard texts. Through the proven question-and-answer format of the Secrets Series®, we have attempted to pass down hundreds of the most valuable radiology pearls and concepts we have learned over the years that will prove useful in any medical specialty. Since radiology is a visual field, a large number of illustrative images and diagrams are included. Clinical and therapeutic concepts, as they pertain to radiology, are also included throughout the book. In radiology, more than any other field, the eye does not see what the mind does not know. It is our hope that reading this book will allow you to know more, see more, and as a result, be able to provide better patient care.

Douglas S. Katz, M.D.
Kevin R. Math, M.D.
Stuart A. Groskin, M.D.

ACKNOWLEDGMENTS

Douglas Katz would like to acknowledge Dr. Kevin Math, who initiated this book, and without whose work this book would not have been possible; Drs. Murphy and Groskin, for their contributions to the interventional and chest sections, respectively; Drs. Gold and Perlmutter, for their editorial assistance with the gastroenterology and genitourinary sections (without their teaching files, these sections could not have been completed); and Dr. R. Brooke Jeffrey, for his general guidance during my fellowship at Stanford University Hospital. Many of the cases in this book (too many to individually acknowledge) were obtained during my fellowship, and I am much indebted to Dr. Jeffrey and to the Radiology Department at Stanford.

Kevin Math would like to acknowledge all radiologists at the Hospital for Special Surgery, New York City, for their teaching and continued collegiality (many of the radiographs in the musculoskeletal section were collected during my fellowship at HSS, and some are from their teaching files); Mrs. Jewel Ann Kramer for outstanding secretarial assistance; Seuk Ky Kim, M.D., Syracuse, New York, for providing all images in the chapter on Peptic Ulcer Disease; and Mr. Richard Matthias for high-quality medical photography.

I. Principles of Diagnostic Imaging

1. PHYSICS OF CONVENTIONAL RADIOGRAPHY

Eric L. Gingold, Ph.D.

1. How is a radiograph produced?

X-rays emanate from a small point source and pass through a portion of the body and onto a detector that records the x-rays that reach the detector as an image.

2. What are x-rays?

X-radiation is electromagnetic radiation that is capable of causing ionization in matter due to its high energy content. In human tissue, the ionization can cause damage to DNA and cells, but it can also penetrate the body to allow noninvasive visualization of the internal anatomy. X-rays can exhibit particle-like behavior, and the individual x-ray "particles," which are discrete packets of pure energy, are called photons.

3. Where do x-rays come from?

When an electron in an atom makes a transition from an outer orbital to an inner orbital, radiation is emitted. Such a transition will occur if the atom has a vacancy in an inner electron shell and is thus in an excited or unstable state. The emitted radiation can be in the visible, ultraviolet, or x-ray portions of the electromagnetic spectrum and is known as characteristic radiation because its energy content is uniquely characteristic of the atomic species that produced it.

4. What is a second mechanism by which x-rays can be produced?

If an electron beam is accelerated toward and hits a metal target, a shower of radiation is produced by the interaction. If the electrons that compose the beam are accelerated with enough voltage, the radiation produced will be in the x-ray portion of the electromagnetic spectrum. Such x-radiation is known as "bremsstrahlung," a German term meaning "braking radiation."

5. How are x-rays produced in diagnostic radiology?

By a vacuum tube device called the x-ray tube (Fig. 1). The tube contains a tungsten filament (the cathode) and a metal target (the anode), also usually made of tungsten. The filament is heated with an electric current, and a high voltage is placed between the anode and the cathode. The high voltage causes electrons in the filament to be drawn off and accelerated toward the anode. When

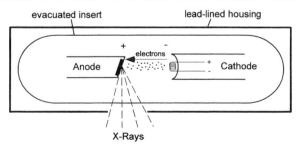

FIGURE 1. The basic components of a diagnostic x-ray tube.

they strike the anode, bremsstrahlung and characteristic x-rays (characteristic of the anode metal) are produced. The x-ray tube is completely surrounded by lead on all sides, except for a small exit port. The lead absorbs most of the emitted x-rays except for the portion that escapes through the port. These x-rays are used to create the radiograph.

6. What ancillary components are required to complete a radiography system?

A high-voltage generator supplies the required power to the x-ray tube (Fig. 2). A collimator is placed at the tube exit port to limit the extent of the x-ray field. An electronic timer is used to keep the x-ray exposure to a precise, finite duration. Phototiming circuits are used to automatically terminate exposures after a certain amount of radiation has been received by the image receptor (the "automatic exposure control"). The technologist selects all operating parameters and initiates the exposure at a control console.

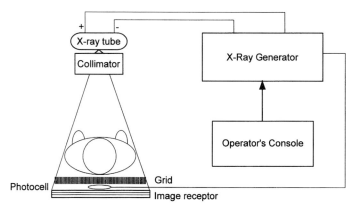

FIGURE 2. The basic components and layout of an x-ray imaging system.

7. What is an image receptor, and how does it record the radiographic image?

An image receptor is a device that can detect and record an x-ray image. It is placed on the opposite side of the patient as the x-ray tube. The patient's anatomy modulates the intensity of the x-ray field as it passes through. That is, differential radiation absorption and transmission by various tissue types results in an exit beam that varies in intensity in two dimensions. This x-ray field reaches a detector that absorbs and records the the two-dimensional intensity distribution.

8. What types of image receptors are used in diagnostic radiology?
- Photographic film, coupled with an intensifying phosphor screen
- Storage phosphor screens
- Direct digital readout devices

9. How does the intensifying screen-radiographic film combination work?

An intensifying, or fluorescent, screen consists of a sheet of polyester plastic coated with a phosphor layer that absorbs x-rays and emits visible light (blue or green) in response. A typical radiographic cassette consists of a pair of intensifying screens, with a sheet of double emulsion film sandwiched between. The double emulsion film is also a sheet of polyester plastic, coated on both sides with a photosensitive emulsion of silver halide (bromide and iodide) and gelatin. The film records the visible light image emitted by the intensifying screens in response to irradiation by x-rays. Photographic x-ray film also is used to store the image and as a display device when used in conjunction with a viewbox light source. Modern x-ray film can be stored for decades without loss of image quality.

10. Why are two intensifying (phosphor) screens used rather than one?

Two phosphor screens are more efficient at detecting x-rays than a single screen, but this improved efficiency comes at the expense of sharpness.

11. For what radiographic procedure are single screen/film combinations used?

Because sharpness is of paramount importance in mammography, specialized single screen/emulsion cassettes are used exclusively for mammography.

12. What is a storage phosphor system?

Photostimulable phosphor, or storage phosphor, technology was introduced in the early 1980s as a means to obtain radiographs in digital form, suitable for computer-based storage and processing. This technology is known commercially as computed radiography (CR). Like conventional screen-film imaging, a photostimulable phosphor (PSP) system also uses a cassette containing a screen coated with phosphor.

13. How does the storage phosphor differ from the phosphor used for generating conventional radiographs?

Unlike the phosphor used in intensifying screens that emits visible light immediately upon absorption of x-rays (fluorescence), the phosphor in PSP systems responds to irradiation with x-rays by storing electrical charge in a pattern corresponding to the pattern of absorbed x-ray intensity. This pattern is read later by a scanning laser device that causes localized heating of the phosphor and stimulation of the meta-stable trapped charge. Upon heating, the trapped charge is converted to visible light (delayed luminescence), which is then converted to electrical current by a photomultiplier tube, and is digitized and stored as a digital image in a computer.

14. How does the direct digital detector work?

The direct electronic capture of the radiographic image, without the need for storage phosphor cassettes and subsequent laser readout or digitization of photographic film, is the future direction of digital radiography. Several investigators have reported building successful prototype devices with a variety of technologies. These detectors convert the radiographic image (the two-dimensional distribution of x-ray intensities) into an electrical signal that can be digitized. Detectors of this design have the potential for having better spatial resolution and less noise than storage phosphor systems and can be mounted permanently in x-ray tables to eliminate cassette handling by technologists.

15. What else is needed to generate high quality diagnostic radiographs?

• Scatter control
• Proper radiographic technique
• Technical image quality control program

16. What is scatter?

In addition to the x-rays that pass straight through the body and contribute to the radiographic image, other x-rays are absorbed or scattered by the tissue. The scattered x-rays are deflected from their original path but can still strike the image receptor. These x-ray photons blur the image, reduce contrast, and increase image noise, which is unwanted background "fog" that does not contain useful information.

17. How can scatter be controlled?

Grids are the most common method. A grid, a device placed directly in front of the image receptor, consists of a series of closely-spaced lead strips that are oriented such that x-rays that are scattered in the patient are absorbed preferentially and unscattered photons pass through. The grid thus filters out a fraction of the scattered radiation and improves image quality (see Fig. 2).

18. What contributes to proper radiographic technique?

Selection of the appropriate parameters by the technologist, sometimes with the aid of an automatic exposure control system. The technique must be chosen carefully to produce an optimally exposed radiograph with acceptable image contrast.

19. What are the components of a technical quality control program?

Quality control is but one component of a radiology department's overall quality assurance program. Image quality is optimized while radiation exposure to patients and staff is kept minimal. Such a program should include peer review of film interpretation by other radiologists in the department, monitoring of patient service times, evaluation of the time it takes to complete a report, and other performance measures. Technical image quality control includes continual tracking of film processor stability, regular performance evaluations of imaging equipment, and monitoring of radiation doses to patients and staff.

20. What is fluoroscopy?

Fluoroscopy is real-time radiography. Fluoroscopic systems allow continuous viewing of a time-varying x-ray image and permit live visual evaluation of dynamic events. The original fluoroscopy systems used fluorescent screens like those used in radiographic cassettes. Radiologists would view the light image emitted from the screens directly, as the patient was exposed. Modern fluoroscopy systems use an x-ray image intensifier, which converts the x-ray energy to visible light and is coupled optically to a television camera. The fluoroscopic image is viewed on a cathode-ray tube video monitor, located either in the fluoroscopy room beside the patient, or else in a remote location (Fig. 3).

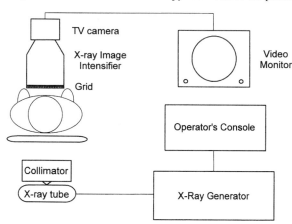

FIGURE 3. The basic components and layout of an intensified fluoroscopy system, with an "undertable" x-ray tube.

21. What are the technical requirements for modern mammography systems?

The need to visualize small, low-contrast details while maintaining a low absorbed radiation dose in the breast has led to a number of technical developments: dose-efficient single screen/single emulsion screen film combinations, small focus x-ray tubes, fine antiscatter grids, and breast compression techniques that control the amount of scatter reaching the image receptor.

22. What is computed tomography?

Computed tomography (CT) allows cross-sectional imaging of anatomy using x-rays. CT has very specialized equipment needs, including linear arrays of electronic radiation detectors, high heat-capacity x-ray tubes, rotating gantries, fast computer hardware, and advanced image reconstruction and image processing algorithms.

23. What are some advantages of a modern angiography system?

Small vessels can be seen using fluoroscopic equipment capable of high spatial resolution, large fields of view, and rapid digital acquisition of images.

24. What is digital subtraction angiography?

Images acquired after the administration of an iodinated contrast agent are subtracted from an image obtained before contrast was injected. This subtraction removes the appearance of stationary anatomy from the resulting images and synthesizes a sequence of images containing only contrast in the blood vessels. Each image in the sequence reveals a different stage in the filling of vessels with contrast.

25. What technical developments have made digital subtraction angiography possible?

Small focus, high-output x-ray tubes, advances in x-ray image intensifier technology, fast computers, and high-speed, large-capacity computer disk drives.

26. What determines image quality?

While image quality can be subjective and its definition may change depending on the information desired from a given image, the three basic components of image quality that can always be applied are contrast, noise, and spatial resolution.

27. What is contrast?

The difference in signal between two regions of an image. In a gray-scale image, where signal differences are represented by varying shades of gray (or brightness), high contrast means that two objects of different composition in the image appear very dark and very light. In a lower contrast image, there is less difference in relative brightness.

28. What are the two components of image contrast?

Subject contrast and film contrast. Subject contrast is the inherent difference in signal (intensity of x-rays passing through) between two objects. Film contrast refers to the ability of the film to record the subject contrast and present it to the viewer on a lightbox. In digital imaging systems, the image receptor and display device are decoupled, and we must consider "detector contrast" and "display contrast" independently. Video display devices allow the viewer to control the display contrast to suit the need.

29. What is noise?

Noise describes any signal component in an image that does not convey useful information. There are two general types of noise: random noise and structured noise. Random noise, also known as quantum noise or quantum mottle, refers to the graininess of an image and depends on the number of photons used to record the image. An image that was recorded with many photons will appear to be less noisy, or have a higher "signal-to-noise" ratio, than an image composed of few photons. The more random noise in an image, the more difficult it is to perceive low-contrast information.

30. What is structured noise?

Nonrandom image components that do not originate with the subject being imaged. Artifacts introduced by the imaging system or film processor are examples.

31. What is spatial resolution?

The ability of an image to faithfully reproduce small details. An image that allows the viewer to see more fine detail and small objects than another image of the same subject is said to have higher spatial resolution, also called sharpness. "Blur" indicates lack of spatial resolution.

BIBLIOGRAPHY

1. Antonuk LE, Boudry J, Huang W, et al: Demonstration of megavoltage and diagnostic x-ray imaging with hydrogenated amorphous silicon arrays. Med Phys 19:1455–1456, 1992.
2. Bushberg JT, Seibert JA, Leidholdt EM Jr, Boone JM: The Essential Physics of Medical Imaging. Baltimore, Williams & Wilkins, 1994.
3. Curry TS III: Christensen's Introduction to the Physics of Diagnostic Radiology, 4th ed. Malvern, PA, Lea & Febiger, 1990.
4. Lee DL, Cheung LK, Jeromin LS: A new digital detector for projection radiography. SPIE 2432:237–249, 1995.
5. Sprawls P Jr: Physical Principles of Medical Imaging, 2nd ed. Gaithersburg, MD, Aspen Publishers, 1993.
6. Zhao W, Rowlands JA: A large area solid-state detector for radiology using amorphous selenium. SPIE 1651:133–134, 1992.

2. RADIATION SAFETY AND PROTECTION

Eric L. Gingold, Ph.D.

1. Is the radiation used in diagnostic radiology harmful?

Potentially, yes. In actual practice, adverse health effects from ionizing radiation used in diagnostic radiology are extremely rare.

2. What are the potential harmful effects of ionizing radiation?

The effects can be classified into two broad categories: stochastic effects and deterministic effects.

3. What are stochastic effects?

Effects in which the probability of occurrence increases with radiation exposure. Examples of stochastic responses are carcinogenesis and genetic effects. An important property of these effects is that the probability, but not the severity of the endpoint condition, is related to the quantity of the radiation dose.

4. What is meant by deterministic effects?

Deterministic effects are associated with a threshold radiation dose, below which the effect is not observed. Above the threshold dose, the probability that the effect will occur is virtually 100%, and the severity of the effect increases with an increased dose.

5. What are examples of deterministic effects?

Skin responses such as erythema, epilation, desquamation, cataracts, fibrosis, and hematopoietic damage.

6. What are the threshold doses for deterministic effects?

The deterministic effect with the lowest dose threshold is early transient erythema, with a threshold dose in the 2–3 Gray range, when delivered acutely. (The Gray, or Gy, is a unit of absorbed dose equal to 1 joule of energy absorbed per kilogram of tissue.) When the radiation exposure is spread over time, the threshold dose is greater than for an acute exposure, due to the ability of cells to repair nonlethal radiation damage.

7. What are some typical entrance skin exposures delivered in common x-ray examinations, such as a chest PA film, an AP cervical spine film, and an abdominal AP film?

Typical doses in milliGrays (mGy) for a PA of the chest, an AP cervical spine film, and an AP abdominal film are 0.15, 0.95, and 3.0 (using a grid and 400 speed film, for an average patient).

8. How many chest radiographs would one need to receive before the erythema dose threshold is reached, if 1 Roentgen of entrance skin exposure results in a skin dose of approximately 1 cGy?

Approximately 10,000 chest x-rays (or 100 CT studies or greater than 30 minutes of fluoroscopy)!

9. Do hospital workers risk receiving an exposure that would result in a deterministic effect?

No. Hospital personnel, in the course of normal clinical work, receive at most only a small radiation exposure, due primarily to scatter.

10. How concerned should we be about stochastic effects?

There is some legitimate reason to be concerned about stochastic effects, since they have no known dose threshold. This implies that even the smallest amount of radiation exposure may increase the probability of the induction of a stochastic effect. However, the most common stochastic effects have a fairly high spontaneous incidence, so there may be a radiation dose below which further reduction in radiation dose does not reduce the likelihood of producing the effect. Since such "negligible risk" levels have not been determined, the conservative approach is to assume that all radiation exposure is potentially harmful.

11. What is ALARA?

"As Low As Reasonably Achievable," which refers to achieving the lowest radiation exposures possible to patients, health care workers, and the general public.

12. What is meant by "background radiation"?

All inhabitants of the Earth receive a certain amount of radiation exposure each year in the form of "natural background" radiation. This comes from rocks and soil, from outer space, from radon gas produced in the ground, and natural isotopes of elements found in living tissue (such as carbon-14 and potassium-40). The background radiation in the United States results in an average annual effective dose equivalent of 3.2 milliSieverts. The Sievert is the SI unit of effective dose, which takes into account partial-body irradiation and the particular type of radiation that results in an absorbed dose.

13. What is the average annual occupational effective dose that radiologists and x-ray technologists are exposed to?

Radiologists, 0.71 milliSieverts; x-ray technologists, 0.96 milliSieverts. These exposures are still below the natural background level.

14. What is the purpose of occupational dose limits?

Although the ALARA principle presumes that there is no absolutely safe level, occupational dose limits are chosen to keep radiation exposures to low levels, based on the following objectives:
- To prevent radiation-induced deterministic effects, by adhering to dose limits that are below the apparent threshold levels.
- To limit the risk of stochastic effects to a reasonable level in relation to social needs, values, benefits gained, and economic factors.

Radiologists and x-ray technologists receive an average annual occupational effective dose well below the occupational limit of 50 milliSieverts/year to the whole body.

15. Which health care workers are most likely to approach the occupational limit?

Angiographers and cardiologists, who perform fluoroscopically guided diagnostic and interventional procedures.

16. What are the main principles in radiation protection?

Time, distance, and shielding. That is, minimize exposure time, maximize the distance between oneself and the source of radiation, and take advantage of protective shielding such as lead garments and lead-lined partitions. The distance rule is particularly effective, since radiation exposure varies inversely with the square of the distance from the radiation source.

17. By what percent do standard 0.5-mm lead aprons reduce radiation exposure?

By 95%.

18. What other principles should be used while working with radiation or around radioactive materials to reduce exposure?
- Exercise proper hygiene (no drinking or eating).
- Limit the x-ray field to only the anatomy of interest.
- Use any dose-saving features such as fast screen-film combinations, pulsed or slow-scan video fluoroscopy, or low-dose fluoroscopy whenever possible.
- Use digital image receptors to reduce the number of radiographic studies that must be repeated because of underexposure or overexposure.

19. What does radiation exposure to a pregnant woman do to the embryo before implantation (first 9 days postconception)?
Either the embryo is lost, or there is no effect and the embryo recovers completely (Fig. 1).

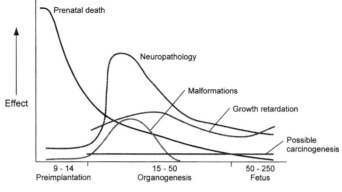

Days Postconception and
Phase of Conceptus Development

FIGURE 1. Adverse effects and relative risks associated with radiation exposure in utero at various stages of gestation. Adapted from Lewis JT, Miller JN: US Public Health Service Monitoring Program, 1977–1983. Rockville, MD, Office of Health Physics, Center for Devices and Radiological Health, Department of Human Services, 1985.

20. When is the fetus most sensitive to the effects of radiation?
During the organogenesis period, 8–15 weeks postconception, exposure to radiation may result in developmental problems such as small head size and mental retardation, with an observed increase in risk above a threshold dose of 40 cGy.

21. What is the risk of developing childhood cancer from radiation exposure in utero?
There is disagreement about the risk of radiation-induced leukemia and other childhood cancers, but a conservative estimate of the increased risk due to in utero exposure is 4–6 per 10,000 children per cGy. The monthly occupational dose limit for pregnant health care workers has been set at 0.5 milliSieverts (50 millirem) to limit these risks.

22. What practical steps can be taken to limit radiation exposure to pregnant patients?
Extra thought should be given to whether an examination that does not use ionizing radiation (e.g., ultrasound) can be used to substitute for a radiographic or fluoroscopic procedure. If ionizing radiation must be used, the field of view and the number of views should be limited as much as possible. These concerns are of greatest importance during the first trimester of pregnancy. Also, the dose to the fetus should be monitored, which can be done by a medical physicist. Only a fraction of radiologic examinations involve doses greater than 1 cGy, so in practice the risk of radiation-induced fetal injury from diagnostic radiology is extremely small. If the information to be obtained from the exam may significantly alter patient management, the small additional risk associated with the radiation exposure should be of less concern. If the results of the imaging study will not affect patient management, it should not be performed.

23. What are the risks of exposure to low levels of ionizing radiation? ("Low levels" are defined as levels of ionizing radiation that are well below levels at which a clear and quantifiable connection is seen between the radiation exposure and a biologic effect.)
There is still disagreement over the risk of biologic injury from low levels of ionizing radiation, delivered over an extended time. Investigators use "dose-response models" to predict the low level dose response from data obtained at higher levels of exposure (Fig. 2). The controversy can be summarized as "which model curve is correct?"

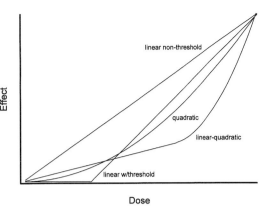

FIGURE 2. Dose-response curves corresponding to various models of radiation damage, used to extrapolate the radiation risk of low-level exposures from data obtained at intermediate-level exposures.

The available data do not provide a definitive answer. Radiation-induced cancers are indistinguishable from nonradiation-induced cancers, so for a given population it is impossible to tell whether an increased cancer incidence is the result of radiation exposures or other factors.

Implicit in the "linear, no threshold model" is the assumption that any amount of radiation is potentially harmful. This is the most conservative of the various dose response models and is the basis of ALARA. If, however, a threshold dose does exist, many of the resources used to protect people against small radiation exposures could be eliminated. Supporting the theory that a negligible risk radiation threshold might exist is the fact that biologic radiation repair mechanisms do exist and are well-understood. At low dose rates, repair mechanisms may be able to keep up with radiation damage, while at higher rates the repair mechanisms may not keep pace with the damage and significant injury may occur.

BIBLIOGRAPHY

1. Conference of Radiation Control Program Directors: Average Patient Exposure Guides, publication 88.5, 1988.
2. Hall EJ: Radiobiology for the Radiologist, 4th ed. Philadelphia, J.B. Lippincott, 1993.
3. Lewis JT, Miller JN: US Public Health Service Monitoring Program, 1977–1983. Rockville, MD, Office of Health Physics, Center for Devices and Radiological Health, Department of Health and Human Services, 1985.
4. Mettler FA, Upton AC: Medical Effects of Ionizing Radiation, 2nd ed. Philadelphia, W.B. Saunders, 1995.
5. National Council on Radiation Protection and Measurements: Ionizing Radiation Exposures of the Population of the United States, report no. 93. Washington, DC, 1987.
6. National Council on Radiation Protection and Measurements: Limitation of Exposure to Ionizing Radiation, report no. 116. Washington, DC, 1993.
7. Shapiro J: Radiation Protection: A Guide for Scientists and Physicians, 3rd ed. Cambridge, MA, Harvard University Press, 1990.
8. Strom DJ: Ten principles and ten commandments of radiation protection. Health Physics 70:388–393, 1996.

3. GASTROINTESTINAL CONTRAST STUDIES

Douglas S. Katz, M.D., and Burton M. Gold, M.D.

1. What are the two major types of contrast agents that are used to image the bowel during fluoroscopic studies?

Barium and water-soluble iodinated contrast, such as Gastrografin, which is an "ionic" contrast agent.

2. What are the advantages of using barium for GI contrast studies versus using water-soluble iodinated contrast?

Barium, an inert substance, can be prepared in a variety of ways—as a suspension that can be diluted or mixed in a paste. Barium is denser than water and is therefore more visible than water-soluble iodinated contrast. Also, barium preparations, especially when "thicker" barium is used, are designated to coat the bowel mucosa, whereas water-soluble contrast just fills the bowel lumen.

3. What is meant by "single" versus "double" contrast studies?

The term "single" contrast usually applies when a single contrast agent is used (typically, barium). A "double" contrast GI study is performed using both air and barium.

4. What type of barium preparation is used for single contrast studies and for double contrast studies?

When single contrast is used for an upper GI study, for example, thinner barium is used so that abnormalities of the mucosa or in the lumen of the bowel will not be obscured by dense overlying barium. For double contrast studies, thicker barium that coats the bowel mucosa is used; air is introduced into the bowel lumen, which distends it and profiles the mucosa.

5. In what situations is water-soluble iodinated contrast contraindicated?

• When a patient has a past history of significant allergy to iodinated contrast
• When contrast is to be administered orally and the patient is at risk of aspirating, because aspirated ionic iodinated contrast can induce pulmonary edema and chemical pneumonitis

6. In what situation is barium contraindicated?

When bowel perforation is suspected. Water-soluble contrast is then indicated. Barium in the peritoneum can cause several problems: it may further add to the contamination of the peritoneum if a bowel perforation is present, and there is the theoretical risk of developing adhesions secondary to the barium in the future, although this is somewhat controversial.

7. Why is a patient kept NPO for upper gastrointestinal contrast studies?

For a variety of reasons but particularly so that food and ingested medications and fluids do not interfere with barium coating of the mucosa and are not confused with true abnormalities.

8. What are some indications for an esophagram?

• To evaluate dysphagia, swallowing problems, and motility disorders
• To search for complications of gastroesophageal reflux
• To examine the esophagus for suspected esophagitis, stricture, varices, or tumor

9. How is an esophagram performed?

In a variety of ways. The specific technique used by the radiologist will depend on institutional and personal preference. The pharynx and cervical and thoracic esophagus are examined. A typical examination includes studying swallowing (in the frontal and lateral positions) in both the supine (to eliminate the effects of gravity on peristalsis in the thoracic esophagus) and the standing positions. The examination is videotaped and reviewed, and fluoroscopic spot films are obtained. Many radiologists obtain images using both single and double contrast; double contrast is ideal to study fine mucosal detail.

10. What is the diameter at which an esophageal narrowing can lead to significant obstruction?

13 mm or less. To test for such a narrowing, a radiopaque tablet measuring 13 mm can be given to the patient to swallow under fluoroscopy.

11. What is a "modified" barium swallow (or swallowing study)?

A specialized study that may be performed in conjunction with a speech pathologist. A variety of substances are swallowed under fluoroscopy; if specific problems are identified during swallowing, the speech pathologist can test a variety of compensatory maneuvers in an attempt to minimize problems such as aspiration.

12. What structures are routinely examined during an upper gastrointestinal series (UGI)?
The thoracic esophagus, the stomach, and the duodenum.

13. What are the indications for UGI series?
The most common indications include:
- Evaluation of upper abdominal pain
- Suspected gastric or duodenal ulcer
- Suspected gastric outlet obstruction or tumor
- Evaluation of the folds of the stomach for gastritis or suspected tumor
- Unexplained weight loss or anorexia

14. How is UGI performed?
This depends on the condition of the patient and the preference of the radiologist/institution. As with most fluoroscopic examinations of the upper GI tract, there is no one correct way to perform a procedure, and the examination should always be tailored to answer the specific question(s) being raised by the referring physician(s). At the same time, a routine series of maneuvers and views should be performed so that a systematic examination is obtained.

For example, if the patient is elderly and cannot easily maneuver on the fluoroscopic table, a UGI series using single contrast is appropriate. The patient swallows thin barium, and a variety of images are obtained. Some of the images are obtained using compression, where the abdomen is compressed—either by the radiologist's hand using a leaded glove or by a compression device—so that lesions are not obscured by the overlying barium.

If the patient is a relatively healthy outpatient, a double contrast study can be performed. The patient swallows effervescent crystals as well as thick barium, and the patient rolls on the fluoroscopy table to coat the stomach with barium. A series of images are then obtained.

15. What are some potential pitfalls of a double contrast UGI series?
The double contrast study provides excellent mucosal detail, but there are some potential pitfalls. It may be difficult to see the anterior wall of the stomach, and ulcers may be missed there. Fortunately, gastric ulcers are much more common on the posterior wall of the stomach. If the stomach is overdistended, mucosal abnormalities may be missed; if the stomach is underdistended, it may be difficult to determine if the folds of the stomach are truly thickened.

16. What are some potential pitfalls of a single contrast UGI series?
If adequate compression is not used, lesions may be missed. Mucosal detail is poor compared to double contrast studies.

17. What are the indications for a small bowel series?
The common indications include:
- To evaluate a known or suspected small bowel obstruction
- To search for a lesion, especially in a patient with significant symptoms and/or lower GI bleeding, in whom evaluation of the lower (and upper) GI tracts has failed to reveal a cause
- To search for causes of diarrhea and malabsorption

18. How is a small bowel series performed?
Also known as a small bowel follow-through, it may be performed as a separate test or at the end of an upper GI series. The patient drinks barium (additional barium if an UGI has just been performed) and serial radiographs are obtained. Periodically during the exam, and when barium reaches the cecum, the radiologist uses a compression paddle and presses on the abdomen while examining the small bowel and the terminal ileal region under fluoroscopy.

19. Is barium or water-soluble contrast preferable as a contrast agent for a small bowel series?
Barium is superior to water-soluble contrast. In fact, many radiologists will not use water-soluble contrast for this study: the contrast gets diluted easily, especially when an obstruction is present, and mucosal detail is not seen.

20. Is there a superior test to a small bowel series, especially when an intermittent or "low-grade" small bowel obstruction is suspected?
  Yes, enteroclysis.

21. How is an enteroclysis performed?
  The radiologist places a long nasogastric tube—often one that is specially made for this procedure—just past the duodenal-jejunal junction and instills barium, often followed by methylcellulose, through the tube, often using a pump that delivers these materials at a standard rate. The bowel is observed under fluoroscopy, and multiple images are obtained. To improve patient tolerance, the patient may be given nasal or oral topical anesthetic, and/or intravenous or oral light sedation can be administered.

22. What are the advantages of enteroclysis over a standard small bowel series?
  Because the small bowel is directly challenged with a bolus of contrast and methylcellulose, subtle transition points may be discovered (e.g., adhesions) that cannot be detected using techniques such as a routine small bowel series or CT. Mucosal detail is outstanding, and unusual lesions such as primary small bowel tumors, which are notoriously difficult to discover by other means, may be identified.

23. What is a major contraindication to enteroclysis?
  "High-grade" small bowel obstruction.

24. What are some of the indications for a barium enema?
  • Evaluation of lower gastrointestinal bleeding
  • Screening for colon cancer or polyps
  • Suspected diverticulitis
  • Rule out obstructing lesion
  • Inflammatory bowel disease
  • Colon incompletely evaluated at endoscopy (i.e., the more proximal colon was not reached)

25. When is a barium enema contraindicated?
  • When there is peritonitis and/or free intraperitoneal air
  • If toxic megacolon is suspected
  (This is why it is extremely useful to obtain scout views of the abdomen and pelvis prior to performing a BE)

26. What are the differences between a single and a double contrast barium enema?
  Double contrast is ideal when evaluating relatively healthy patients who can cooperate with the relatively rigorous examination. To perform a double contrast study, both barium and air are instilled under fluoroscopic observation into the colon. Multiple spot films are obtained during the procedure, as well as multiple "overhead" radiographs. The radiologist also "spots" the terminal ileal region, meaning that he or she uses a compression balloon to press on the right lower quadrant, which spreads the structures in this area apart and allows them to be identified and examined (i.e., the cecum, terminal ileum, ileocecal valve, and appendix). Double contrast provides excellent mucosal detail.
  Single contrast is ideal when the patient cannot tolerate a double contrast exam, when obstruction of the colon needs to be excluded, or to evaluate for the presence of a fistula. If perforation is suspected but there is no free air and no evidence of peritonitis, water-soluble contrast should be utilized, in case a perforation is encountered.

27. Can a barium enema be performed if the patient has an ostomy?
  Yes, the study can be performed through the ostomy; either single or double contrast techniques can be used. However, in contrast to the typical BE where a balloon (which is present near the end of the tip of the enema tube which is inserted into the rectum) may be inflated, this type of apparatus

should not be used in the ostomy, because it may be damaged; special soft enema tips have been devised for this purpose.

28. When is a barium enema diagnostic as well as therapeutic?

When a BE is performed for intussusception in children. However, many radiologists are now using air as the sole contrast medium for intussusception, as opposed to barium or water-soluble contrast. There is some evidence that the results are better when air is used—along with a special device that monitors the pressure generated by the air, ensuring that the colon is not overinflated—and that the risk of complications, which is already low when conventional techniques are used, may be lowered even further. In infants, a water-soluble enema may be therapeutic in cases of meconium ileus. In adults, a barium enema may rarely "reverse" a colonic volvulus.

29. How is a fistulogram used?

When a fistula is present or suspected, water-soluble contrast can be instilled into the abnormal area of the skin, under fluoroscopic control, and a communication with the bowel can be sought. Also, a CT scan can be done immediately after, which can provide additional information.

BIBLIOGRAPHY

1. Ell SR: Handbook of Gastrointestinal and Genitourinary Radiology. St. Louis, Mosby, 1992.
2. Laufer I, Levine MS: Double Contrast Gastrointestinal Radiology, 2nd ed. Philadelphia, W.B. Saunders, 1992.

4. ULTRASOUND

Robert J. Botash, M.D.

1. What is ultrasound?

Ultrasound is a method of imaging that uses high-frequency sound waves beyond the range of human hearing to image structures inside the body. Tissues differ in their ability to transmit sound. When a sound wave encounters a change in tissue, some of the sound is transmitted, and some is reflected to the transducer. The reflected sound is converted into an image. Based on the length of time it takes for the sound waves to return to the transducer, the depth of the tissue interface can be estimated.

2. How are ultrasound waves generated?

By applying an electric field to a piezoelectric crystal in the transducer, the crystal vibrates and generates sound waves. The transducer also functions as a detector, which receives the echoes reflected from within the patient.

3. How is an ultrasound examination performed?

To transmit the sound waves from the hand-held transducer into the patient, a thin layer of gel is placed on the skin to serve as a coupling medium. There is no discomfort for the patient during the examination. No harmful effects of diagnostic ultrasound have been documented to date.

4. How are ultrasound images displayed?

There are several methods for recording ultrasound images. In one of the most commonly used methods, B-mode, the intensity of the echoes reflected to the transducer is proportional to the whitening of the film. Anechoic structures, which have no internal echoes, appear black. Structures containing internal echoes are said to be echogenic and appear as an area of white on the film. Rapid viewing of multiple images on a monitor permits motion of internal body structures to be demonstrated in real time.

5. What is the orientation of transverse images? Of longitudinal images?

Transverse images are oriented as if the viewer were looking upward from the patient's feet. Longitudinal images are displayed with the patient's head toward the left side of the image and the feet to the right.

6. What is Doppler ultrasound?

Doppler ultrasound is based on the principle that sound reflected by a moving target (e.g., blood) has a different frequency from the incident sound wave. This frequency shift is proportional to the velocity of the flowing blood. Doppler ultrasound, therefore, not only allows the detection of flowing blood but also enables the velocity to be quantified. Color-coding the Doppler information and superimposing it on a real-time B-mode image facilitates identification of vessels and abnormal flow.

7. What structures in the body cannot be imaged by ultrasound?

High-frequency sound waves propagate readily through fluid and soft tissues. However, they are stopped by air or calcium. Air-containing structures (such as lung) and bone cannot be imaged with ultrasound.

8. What are the ultrasound characteristics of a fluid-filled structure (e.g., a cyst)?

Fluid-filled structures allow complete transmission of a sound wave without significant absorption or reflection. As a result, the posterior wall of these structures can be well seen. A strong sound wave reaches the tissues deep to fluid-filled structures such as cysts, causing them to appear more echogenic than adjacent tissues, where the sound beam has been attenuated by passing through soft tissue. This process is referred to as "acoustic enhancement" or "increased through-transmission." Fluid-filled structures contain no internal interfaces and therefore appear anechoic (Fig. 1).

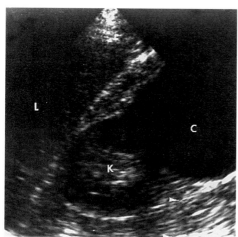

FIGURE 1. This exophytic renal cyst demonstrates (1) a sharply defined posterior wall; (2) absence of internal echoes; (3) posterior acoustic enhancement (*arrowheads*). (K = kidney, C = cyst, L = liver.)

9. What is an acoustic shadow?

A significant density difference between two adjacent structures will result in reflection of sound waves (if all other factors remain constant). For example, there is a great density difference between a gallstone and the surrounding bile within the gallbladder. When sound waves strike the surface of a gallstone, most of the waves are reflected to the transducer, creating intense echoes in the resulting image. Few waves remain to penetrate structures beyond the gallstone, which prevents visualization of deeper anatomy. The absence of echoes deep to the gallstone is referred to as an acoustic shadow (Fig. 2). Any structure that blocks the transmission of sound waves will cast a shadow.

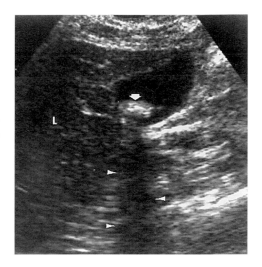

FIGURE 2. Transverse image of the gallbladder demonstrates an acoustic shadow (*arrowheads*) deep to a gallstone (*arrow*). (L = liver.)

10. What are the disadvantages of ultrasound compared with other imaging modalities?

- Ultrasound is an operator-dependent, problem-oriented modality. It should not be used as a total-body survey.
- Ultrasound cannot image air-containing structures or bone.
- Resolution of the ultrasound image is inversely related to depth of penetration. Image quality in obese patients is therefore suboptimal.

11. What are the advantages of ultrasound over other imaging modalities?

Ultrasound is relatively inexpensive, widely available, and noninvasive. It does not expose patients to radiation. It is therefore used frequently in children and pregnant women.

BIBLIOGRAPHY

1. Lewis BD, James EM, Charboneau JW, et al: Current applications of color Doppler imaging in the abdomen and extremities. Radiographics 9:599–631, 1989.
2. Rumack CM, Wilson SR, Charboneau JW: Diagnostic Ultrasound, 2nd ed. St. Louis, Mosby, 1998.
3. Mitchell DG: Color Doppler imaging: Principles, limitations, and artifacts. Radiology 177:1–10, 1990.

5. COMPUTED TOMOGRAPHY

Douglas S. Katz, M.D.

1. What is computed tomography (CT)?

CT is a technology that uses x-rays to generate cross-sectional (axial) images. Any portion of the human body can be imaged by CT. Current CT scanners can obtain an image of a transverse section of the body in 1 second or less.

2. How do modern CT scanners work?

The x-ray beam is swept around the patient; after passing through the body, the radiation strikes a series of detectors that either move with the x-ray tube or are stationary. Relatively advanced mathematical techniques (Fourier transformations, back-projection algorithms) are used to create a two-dimensional image of the cross-sectional volume that is scanned. Although the technology is much more sophisticated than plain film radiography, the basic principle is similar—dense structures in the body block the transmission of x-rays.

3. What is a pixel? What is a voxel?
Each point on a CT image (a pixel) represents a small volume within the patient (a voxel).

4. How are dense structures displayed on CT? How are less dense structures displayed?
Dense structures, such as metal and bone, are displayed as white on CT. Less dense structures are displayed as various shades of gray, with the least dense structures (which contain gas) shown as black.

5. What is a Hounsfield unit?
Named after the inventor of CT, Sir Geoffrey Hounsfield, the Hounsfield Unit (HU) is a measure of the relative density of a structure on CT. By definition, water has an HU of zero. HU measurements are not precise. They have been shown to vary somewhat from scanner to scanner (e.g., when scanning the same patient) and may even vary within the same structure in a patient (e.g., if serial scans of the same patient are obtained using the same machine on different days).

6. Match the approximate HU measurement with the appropriate structure.

Minus 1500	Soft tissue	Positive 400	Air
Minus 40	Bone	Positive 2000	Fat
Positive 80	Metal		

Answers: Minus 1500—air; minus 40—fat; positive 80—soft tissue (e.g., liver, on contrast-enhanced CT); positive 400—calcium/bone; positive 2000—metal.

7. What is meant by a window—for example, a lung window?
Each pixel on a CT image is composed of a shade of gray corresponding to the average HU of the voxel that it represents. The various shades of gray create contrast in the image. The eye can appreciate only a relatively limited number of shades of gray, whereas the CT data span an HU range of several thousand. To compensate for this problem, various windows are created to view optimally different structures in the body.

8. What are the standard types of windows?
To look at the lungs, a wide window is used, in which a large range of densities (i.e., a large range of HUs) is examined, but subtle density differences are obscured. This technique is good for examining the lungs because the low density air in the lungs is contrasted sharply with the much higher-density vessels, airways, and other interstitial structures. For looking at abdominal structures, a much narrower window is used so that subtle differences in density are seen. The center of the window (the level) is also set by the CT operator. For example, a typical abdominal window setting would be a level of +40 (the center HU value) and a range or width of 400 so that the CT demonstrates all HUs between −160 and +240 as a series of shades of gray, with all pixels above 240 HU shown in white and all pixels below −160 shown in black.

9. What is the typical slice thickness for CT?
Depending on the particular CT unit, a typical slice thickness is 7–10 mm. This thickness is fine for most routine imaging. To resolve smaller details—for example, to image the temporal bone or to obtain high-resolution CT images of the lungs—slices as thin as 1 mm can be obtained. Because a much thinner slice is imaged, much less signal is obtained by the detectors. This trade-off means that a higher dose of radiation must be administered to acquire high-quality images.

10. Why is CT a major advance over plain films?
With CT, the body is imaged cross-sectionally so that complex structures can be imaged. A plain radiograph is the two-dimensional representation of a three-dimensional structure. It is often difficult

to sort out overlapping structures on plain films (e.g., in the chest), and CT effectively eliminates this problem. In addition, CT is much more sensitive to differences in density than plain films are; thus it can reveal abnormalities that plain films cannot.

11. A patient just had a barium enema, and the referring physician now requests a CT scan of the abdomen and pelvis. Is this a problem?

Yes. Retained barium in the colon is of much higher density than the dilute barium that is used as an oral contrast agent. The higher-density barium causes significant "streak" artifacts on the CT images, obscuring the anatomy.

12. Can the CT scan obtain only true axial images (images perpendicular to the CT table on which the patient rests)?

No. The gantry (which contains the CT x-ray tube and detectors and through which the table moves) can tilt so that a certain degree of angulation off the true perpendicular can be obtained. For instance, CT images of the head are angled so that the front of the brain on each image is at a slightly higher level than the back of the brain. For imaging the paranasal sinuses, the neck of the patient is tilted backward and the gantry is angled forward so that true coronal images (slices obtained from the top of the sinuses to the bottom of the sinuses, at 90° to the axial images) are produced.

13. What is meant by the "scout" image?

The scout image is a digital radiograph obtained at the start of a CT examination. It is used by the CT technologist to pick the levels at which to obtain the axial images. It is important to look at this image, which contains important information (e.g., when imaging the abdomen, the bowel gas pattern should always be examined).

14. When is intravenous contrast given?

Intravenous contrast is used for most abdominal and pelvic CT scans and is often administered as part of many brain and lung CTs. The contrast is an iodine-based dye which comes in two basic forms—ionic and nonionic. The nonionic form is significantly more expensive. Because of cost considerations, many radiologists use the ionic form in most patients for routine CT applications and reserve the use of nonionic low osmolar contrast for the following situations:

- Patients with a history of previous contrast reaction
- Patients with asthma, hay fever, or food and environmental allergies
- Patients with significant heart and lung conditions
- Patients with mild renal insufficiency (typically creatinine < 2)
- Young children

Indications vary, and the scientific principles behind many of these recommendations are not especially well founded. The American College of Radiology has published specific guidelines for nonionic contrast administration; since this is the "party line," for medicolegal reasons it is a good idea to follow them fairly closely.

15. What if you are not sure whether a particular patient should receive intravenous or oral contrast?

Ask the radiologist! The radiologist should be liberally consulted, because in certain situations it may be desirable not to give contrast—for example, to exclude a hematoma or to look for calcification.

16. A CT scan of the abdomen is ordered for a patient who developed hives in response to intravenous ionic contrast in the past. What should be done?

Nonionic contrast should be given, and it may be beneficial for the patient to receive prophylactic premedication with a series of oral doses of prednisone (typically 50 mg orally 13, 7, and 1 hour before the scan), along with 50 mg of oral diphenhydramine (Benadryl) 1 hour before the scan. Various premedication regimens may be used. Some evidence suggests that this type of preparation reduces the risk of a contrast reaction. The radiologist performing the scan should be consulted when the study is ordered.

17. What if the patient had a more serious reaction to intravenous contrast in the past, such as laryngospasm, bronchospasm, or a hypotensive reaction that required resuscitation?

An alternative test (e.g., ultrasound, MRI) should be considered, or the study should be performed without intravenous contrast. An unenhanced CT may still be useful, depending on the clinical question.

18. Can reactions to intravenous contrast be predicted?

Unfortunately, no. Even patients who are given nonionic contrast (and who are premedicated if appropriate) may develop life-threatening reactions in rare instances. In addition, because reactions are not predictable, a patient may have received intravenous contrast 10 times with no problem, yet on the 11th time experience a life-threatening reaction. The likelihood of a serious contrast reaction is low and probably significantly less if nonionic contrast is used, although deaths may occur from both ionic and nonionic contrast agents.

19. A patient has significant renal failure, and a CT scan is requested for which intravenous contrast is needed. What can be done?

Because intravenous contrast may worsen renal function in a small percentage of patients, alternative testing should be used if at all possible—for instance, MRI. Alternatively, if the patient is already on dialysis and intravenous contrast is administered, the patient should undergo dialysis just before or after the CT.

20. What other types of contrast can be given for a CT?

There are various specialized uses of contrast. For example, contrast can be injected through a Foley catheter into the bladder in a patient with a suspected bladder rupture. Rectal contrast, in the form of dilute iodine, dilute barium, water, or air can be injected through an enema tube or a small red rubber catheter to opacify the colon; this can be helpful in various situations, such as in a patient with a suspected colonic mass or to determine whether a collection communicates with the colon.

21. Does the CT table have a weight limit?

Yes. Check with the radiologist/CT technologist at your institution, but many CT tables have a weight limit of 300–350 pounds. The table may be seriously damaged (and require tens of thousands of dollars to be replaced, often not under warranty) if patients significantly over this weight limit are imaged.

22. What is a spiral CT?

Spiral (also known as helical) CT is a major recent advance in CT technology. With conventional CT, when the chest, abdomen, and pelvis are imaged, the patient has to hold his or her breath as each image is acquired. Then the CT tube resets, and the table is moved to the next location to acquire the next slice. The patient is asked to hold his or her breath again as the next image is taken.

23. So what?

Problems may arise due to misregistration of the images—for example, if a patient did not hold his or her breath in exactly the same way each time, a portion of the scanned organ (e.g., the liver) may be missed completely and small lesions may not be identified. Spiral CT eliminates this problem because the machine does not need to reset itself. There are no constricting cables in the gantry that need to be unwound before the next image is taken. Because of electrical "slip-ring" contacts, the need for these cables is removed, and the x-ray tube can continuously rotate around the patient and acquire data while the patient holds his or her breath.

24. Where does the term *spiral* (or even better, *helical*) come from?

As the x-ray tube moves around the patient and the patient is holding his or her breath, the table is moved through the gantry. The x-ray tube movement describes a helix in space. A three-dimensional data set is acquired and then reconstructed into images representing transverse sections of the body. An entire scan can be obtained while the patient holds his or her breath (or several smaller spirals can be obtained, each during a breath hold, which is easier for the patient), essentially eliminating the problem of misregistration.

25. How is intravenous contrast given for a spiral CT of the chest, abdomen, or pelvis?
Routinely, a mechanical power injector is used to deliver contrast at a uniform rate into an intravenous catheter. This mechanical device is monitored by the CT technologist and the radiologist.

26. What specialized applications can be performed with a spiral CT scanner?
Images can be easily reconstructed into different planes, especially if thin sections were initially obtained. Alternatively, with work stations that are connected to the CT scanner, the CT data also can be used to create more elaborate three-dimensional images.

27. What is CT angiography?
CT angiography is a relatively new technique that can be used to study the vasculature and can be performed fairly easily and routinely with a spiral CT scanner. A large-gauge peripheral intravenous line is inserted, and contrast is given at a fairly rapid rate to image, for example, an abdominal aortic aneurysm. Relatively thin sections are obtained so that the vessels originating off the aneurysm (e.g., the renal arteries) can be imaged accurately. Reconstructions can then be performed for surgical planning.

28. Is a CAT scan the same thing as a CT scan?
Yes. The abbreviation CAT (computerized axial tomography) has been replaced by the preferred abbreviation CT (computed or computerized tomography). This may have been in response to dopey managed care cartoons of the new and improved (and much cheaper) CAT scan—a furry animal held next to someone's head.

BIBLIOGRAPHY

1. Haaga JR, Lanzieri CF, Sartoris DJ, Zerhouni EA (eds): Computed Tomography and Magnetic Resonance Imaging of the Whole Body. St. Louis, Mosby, 1994.

---

6. MAGNETIC RESONANCE IMAGING

Kevin R. Math, M.D.

---

1. What is the difference between MRI and NMR?
There is no difference. The physical principles of nuclear magnetic resonance (NMR) are the basis for magnetic resonance imaging (MRI). The term NMR was replaced with MRI because of potential public concern over the word "nuclear."

2. How is an MR image generated?
The basic principles are as follows. The patient or body part is placed in a superconducting magnet. A strong magnetic field is created by movement of current through a series of helical coils. An electromagnetic wave or radiofrequency pulse is created through the brief application of an alternating electric current, and this "pulse" causes the hydrogen nuclei of protons in the body tissues to resonate to varying degrees, thus generating a signal or an electromagnetic wave. The generated signal is based on the properties of the tissue and the settings of the magnet. This signal is detected by the receiving coil, and after complex data processing an image is displayed on the monitor.

3. How does the MRI unit know where in the body the signal originated?

Special coils called gradient coils vary the strength of the magnetic field and the frequency and phase of the electromagnetic wave in the transverse (x and y axes) and longitudinal (z axis) planes. This permits the detectors to calculate exactly where on the image to plot a signal received from a site in the body.

4. What is the cause of the loud banging noises during an MR study?

The continuous movement of the gradient coils during the examination is very loud. Patients are given earplugs or stereo headphones during the examination to make it more tolerable.

5. What is a Tesla?

The Tesla is a unit of measurement of a magnetic field strength (meter-kilogram-second system). Gauss is the unit of measurement for the centimeter-gram-second system. One Tesla (T) = 10,000 Gauss.

6. What is meant by high- and low-field strength MRI?

Manufacturers produce magnets of varying strengths. The most common magnet field strengths used clinically are 0.3, 0.5, 1.0, and 1.5 Tesla. Magnets of 1.0 T or greater are considered high-field strength and generate greater signal and usually more appealing images than lower-field strength units.

7. What is the strength of the earth's magnetic field?

About 1 Gauss. Therefore, most MR units generate a magnetic field strength more than 10,000 times the earth's magnetic field.

8. What is meant by T1 and T2?

T1 and T2 refer to physical properties of the tissues after exposure to a series of pulses at predetermined time intervals. Different tissues have different T1 and T2 properties, based on the response of their hydrogen nuclei to radiofrequency pulses imposed by the magnet. These differential properties are exploited by setting equipment parameters (TR and TE) that elicit images based on either the T1 or T2 properties of the tissues (T1- or T2-weighted). TR is the time to repeat, or the time between radiofrequency pulses; TE is the time to echo, or the time interval between applying the pulse and listening for the signal. TR and TE are both expressed in milliseconds (ms). Equipment settings that elicit images that are a combination of T1 and T2 properties are called balanced or proton density images.

9. What is signal intensity?

Signal intensity refers to the brightness of signal generated by specific tissues. Tissues that are bright (whiter) are hyperintense, whereas darker signal tissues are hypointense. Tissues that are somewhere in the middle are isointense. These terms usually refer to the signal of a pathologic process relative to surrounding tissues (e.g., the mass is hyperintense to the adjacent muscle). Note that the term *intensity* is used rather than the term *density*, which is used when referring to CT or plain films.

10. Describe the signal intensity of fat and water on T1- and T2-weighted images.

Fat is bright (hyperintense) on T1-weighted images and less bright on T2-weighted images (Fig. 1). Water is dark on T1-weighted images and bright on T2-weighted images. These principles are important to remember because most pathologic processes are associated with increased water content and therefore are hyperintense on T2-weighted images and hypointense on T1. A mnemonic that may be helpful is **W**orld **W**ar **II** (water is white on T2).

11. Aside from fat, what other tissues are bright on T1-weighted images?

Blood (methemoglobin in subacute hemorrhage), proteinaceous material, melanin, and gadolinium (MR contrast agent).

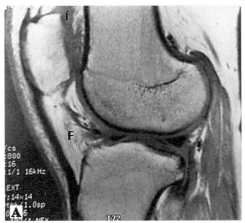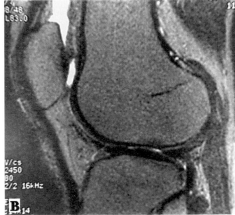

FIGURE 1. Signal intensity on MRI. *A*, T1- and *B*, T2-weighted sagittal images of the knee showing the relative signal intensity of fat (F) and joint fluid (f) on these pulse sequences. Note that the fluid gets brighter and fat becomes less bright on the T2-weighted images.

12. List four things that are dark on T2-weighted images.

Calcium, gas, chronic hemorrhage (hemosiderin), mature fibrous tissue.

13. What is unique about the signal intensity of a hematoma?

The signal intensity of blood changes over time as the hemoglobin properties change (i.e., oxy-hemoglobin conversion to deoxyhemoglobin and methemoglobin). These principles are helpful in attempting to determine the age of a hemorrhagic process. Acute hemorrhage (oxy- or deoxyhemoglobin) is hypointense or isointense on T1-weighted images, whereas subacute hemorrhage is hyperintense. Hemosiderin deposition in a chronic hematoma is hypointense on all pulse sequences.

14. Describe the appearance of blood vessels on MRI.

Vessels with flowing blood appear as signal voids, which result in a dark circular or tubular appearance on transverse or longitudinal images, respectively. Exceptions to this rule include vessels with slow flowing blood and special types of pulse sequences (gradient-echo), in which blood vessels appear bright.

15. How can you tell if you are looking at a T1- or T2-weighted image?

Looking for the TE and TR numbers on the images is the more difficult approach. A relatively low TE is about 20 ms, and a high TE is about 80 ms. A low TR is about 600 ms, and a high TR is around 3000 ms. T1-weighted images have a low TE and low TR, whereas both are high for T2-weighted images. Proton density images have a low TE and high TR.

Knowledge of the signal characteristics of water and fat are more helpful and are especially useful when the specific TR and TE are not indicated on the images. Look for fluid containing structures such as cerebral ventricles, urinary bladder, or cerebrospinal fluid. If fluid is bright, it is most likely a T2-weighted image, and if it is dark, it is probably T1-weighted. If fluid looks bright, but the rest of the image does not look T2-weighted and the TE and TR are low, you are probably dealing with a gradient echo image.

16. What is MRA?

Magnetic resonance angiography. MRI principles are used to exploit the unique properties of flowing blood. Images are generated in which only structures containing flowing blood are visualized; all other structures are suppressed (Fig. 2). These principles can be further modified so that only vessels with flow in a specific direction (i.e., arteries vs. veins) are visualized. MRA is useful for evaluating patients with suspected cerebrovascular disease (circle of Willis or carotid arteries), and also may be applied to the venous system for evaluating suspected deep venous thrombosis. Definite limitations and artifacts are associated with MRA, particularly with applications outside the central nervous system.

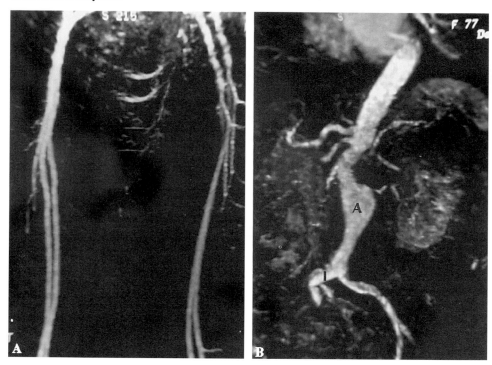

FIGURE 2.   *A*, Normal MR angiogram of the lower extremity arteries (courtesy of Dr. D. DeCorato). *B*, MR angiogram of the abdominal aorta shows an infrarenal abdominal aortic aneurysm (A). The aneurysm does not involve the common iliac arteries (I).

17. What are the advantages of MRI over CT?
  • No ionizing radiation
  • Multiplanar imaging capability (axial, coronal, sagittal, oblique)
  • Better anatomic detail
  • More sensitive in detecting subtle pathologic tissue alterations (e.g., bone marrow infiltration, cerebral edema)
  • Ability to characterize specific types of tissues based on signal intensity (fat, blood, water)
  • Improved tissue contrast compared with CT

18. What are the advantages of CT over MR?
    CT is superior to MR for evaluating calcified or ossified abnormalities of the musculoskeletal system. This superiority is due to the lack of signal of calcium on MR and the optimal visualization of calcium and cortical and trabecular bone on CT. Whereas CT can demonstrate the classic bony findings of Paget's disease or myositis ossificans better than MR, MR remains superior for evaluation of bone marrow diseases and bone and soft tissue tumors. CT is considered the modality of choice for initial evaluation of the chest, abdomen, and pelvic organs, providing high-resolution anatomic images. MRI is helpful for clarifying abnormal findings detected on CT. CT is currently less expensive than MR, increasing its appeal in our cost-conscious environment. Current CT technology allows most studies to be completed within a few minutes, compared with 30–60+ minutes

for MR. Claustrophobia is rarely a problem with the large gantry used in CT as opposed to the 10% claustrophobia rate for MR (due to the small bore opening of the magnet).

19. Is MRI safe for pregnant women?

The safety of MRI for the unborn fetus has not yet been established. Concern still remains that exposure of the fetus to the strong magnetic field and electromagnetic radiation may be potentially harmful, especially in the first trimester. Therefore, except for emergency situations (e.g., spinal cord compression), MRI is not routinely done on pregnant women. Furthermore, intravenous MR contrast agents have been shown to cross the placenta readily; administration to pregnant women is ill-advised because contrast agents may have a negative effect on the fetus and pregnancy, although no such effect has been proved.

20. Are there any contraindications to MRI?

Yes. Contraindications apply to patients with magnetically susceptible devices or materials in their bodies whose movement or loss of function can have deleterious consequences:

- Cardiac pacemakers
- Cochlear implants
- Some prosthetic heart valves
- Bone growth or neurostimulator (TENS)
- Brain aneurysm clips or coils
- Metal fragments (periorbital)
- Some penile prostheses

It is crucial to screen each and every patient for these contraindications before any MR study. Some manufacturers now produce surgical clips and other devices that are nonferromagnetic and safe for MR. The radiologist must be consulted if there is any question about safety.

21. What is fat suppression? How is it helpful in MR imaging?

Fat suppression has nothing to do with a weight reduction program. Rather, special MR techniques are used to eliminate the bright signal imparted by fat. The most common technique uses selective saturation of fat protons (chemical saturation); protons associated with fat behave slightly differently from water protons when exposed to a magnetic field. Repetitive radiofrequency pulses targeting fat protons result in relative absence of signal from fatty tissues.

The primary usefulness of fat suppression is based on the following facts. Most pathologic processes are associated with increased water content and therefore are bright on T2-weighted images; fat also remains somewhat bright on T2-weighted images and may mask the abnormal pathologic signal. Suppression of fat serves to make the pathologic bright T2 signal more conspicuous and more easily detectable. These techniques are also useful after intravenous contrast administration: postcontrast images are usually T1-weighted, and the tissue enhancement sought on these images may be difficult to appreciate, particularly if the abnormality is adjacent to epidural or subcutaneous fat.

22. What two gases are used to cool the superconducting magnet?

Helium and/or nitrogen.

23. Does the MR technologist turn off the magnet at the end of the day?

No. The superconducting magnet is always left on.

24. What is an open MRI? What are its advantages and disadvantages?

Open MRI units have two advantages: they can be used for claustrophobic patients, and they provide imaging guidance for interventional procedures (this is a new application). Open units image the patient in larger-bore or C-shaped magnets rather than the closed narrow tunnel used in conventional units. Unfortunately, these magnets are weaker (0.1–0.3 T) than the closed units, and their basic construct results in some limitation in anatomic and spatial resolution. Therefore, the high-field strength units generally offer more esthetic and diagnostic images than the open units and should be preferentially used whenever possible. Often, administration of an anxiolytic medication before the study will permit a claustrophobic patient to tolerate an examination in a high field-strength unit.

25. What are "wraparound" and chemical shift?
If you guessed that they are modern dances, you are wrong. Both are MR artifacts; discussion of the physics involved is beyond the scope of this book.

BIBLIOGRAPHY

1. Horowitz AL: MRI Physics for Radiologists, 3rd ed. New York, Springer Verlag, 1995.
2. Hashemi RH, Bradley WG: Essentials of MRI Physics. Baltimore, Williams & Wilkins, 1996.
3. Stark DD, Bradley WG: Magnetic Resonance Imaging, 2nd ed. St. Louis, Mosby, 1992.

7. NUCLEAR IMAGING

Zachary D. Grossman, M.D.

1. How does nuclear imaging differ from CT, ultrasound, and MR?
CT, ultrasound, and MR provide anatomic or structural information, whereas the primary purpose of nuclear imaging is to provide functional data.

2. Has this changed recently?
Yes, to some extent. Color Doppler ultrasound now provides excellent images revealing blood flow; dynamic CT, especially when performed with spiral technology, and MR, if done dynamically, reveal contrast enhancement in various lesions.

3. How are nuclear images generated?
Gamma rays that originate from within a patient after a radiopharmaceutical has been administered (usually intravenously) are used to form images on a gamma camera.

4. Of what are radiopharmaceuticals made?
Some may consist of a single radioactive species in its elemental atomic form, such as iodine-131, but more often they are composed of two parts—a radioactive species and an organ-specific molecule to which the radioactive species is bound. For example, a renal scan can be produced after injecting technetium-99m-diethylenetriamine pentaacetic acid (Tc-99m-DTPA). Tc-99m is a radioactive atom, and DTPA is a small molecule that is excreted by glomerular filtration. The combination, Tc-99m-DTPA, is a radioactive small molecule that undergoes rapid renal excretion; thus, almost immediately after intravenous injection of this radiopharmaceutical, the kidney, ureters, and bladder become more radioactive.

5. How does a gamma camera work?
A nuclear or gamma camera is positioned over the patient. The camera consists of a collimator, a sodium iodide crystal, and photomultiplier tubes. The collimator, which is located on the face of the camera, excludes unwanted radioactive emissions; the crystal emits a tiny flash of light or a scintillation when impacted by a photon (i.e., the gamma ray). This scintillation is amplified, exposing a radiographic film. The sum of hundreds of thousands of scintillations creates an image that represents the distribution of radioactivity within an organ or system.

6. What is SPECT?

SPECT, single photon emission computed tomography, uses the radionuclides of standard nuclear imaging—i.e., those that emit a single photon with each radioactive decay event. The term *emission* differentiates the technique from computed x-ray tomography (CT), in which x-rays are transmitted from the x-ray tube through the patient to the detectors. The term *computed tomography* indicates that slices through the body are generated by the computer-aided gamma camera.

7. What is the advantage of adding computed tomography?

Cross-sectional images allow the radiologist to focus on findings at a given section within the body. In addition, interference of overlying tissue is minimized.

8. When is SPECT indicated?

Usually SPECT images are performed immediately after standard planar images (e.g., to evaluate further abnormalities in the spine as part of a bone scan) or as the primary procedure (e.g., for a brain scan). SPECT is usually performed at the discretion of the radiologist.

9. What is PET?

PET is an acronym for positron emission tomography. Fewer than 20 centers in the United States have this technology. PET is a form of nuclear medicine that uses cyclotron-produced positron emitters and a special camera to detect them by virtue of the concurrent production of a pair of photons traveling away from each other at 180° after each positron undergoes an annihilation reaction.

10. What is the advantage of PET over conventional SPECT imaging?

The cyclotron can produce isotopes of carbon, oxygen, and nitrogen—key elements of life. No isotopes of carbon, oxygen, and nitrogen are suitable to standard nuclear gamma camera detection. The special requirements of PET scanning are balanced by the potential of actually following the biodistribution and fate of key molecules in many metabolic processes. PET is expensive; it is primarily a research tool.

11. What are some clinical uses of PET?

Examples include characterizing pulmonary nodules as benign (not active) vs. malignant (actively taking up a pharmaceutical such as 18-fluorodeoxyglucose) and distinguishing between recurrent or residual brain tumor (metabolically active) and postradiation therapy change (not metabolically active).

12. For what is a bone scan useful?

Still the most commonly performed nuclear scan, bone scans reveal areas that have increased blood flow to bone as "hot spots," i.e., foci of increased radiopharmaceutical uptake. This technique is sensitive to a wide variety of diseases, including osteomyelitis, primary and secondary bone tumors, arthritis, metabolic bone disease, trauma, and avascular necrosis. This sensitivity is also a major weakness, because the specificity of a bone scan is limited; however, in the proper clinical context, a firm diagnosis is often possible. In current practice, two chief applications are (1) detection of metastatic disease and (2) detection of osteomyelitis.

13. Which is more sensitive for detecting metastatic disease—a bone scan or plain films? What about for osteomyelitis?

A bone scan is far more sensitive than plain films for detecting metastatic disease, except for multiple myeloma. Bone scan is highly sensitive for detecting early osteomyelitis and may precede plain film findings by a week or more.

14. How do nuclear medicine agents that image the kidney work?

Radiopharmaceuticals excreted by either glomerular filtration or tubular mechanisms are available. When a filtered agent is used, each kidney's glomerular filtration or effective renal plasma flow is calculated, and images are also obtained showing blood flow to and in the kidneys and excretion of the radiopharmaceutical by the kidneys into the renal pelvis, ureters, and bladder. If a tubular agent is used, the renal cortex can be imaged.

15. What are some common uses of a renal scan?
- To assess differential renal function (i.e., the exact glomerular filtration rate of each kidney), as in renal failure
- To determine whether renal obstruction is present (furosemide [Lasix] is given in the middle of the test and washes the pharmaceutical from a dilated but nonobstructed renal collecting system but does not washout the pharmaceutical if true obstruction is present)
- To image the transplanted kidney
- To screen for renovascular hypertension (before and after an oral dose of an angiotensin-converting enzyme inhibitor, e.g., captopril)

16. How does a lung scan (performed to rule out pulmonary embolism) work?
Both ventilation and perfusion studies are performed at the same setting. For the ventilation study, the patient inhales radioactive gas (typically xenon) or aerosolized radioactive particles, whose distribution in the lungs is then mapped by images obtained with the gamma camera. For the perfusion study of the lungs, radioactive microaggregated albumin particles are injected intravenously; they are trapped in the pulmonary capillary bed so that their distribution mirrors perfusion.

17. Is there any use for a ventilation scan other than to rule out pulmonary embolism?
Yes. On occasion, it is useful to know differential ventilation in the lungs (for example, before pulmonary resection for a primary lung tumor).

18. For what is a cardiac ventriculogram useful?
This study (also known as a multigated acquisition [MUGA]) images the intracardiac blood pool during the cardiac cycle, using red blood cells that have been tagged with radioactivity. Imaging may be performed at rest and after stress (exercise). The cardiac ejection fraction is calculated; this is most useful in patients undergoing chemotherapy to monitor cardiotoxicity.

19. What other nuclear medicine examination is performed before and after exercise?
A stress cardiac study, which is a test of myocardial perfusion. The uptake of radiopharmaceutical in the myocardium is compared during rest and immediately after exercise. Areas of decreased uptake during both rest and exercise usually represent scar (i.e., dead myocardium), whereas areas of decreased uptake during exercise only, with normal uptake at rest, usually represent areas experiencing exercise-induced transient ischemia.

20. For what is a radiolabeled white blood cell scan useful?
White blood cells are radiolabeled and then reinjected into the patient. The white blood cells then migrate to areas of infection, where they form "hot spots" or areas of increased activity on the gamma camera. The primary uses are to detect areas of infection or abscess, especially when CT is equivocal or normal, and to detect osteomyelitis when three-phase bone scans are equivocal.

21. What is the purpose of a gallium scan?
Gallium is concentrated in areas of active infection or inflammation and in various tumors, especially in non-Hodgkin's lymphomas. For the detection of abscess or infection, gallium has been largely replaced by radiolabeled leukocytes, but for lymphoma, especially to differentiate active residual disease from areas of scar, gallium remains quite useful.

22. What is the purpose of a thyroid scan?
The thyroid gland is imaged to reveal hyperfunctioning and/or hypofunctioning areas such as nodules and masses. The study can establish that a clinically prominent gland is consistent with the

diagnosis of Graves' disease (large, homogeneous, hyperfunctioning gland). Other conditions, such as subacute thyroiditis (barely visible gland) and colloid goiter (large, inhomogeneous, irregular gland), also have typical imaging patterns.

23. What is the clinical significance of a "hot" thyroid nodule? A "cold" thyroid nodule?

Traditionally, thyroid scanning has been applied to palpable nodules on the grounds that "hot" nodules are always benign (hyperfunctioning adenomas), whereas "cold" nodules may be nonfunctioning adenomas, cysts, or cancer. Recently, the trend has been to substitute fine-needle aspiration biopsy for thyroid scanning in the analysis of a single palpable thyroid nodule.

24. Do all of the above studies use the same radionuclide, Tc-99m?

No, although Tc-99m (technetium) is the most common nuclide in clinical practice.

25. Is "technetium scan" a meaningful phrase?

No. Never ask for a technetium scan. Order a scan by organ system; consult with the nuclear imager, if necessary.

26. What are the most common uses for technetium?

Tc-99m-DTPA—a renal agent filtered by the glomeruli.
Tc-99m-MAA—macroaggregated albumin used in the perfusion portion of the lung scan.
Tc-99m-MDP (methylene diphosphonate)—the bone scan agent.
TcO_4- (pertechnetate, a free state of technetium)—used for thyroid and testicular scans.
Tc99m-Sestamibi—used for myocardial perfusion imaging.

27. What other common radiopharmaceuticals are in use?

I-131 (radioiodine) and I-123—used for thyroid imaging; I-131 is used for therapy of hyperthyroidism and thyroid cancer.
Tl-201 (thallium)—used for myocardial perfusion imaging.
In-111 (indium)—used to tag white blood cells.

28. Have any new agents found clinical uses in nuclear medicine?

Yes. A radiolabeled antibody marketed as Oncoscint is directed against the cell surface antigens of certain ovarian and colon cancers. It has been available for a few years but has seen limited acceptance, largely because it is very expensive. Similarly, new brain imaging agents that cross the blood-brain barrier, producing superb images that reflect blood flow in the brain, have seen limited acceptance because of the competition from magnetic resonance imaging. Octreotide, a somatostatin receptor agent, is the newest entry; it is used for imaging neuroendocrine tumors (e.g., carcinoid).

29. How risky is the intravenous injection of a radiopharmaceutical?

Severe reactions are extraordinarily rare; many busy nuclear medicine departments have never seen one. The doses of radiopharmaceuticals are so small that they are not pharmacologically active; deaths are virtually unheard of. Even minor reactions are highly unusual.

30. Is the dose from diagnostic nuclear scans higher than the doses received from x-ray examinations?

No. In fact, the radiation doses from nuclear scans are typically on the order of one-tenth to one-hundredth of the dose from x-ray studies.

31. All this sounds too good to be true. Why doesn't nuclear medicine dominate medical imaging?

There are three reasons: spatial resolution, spatial resolution, and spatial resolution.

32. How so?

Medical imagers like to see what they are looking at, and both CT and MR can usually detect (spatially resolve) much smaller lesions than nuclear medicine studies, and examine normal organs in much greater detail. In addition, nuclear scans are usually single-organ, single-system, or single-condition examinations, because the radiopharmaceuticals target one system or organ only. Nuclear medicine, however, is sensitive to functional changes that reflect some diseases long before anatomic changes are seen on other imaging studies.

BIBLIOGRAPHY

1. Henkin RE, Boles MA, Dillehay GL, et al (eds): Nuclear Medicine. St. Louis, Mosby, 1996.

8. RADIOGRAPHIC CONTRAST MEDIA

Mark A. Westcott, M.D.

1. Why is intravenous contrast media injected during radiologic examinations?

- Abnormal tissues (e.g., tumor, inflammation) enhance differently than normal tissues with intravenous contrast; this enables the abnormal tissues to be identified and characterized.
- Contrast media opacify specific structures (e.g., blood vessels, the urinary tract) in order to detect abnormalities in them (e.g., filling defects, contour abnormalities).

2. What are the two major types of iodinated contrast media?

Ionic or high osmolar contrast media (HOCM) and nonionic or low osmolar contrast media (LOCM).

HOCM are composed of salts which dissociate into cations (sodium, meglumine) and anions (diatrizoate, iothalamate, and metrizoate). The osmolarity of HOCM is five times that of serum. LOCM are made of monomers which are not salts and do not dissociate. They are less osmolar than the hyperosmolar agents (they are only about twice the osmolality of serum).

3. What are some of the advantages of LOCM compared with HOCM?

There are fewer side effects following the administration of LOCM. LOCM are less nephrotoxic than HOCM in patients with renal insufficiency.

4. What are some disadvantages of LOCM compared with HOCM?

LOCM are much more expensive than HOCM (five to ten times more). LOCM are weak anticoagulants; HOCM have more anticoagulant activity (this is potentially important when performing invasive vascular procedures).

5. What is the primary difference between the sodium and meglumine forms of ionic contrast?

In the renal tubules, there is resorption of sodium and water, which leads to greater concentration of iodine-containing anions in the excreted urine. Meglumine is not resorbed and therefore causes some diuresis with resultant distention of the renal collecting systems and the ureters (there may be some advantage to using meglumine salts for intravenous urography).

6. What are the three major types of reactions to iodinated contrast media?

Anaphylactoid (idiosyncratic), nonidiosyncratic, and local reactions. All three types may occur with both HOCM and LOCM.

7. What are anaphylactoid reactions?

Anaphylactoid, or idiosyncratic, reactions are so called because the exact mechanism of action is unknown; these reactions occur unpredictably, although certain conditions increase the risk. The etiology is probably multifactorial, involving the release of serotonin and histamine, with resultant increased capillary permeability and constriction of bronchial smooth muscle cells. Anaphylactoid reactions include urticaria, facial and laryngeal edema, bronchospasm, and hypotension; such reactions may be life-threatening.

8. What are nonidiosyncratic reactions to contrast media?
These involve the direct effect of the contrast agent on an organ (e.g., nephrotoxicity, cardiac arrhythmia, myocardial ischemia, and vasovagal reactions).

9. What are local reactions to contrast media?
When contrast extravasates from the venous or arterial system into the adjacent soft-tissues, in a small percentage of cases local necrosis may occur. This appears to occur more frequently with ionic than with nonionic contrast. Other types of local reactions include phlebitis secondary to endothelial damage following lower extremity venography.

10. How are contrast reactions categorized as to their severity?
Mild, moderate, or severe. Mild reactions require no therapy; these include reactions such as hives. Moderate reactions require therapy but are not life-threatening. Severe reactions are life-threatening and require immediate therapy. Most reactions occur within 20 minutes of intravenous contrast administration. Delayed reactions are rare and usually require no treatment.

11. What distinguishes hypotension due to an idiosyncratic reaction from hypotension due to a vasovagal episode?
If the patient has tachycardia, it is likely that the cause is an idiosyncratic reaction. Patients experiencing a vasovagal reaction will be bradycardic. It is critical to distinguish the two types of reactions because the treatment for a vasovagal reaction is different from the treatment for an idiosyncratic reaction.

12. How is hypotension due to a vasovagal episode treated?
With atropine and intravenous fluids.

13. In what situation will a patient experiencing an idiosyncratic contrast reaction have bradycardia?
When the patient is taking a beta blocker.

14. What is the overall incidence of contrast reactions for HOCM and LOCM?
5–12% for HOCM and 1–3% for LOCM.

15. What are the radiographic findings of contrast-induced nephrotoxicity?
A persistent nephrogram (retained contrast in the kidneys, which is visible on plain films and CT) for 24–48 hours, and evidence of "vicarious excretion" of contrast by the liver and biliary system and small bowel (contrast is seen in the gallbladder).

16. Which conditions appear to increase the risk of a reaction to iodinated contrast media?
While some factors are controversial and based on anecdotal reports, some of the better-established risk factors included:
- Diabetes, when renal disease is present (elevated creatinine)
- Renal insufficiency
- Severe cardiac or pulmonary disease
- Asthma
- Previous reaction to contrast media
- Significant history of allergies
- Very young and very old patients

Other less well established and controversial risk factors that have been identified in the literature include:

- Sickle cell disease (iodinated contrast appears to promote sickling of erythrocytes)
- Myasthenia gravis
- Lupus
- Multiple myeloma (especially if there is concurrent dehydration)
- Hyperthyroidism
- Pheochromocytoma

17. Which patients should receive LOCM?

This is not an easy question to answer. Protocols vary widely among institutions. Due to cost considerations, many radiology departments and practices "triage" patients depending on the risk factors for a contrast reaction. Patients for whom LOCM should be considered include those with the better-established risk factors noted above.

18. What patients should be premedicated with steroids before intravenous contrast is given?

Several clinical trials have shown a decrease in frequency of contrast reactions if steroids are administered prior to HOCM administration. It is not as clear if steroid prophylaxis offers any added benefit if LOCM are being used in patients at risk for a contrast reaction. However, since there is basically no risk from giving a few doses of steroids and there is no significant expense, many radiology practices will premedicate patients who have had a prior reaction to HOCM (e.g., hives) with steroids as well as administering LOCM. If there has been a serious contrast reaction to either LOCM or HOCM, alternative imaging strategies that do not require iodinated contrast should be pursued (e.g., MR, MR angiography, etc.).

19. What is a typical premedication regimen?

Prednisone 50 mg orally 13, 5, and 1 hour before contrast administration

Diphenhydramine 50 mg orally 1 hour before contrast administration (if this is given, it is important to ensure that someone will be taking the patient to and from the radiology department, due to drowsiness induced by this medication)

20. What is the mortality rate from iodinated contrast?

The incidence of fatal contrast reactions is approximately 1 per 100,000 administrations, for both LOCM and HOCM. The Food and Drug Administration reported a slightly higher number of deaths from LOCM as compared with HOCM from 1990–1994 (138 versus 82). This may be due to the widespread use of LOCM during this period.

21. Does the administration of intravenous mannitol decrease the incidence of nephrotoxicity in patients with chronic insufficiency who receive iodinated contrast media?

No. Recent studies have shown that the incidence of nephrotoxicity is actually slightly higher in patients receiving mannitol when compared with patients who receive hydration with saline. This regimen is therefore not recommended.

22. What are the early interventions that should be performed when treating a serious anaphylactoid reaction?

Specific treatments will depend on the exact clinical circumstances (e.g., bronchospasm can be treated initially with inhaled bronchodilators), but in general oxygen and intravenous fluids should be administered. To treat unresponsive bronchospasm, facial and laryngeal edema, and hypotension with tachycardia, give epinephrine 1:1000, 0.1–0.3 ml, subcutaneously (can repeat up to three times); if ineffective or peripheral vascular collapse occurs, give 1:10,000, 1.0–3.0 ml intravenously; also call code team. (For more detailed treatment information, refer to the Manual on Iodinated Contrast Media issued by the American College of Radiology.)

23. What type of contrast media should be used for myelography?

Nonionic contrast agents only. Lethal reactions have been reported following myelography performed with ionic contrast.

24. What is gadolinium?

A rare, heavy-earth metal that, when linked to ligands such as DTPA, is used as the intravenous contrast agent for MR.

25. What are the contraindications to gadolinium administration?

Other than a history of a prior reaction to gadolinium, there are no contraindications.

26. Have reactions been reported to gadolinium?

Yes, including serious and lethal reactions; fortunately, such reactions are rare. Reactions to gadolinium are believed to be anaphylactoid and are treated in a manner similar to reactions to iodinated contrast.

27. What is the recommended dose of gadolinium?

The standard adult dose of gadolinium for most MR applications is 0.1 mmol/kg (0.2 ml/kg) intravenously. A 70 kg patient should receive approximately 14 ml. Some imaging protocols (e.g., MR angiography) call for administration of a double dose of gadolinium.

28. How does gadolinium work?

Gadolinium is a paramagnetic agent that produces increased signal intensity on T1-weighted images.

29. Are there any other intravenous contrast agents that can be given during an MR examination?

There are iron oxide particles, which produce decreased signal intensity (e.g., in the liver) on T2-weighted images.

BIBLIOGRAPHY

1. Mishkin MM, Bettmann MA, Buenger RE, et al: Manual on Iodinated Contrast Media. American College of Radiology, 1991.
2. Solomon R, Werner C, Mann D, et al: Effects of saline, mannitol, and furosemide on acute decreases in renal function induced by radiocontrast agents. N Engl J Med 331:1416–1420, 1994.
3. Deray G, Jacobs C: Renal tolerance of nonionic dimers. Invest Radiol 31:372–377, 1996.

II. Thoracic Radiology

9. GENERAL PRINCIPLES AND PATTERN RECOGNITION

Stuart A. Groskin, M.D.

1. What technical factors should always be checked before interpreting a frontal chest radiograph?

Before doing anything, check the identifying information on the film to make sure it is the correct film and the correct patient. Then check the following:

- Inspiration
- Penetration (exposure)
- Position
- Rotation

2. How is inspiration checked?

Frontal chest radiographs are usually made at the end of a full, deep inspiration. From 9–10 posterior ribs or 5–6 anterior ribs should be visible on the right, above the dome of the right hemidiaphragm, if the patient has taken an adequately deep breath (Fig. 1).

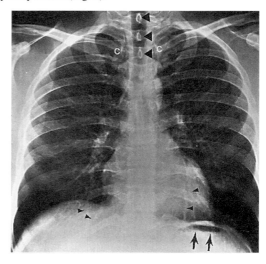

FIGURE 1. Normal frontal chest radiograph. This film demonstrates the technical factors that should be checked on all chest radiographs. A vertical line connecting several spinous processes (large arrowheads) should bisect a horizontal line connecting the clavicular heads (C) if the patient is not rotated. Bronchovascular structures (small arrowheads) should be visible behind the heart and through the dome of the right hemidiaphragm if exposure is adequate, and the intervertebral spaces should be visible. Nine to ten posterior ribs should be visible above the dome of the right hemidiaphragm when the lungs are well inflated (ten on this film). An air-fluid level (arrows), in this case in the stomach, indicates that the patient was upright when the film was made.

3. How is patient position checked?

Patients routinely stand or sit upright when chest radiographs are made. Although the patient's position when the film was made is often marked on the radiograph, it is always wise to determine if the patient was upright when the chest radiograph was made. This information can substantially alter the interpretation of the chest radiograph, particularly the distribution of free air and fluid in the pleural space, the size and distribution of pulmonary blood vessels, and the size of the cardiac silhouette.

4. How can one determine that a film was made with the patient upright?

If an air-fluid level is visible anywhere on the frontal chest radiograph—stomach, hiatal hernia, abscess, bowel—the patient was almost certainly erect when the film was exposed (see Fig. 1). Simply being able to see the gastric air bubble does not indicate the patient's position. Also, failure to seen an air-fluid level does not necessarily mean that the patient was not upright when the film was made; there simply may not have been enough gas and fluid in an appropriate hollow viscus to produce a radiographically visible air-fluid interface.

5. How does one check for correct exposure?

A well-exposed chest radiograph should provide information about the status of the patient's lung, mediastinal structures, bony thorax, and upper abdominal organs. To do so, the film must be made with a relatively high energy beam of photons. A properly exposed film should show branching, tapering bronchovascular structures through the right and left heart shadows and beneath the right hemidiaphragm as well as the intervertebral disc spaces in the midthoracic spine (see Fig. 1).

6. How is patient rotation checked?

The patient should be facing the x-ray cassette straight on when the frontal chest radiograph is made. Barring major deformities of the chest wall, if the patient is well centered, a vertical line connecting the 2–3 upper thoracic spinous processes should bisect almost exactly a horizontal line drawn between the two clavicular heads (see Fig. 1).

7. How important are these factors in daily practice?

Very important! For example, pleural effusions and pneumothoraces that are easily seen on erect frontal chest radiographs may be virtually invisible on semierect or supine chest radiographs. Also, the cardiac silhouette frequently appears enlarged on AP supine chest radiographs, particularly if the patient did not take an adequately deep breath when the film was made. These same technical factors can produce an increase in the size of the upper lobe pulmonary vessels. The combination of artifactual changes in the appearance of the heart and the pulmonary vessels can simulate the appearance of cardiomegaly and pulmonary venous hypertension/pulmonary edema and may lead to the institution of inappropriate and possibly dangerous treatments, while delaying the correct diagnosis and treatment (Fig. 2).

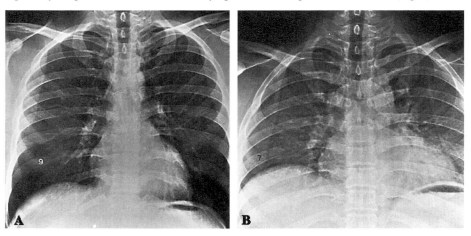

FIGURE 2. Inspiratory-expiratory frontal chest radiographs. Note the changes produced when the patient inspires deeply *(A)* and then exhales *(B)* before frontal films are obtained. Cardiomegaly and pulmonary edema are simulated on the expiratory film.

8. What is the difference between a PA and an AP chest radiograph?

Most frontal chest radiographs are made PA (posteroanterior), meaning that the patient faces the cassette holding the radiographic film; the x-ray beam enters the patient's back, traverses the thorax, and exits the anterior chest wall before striking the film. An AP (anteroposterior) frontal radiograph is made with the patient facing the opposite direction.

9. Why are PA chest radiographs preferable to AP radiographs?

Because, when the patient faces the x-ray film, the heart is closer to the film. This diminishes the extent to which the heart is magnified on the x-ray and allows more precise measurements of cardiac size. Knowing whether a series of chest radiographs was obtained with the patient in the AP or PA position helps to determine if there has been a change in the size of the heart over time. Realistically, to measure the size of the heart precisely and to assess the size of the cardiac chambers, ultrasound, MR, and even CT are much better than plain chest radiographs.

10. Other than differences in magnification, are there other reasons that PA films are preferable to AP films?

No. However, PA films are generally of better quality than AP films because most patients who have AP frontal chest radiographs are too ill to be positioned for a PA film. They are often unable to take and hold a deep breath during film exposure, are often too ill to sit or stand upright, and are therefore filmed in a supine or semirecumbent position using portable radiographic equipment. Portable radiographic equipment imposes a further technical limitation on most AP chest radiographs because it is not able to generate as high energy an x-ray beam as conventional chest radiographic units.

11. Are radiographic techniques ever intentionally altered to improve the diagnostic usefulness of a chest radiograph?

Yes. For example, a pneumothorax (free air in the pleural space) is often easier to see on a frontal chest radiograph made at the end of expiration than on a film exposed at the end of a deep inspiration for at least two reasons: (1) because the volume of the lung is decreased at the end of expiration but the volume of a pneumothorax is relatively unchanged, the pneumothorax occupies a greater total percentage of the volume of the thorax at the end of expiration and appears larger, and (2) the radiographic density of the lung is increased at the end of expiration while the radiographic density of a pneumothorax remains unchanged; this increases the difference in density between the lung and the adjacent pneumothorax and increases the visibility of the pneumothorax.

12. How are oblique and apical lordotic views of the chest useful?

They can help to show lesions that are obscured by overlying bony or soft-tissue structures on conventional frontal chest radiographs. Lateral decubitus views of the chest can aid in detecting pneumothoraces and pleural effusions (Fig. 3).

13. Why do clinicians prefer frontal chest x-rays to lateral chest x-rays?

Clinicians and some radiologists erroneously believe that all the important information about chest disease is contained on frontal radiographs. Lateral chest radiographs also can be very confusing to the observer because the right and left lungs are superimposed.

14. So why are lateral chest x-rays so important?

- Objects can be localized in three dimensions.
- About 10% of all pulmonary pathology is seen better or exclusively on lateral chest films.
- Lateral views of the chest can confirm the presence of a lesion that was suspected after viewing a frontal radiograph.

15. How do lateral chest radiographs allow localization of objects in space?

Because a radiograph is a two-dimensional representation of a three-dimensional object, two dimensions have to be collapsed onto each other, creating problems with depth perception. For example, if a nodule appears to be next to the right atrial border on a frontal chest radiograph, the clinician cannot determine where the lesion is in the patient's sagittal plane; it could be on the patient's skin (front or back), in the soft tissues or bones of the chest wall (front or back), in the pleural

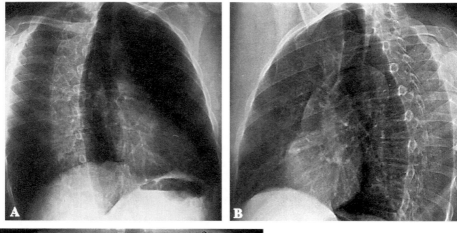

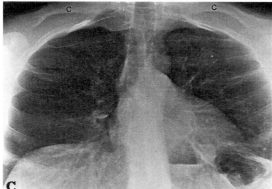

FIGURE 3. Oblique and apical lordotic views of the chest. *A,* Right anterior oblique view of the chest shows the heart rotated to the left, and the right clavicle projects across the spine. *B,* Left anterior view of the chest shows the heart rotated to the right, and the left clavicle projects across the spine. *C,* Apical lordotic view of the chest shows the clavicles (C) projected above the lung apices.

space, or in the right middle or right lower lobe. A lateral radiograph allows localization in the sagittal plane. Precise three-dimensional localization is very important for differential diagnosis and is a must if a percutaneous biopsy or bronchoscopy for biopsy is contemplated.

16. Why is some pulmonary pathology seen better or exclusively on lateral chest films?

There are significant "blind spots" on frontal chest radiographs, where soft-tissue or bony structures overlie and obscure underlying lung tissue. The left lower lobe is particularly notorious in this respect, since much of the basilar segments are masked by the bulk of the left ventricle. Also, a lateral view of the chest is the best plain film view to evaluate the sternum—the only better radiographic examination is a CT scan (Fig. 4).

17. What is the pulmonary interstitium?

An interconnected series of fibrous tissue compartments that acts as the skeleton of the lungs. The interstitium can be subdivided into (1) an axial compartment—the connective tissue sheaths that surround branches of the pulmonary arteries and bronchi as they course from their origins into the substance of the lung; (2) the interlobular septa—fibrous tissue bands that separate individual secondary pulmonary lobules and contain lymphatics and branches of the pulmonary veins; (3) the subpleural space—an extension of the interlobular septa that is found just deep to the visceral pleura; and (4) the alveolar walls. Involvement of any or all of these compartments by pathologic processes (tumors, edema, fibrosis) can accentuate and increase the visibility of these structures and produce a radiographic pattern of interstitial lung disease.

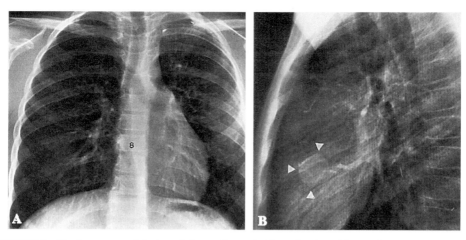

FIGURE 4. The importance of the lateral chest radiograph. The patient has a history of neuroblastoma at the apex of the left chest (note surgical clips). A frontal view of the chest *(A)* does not suggest the presence of metastases. A lateral view of the chest *(B)* shows a large pulmonary nodule (arrowheads) projecting over the cardiac silhouette that was subsequently shown to be a pulmonary nodule. Close examination of the right lateral border of the T8 vertebral body in the frontal chest film shows that the apparently convex border of the vertebral body really is the lateral margin of the pulmonary metastasis.

18. What are the alveoli? What is alveolar or airspace disease?

Alveoli are normally gas-filled sacs that form the grape-like clusters at the ends of the distal airways. When the alveoli are filled with fluid or cellular material, or when they collapse and become airless, they become opaque and produce poorly marginated, inhomogeneous areas of increased density on chest radiographs that are called areas of airspace or alveolar disease.

19. What are the radiographic features of interstitial disease?

Radiographic Findings Most Commonly Associated with Disease Processes Affecting Various Portions of the Pulmonary Interstitium

INTERSTITIAL COMPONENT	RADIOGRAPHIC SIGN
Axial	Peribronchial thickening
Interlobular septum	Kerley A, B, and C lines (Fig. 5)
Subpleural space	Thickening of the interlobar fissures
Alveolar wall	Perihilar "haze"

20. What are the radiographic features of alveolar disease?

Disease processes that primarily affect the alveoli produce inhomogeneous, patchy, poorly marginated radiographic opacities (Fig. 6). Air-bronchograms are a classic radiographic hallmark of alveolar disease. They represent gas-filled bronchi that become radiographically visible when they are surrounded by radiopaque alveoli.

21. Can interstitial disease mimic alveolar disease?

Yes. Although air-bronchograms usually indicate the presence of an alveolar process that fills the alveoli with fluid (pus, edema, or blood) or tumor (lymphoma, bronchoalveolar cell carcinoma), on rare occasions extensive interstitial lung disease can compress the alveoli, causing them to become gasless and air-bronchograms can be seen. Sarcoidosis is notorious for producing this "pseudoalveolar" appearance. Atelectasis also can produce air-bronchograms, as long as the airway remains gas-filled.

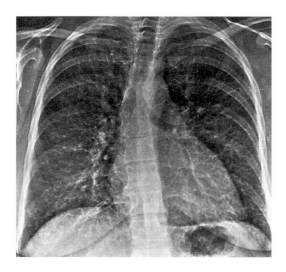

FIGURE 5. Interstitial lung disease—Kerley's lines. The patient has interstitial pulmonary edema. The myriad linear opacities that do not branch or taper represent Kerley B (peripheral, short and horizontal) and C (more central, forming a cobweb pattern) lines.

22. Is it important to determine if a radiographic density is interstitial or alveolar?

Although many pulmonary diseases have both an interstitial and an alveolar component (pneumonia, pulmonary edema, ARDS), determining the dominant radiographic pattern is worthwhile for the differential diagnosis.

23. Which diseases present with an alveolar pattern?

The diseases are usually acute or subacute and include bacterial pneumonia, cardiogenic and noncardiogenic pulmonary edema, aspiration, and pulmonary hemorrhage.

24. Which diseases present with an interstitial pattern?

Interstitial lung disease is usually subacute or chronic and includes pulmonary fibrosis, sarcoidosis, metastatic carcinoma (lymphangitic spread), and occupationally related lung disease such as asbestosis and silicosis. Interstitial cardiogenic pulmonary edema, typically an acute process, is a notable exception to this rule, as is atypical pneumonia (viral, mycoplasma, miliary tuberculosis, and histoplasmosis).

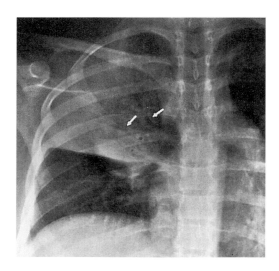

FIGURE 6. Alveolar lung disease—air bronchograms. Note black, air-filled airways (arrows) surrounded by white, fluid-filled airspaces in this patient with right upper lobe pneumococcal pneumonia. The sharply defined lower margin of the area of pneumonia is produced by the minor, or horizontal, fissure.

25. What happens when interstitial and alveolar abnormalities coexist?
The interstitial component of the process is frequently obscured by the adjacent alveolar opacities.

BIBLIOGRAPHY

1. Fraser RG, Pare JA, Pare PD, et al: Diagnosis of Diseases of the Chest, 3rd ed. Philadelphia, W.B. Saunders, 1988.
2. Groskin SA: Heitzman's The Lung. Radiologic-Pathologic Correlations, 3rd ed. St. Louis, Mosby-Year Book, 1993.
3. Proto AV, Speckman JM: The left lateral radiograph of the chest. Med Radiogr Photogr 55:30–74, 1979.
4. Proto AV, Speckman JM: The left lateral radiograph of the chest. Med Radiogr Photogr 56:38–64, 1980.

10. TUBES, LINES, AND CATHETERS

Stuart A. Groskin, M.D.

1. When should all lines, tubes, and extraneous devices be accounted for in reviewing a chest radiograph?
As soon as the technical adequacy of a chest film has been assessed.

2. Why is it important to inventory all lines and tubes on a chest radiograph?
Such inventory will:
- Give valuable information about the patient's general health or lack thereof
- Alert the person reviewing the radiograph to look for complications associated with the lines and tubes
- Keep the person reviewing the film from mistaking a line or tube for pathology (e.g., oxygen rebreather masks have been mistaken for pneumothoraces)

3. How can the location of the tip of an endotracheal tube be confirmed?
On a frontal chest film, an endotracheal tube that projects over the trachea could actually be on or under the patient or in the esophagus. If there is reason to believe that the endotracheal tube is not in the trachea, i.e., progressive gaseous distention of the stomach while the lung volumes remain low, shallow oblique or lateral chest radiographs can help to define its location in three dimensions.

4. Exactly where should the tip of an endotracheal tube be?
Ideally the tip should be about 4 cm above the tracheal carina. The endotracheal tube tip position is not fixed in the trachea; during flexion and extension of the neck, the tip of the tube can move about 4 cm. By positioning the tube tip at least 4 cm (usually 6–8 cm) above the carina, inadvertent selective intubation of the right or, less commonly, the left mainstem bronchus as the patient's neck moves can be avoided. This position is also low enough to keep the endotracheal tube balloon from rubbing against the vocal cords, decreasing the incidence of cord trauma. In most adults, if the tube tip projects at the level of the clavicular heads, it is in acceptable position (Fig. 1).

5. How can the endotracheal tube move up and down in the trachea when the tube cuff (balloon) is inflated?
The cuff, or balloon, of an endotracheal tube should never be inflated to the point that it continuously and completely occludes the tracheal lumen. The position of the endotracheal tube tip is largely maintained by anchoring the tube externally to the patient's nose or mouth. The endotracheal tube cuff itself primarily prevents retrograde flow of the ventilator-delivered tidal volume up the trachea and out the patient's mouth and nose. If the cuff is inflated to the point that it fixes the endotracheal tube within the trachea, it could cause pressure-induced necrosis of the tracheal mucosa and predispose to tracheal rupture or eventual tracheal stenosis.

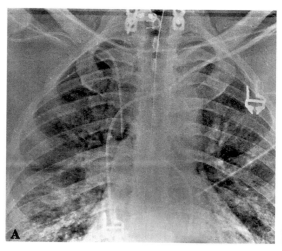
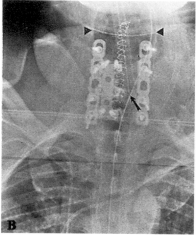

FIGURE 1. Malpositioned endotracheal tube. *A,* No endotracheal tube can be seen on a frontal chest radiograph made to localize the tip of the patient's endotracheal tube. *B,* A frontal film of the neck shows the endotracheal tip within the cervical trachea (arrow) and reveals a markedly overinflated endotracheal tube cuff (arrowheads).

6. What is the maximal diameter to which an endotracheal cuff should be inflated?

The maximal coronal diameter of the adult trachea is 2.5–3.0 cm. If the cuff of an endotracheal tube equals or exceeds 3.0 cm in diameter on radiographs, the pressure in the cuff should be checked to make sure that it is not hyperinflated. An even easier way to gauge overinflation is to note whether the diameter of the balloon is greater than the diameter of the trachea above and/or below the balloon. If the balloon creates a focal bulge in the contour of the tracheal wall, it is time to be concerned.

7. Does an endotracheal tube protect a patient against aspiration?

No. Occasionally a nasogastric tube placed in a patient who already has an endotracheal tube with an inflated cuff in place can slip by the cuff and enter the bronchial tree, usually on the right side. For this reason, a chest film should be obtained after passing a nasogastric tube even if the patient already has an endotracheal tube or tracheostomy tube (Fig. 2).

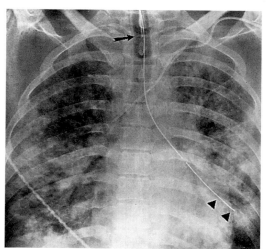

FIGURE 2. Aberrant placement of a nasogastric tube. Despite the prior placement of an endotracheal tube (arrow) with an inflated cuff, a newly inserted nasogastric tube entered the trachea and terminated in the left lower lobe bronchus (arrowheads).

8. Is there an ideal location for the tip of a nasogastric tube?

It depends on the intended purpose of the tube. Generally, the tip and the sideport of a nasogastric tube should be positioned distal to the esophagogastric junction and proximal to the gastric pylorus. Radiographic confirmation of the position of the nasogastric tube is mandatory, because clinical techniques for assessing tip position may be unreliable and are certainly inadequate for determining the location of the sideport of the tube.

9. What is the ideal position of a chest tube?

Chest tubes are usually placed to evacuate gas or fluid from the pleural space. Gas in the pleural space tends to collect in the most nondependent portion of the pleural space, while fluid puddles in the most dependent part of the space. Consequently, a chest tube placed to evacuate a pneumothorax should ideally be placed with its tip in the nondependent part of the pleural space, and a chest tube placed to evacuate pleural fluid such as blood should be positioned in a dependent portion of the pleural space. Of course, the nondependent and dependent portions of the pleural change as the patient's position changes, and it is simply not practical to reposition chest tubes each time a patient rolls over or sits up.

10. Exactly where are chest tubes usually positioned to drain fluid in the pleural space versus air in the pleural space?

Usually in the dorsal and caudad portion of the pleural space. Tubes placed to evacuate pneumothoraces are usually placed in the ventral and cephalad portions of the pleural space.

11. Is there a problem if a chest tube ends up positioned in a fissure?

Although there has been a great deal of controversy about whether chest tubes inadvertently placed in an interlobar fissure (an extension of the pleural space) should be repositioned, it appears that they generally work fine and and should not be relocated unless there is clinical evidence that they are not fulfilling their function.

12. What is the best position for the tip of a central venous catheter? Why?

Central venous catheters are used primarily to administer fluids and medications and to provide vascular access for hemodialysis; they are also occasionally used to monitor central venous pressure. If pressure measurements are going to be obtained, the tip of the catheter must be proximal to the venous valves. Under all circumstances the tip of the catheter must be located distal to (above) the right atrium; this prevents the catheter tip from producing arrhythmias or perforating the wall of the right atrium. The tip of a well-positioned central venous catheter projects over the silhouette of the superior vena cava, in a zone demarcated superiorly by the anterior first rib end and clavicle and inferiorly by the top of the right atrium. The course of the catheter should parallel the course of the superior vena cava; if the catheter appears to bend as it approaches the wall of the superior vena cava, or its path is perpendicular, not parallel to the path of the superior vena cava, the possibility of the catheter damaging and ultimately perforating the wall of the superior vena cava should be considered and the catheter should be repositioned.

13. Where should the tip of a Swan-Ganz catheter be located?

A Swan-Ganz catheter is used to monitor the pulmonary capillary wedge pressure (usually a reasonable approximation of the left atrial end-diastolic pressure) and to measure cardiac output in patients suspected of having left ventricular dysfunction. The tip of a Swan-Ganz catheter should be positioned within the right or left main pulmonary arteries or in one of their large, lobar branches. If the tip is located more distally, there is an increased risk of the catheter producing prolonged pulmonary artery occlusion, resulting in pulmonary infarction or, rarely, pulmonary artery rupture (Fig. 3).

14. What should be routinely checked when a cardiac pacemaker is seen on a chest radiograph?

Check the **L.E.A.D.**

Location refers to the location and appearance of the pacemaker's generator. Note the site of generator placement and the appearance of the lead wire(s) around the generator. In particular, look

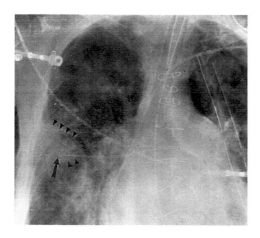

FIGURE 3. Pulmonary infarction related to distal placement of a Swan-Ganz catheter. The tip of the Swan-Ganz catheter is very distally positioned (arrow). The surrounding area of airspace opacity (arrowheads) represents an area of pulmonary infarction produced by interruption of blood supply to the area of lung distal to the catheter tip.

for an unusually large tangle of wire around the generator that may suggest that the patient has been twirling the pacemaker generator in its subcutaneous pocket, "reeling in" the pacer lead in the process (the Twiddler's syndrome) (Fig. 4).

Exit refers to the direction in which the pacer wires exit the generator. The insulation around most pacemakers is configured so that when the pacer generator is appropriately positioned, the pacer wires appear to exit the generator in a clockwise direction (Fig. 5). Appropriate generator placement is important in preventing the pacemaker from (1) sensing (and being shut down by) electrical activity generated in the pectoralis muscle and (2) stimulating contraction of the pectoralis muscle.

Alignment refers to the alignment of the various portions of the pacer lead(s). Areas of discontinuity could indicate the presence of a broken lead. To assess adequately the integrity and location of a pacing lead, at least two different, preferably orthogonal, radiographic views are needed (Fig. 6).

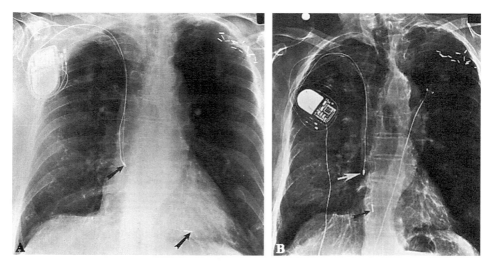

FIGURE 4. Twiddler's syndrome. *A,* Frontal chest radiograph shows normal positioning of the patient's proximal and distal pacemaker leads (arrows). *B,* The patient returned for evaluation of pacemaker malfunction. A repeat frontal chest radiograph shows that the pacemaker generator has changed position and that the most distal lead tip (black arrow) has been retracted into the right atrium. The proximal lead tip (white arrow) is at the cavoatrial junction.

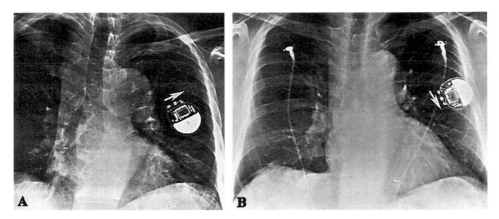

FIGURE 5. Flipped pacemaker generator. *A,* Frontal chest radiograph shows a pacemaker generator. The single lead exits the generator in a clockwise direction (arrow). *B,* The patient returned for evaluation when his left chest muscles began to twitch at a rate of 60/min. The pacemaker has flipped over and the lead now exits the generator in a counterclockwise direction (arrow).

Destination refers to the final destination of the pacer lead(s). If there is only a single pacer lead, the tip of the lead should project within the right ventricle; if there are two leads, one lead should project within the right ventricle and the other lead should terminate in the right atrium. Pacemaker leads can perforate the wall of the chamber they are in; this should be a consideration whenever the tip of the lead projects within 3 mm of the outer wall of the heart. If the lead tip projects beyond the outer border of the heart, perforation of the heart should be the leading concern.

15. What is an IABP device?

IABP stands for intraaortic balloon pump, a cardiac assist device positioned in the descending thoracic aorta via a femoral arterial approach. The radiopaque distal tip of the IABP should be seen at the junction of the aortic arch and descending thoracic aorta, just distal to the origin of the left subclavian artery. A balloon on the catheter inflates during diastole, improving myocardial perfusion by increasing blood flow through the coronary arteries; the balloon deflates during systole.

16. Review the major complications associated with line and tube placement.

The table on the next page is a partial list of the complications of line and tube placement and the problems associated with inappropriate positioning. The resultant radiographic findings are listed in parentheses. The findings in the second and third columns are not related.

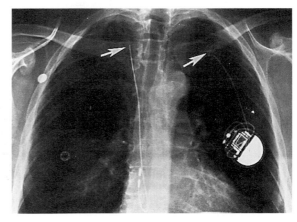

FIGURE 6. Fractured pacemaker lead. Frontal chest radiograph shows fracture of the pacemaker lead with distraction of the ends of the wire (arrows).

Device	Complications of Placement	Inappropriate Positioning
Endotracheal tube	Aspiration (parenchymal opacities) Pharyngeal perforation (subcutaneous emphysema, pneumomediastinum, mediastinitis)	Esophageal intubation (hypoventilation, gastric distention, aspiration) Selective mainstem bronchus intubation (atelectasis of the nonventilated lung) Too high (laryngeal injury, inadequate ventilation) Balloon too big (tracheal rupture, tracheal stenosis)
Nasogastric tube	Aspiration (parenchymal opacities) Intracranial perforation Pneumothorax	Intratracheal intubation (aspiration, hypoventilation) Intraesophageal position (aspiration) Intraduodenal placement (metabolic disturbances if on suction)
Chest tube	Lung perforation (mediastinal opacity)	Extrathoracic position (refractory pneumothorax, effusion) Apical positioning (Horner's syndrome) Intrafissural positioning (usually no problems)
Central venous catheter	Pneumothorax Bleeding (mediastinal, pleural)	Extravascular placement (pleural effusion, extrapleural hematoma) (Fig. 7)

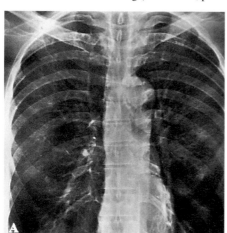
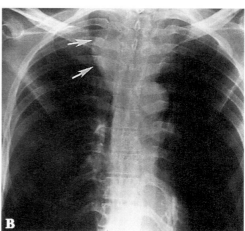

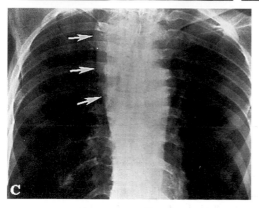

FIGURE 7.   Subclavian artery laceration during attempted central venous catheter placement. *A,* Frontal chest radiograph prior to CVP placement shows normal mediastinal contours. *B,* Mediastinal widening (arrows) occurred shortly after an abortive attempt to place a right subclavian central venous catheter. *C,* The patient became hypotensive, and a repeat chest radiograph showed increasing mediastinal widening (arrows) produced by an expanding mediastinal hematoma. Operative repair of this lacerated right subclavian artery was attempted.

Device	Complications of Placement	Inappropriate Positioning
Central venous catheter *(cont.)*	Air embolism	Peripheral placement (inaccurate pressure readings, inadequate mixing volume)
		Intracardiac placement (arrhythmia, atrial perforation)
Swan-Ganz catheter	Pneumothorax	Proximal placement (inaccurate pressure reading)
	Bleeding (mediastinal, pleural)	
	Air embolism	Distal placement (pulmonary artery perforation, pulmonary infarction)
Intraaortic balloon pump	Pneumothorax	Distal placement (inadequate coronary artery perfusion)
	Bleeding (mediastinal, pleural)	
	Air embolism	Proximal placement (inadequate cerebral perfusion)

BIBLIOGRAPHY

1. Curtin JJ, Goodman LR, Quebbeman EJ, Haasler GB: Thoracostomy tubes after acute chest injury: Relationship between location in a pleural fissure and function. AJR 163:1339–1342, 1994.
2. Gallagher TJ: Endotracheal intubation. Crit Care Clin 8:665–676, 1992.
3. Rosado LJ, Arabia FA, Smith RG, Copeland JG: Cardiovascular assist devices. Acad Radiol 2:418–427, 1995.
4. Templeton PA, Diaconis JN: Critical care chest imaging. In Mirvis SE, Joung JWR (eds): Imaging in Trauma and Critical Care. Baltimore, Williams & Wilkins, 1992, pp 516–568.
5. Wechsler RJ, Steiner RM, Kinori I: Monitoring the monitors: The radiology of thoracic catheters, wires, and tubes. Semin Roentgenol 23:61–84, 1988.
6. Zarshenas Z, Sparschu RA: Catheter placement and misplacement. Crit Care Clin 10:417–436, 1994.

11. MEDIASTINAL AND HILAR ABNORMALITIES

Stuart A. Groskin, M.D.

1. How are mediastinal and hilar abnormalities recognized on chest radiographs?

By the way in which they change the shape, size, density (opacity), and position of normal mediastinal and hilar structures.

2. What are the anterior and posterior junction lines?

Vertical lines that may be seen over the upper, central portion of a frontal chest radiograph (Fig. 1). They represent, respectively, the anterior and posterior conjunction of the right and left visceral and parietal pleural layers at the midline of the thorax. Recognition of deviation or distortion of the junction lines can make localization of mediastinal masses easier. For example, widening of the anterior junction line in a patient complaining of dysphagia and diplopia should suggest the presence of an anterior mediastinal mass—specifically, a thymoma.

3. What percentage of thymomas are associated with myasthenia gravis?

About 30%.

4. When does the thymus reach its maximum size and weight?

Although the thymus is most easily seen on chest radiographs of children under age 2, it does not reach its maximum size and weight until the ages of 12–19. The size then regresses until, at the age of 60, it is approximately half the size it was at age 20. The thymus is composed of epithelial and lymphocytic cells and is the source of T-cells that take part in cell-mediated immunity.

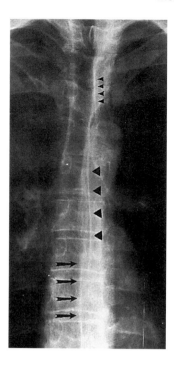

FIGURE 1. Normal mediastinal lines and interfaces. Coned-down frontal views of the chest shows the anterior junction line (large arrowheads), posterior junction line (small arrowheads), and the azygoesophageal recess (arrows).

5. What are the most common thymic tumors?

Thymomas, which are derived from thymic epithelial cells. They are also the most common surgical tumors of the anterior mediastinum, accounting for 20% of all mediastinal tumors. Up to 70% of patients with thymomas have associated syndromes or clinical abnormalities. About 30% of patients with thymomas have myasthenia gravis, but only 10–15% of patients with myasthenia gravis also have thymomas; 5% have red cell aplasia and 5% have hypogammaglobulinemia.

6. What is the prognosis for a patient with a thymoma?

It depends on the stage of the thymoma, which is determined not by the cell type or degree of cellular atypia but by the presence or absence of invasion of adjacent tissues. Patients with noninvasive, encapsulated thymomas have an excellent prognosis, with only a 2% recurrence rate and greater than 85% 10-year survival after surgical resection. Thymomas that invade adjacent tissues such as the pericardium or lung are more difficult to resect and have a 30% recurrence rate after surgery. They are associated with only a 65% 10-year survival; if systemic dissemination occurs, the 10-year survival drops to about 40%.

7. Are there any other primary neoplasms of the thymus?

Although thymomas arc by far the most common primary thymic neoplasm, other tumors can evolve from the thymus, including thymic carcinoma, thymic carcinoid, thymolipoma, small-cell carcinoma of the thymus, and Hodgkin's and non-Hodgkin's lymphoma.

8. What is the cervicothoracic sign, and what does it mean?

The cervicothoracic sign uses the sharpness of definition of the lateral margins of a mediastinal mass that projects above the level of the clavicles to determine whether the mass is located in the anterior or posterior mediastinal compartment (Fig. 2). Lesions in the anterior or posterior mediastinum have sharply defined lateral margins below the level of the clavicles since they are bordered laterally by aerated lung. As anterior masses (e.g., thyroid goiters) extend superiorly into the neck, definition of their lateral margins blurs above the clavicles, since the mass is no longer intrathoracic

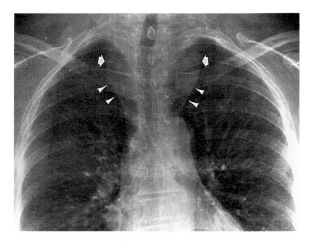

FIGURE 2. Cervicothoracic sign. Frontal chest radiograph demonstrates a large upper mediastinal mass. The interface between the lower portion of the mass and the adjacent lung (arrowheads) is sharply marginated, while the interface between the upper portion of the mass and the adjacent tissues (arrows) is poorly defined.

and is now bordered by the soft tissues of the neck, not by air. Since the posterior portions of the lungs extend superiorly above the levels of the clavicles (and above the anterior portions of the lungs) to the apex of the thorax, posterior mediastinal masses are bordered laterally by aerated lung over their entire course and, therefore, have clearly defined lateral margins both below and above the level of the clavicles.

9. What is the aortic "nipple"?

A small convex bump that protrudes from the left lateral wall of the aortic knob (Fig. 3). It is seen in 1.4–9.5% of PA chest radiographs and represents the left superior intercostal vein. This vein drains the second, third, and fourth intercostal spaces on the left and then courses anteriorly adjacent to the aortic arch, before emptying into the left brachiocephalic vein. The aortic nipple may be seen more easily in recumbent patients and in patients with obstruction of the superior or inferior vena cava or left brachiocephalic vein; it may disappear on films obtained while the patient performs a Valsalva maneuver.

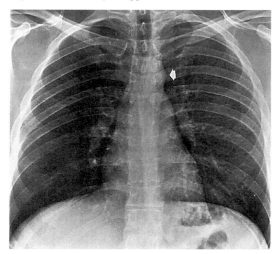

FIGURE 3. Aortic "nipple." The aortic nipple is a focal bulge in the lateral aspect of the aortic knob (arrow) produced by the left superior intercostal vein.

10. What is the significance of the aortic nipple?

That it should not be confused with pathology. On plain chest radiographs, the aortic nipple may be mistaken for mediastinal adenopathy, while on CT scans of the chest, the left superior intercostal vein may be mistaken for aortic dissection.

11. How big does a mediastinal lymph node have to be before it is considered enlarged?

Most normal mediastinal lymph nodes are less than 1 cm in diameter when measured along the short axis. Lymph nodes greater than 2 cm in diameter are usually abnormal. Lymph nodes between 1–2 cm in diameter have an intermediate probability of being abnormal.

12. What is the significance of enlarged lymph nodes seen on CT examinations of the chest?

In patients who have an underlying bronchogenic carcinoma, enlarged lymph nodes likely contain metastases from the lung cancer. Abnormally enlarged lymph nodes in patients who do not have a previously diagnosed cancer also may represent the site of metastatic disease, from either a previously occult lung cancer or an extrathoracic primary tumor. However, enlarged lymph nodes in a patient who does not have a documented malignancy are equally or more likely to be enlarged because of an infection such as tuberculosis or another inflammatory process.

13. What does dense calcification within an enlarged node favor?

The presence of infection, usually old granulomatous disease such as tuberculosis and histoplasmosis, although nodal metastases from carcinoid tumors and from osteogenic sarcoma may calcify or ossify.

14. Since the size of a lymph node can only indicate the probability that the node is abnormal and cannot reveal exactly what is making it too big, how can a definite diagnosis be established?

Node biopsy is the most widely accepted way to determine if enlarged lymph nodes contain tumor. This question is of particular importance in patients who have bronchogenic cancer, since surgery represents the only reasonable chance for a patient with lung cancer to be cured. Before attempting a curative surgical resection, it is important to determine whether the lung cancer has metastasized, because extrathoracic metastases and spread to certain mediastinal node groups can influence prognosis and may preclude an aggressive attempt at tumor resection.

15. What is the specific approach to lymph node sampling?

Patients who have no evidence of enlarged mediastinal lymph nodes on preoperative CT scans do not need to undergo preoperative node biopsy but should have nodes sampled at the time of thoracotomy. Patients who have enlarged nodes as seen on staging on CT scans need to have their abnormal nodes biopsied to determine if tumor is present before a decision is made regarding the advisability of thoracotomy and surgical resection of the primary tumor.

16. How is mediastinoscopy performed?

Mediastinoscopy is an invasive surgical procedure that requires the use of general anesthesia. An incision is made at the base of the neck and a rigid tube inserted into the visceral compartment of the neck and mediastinum. Paratracheal, anterior carinal, and tracheobronchial angle lymph nodes can be directly visualized and biopsied using this technique, and the presence or absence of metastases can be confirmed. Complications are uncommon, but in cases with enlarged left-sided mediastinal lymph nodes, access by mediastinoscopy may be limited.

17. What is the Chamberlain procedure?

Also called parasternal mediastinotomy, it is a limited, anterior parasternal thoracotomy usually performed on the left to allow evaluation of node groups that cannot be assessed by mediastinoscopy. The Chamberlain procedure is a very effective means of evaluating mediastinal nodes, but like mediastonoscopy, it is an invasive procedure that requires the use of general anesthesia.

18. Can percutaneous lymph node biopsy be performed?

Yes, using CT or fluoroscopic guidance, percutaneous fine needle aspiration is an extremely valuable technique for biopsying enlarged mediastinal lymph nodes. In experienced hands, the sensitivity of percutaneous lymph node biopsy in detecting mediastinal lymph node metastases is about 90%. Pneumothorax occurs in 15–40% of patients, but only rarely is chest tube drainage necessary.

19. Is bronchoscopy useful in evaluating mediastinal lymph nodes?

Not particularly; however, if imaging-guided transtracheal or transbronchial needle aspiration is performed via the bronchoscope, adjacent lymph nodes can be sampled and metastatic disease can be detected.

20. Are there any other promising examinations for evaluating mediastinal lymph nodes?

Positron emission tomography (PET) shows promise for providing a noninvasive diagnostic alternative in evaluating enlarged mediastinal and hilar lymph nodes.

21. Are there any primary tumors of the thoracic duct?

They are extremely rare—probably the closest thing to a primary tumor of the thoracic duct is a lymphangioma—but it is not uncommon for the thoracic duct to be involved by other intrathoracic malignancies, including lymphoma and bronchogenic carcinoma. Adenopathy associated with sarcoidosis has also been implicated as a source of thoracic duct dysfunction.

22. Describe the course of the thoracic duct.

The thoracic duct arises from the cisterna chyli and ascends in the thorax between the azygous vein and the aorta, just to the right of midline. In the mid to upper thorax, it crosses to the left, swings anteriorly at the level of the aortic arch, and enters the root of the neck where it terminates by emptying into the junction of the subclavian and internal jugular veins. Sixty to one hundred and ten milliliters of chyle flow through the thoracic duct per hour, for a total daily output of up to 2,500 ml.

23. What happens when the thoracic duct is disrupted by tumor or blunt trauma?

Chyle can accumulate in the pleural space (chylothorax). If the duct is interrupted in the lower part of the thorax, a right chylothorax usually occurs, while if the disruption involves the upper part of the duct, chyle accumulates in the left pleural space. The diagnosis of chylothorax is made by thoracentesis followed by lipid analysis of the aspirated fluid. Treatment usually focuses on the process that produced the thoracic duct disruption, but can also include ligation of the thoracic duct, dietary manipulation, and sclerosis of the affected pleural space.

24. What is the significance of a focal bulge in the left paraspinal line?

The left paraspinal line is not really a line but an interface between the aerated left lower lobe and the paraspinal soft tissues. Any disease which affects the vertebral bodies, the sympathetic nerve trunks, the hemizygous vein, the intercostal arteries and veins, the lymph nodes, and the pleura and adipose and connective tissues can distort the usual contour of the lung-paraspinal soft tissue interface.

25. What accounts for 90% of all localized paraspinal masses?

Neurogenic tumors, particularly neurofibromas and ganglioneuromas. Tumors arising from ganglion cells tend to be fusiform in appearance and extend vertically over several vertebral body levels. All neurogenic tumors can erode and separate the adjacent ribs (Fig. 4).

26. What can an abnormality in the paraspinal-lung interface in a trauma patient be a sign of?

Always examine the paraspinal-lung interface carefully in trauma patients, since a focal bulge in this interface may be the only or most visible sign of an underlying thoracic spine fracture and its associated paraspinal hematoma.

27. When should extramedullary hematopoiesis be suspected as the cause of paraspinal soft tissue masses?

In patients with hemolytic anemias, particularly if the masses occur between the T6 and T12 levels.

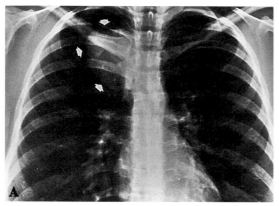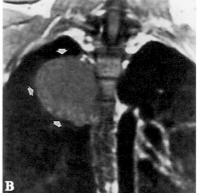

FIGURE 4.   Posterior mediastinal mass. *A,* Frontal chest radiograph shows right paraspinal mass sharply mar-ginated both below and above the level of the clavicles (arrows) indicating its posterior location. *B,* MR examina-tion confirmed the posterior location of the lesion (arrows) that was subsequently shown to be a schwannoma.

28. Can free fluid in the pleural space simulate a paraspinal soft-tissue mass?

Yes. Free pleural fluid can accumulate in the medial pleural space, producing a paraspinal soft-tissue mass. These collections are usually triangular in shape, with the apex of the triangle directed cephalad. Their true nature can usually be confirmed by obtaining the appropriate lateral decubitus chest radiograph; sonography and CT can also be helpful.

BIBLIOGRAPHY

1. Brown K, Aberle DR, Batra P, Steckel RJ: Current use of imaging in the evaluation of primary mediastinal masses. Chest 98:466–473, 1990.
2. McLoud TC, Bourgouin PM, Greenberg RW, et al: Bronchogenic carcinoma: Analysis of staging in the medi-astinum with CT by correlative lymph node mapping and sampling. Radiology 182:319–323, 1992.
3. Meza MP, Benson M, Slovis TL: Imaging of mediastinal masses in children. Radiol Clin North Am 31:583–604, 1993.
4. Morgenthaler TL, Brown LR, Colby TV, et al: Thymoma. Mayo Clin Proc 68:1110–1123, 1993.
5. Patz EF, Goodman PC: Positron emission tomography imaging of the thorax. Radiol Clin North Am 32:811–823, 1994.
6. Quagliano PV: Thymic carcinomas: Case reports and review. J Thorac Imag 11:66–74, 1996.
7. Rosado-de-Christensen ML, Galobardes J, Moran CA: Thymoma: Radiologic-pathologic correlation. Radio-graphics 12:151–168, 1992.

12. PNEUMONIA

Stuart A. Groskin, M.D.

1. How prevalent is pneumonia now that we have powerful antibiotics?

Pneumonias are responsible for more than 500,000 hospitalizations each year, which costs more than $15 billion dollars to treat. Pneumonia is the sixth most common cause of death in the United States.

2. How specific are the radiographic findings associated with different forms of pneumonia?

Although certain radiographic findings may suggest a specific organism as the cause of a given episode of pneumonia, microbiologic or immunologic examination of the sputum, lung tissue, or blood is the only certain way to establish a specific diagnosis. Not only can a wide variety of bacterial organisms produce similar changes on chest radiographs, but even the radiographic changes produced by viral and bacterial infections can be remarkably similar and and cannot usually be reliably distinguished.

3. What is the difference between pneumonia and pneumonitis?

There is really no difference. These terms can be used interchangeably. Some clinicians prefer to use the term *pneumonitis* when they are not sure that a parenchymal opacity is caused by an infection because they feel that this term is nonspecific.

4. Why should repeat chest radiographs be obtained in a patient with confirmed bacterial pneumonia?

To make sure that the pneumonia is going away.

5. If a pneumonia is not resolving radiographically in the usual anticipated manner, what are the possibilities?

- The wrong antibiotic is being used.
- The patient is not taking the prescribed medication or is taking it sporadically (the latter is probably worse than not taking the antibiotic at all, because organisms that are resistant to the specific antibiotic may be selected, leading to a truly difficult treatment problem).
- The patient may have difficulty absorbing the antibiotic.
- There is a problem with the patient's defense mechanisms.
- The patient has an intrinsic airways problem, such as a neoplasm; airways obstruction severely retards the resolution of pneumonia.
- Maybe it isn't pneumonia!

6. What examinations should be considered in patients with pneumonia that does not resolve as promptly as it should?

- Fiberoptic bronchoscopy, to exclude an underlying aspirated foreign body or an endobronchial neoplasm
- CT, which allows the airways to be visualized noninvasively and enables both extraluminal and intraluminal abnormalities to be identified

7. When should bacterial pneumonia resolve on radiographs?

In otherwise normal hosts, all radiographic abnormalities should disappear after 6 weeks of appropriate antibiotic therapy.

8. Why would a bacterial pneumonia not resolve by 6 weeks?

- The patient is elderly.
- There is underlying COPD.
- The patient is an alcoholic.

Patients who respond clinically in an appropriate fashion with prompt resolution of fever and leukocytosis should have a chest radiograph repeated in 4–6 weeks. Patients who do not respond to apparently adequate treatment in a timely fashion may warrant earlier and more frequent repetition of the chest films. Failure of a pneumonia to significantly improve after 4–6 weeks of therapy usually indicates the need for further evaluation with fiberoptic bronchoscopy, CT, or both.

9. Is it true that a dehydrated patient may have a pneumonia that cannot be seen on radiographs and that the pneumonia may become visible only after the patient is rehydrated?

Although this is not usually a major problem, a patient's state of hydration probably can influence the radiographic visibility of a pneumonia. Dehydration can make a pneumonia more difficult to see on a chest radiograph, while hydration can increase the visibility (and the weight) of an infected pulmonary lobe or segment.

10. What is the effect of neutropenia on the radiographic visibility of pneumonia?

This is a greater clinical and radiographic concern than the hydration status of the patient. Neutropenic patients may have clinical evidence of pneumonia without corresponding radiographic abnormalities. As the granulocyte count increases, radiographic opacities may appear, and in some cases, particularly in patients with invasive pulmonary aspergillosis, cavitation may be noted. A normal chest radiograph, therefore, does not exclude pneumonia in a neutropenic patient.

11. Does the radiographic appearance of pneumonia in young children differ from that in adults?

Most pneumonias in children under age 2 are caused by viruses. Histologically they show extensive, inhomogeneous airway wall edema and necrosis and sloughing of the airway mucosa. These processes produce intermixed areas of atelectasis and air-trapping that are seen on chest radiographs as coarse, linear opacities and generalized pulmonary hyperinflation. Lobar areas of airspace opacification are relatively uncommon in young children.

12. What is a "round" pneumonia?

A spherical pulmonary mass that is caused by a pneumonia, usually by pneumococcus. While this peculiar finding may be rare in adults, it is more common, although still unusual, in children. The reason the pneumonia assumes this shape is unclear, but in all other respects it behaves like a normal pulmonary infection. Over several days, if appropriate antibiotic therapy is begun, the margins of the mass become indistinct, air-bronchograms appear, and the lesion assumes the more characteristic appearance of a pneumonia.

13. What is the radiographic appearance of atypical measles pneumonia?

Multiple pulmonary nodules.

14. Can other diseases look like pneumonia on chest radiograph?

Yes. Lung cancer can mimic pneumonia by producing a postobstructive pneumonia or a "drowned" lobe or lung. When a neoplasm occludes a bronchus, sloughed cells, secretions, and transuded fluid accumulate distal to the site of obstruction, producing a radiographic opacity called a post-obstructive pneumonia. Infection is usually absent, and if the obstruction occurs slowly, the volume of the affected lobe or segment may be maintained or may increase.

15. What other types of neoplasms can mimic pneumonia on chest radiographs?

Bronchoalveolar lung cancer, a type of adenocarcinoma of the lung, mimics pneumonia by filling airspaces with malignant cells instead of infected edema fluid. The neoplastic cells fill the alveoli without invading or destroying their walls, and they percolate through the airways, spilling into and filling adjacent airspaces to create a radiographic picture that is identical to an alveolar pneumonia. Pulmonary lymphoma can also present with a radiographic picture that is indistinguishable from an alveolar pneumonia.

16. What are some non-neoplastic diseases that can simulate pneumonia on chest radiographs?

- Aspiration
- Hemorrhage
- Pulmonary edema (cardiogenic or non-cardiogenic)
- Sarcoidosis
- Lipoid pneumonia
- Alveolar proteinosis

17. How can the above entities be distinguished from pneumonia?

Clinical findings such as lack of fever or leukocytosis, may be helpful in distinguishing these disorders from pneumonia. The chronologic evolution of the process can be of great diagnostic value. Neoplasms change slowly and rarely, if ever, spontaneously improve; pulmonary edema can change very rapidly, often appearing or clearing in hours. Lipoid pneumonia is usually an indolent process that may improve with the administration of glucocorticoids but is not affected by antibiotics.

18. What is the radiographic appearance of *Pneumocystis carinii* pneumonia (PCP) in patients with AIDS?

PCP is the most common cause of morbidity and mortality in patients who have AIDS. PCP has been recognized as a cause of illness in HIV-infected patients for years. Typically it caused bilateral symmetric perihilar opacities, and death resulted or the pneumonia cleared completely. Although bilateral symmetric opacities are the most common radiographic findings in HIV-positive patients with PCP, an impressive array of varied radiographic abnormalities have been demonstrated: focal airspace opacities, hilar and/or mediastinal lymphadenopathy (which is occasionally calcified), pleural effusions, cavities, and bilateral upper lobe cysts (usually attributed to the prior prophylactic administration of aerosolized pentamidine).

19. What is the radiographic appearance of mycobacterial infections in HIV-positive patients?

Mycobacterial infections, especially tuberculosis, occur with increased frequency in HIV-positive patients. Although most of these infections represent reactivation or postprimary disease, the findings on chest radiographs and CT scans more closely resemble the abnormalities usually seen in patients who have primary mycobacterial infection: airspace opacities and lymphadenopathy predominate, and cavitation, the radiographic hallmark of reactivation, is less common.

20. Why is cavitation less common in HIV-positive patients who have tuberculosis?

Cavitation requires the presence of relatively intact cell-mediated immunity. HIV-positive patients whose CD4 counts are above 200/mm³ may develop cavitation, while patients whose CD4 counts are below 200/mm³ are much less likely to develop cavitation.

21. Is bacterial pneumonia common in HIV-positive patients?

Attention initially was focused on the high incidence and atypical appearance of opportunistic pulmonary infections in HIV-positive patients. Gradually, it became apparent that about 30% of pulmonary infections in these patients were caused by ordinary bacterial pathogens. *Streptococcus pneumoniae, Hemophilus influenzae, Legionella pneumophila,* and *Mycoplasma pneumoniae* are common offenders. Focal airspace opacities in HIV-positive patients, particularly in outpatients, should be considered to represent bacterial pneumonias until proven otherwise.

BIBLIOGRAPHY

1. Bettenay FA, deCampp JF, McCrossin DB: Differentiating bacterial from viral pneumonias in children. Pediatr Radiol 18:453–454, 1988.
2. Bowton DL, Bass DA: Community-acquired pneumonia: The clinical dilemma. J Thorac Imag 6:1–5, 1991.
3. Burke M, Fraser R: Obstructive pneumonitis: A pathologic and pathogenetic reappraisal. Radiology 166: 699–704, 1988.
4. DeLorenzo LJ, Huang CT, Maguire GP, Stone DJ: Roentgenographic patterns of Pneumocystis carinii pneumonia in 104 patients with AIDS. Chest 91:323–327, 1987.
5. Donowitz G, Harman C, Pope T, Stewart F: The role of the chest roentgenogram in febrile neutropenic patients. Arch Intern Med 151:701–704, 1991.
6. Goodman PC: Pneumocystis carinii pneumonia. J Thorac Imag 6:16–21, 1991.
7. Groskin SA: Heitzman's The Lung, 3rd ed. St. Louis, Mosby-Year Book, 1993.
8. Hill CA: Bronchoalveolar carcinoma: A review. Radiology 150:15–20, 1984.

13. PULMONARY EMBOLISM

Stuart A. Groskin, M.D.

1. How common are pulmonary emboli (PE)?

Almost 750,000 Americans have pulmonary emboli each year; 150,000 people die as a direct result.

2. Is pulmonary embolism the same thing as pulmonary infarction?

No. A pulmonary embolus is a blood clot that is carried by the systemic venous circulation to the right side of the heart and is then ejected into the pulmonary arterial bed. The embolus becomes impacted in a branch of the pulmonary artery, obstructing it, which leads to diminished perfusion of the distal vessels that the artery supplies. Pulmonary infarction is necrosis of lung tissue caused by insufficient blood supply.

3. How often does pulmonary infarction occur when a pulmonary embolus is present?

In less than 10% of all episodes of pulmonary embolism.

4. Why is the incidence of pulmonary infarction so low?

The most likely explanation is that the lung has a dual blood supply. The pulmonary parenchyma is perfused by systemic venous blood carried by the pulmonary artery, which arises from the right ventricle, and by oxygenated systemic arterial blood carried by the bronchial arteries, which originate from the aorta. When an embolus stops the flow of pulmonary arterial blood to a portion of the lung, the flow of bronchial arterial blood to the same portion of lung increases up to 300%, which allows the lung tissue to survive.

5. How accurate is the physical examination in suggesting the diagnosis of pulmonary embolism?

The physical examination and the clinical history are of limited value in diagnosing pulmonary embolism.

6. What are the signs and symptoms associated with pulmonary embolism?

They are nonspecific and include dyspnea, chest pain or tightness, cough, hemoptysis, hypoxia, arrhythmia, and hypotension. Although all of these findings may occur in patients who have PE, they are just as likely to be found in patients who have other cardiopulmonary diseases.

7. Where do most PE originate?

From thrombi, which occur in the deep veins of the legs and pelvis.

8. Are physical findings reliable in diagnosing deep venous thrombosis?

No. These findings (e.g,. leg swelling/tenderness) are extremely unreliable indicators of the presence of deep venous thrombosis and, therefore, pulmonary embolism.

9. What are the risk factors for deep venous thrombosis?

- Venous stasis—prolonged immobilization, recent surgery, long car/airplane ride
- Vascular injury: trauma, indwelling vascular catheters
- Hypercoagulable state: malignancy, antibodies to cardiolipin, antithrombin III deficiency, protein C deficiency, homocystinuria, oral contraceptives
- Past history of PE

Despite the degree of clinical suspicion, the diagnosis of pulmonary embolism requires confirmation with more specific testing.

10. What do chest radiographs usually show in patients who have PE?

About 80–90% of patients with PE have abnormalities on their chest radiographs. Unfortunately, these findings are usually nonspecific (subsegmental atelectasis, ill-defined opacities) and are of little or no diagnostic use. More suggestive radiographic abnormalities such as a Hampton's hump and Westermark's sign are rarely seen and, when present, may be mistaken for pneumonia, bullous emphysema, or artifact.

11. What is a Hampton's hump?

A peripheral, pleural-based wedge-shaped opacity that represents an area of pulmonary infarction (Fig. 1).

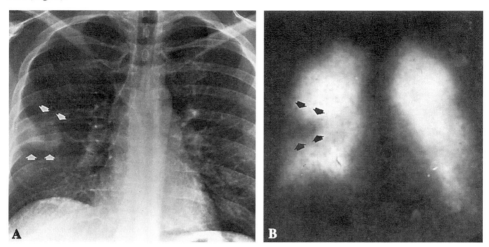

FIGURE 1. Hampton's hump. *A,* Frontal chest radiograph reveals a peripheral, pleural-based opacity, shaped like a truncated cone (arrows). *B,* Frontal image from subsequent perfusion lung scan shows a corresponding peripheral, pleural-based area of absent perfusion in the right mid-lung. The ventilation study showed diminished ventilation in this area, consistent with pulmonary embolus with infarction, and multiple unmatched perfusion defects were seen in the left lung, indicating that the probability of pulmonary embolism is high.

12. What is Westermark's sign?

An area of hyperlucent lung caused by diminished pulmonary arterial flow in lung distal to an embolus.

13. What is the best way to establish or exclude the diagnosis of pulmonary embolism?

This question has plagued clinicians and radiologists for over 30 years. Although the clinical features of PE were described by Laennec over 175 years ago, the first real objective diagnostic test did not exist until 1931, when Moniz performed the first pulmonary angiogram. Even then, it took 30 years for the medical community to recognize the clinical usefulness of pulmonary angiography in detecting pulmonary emboli. At the present time, pulmonary angiography is considered to be the "gold standard" against which all other tests designed to diagnose pulmonary emboli are measured.

14. How is a pulmonary angiogram performed?

A catheter is placed into the femoral vein and is fed through the inferior vena cava into the right heart ventricle and out into the pulmonary artery. The procedure is performed using fluoroscopic guidance. The right and left lungs are individually imaged in multiple projections as contrast is injected through the catheter.

15. Is pulmonary angiography safe?

In experienced hands, pulmonary angiography is relatively safe (0.5% mortality, 1% major nonfatal complications, 5% minor complications) and is sensitive (false negative rate less than 1%) and specific (Fig. 2). Because it is an invasive procedure, it is usually reserved for patients in whom noninvasive examinations, including nuclear medicine ventilation-perfusion scans and ultrasound examination of the deep veins of the legs, fail to determine whether pulmonary emboli are likely.

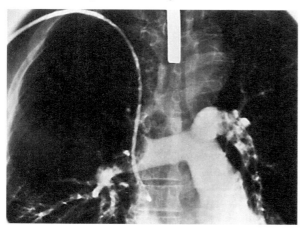

FIGURE 2. Positive pulmonary angiogram. Frontal view of the main pulmonary outflow tract and central pulmonary arteries made during the injection of contrast reveals multiple intraluminal filling defects produced by pulmonary emboli.

16. What are the indications for performing a pulmonary angiogram in a patient with a suspected PE?

Angiography should be considered when:
- There is a high clinical suspicion of PE but noninvasive diagnostic tests are inconclusive.
- Anticoagulation is contraindicated or more aggressive treatment, such as IVC filter placement, is being considered.
- In a hemodynamically unstable patient suspected of having massive PE who is being considered for emergency embolectomy.
- Any time the diagnosis of PE needs to be conclusively established.

17. What are the relative contraindications to pulmonary angiography?

- Previous history of a major reaction to intravenous contrast
- Pulmonary arterial hypertension (> 70 mmHg) or elevated right ventricular end diastolic pressure (> 20 mmHg)
- History of a bleeding disorder
- Left bundle branch block, which usually requires placement of a temporary transvenous pacemaker prior to angiography

18. How accurate are nuclear ventilation-perfusion (V/Q) scans in diagnosing pulmonary embolism?

It depends on what is meant by "diagnosing" PE. V/Q scans provide excellent information regarding the distribution of ventilation and perfusion to all portions of the lungs. They can easily demonstrate areas where pulmonary arterial perfusion is deficient and can also indicate what portions of the lungs are inadequately ventilated.

19. How is a ventilation-perfusion study performed?

The patient inhales a radioactive gas (typically xenon) and images of the lungs are obtained with a gamma camera. The perfusion portion of the study is then performed. A solution of albumin particles that have been tagged with a radioactive tracer is injected intravenously, and images of the lung are again obtained with a gamma camera. The ventilation and perfusion images are compared in conjunction with a recent chest radiograph.

20. Why is it critical to have a recent chest radiograph when interpreting a V/Q scan?

To use one of the described algorithms (i.e., modified Biello or modified PIOPED) to interpret a V/Q scan—that is, to categorize it as normal, low probability for PE, intermediate or indeterminate probability, or high probability—a chest radiograph obtained within the last 24 hours, and preferably more recently, is required. The presence of a variety of findings on the chest radiograph, such as an enlarged heart, a pleural effusion, evidence of COPD, parenchymal abnormalities, changes the interpretation of the V/Q scan.

21. What is the classic appearance of a PE on a V/Q scan?

Pulmonary emboli produce regional deficiencies in pulmonary arterial perfusion that are easily seen as cold areas on nuclear perfusion scans. Classically, ventilation is normal in the affected lung, producing an imaging pattern known as ventilation perfusion mismatch (diminished or absent perfusion in an area of normally ventilated lung) that is virtually diagnostic for pulmonary embolism ("high probability" V/Q scan). Unfortunately, it is not uncommon to find diminished ventilation as well as diminished perfusion in areas of the lung with emboli.

22. What is the probable cause of "matching" ventilation and perfusion defects on a V/Q scan of a patient with pulmonary emboli?

Impaired ventilation may be the result of reflex bronchoconstriction triggered by the embolus or, probably more commonly, it reflects an underlying comorbid problem with airway obstruction. Although ventilation-perfusion abnormalities (areas of diminished ventilation as well as perfusion in a given area of lung) are common in patients who have PE, they are more common in patients who have COPD without pulmonary emboli. In these patients, the primary abnormality is airflow obstruction, which produces regional alveolar hypoxia, which in turn induces local hypoxic vasoconstriction; the result is a V/Q scan with matched V/Q abnormalities.

23. Why are patients with COPD at increased risk of developing pulmonary emboli?

Because they are frequently sedentary and because their chronic hypoxia may induce polycythemia and a hypercoagulable state.

24. Does a normal V/Q scan effectively exclude a pulmonary embolus?

Yes, and the workup for pulmonary embolic disease usually stops.

25. What percentage of patients with pulmonary emboli have a high-probability scan?

Only 15%. A high-probability scan is associated with a 90% incidence of pulmonary emboli on pulmonary angiography; usually, however, the V/Q scan is initially performed and, if high probability, the diagnostic workup usually stops.

26. What percentage of V/Q scans are indeterminate for PE?

Between 40–66% of patients with PE have matching areas of diminished perfusion and ventilation; these scans are indeterminate or are of intermediate probability for PE. An indeterminate or intermediate V/Q scan result usually mandates the performance of another test, such as pulmonary angiography, to establish or exclude the diagnosis of pulmonary embolism.

27. Is there any role for computed tomography in diagnosing pulmonary emboli?

Preliminary studies have demonstrated that dynamic contrast-enhanced helical (and also electron beam) CT scans reliably demonstrate pulmonary emboli in main, lobar, and segmental pulmonary artery branches. It seems likely that modern fast CT techniques will soon be used to screen patients suspected of having pulmonary emboli. The advantages of CT over other techniques are that the examination is noninvasive (only a peripheral i.v. is needed) and the emboli are seen directly, whereas on a V/Q scan their presence can only be inferred. The major questions regarding the use of CT as a substitute for the V/Q scan are (1) how often emboli in the more peripheral branches will be missed on CT and (2) what are the clinical implications of missing such a finding (in the absence of central emboli, which will be detected).

28. What is the role of imaging studies in demonstrating deep venous thrombosis in the legs of patients suspected of having pulmonary emboli?

About 80% of pulmonary emboli are thought to originate from venous thromboses that occur in the deep veins of the legs. Investigators have reasoned that if deep venous thrombosis can be demonstrated in patients clinically suspected of having pulmonary emboli or who have low or intermediate probability V/Q scans, the probability that the patient actually has pulmonary emboli should be very high. Since the treatment for both disorders is anticoagulation, appropriate therapy can be initiated.

29. Can an ultrasound of the deep veins of the legs be negative for thrombosis and a PE be present?

Unfortunately, yes. Ultrasound can be negative in patients who have no clinical evidence or risk factors for deep venous thrombosis, but pulmonary emboli can still be present. Even in symptomatic patients who are at risk for developing deep venous thrombosis, the incidence of sonographically documented clots is quite small. The exact role of ultrasound in the diagnosis of deep venous thrombosis and PE is still undefined, but computed tomography and MRI may soon change the approach to the patient suspected of having a pulmonary embolus, making the question of whether to do an ultrasound of the legs moot.

BIBLIOGRAPHY

1. Carson JL, Kelley MA, Duff A, et al: The clinical course of pulmonary embolism. N Engl J Med 326:1240–1245, 1992.
2. Cronan JJ: Venous thromboembolic disease: The role of US. Radiology 186:619–630, 1993.
3. Gefter WB, Hatabu H, Holland GA, et al: Pulmonary thromboembolism: Recent developments in diagnosis with CT and MR imaging. Radiology 197:561–574, 1995.
4. Goodman LR, Curtin JJ, Mewissen MW, et al: Detection of pulmonary embolism in patients with unresolved clinical and scintigraphic diagnosis: Helical CT versus angiography. AJR 164:1369–1374, 1995.
5. Goodman LR, Lipchik RJ: Diagnosis of acute pulmonary embolism: Time for a new approach. Radiology 199:25–27, 1996.
6. Matsumoto AH, Tegtmeyer CJ: Contemporary diagnostic approaches to acute pulmonary emboli. Radiol Clin North Am 33:167–183, 1995.
7. Oser RF, Zuckerman DA, Gutierrez FR, Brink JA: Anatomic distribution of pulmonary emboli at pulmonary angiography: Implications for cross-sectional imaging. Radiology 199:31–35, 1996.
8. PIOPED investigators: Value of the ventilation/perfusion scan in acute pulmonary embolism: Results of the Prospective Investigation of Pulmonary Embolism Diagnosis (PIOPED). JAMA 263:2753–2759, 1990.
9. Rosen MP, Sheiman RG, Weintraub J, McArdle C: Compression sonography in patients with indeterminate or low-probability lung scans: Lack of usefulness in the absence of both symptoms of deep-vein thrombosis and thromboembolic risk factors. AJR 166:285–289, 1996.
10. Stein PD, Alavi A, Gottschalk A, et al: Usefulness of noninvasive diagnostic tools for diagnosis of acute pulmonary embolism in patients with a normal chest radiograph. Am J Cardiol 67:1117–1120, 1991.
11. Stein PD, Terrin ML, Hales CA, et al: Clinical, laboratory, roentgenographic, and electrocardiographic findings in patients with acute pulmonary embolism and no pre-existing cardiac or pulmonary disease. Chest 100:598–603, 1991.

14. PNEUMOTHORAX

Stuart A. Groskin, M.D.

1. What is a pneumothorax?
Free air in the pleural space. Normally, there is 5–10 ml of fluid in the space between the visceral and parietal pleural layers, but there is no air.

2. How does air get into the pleural space?
In a number of different ways. It can get into the pleural space through an opening in the chest wall created by blunt or penetrating trauma (for instance, as a result of thoracentesis) or from rupture of a portion of the lung with associated disruption of the visceral pleura.

3. What happens to air once it gets into the pleural space?
It is gradually resorbed by pleural capillaries. So long as the process that leads to the development of the pneumothorax is self-limited—i.e., the pleural air leak has been sealed—and the patient is oxygenating adequately and is hemodynamically stable, observation is usually all the treatment that is needed.

4. What is spontaneous pneumothorax?
A pneumothorax (PTX) that occurs without an inciting event. There are two types of spontaneous PTX, primary and secondary. A primary spontaneous PTX occurs in the absence of underlying pleuropulmonary pathology, while a secondary spontaneous PTX occurs without provocation in a patient who has underlying pulmonary disease that may predispose him or her to develop a PTX.

5. Name some diseases associated with secondary spontaneous pneumothorax.
• COPD
• Pulmonary fibrosis
• Langerhans cell histiocytosis (eosinophilic granuloma of the lung)
• Primary and secondary neoplasm, particularly metastatic osteogenic sarcoma

6. What has been implicated in the pathogenesis of primary spontaneous pneumothorax?
Apical blebs.

7. Does spontaneous pneumothorax commonly recur?
Yes, both primary and secondary spontaneous PTX have a tendency to recur. Almost 50% of patients will have an ipsilateral PTX, often within 2 years of the initial episode.

8. What are some of the causes of pneumothorax in hospitalized patients?
Thoracentesis, mechanical ventilation, and successful or unsuccessful attempts at central venous catheter placement are common causes. Uncommon causes include nephrectomy, fiberoptic bronchoscopy, and liver biopsy.

9. What is a tension pneumothorax?
A PTX in which the intrapleural pressure becomes supraatmospheric, at least during expiration. Tension pneumothoraces are usually large and continue to expand until appropriate measures are taken to evacuate them.

10. What can happen if a tension pneumothorax is not promptly decompressed?
If it is not promptly decompressed with a needle, catheter, or chest tube, death from cardiorespiratory collapse usually rapidly ensues.

11. When is tension pneumothorax most common?

In patients on positive pressure mechanical ventilators; a tension PTX constitutes a true medical/surgical emergency. It can also be seen in patients who have penetrating chest wounds.

12. What are clinical clues that tension pneumothorax is present?

• Rapid hemodynamic and respiratory deterioration, particularly in a patient on a positive pressure ventilator
• The above findings in a patient with blunt or penetrating thoracoabdominal trauma
• Hyperresonant ipsilateral hemithorax, with diminished breath sounds and contralateral displacement of the trachea and the cardiac apex

13. Should a chest radiograph be taken in a patient suspected of having a tension pneumothorax?

No, because a tension pneumothorax can rapidly produce life-threatening cardiopulmonary instability. Instead, a diagnostic and therapeutic attempt to decompress the PTX should be made with a large-bore needle. If the desired response is achieved, a chest tube should be inserted to provide more definitive treatment. A chest radiograph can then be obtained to confirm the position of the chest tube, to determine the extent of the residual PTX, and to search for other abnormalities that may have contributed to or been associated with the PTX.

14. What is the best way to diagnose a pneumothorax?

The clinical findings associated with a simple PTX are nonspecific and are rarely diagnostic (except in the case of very large pneumothoraces or when tension is present). Patients complain of the acute onset of chest pain, which may be pleuritic, and dyspnea. These symptoms, however, may be seen in a wide variety of disorders. A history of chest trauma or a previous PTX can be helpful, as can a history of other predisposing conditions such as asthma, emphysema, cystic fibrosis, or interstitial fibrosis, but such historical information cannot be regarded as diagnostic. Physical examination findings of hyperresonance to percussion, distant heart sounds, diminished breath sounds, and contralateral shift of mediastinal structures are not commonly encountered in patients with small or moderate pneumothoraces and may not be readily detectable even in patients with large pneumothoraces.

15. Are laboratory tests of any value in diagnosing a pneumothorax?

No. Both the pO_2 and the pCO_2 may be low as a result of ventilation-perfusion mismatch and hyperventilation, respectively. If formal pulmonary function testing is performed, a restrictive ventilatory defect may be noted. It is difficult to imagine diagnosing a PTX on the basis of pulmonary function testing or arterial blood gas analysis.

16. So how is the diagnosis of a pneumothorax usually made?

With a chest radiograph. An upright, frontal chest x-ray is highly sensitive for detecting pneumothoraces. If the film is made during expiration, the relative increase in the percent of the thorax occupied by the PTX, and the increased contrast between the lucent PTX and the more opaque, adjacent degassed lung, increase the sensitivity of this test.

17. How is a pneumothorax diagnosed on a chest radiograph?

The sharp line of the visceral pleura is highlighted on one side by the aerated lung and on the other side by free air in the pleural space (Fig. 1). A hyperlucent area devoid of bronchovascular markings is not enough to diagnose a PTX.

18. What is the best test for a pneumothorax?

Usually, only an erect frontal chest radiograph. However, a PTX is sometimes difficult to see on a chest radiograph. Overlying clothing, subcutaneous emphysema, and normal anatomic structures such as ribs may occasionally obscure a PTX. In these situations, the best test is a CT scan.

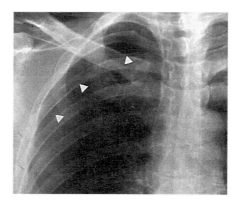

FIGURE 1. Pneumothorax in a patient who was stabbed in the right chest. Arrowheads point to the visceral pleural line, which is separated from the parietal pleura and the chest wall by the patient's right pneumothorax.

19. Where should a pneumothorax be looked for on chest films?

Free air in the pleural space usually migrates to the most nondependent portion of the pleural space. In an upright patient, a PTX is usually most easily seen at the apex of the chest.

20. How is a pneumothorax diagnosed in a patient who has been radiographed in the supine position?

This poses a special challenge. In a supine patient, the anterior, inferior, and medial portions of the pleural space are the most nondependent. Unfortunately, this means that free pleural air is positioned directly over the aerated lung and that the interface between the PTX and the underlying lung is perpendicular, not parallel to the incident x-ray beam, and cannot be easily seen.

21. What are some clues to the presence of a pneumothorax on a supine chest radiograph?

- Hyperlucency of the lung base
- Apparent deepening of the costophrenic angle (the "deep sulcus sign") (Fig. 2)
- Apparent presence of two diaphragm-lung interfaces (the "double diaphragm sign")

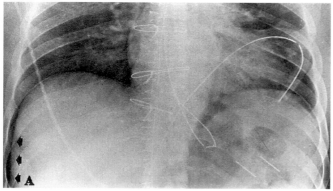
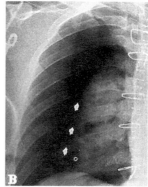

FIGURE 2. The deep sulcus sign of pneumothorax in a supine patient. *A,* Coned-down view of the lower thorax obtained with the patient supine shows apparent deepening of the right costophrenic angle (arrowheads); compare with the normal appearance of the left costophrenic angle. *B,* A repeat frontal chest radiograph obtained several hours later shows an obvious, large right pneumothorax (arrows demarcate the lateral lung edge).

22. What can be done if the diagnosis of pneumothorax must be conclusively established or excluded in a patient who cannot be placed upright?

Consider obtaining a lateral decubitus chest radiograph with the side of interest placed up; if this fails or cannot be done, consider a CT scan.

23. How commonly are occult pneumothoraces detected in trauma patients undergoing CT scans of the abdomen?

Trauma patients frequently have CT scans of the abdomen to exclude visceral injury. The uppermost images from an abdominal CT scan should include the lower portions of the chest, and these images should always be viewed on lung settings and soft-tissue settings, since in about 20% of trauma patients, previously unsuspected pneumothoraces can be seen. Up to 75% of these occult pneumothoraces ultimately require chest tube placement (Fig. 3).

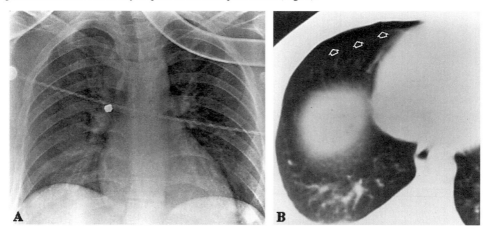

FIGURE 3. Occult pneumothorax seen on CT. *A,* Supine frontal chest radiograph of a patient who sustained a gunshot wound to the upper abdomen and thorax. The retained bullet is seen in the right chest.No pneumothorax was seen. *B,* A CT image through the base of the chest shows a small right pneumothorax (open arrows).

24. How do you determine the "percent pneumothorax"?

You don't! "Why would anyone want to determine what percent of the total volume of a hemithorax is occupied by a pneumothorax?" is a more rational question. Some individuals have proposed that the percent pneumothorax can be used to determine which patients with PTX should receive a chest tube and which patients should simply be observed until the PTX resolves on its own. This approach does not make such sense, because a young, otherwise healthy person can easily accommodate a 100% PTX with few symptoms and would probably suffer much more discomfort from placement of a chest tube, while a person with underlying cardiopulmonary disease and limited reserve can develop life-threatening physiologic alterations with as little as 3–5% PTX, a PTX that by numbers alone would not merit consideration of chest tube placement. It is much more appropriate to consider the effect of the PTX on the individual patient and the severity of the patient's physiologic disability when considering the need for tube thoracostomy and whether to treat.

25. What if the patient is an outpatient?

The availability of emergency medical care should be considered when deciding what action should be taken with an outpatient who has a PTX. A patient who has the potential for rapid cardiopulmonary decompensation if the pneumothorax expands and who does not have ready access to emergency medical services may merit a longer observation before discharge or may benefit from the insertion of a chest tube for a short time.

26. When should a pneumothorax be treated?

Tube drainage of a PTX should be performed whenever there is associated life-threatening cardiorespiratory dysfunction. Patients who cannot inform others of the presence of increasing respiratory distress, such as comatose patients, also should probably have aggressive management, as should patients with a PTX who are on positive pressure mechanical ventilators. A rapid, catastrophic increase in the size of PTX is particularly possible in this last group of patients, and, since they are intubated, they may not be able to tell anyone about their worsening respiratory status.

BIBLIOGRAPHY

1. Enderson BL, Abdalla R, Frame SB, et al: Tube thoracostomy for occult pneumothorax: A prospective randomized study of its use. J Trauma 35:726–729, 1993.
2. Sassoon CS, Light RW, O'Hara VS, Mortiz TE: Iatrogenic pneumothorax: Etiology and morbidity. Results of a Department of Veterans Affairs cooperative study. Respiration 59:215–220, 1992.
3. Wolfman NT, Gilpin JW, Bechtold RE, et al: Occult pneumothorax in patients with abdominal trauma: CT studies. J Comput Assist Tomogr 17:59–69, 1993.

15. PLEURAL EFFUSION

Stuart A. Groskin, M.D.

1. How many kinds of pleural effusions are there?

A wide variety of fluids can collect in the pleural space and produce pleural effusions: plasma ultrafiltrate, pus, blood, chyle, urine, ascitic fluid, and bile.

2. What is the difference between a transudate and an exudate?

Pleural effusions are often divided into transudates and exudates based on their biochemical composition. Transudative pleural effusions are plasma ultrafiltrates. They form when a shift in the Starling forces (increase in hydrostatic pressure or decrease in colloid osmotic pressure) leads to an increase in the transudation of fluid from pleural capillaries (usually parietal pleural capillaries) into the pleural space. Decreased absorption of fluid from the pleural space, because of increased visceral pleural capillary hydrostatic pressure or lymphatic obstruction, also leads to the accumulation of transuded fluid in the pleural space. Exudative effusions form whenever the permeability of the pleural capillaries increases because of inflammatory or malignant processes.

3. How can transudates and exudates be distinguished biochemically?

Transudative effusions have a low protein content (pleural protein is ≤ 50% of the serum protein) and low LDH (pleural protein ≤ 60% of serum LDH or less than 200 IU). Exudative effusions have high protein and LDH contents.

4. How can pleural effusions form in patients with ascites?

Pleural effusions in patients with ascites can actually be composed of ascitic fluid that finds its way into the pleural space through openings in the diaphragm. These openings seem to function as one-way valves because migration of pleural effusions into the peritoneal space has not been documented.

5. Can transudative pleural effusions be distinguished on chest radiographs from exudative pleural effusions?

No. All pleural fluid looks the same on chest radiographs regardless of its cellular composition or its protein/LDH content.

6. Can CT determine the content of a pleural effusion?

CT may be able to suggest the composition of a pleural effusion. Blood (hemothorax) is usually high in density, while chylothorax (the accumulation of chyle in the thorax, usually as a result of disruption of the thoracic duct) may be of low density because of the high lipid content of the fluid. However, if the composition of a pleural effusion must be known with certainty, a thoracentesis must be performed and the aspirated fluid sent for biochemical, cytologic, and microbiologic tests.

7. What can chest radiographs reveal about the nature of pleural effusions?

Chest radiographs give information about the quantity of fluid in the pleural space and can help determine whether the fluid is free-flowing or loculated and whether there are associated abnormalities of the pleura, lung, mediastinum, chest wall, or abdomen that may indicate the possible source of the effusion (Fig. 1).

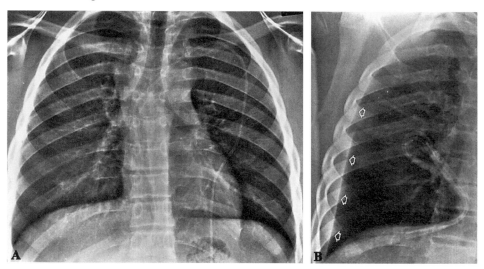

FIGURE 1. Utility of lateral decubitus radiographs in detecting pleural effusions. *A,* An erect frontal chest radiograph reveals no definite evidence of pleural effusion. *B,* Right lateral decubitus chest radiograph shows a moderate right pleural effusion (open arrows).

8. How much fluid must be present in the pleural space before an effusion can be seen on a standard erect frontal chest radiograph?

About 150–300 ml.

9. How can smaller amounts of pleural fluid be detected?

Lateral decubitus radiographs, made with the side suspected to contain an effusion in the dependent position, can be used to detect smaller amounts of free-flowing fluid. CT and ultrasound are the most sensitive tests available for detecting pleural effusions.

10. Is it important to determine if an effusion is free-flowing?

Whether a pleural effusion is free-flowing or loculated is generally not of much specific diagnostic importance, but it can be helpful if a thoracentesis is planned. The lateral decubitus position also can be used to change the location of pleural fluid so that underlying lung tissue and pathology are revealed.

11. What is a loculated pleural effusion?

An effusion that does not flow freely throughout the pleural space, because fibrous bands divide the pleural space into multiple noncommunicating compartments. These bands are usually the result of pleural inflammation associated with empyema or hemothorax.

12. What is a subpulmonic effusion?

An effusion that occupies the pleural space between the base of the lung and the diaphragm. Since this is the most dependent portion of the pleural space in an upright patient, the accumulation of fluid here is not really surprising or unusual; indeed, subpulmonic effusions are not uncommon.

13. Why is a subpulmonic effusion tricky to diagnose on a frontal erect chest radiograph?

The confusing feature of a subpulmonic effusion is that a lateral meniscus, i.e., blunting of the costophrenic angle, cannot be seen on an erect frontal radiograph. The reason is uncertain, and this finding has been attributed to the overlying lung being normal or abnormal.

14. What are some specific features of a subpulmonic effusion on chest radiographs?

- There is lateral displacement of the apparent apex of the diaphragm. In patients with subpulmonic effusions, the apparent interface between the lung and the diaphragm is actually an interface between the lung and the subpulmonic fluid; the diaphragm is actually displaced inferiorly and is separated from the lung by the effusion.
- There are no visible bronchovascular structures behind the "pseudodiaphragm," meaning that the lung is floating on top of the subpulmonic effusion.
- If the effusion is on the left side, there may be an increase in the distance between the top of the gastric air bubble and the top of the pseudodiaphragm. Normally the distance is less than 2 cm.
- An erect lateral chest radiograph often reveals a meniscus in the posterior portion of the pleural space, although the frontal chest film does not have such a meniscus (Figs. 2 and 3).

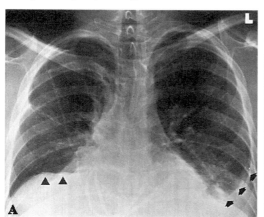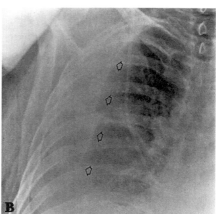

FIGURE 2. Subpulmonic and "conventional" pleural effusions. *A,* An erect frontal chest radiograph shows a meniscus blunting the left costophrenic angle (arrows) and flattening of the apparent right hemidiaphragm-lung interface (arrows). Note the lack of visible bronchovascular structures behind the dome of the apparent right diaphragm. *B,* A right lateral decubitus chest radiograph reveals a large free-flowing right pleural effusion (open arrows) that had been responsible for the distortion of the apparent right lung-hemidiaphragm interface.

15. What is a pleural pseudotumor?

A pleural effusion that has found its way into a fissure. The interlobar pulmonary fissures are really only extensions of the pleural space. Fluid, or gas, that accumulates in the pleural space often enters the fissures, where it can create confusing shadows on chest radiographs. Fluid that enters the minor (horizontal) fissure can produce an oval opacity in the midportion of the right lung that can be seen on both frontal and lateral radiographs. Superficially, this opacity resembles a lung mass or tumor.

16. What are some clues that a pleural pseudotumor is present?

- Evidence of pleural fluid in other portions of the pleural space.
- The position of the mass corresponds precisely to the position of the minor fissure; often, the minor fissure can be seen extending medially, laterally, anteriorly, and posteriorly from the tumor.
- The mass has tapering ends; it is not truly spherical but is instead more elliptical.

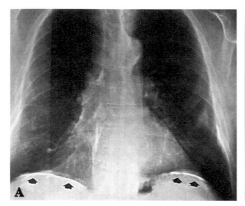 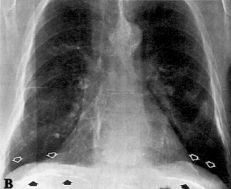

FIGURE 3. Subpulmonic pleural effusion. *A,* An erect frontal chest radiograph shows bilateral calcified pleural plaques (arrows). *B,* An erect frontal chest radiograph made several months later shows apparent inferior displacement of the calcified diaphragmatic parietal pleural plaques (open arrows indicate the lung-effusion interface; black arrows indicate the position of the calcified pleural plaques). The space between the open and closed arrows represents bilateral subpulmonic pleural effusions.

- Fluid in the major fissure produces a poorly marginated, crescentic opacity on frontal films, which is denser and broader inferiorly and tapers and becomes less opaque as it proceeds superiorly and medially; because of the orientation of the major fissures, fluid in this location does not usually produce a mass on frontal films. But an oval density similar to the one seen when there is fluid in the minor fissure may be seen on lateral radiographs.
- Fluid in the fissure is not necessarily loculated, but may be freely mobile.

17. How well do supine or semierect chest radiographs demonstrate pleural effusions?
Not very well. When a patient is supine, free fluid in the pleural space distributes itself throughout the dorsal portion of the pleural space, producing a veiling density on chest radiographs. This increases the overall opacity of the structures without completely obscuring them. The interface between the lung and the underlying effusion is perpendicular to the incident x-ray beam and cannot be seen on a frontal radiograph.

18. What are clues to the presence of a pleural effusion on a supine chest film?
- Blunting of the costophrenic angle
- Loss of definition of the hemidiaphragm
- Generalized increase in the density of the hemithorax

19. If a supine chest radiograph is normal, and it is important to exclude a pleural effusion in a patient who cannot be placed upright, what view should be obtained?
A lateral decubitus radiograph with the suspect side dependent. A cross-table lateral radiograph can be extremely helpful, as can oblique semi-erect radiographs. If all else fails, CT and ultrasonography are excellent techniques for detecting pleural effusions in supine patients.

20. What role do radiologists play in the management of patients who have pleural effusions?
Radiologists are often the first physicians to suggest that a patient has a pleural effusion and are usually the ones responsible for definitively establishing the presence of fluid in the pleural space. Interventional radiologists are now also often asked to drain pleural effusions. By using ultrasound or CT to provide guidance, radiologists can often drain complex or loculated pleural fluid collections that have been refractory to conventional tube thoracostomy, sparing patients thoracotomy and open pleural drainage.

BIBLIOGRAPHY

1. Bartter T, Santarelli R, Akers SM, Pratter MR: The evaluation of pleural effusion. Chest 106:1209–1214, 1994.
2. Heitzman ER, Raasch BN: Diseases of the pleura. In Groskin SA (ed): Heitzman's The Lung, 3rd ed. St. Louis, Mosby-Year Book, 1993, pp 575–614.
3. Klein JS, Schultz S, Heffner JE: Interventional radiology of the chest: Image-guided percutaneous drainage of pleural effusions, lung abscess, and pneumothorax. AJR 164:581–585, 1995.
4. Light RW: Pleural Diseases, 3rd ed. Baltimore, Williams & Wilkins, 1995.

16. AORTIC DISSECTION AND THORACIC AORTIC ANEURYSM

Stuart A. Groskin, M.D.

1. What is an aortic aneurysm?

A focal bulge in the aorta that involves all layers of the aortic wall. Aneurysms are typically fusiform in shape and involve the entire circumference of the affected aortic segment. Occasionally, aneurysms can be eccentric, appearing to bud off of the aorta (saccular aneurysm); even in this circumstance, all layers of the aortic wall are found in the aneurysm.

2. What is an aortic dissection?

Unlike an aortic aneurysm, aortic dissections may or may not produce a bulge in the aortic wall. A dissection occurs when a tear in the intimal layer of the aorta allows blood from the aortic lumen to dissect into the medial layer of the aorta. The dissecting blood creates a second channel for blood flow in the wall of the aorta. Usually this second channel rejoins the main aortic lumen downstream and the two bloodstreams merge. Flow in the second, or false channel, is usually but not always slower and of smaller volume than flow in the true lumen. It is not uncommon for the slowly flowing blood in the false channel to clot, effectively ending the dissection. Dissections usually involve a longer segment of the aorta than aneurysms.

3. What are the critical differences between aortic aneurysms and aortic dissections?

	Aneurysm (Fig. 1)	*Dissection* (Fig. 2)
Shape	Fusiform or saccular	Fusiform or normal
Extent	Focal	Diffuse
Histology	All layers of the wall	Intimal tear with medial dissection

4. What is a thoracic aortic pseudoaneurysm?

A focal outpouching of the aorta, often eccentrically located, whose wall consists only of the aortic adventitia and adjacent fibrous tissue. Pseudoaneurysms are often the result of trauma.

5. Where are traumatic aortic pseudoaneurysms most commonly located?

At the junction of the aortic arch and the proximal descending thoracic aorta, just distal to the origin of the left subclavian artery.

6. What are the important factors to consider when deciding whether a patient with a thoracic aortic dissection or a thoracic aortic aneurysm needs immediate treatment?

Clinical signs and symptoms and radiographic evidence of interval change in aortic size or shape. Hypotension and chest pain are obvious clinical red flags.

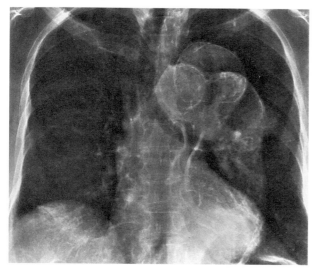 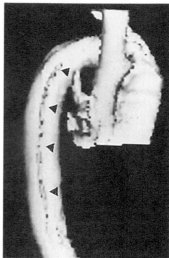

FIGURE 1 *(Left).*   Aortic aneurysm. Frontal chest radiograph demonstrates at least two calcified aortic aneurysms of the aortic arch or proximal descending thoracic aorta.

FIGURE 2 *(Right).*   Aortic dissection. A three-dimensional image of the aorta (shaded surface display) reconstructed from axial helical CT images shows a type III aortic dissection. The arrowheads point to the intimal flap separating the true and false lumens. (Contributed by Dr. Jeffrey Buran).

7. **What radiographic signs may indicate the need for urgent surgery in patients with thoracic aortic aneurysms and aortic dissections?**
   • Mediastinal widening (a sign of possible hemorrhage into the mediastinum)
   • Increase in the size of the aorta
   • Increase in the size of the cardiac silhouette, indicating the possible presence of hemopericardium, or chamber dilatation because of aortic regurgitation
   • New pleural effusions
   • Extrapleural fluid collections, e.g, the apical cap, which may represent extrapleural dissection of mediastinal blood

The presence of any of these abnormalities should usually prompt a more specific urgent diagnostic evaluation unless the patient is hemodynamically unstable, in which case a trip to the operating room is in order. Transesophageal echocardiography can be done in the operating room prior to and during thoracotomy.

8. **What is the DeBakey classification for aortic dissection?**
   • Type I: dissection starts in the ascending aorta and extends into the descending aorta
   • Type II: dissection starts in the ascending aorta and stops before the origin of the great vessels
   • Type III: dissection starts distal to the origin of the left subclavian artery and extends into the distal descending aorta

9. **What is the Stanford classification for aortic dissection?**
   • Type A: any dissection that involves the ascending aorta
   • Type B: any dissection that spares the ascending aorta

10. **What important distinction do these two classification systems make from a therapeutic viewpoint?**
   To distinguish dissections involving the ascending aorta from those that spare the ascending aorta. Only 5% of patients with dissections of the ascending aorta survive 1 year without surgical

treatment, but over 70% of patients with dissections that spare the ascending aorta survive for 1 or more years without surgical intervention. Type I, II, and A dissections are therefore usually considered surgical emergencies, while medical treatment (reduction of systemic blood pressure) is often employed first in patients with type III or B dissections.

11. Is surgery always mandatory when an aortic aneurysm reaches a certain size?

No. The larger the aneurysm, however, the greater the likelihood of rupture. The law of Laplace states that the wall tension of a sphere increases as the radius of a sphere increases; the bigger the aneurysm, the greater the wall tension. But there is no absolute size at or above which surgery must be performed. Patients who have atherosclerotic aortic aneurysms often have generalized vascular disease and many die from complications of their systemic vascular problem before their focal aortic aneurysms have an opportunity to rupture.

12. What is a penetrating aortic ulcer?

An atheromatous plaque in the wall of the aorta that erodes through the aortic intima, creating a communication between the aortic lumen and the deeper structures of the aortic wall. Blood entering the ulcerated area can form a localized saccular collection in the aortic wall and/or periaortic connective tissue (penetrating ulcer or pseudoaneurysm) or may dissect distally or proximally in the aortic wall.

13. How do patients present with penetrating aortic ulcers?

With acute chest pain that may mimic myocardial infarction or a classic aortic dissection.

14. What is the radiographic appearance of a penetrating aortic ulcer?

Most penetrating ulcers occur in the descending thoracic aorta, involve aortas that have extensive atherosclerotic disease, and, if they dissect within the aortic wall, the flap separating the true and false aortic lumens is usually thicker and more irregular than the intimal flap seen in patients who have true aortic dissections.

15. What is the best way to diagnose an aortic dissection?

This is difficult to answer, because many good imaging modalities are available to make this diagnosis. Plain films of the chest, however, are not very useful in establishing or excluding this diagnosis.

16. What chest radiographic findings suggest an aortic dissection?

Progressive enlargement of the aorta on sequential chest films, or medial displacement of intimal calcification in the aorta, may suggest the diagnosis, but chest films are rarely diagnostic and are not uncommonly normal.

17. What has been the traditional examination for establishing the diagnosis of aortic dissection?

Aortography. It is very—but not absolutely—sensitive and specific, but it is also time-consuming to perform, should be done only by angiographers, is invasive, and requires the use of intravascular contrast.

18. What less invasive tests are used to image patients with suspected aortic dissection?

Dynamic enhanced CT, transesophageal echocardiography, and MRI. All of these techniques are at least as sensitive and specific as aortography in detecting aortic dissections and are less invasive. All of these examinations, however, are less reliable in evaluating extension of dissection into the great vessels.

19. What are the advantages and disadvantages of CT for diagnosing aortic dissection?

Intravenous contrast must be administered, but imaging can be performed very rapidly using equipment found in most radiology departments. An angiography team is not required, nor does a central catheter need to be placed.

20. What are the advantages and disadvantages of transesophageal sonography for diagnosing aortic dissection?

This examination must be performed by a trained operator and cannot always evaluate the entire aortic arch because of intervening structures like the trachea and the left mainstem bronchus. Also, a small percentage of patients cannot tolerate placement of the ultrasound transducer in the esophagus. The advantages include the fact that it does not require the administration of intravenous contrast material, and it can be done at the bedside or in the operating room with portable equipment.

21. What are the advantages and disadvantages of MRI for diagnosing aortic dissection?

MRI usually requires more time to perform than CT or transesophageal sonography, and monitoring critically ill patients in a high-field strength magnetic field remains something of a challenge. On the plus side, vascular contrast is not necessary for MRI of the aorta, although in some instances it may be helpful. Nor is an angiography team required, and cine images of the aorta in different phases of the cardiac cycle can be obtained, which helps determine whether blood is flowing in the false lumen. Considerable expertise, however, is often required to interpret magnetic resonance studies of thoracic aorta, because of the high frequency of artifacts induced by motion (respiratory and cardiac) and by the variable, unpredictable velocity of blood flow in the false lumen.

BIBLIOGRAPHY

1. Bansal RC, Chandrasekaran K, Ayala K, Smith DC: Frequency and explanation of false negative diagnosis of aortic dissection by aortography and transesophageal echocardiography. J Am Coll Cardiol 25:1393–1401, 1995.
2. Chen JTT: Plain radiographic evaluation of the aorta. J Thorac Imag 5:1–17, 1990.
3. Guilmet D, Bachet J, Goudot B, et al: Aortic dissection: Anatomic types and surgical approaches. J Cardiovasc Surg 34:23–32, 1993.
4. Harris JA, Bis KG, Glover JL, et al: Penetrating atherosclerotic ulcers of the aorta. J Vasc Surg 19:90–98, 1994.
5. Miller SW: Cardiac Radiology: The Requisites. St. Louis, Mosby-Year Book, 1996.
6. Movsowitz HD, Lampert C, Jacobs LE, Kotler MN: Penetrating atherosclerotic aortic ulcers. Am Heart J 128:1210–1217, 1994.
7. Sommer T, Fehske W, Holzknecht N, et al: Aortic dissection: A comparative study of diagnosis with spiral CT, multiplanar transesophageal echocardiography, and MR imaging. Radiology 199:347–352, 1996.

17. CONGESTIVE HEART FAILURE AND PULMONARY EDEMA

Stuart A. Groskin, M.D.

1. Are congestive heart failure and pulmonary edema the same thing?

No, although the terms are often used as though they were synonyms. Pulmonary edema refers to increased fluid in the extravascular space of the lungs, and congestive heart failure is an imprecise term that refers to cardiac decompensation accompanied by peripheral or pulmonary edema.

2. What can cause pulmonary edema?
- Increased hydrostatic pressure
- Decreased plasma oncotic pressure
- Impaired capillary integrity

3. Can increased negative intrapleural pressure lead to pulmonary edema? If so, how?

Rarely, increased negative intrapleural pressure can also lead to the formation of pulmonary edema. This has been seen in patients who develop pulmonary edema after relief of upper airway obstruction or after the evacuation of a large, usually chronic pleural effusion.

4. **What processes increase the hydrostatic pressure in the pulmonary veins?**
   - Left ventricular failure
   - Mitral stenosis
   - Atresia of the pulmonary veins (rare)
   - Anomalous pulmonary venous return (usually infradiaphragmatic, also fairly rare)
   - Pulmonary veno-occlusive disease (rare)

   All of these conditions can cause hydrostatic pulmonary edema. Any process that increases the hydrostatic pressure in the pulmonary veins can lead to the transudation of fluid from the pulmonary capillaries into the pulmonary interstitium, which causes the pulmonary edema.

5. **What is high-altitude pulmonary edema?**
   This affects people who abruptly ascend to heights in excess of 2500 meters. It is probably a form of hydrostatic edema caused by hyperperfusion of a limited number of pulmonary artery branches that do not constrict under the influence of the alveolar hypoxia that occurs at high altitudes.

6. **How does pulmonary edema occur when the plasma oncotic pressure decreases?**
   Under normal circumstances, the plasma oncotic pressure counteracts the hydrostatic forces that favor the movement of fluid from the pulmonary capillaries into the interstitial space. When plasma oncotic pressure falls, as in nephrotic syndrome, fluid seeps from the vessels into the interstitium even if intravascular pressures are normal.

7. **How does pulmonary edema occur when capillary integrity in the lungs is impaired?**
   A variety of processes make the pulmonary capillaries leaky, leading to pulmonary edema. These include infections, aspiration of acid material (gastric contents), and inhalation of toxic gases. They loosen the capillary endothelial junctions and allow fluid and protein to seep into the perivascular interstitial space.

8. **What is cephalization of blood flow and what does it mean?**
   Cephalization of blood flow, also known as redistribution of blood flow, is one of the earliest radiographic signs of pulmonary venous hypertension. When the left ventricle fails, it does not empty effectively during systole. The residual ventricular blood leaves less room for incoming left atrial blood during the next diastole. This leads to an increase in left atrial end-diastolic volume and pressure. As left atrial pressure increases, pulmonary venous pressure must also increase, since blood continues to flow from the right ventricle into the pulmonary vascular bed. Eventually, the hydrostatic pressure in the pulmonary capillaries increases to a point where the osmotic pressure of the capillary blood is no longer sufficient to prevent transudation of fluid from the capillaries into the pulmonary interstitial tissues, and interstitial pulmonary edema begins.

9. **What are the radiographic manifestations of this pathophysiologic sequence?**
   Initially, edema fluid collects in the extraalveolar interstitium of the lower lobes, where the hydrostatic pressure is the greatest. This fluid decreases pulmonary compliance and compresses small extraalveolar blood vessels, leading to an increase in vascular resistance. The combination of decreased compliance and increased vascular resistance leads to a decrease in blood flow to the lower lobes and, accordingly, since the right ventricular output has to go somewhere, to an increase in blood flow to the upper lobes. On radiographs, there is blunting or lack of definition of the margins of the lower lobe blood vessels (caused by dependent, perivascular interstitial edema) and equalization of the size of the blood vessels in the upper and lower portions of the lungs. As pulmonary venous pressure continues to increase, the diameter of the upper lobe pulmonary arteries actually surpasses the diameter of the lower lobe vessels, producing the classic radiographic picture of redistribution or cephalization of blood flow.

10. **What conditions other than pulmonary edema produce cephalization of blood flow?**
    Obstruction or destruction of the pulmonary arteries in the lower lobes, i.e., in patients with panacinar emphysema associated with alpha-1 antitrypsin deficiency or patients with multiple or

recurrent pulmonary emboli. The size of the upper and lower lobe pulmonary vessels equalizes when patients are supine, since the normal hydrostatic gradient is redistributed from the "typical" cephalo-caudad direction to a ventrodorsal direction, when patients assume this position.

11. What are Kerley B lines?

Histologically, they are the same as Kerley A or C lines. Kerley's lines—also and perhaps more appropriately known as septal lines—represent thickened interlobular septa. Interlobular septa are connective tissue bands that divide the lung into secondary pulmonary lobules. Branches of the pulmonary veins and lymphatics travel in the interlobular septa. When the surface of the lung is examined, the cobblestone appearance is produced by secondary pulmonary lobules; each cobblestone represents one secondary lobule and each facet of each cobblestone represents an interlobular septum.

After redistribution of pulmonary blood flow occurs, continued increases in left atrial end-diastolic pressure leads to the accumulation of transuded fluid in the pulmonary interstitium (interstitial edema). Edema fluid that collects in the perivascular axial connective tissue sheaths surrounding pulmonary and bronchial branches produces the radiographic finding of peribronchial thickening and lack of definition of vascular margins. Fluid that collects in the subpleural interstitial space produces thickening of the interlobar fissures, not to be confused with pleural effusion in the interlobar fissures. Fluid that collects in the interlobular septa produces the Kerley's lines.

12. What distinguishes a Kerley B from a Kerley A or C line?

If the fluid fills peripheral interlobular septa, on radiographs multiple short, horizontal linear densities that abut the pleural space are seen, which are termed Kerley B lines. If more central interlobular septa become fluid-filled and radiographically apparent, Kerley A lines, arcuate lines that radiate outward from the hila, are seen. Kerley C lines refer to a cobweb mesh of linear opacities in the middle portion of the lungs.

13. Do Kerley lines always indicate the presence of pulmonary edema?

No. Any process that involves the pulmonary interstitium can produce Kerley lines; interstitial fibrosis, pulmonary hemorrhage, and even lymphangitic spread of tumor can cause interlobular septal thickening and Kerley lines. When Kerley's lines are seen on a chest radiograph, look for other signs of interstitial or alveolar fluid accumulation before concluding that the patient has pulmonary edema; correlation of the radiographic findings with the patient's clinical status can also be helpful (Figs. 1 and 2).

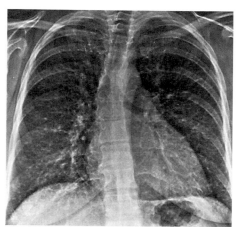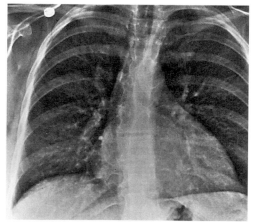

FIGURE 1 *(Left).*   Frontal chest radiograph of patient presenting with dyspnea. Kerley B and C lines and peribronchial thickening are noted, all of which are compatible with, but not diagnostic of, interstitial pulmonary edema.

FIGURE 2 *(Right).*   Repeat frontal chest radiograph obtained 1 day later, after diuretic therapy, shows resolution of interstitial abnormalities, making the radiographic diagnosis of interstitial pulmonary edema virtually certain.

14. How can cardiogenic pulmonary edema be distinguished from noncardiogenic pulmonary edema?

Clinical, physiologic, and radiologic clues may be useful. Clinical history, such as recent myocardial infarction, and the recent administration of a large amount of intravenous fluid may favor a hydrostatic, cardiac source for the patient's edema or may instead indicate that noncardiogenic, increased permeability edema or neurogenic edema is present. Decreased plasma oncotic pressure is rarely the sole cause of pulmonary edema. Direct physiologic measurements also can help to make this distinction; pulmonary capillary wedge pressure readings below 12 mmHg suggest a noncardiogenic cause of edema, while pressures above 18–25 mmHg are consistent with alveolar cardiogenic edema.

15. What are radiographic clues that cardiogenic pulmonary edema is present, as opposed to noncardiogenic edema?

Enlargement of the upper lobe pulmonary vessels and widening of the upper mediastinum (the "vascular pedicle") by engorged mediastinal venous structures (azygous vein, superior vena cava). Kerley's lines may be seen in cardiogenic pulmonary edema but are uncommon, if they occur at all, in patients who have increased permeability pulmonary edema. Also, alveolar cardiogenic pulmonary edema usually involves both lungs symmetrically, with a basilar predominance, while noncardiogenic, increased permeability pulmonary edema usually produces a patchy, inhomogeneous pattern of airspace opacities in both lungs.

16. Can the heart size reliably be used to separate cardiogenic from noncardiogenic pulmonary edema?

No. Patients who develop cardiogenic pulmonary edema after an acute myocardial infarction may have a normal heart size, while patients who develop increased permeability pulmonary edema may have an enlarged cardiac shadow because of unrelated cardiac disease or because of a concomitant pericardial effusion that mimics cardiomegaly.

17. What is atypical pulmonary edema?

Cardiogenic pulmonary edema that has a radiographic picture of asymmetric, inhomogeneous airspace opacities; the atypical distribution is probably most common in patients who have underlying chronic obstructive pulmonary disease and associated patchy destruction of the pulmonary vascular bed (if a portion of the lung does not contain blood vessels, pulmonary edema cannot develop). Obstruction of pulmonary artery branches by pulmonary emboli (usually recurrent) can also produce radiographically atypical pulmonary edema, for the same reason. Patients who preferentially lie on one side may develop unilateral pulmonary edema in the chronically dependent lung on the basis of redistribution of their hydrostastic gradient.

BIBLIOGRAPHY

1. Aronchick JM, Gefter WB: Drug-induced pulmonary disorders. Semin Roentgenol 30:18–34, 1995.
2. Eli SR: Neurogenic pulmonary edema. A review of the literature and a perspective. Invest Radiol 26:499–506, 1991.
3. Gropper MA, Wiener-Kronish JP, Hashimoto S: Acute cardiogenic pulmonary edema. Clin Chest Med 15:501–515, 1994.
4. Groskin SA: Heitzman's The Lung, 3rd ed. St. Louis, Mosby-Year Book, 1993.
5. Hutgren HN: High-altitude pulmonary edema: Current concepts. Annu Rev Med 47:267–284, 1996.
6. Kollef MH, Pluss J: Noncardiogenic pulmonary edema following upper airway obstruction. Seven cases and a review of the literature. Medicine 70:91–98, 1991.
7. Morgan PW, Goodman LR: Pulmonary edema and adult respiratory distress syndrome. Radiol Clin North Am 29:943–963, 1991.

18. CARDIAC RADIOLOGY

Ernest M. Scalzetti, M.D.

1. How is the size of the heart estimated on a chest radiograph?

The subjective impression of an experienced reader is the best indication of heart size. Many objective measures have been tried and discarded. However, one of the simplest ways to measure heart size is to measure the distance between the right-most extent of the right heart border and the left-most extent of the left heart border and then measure the width of the chest at its widest point, from the inner margin of the right ribs to the inner margin of the left ribs.

2. What is this measurement called?

The cardiothoracic ratio. Between 25–50% is considered normal; 50–60% is a gray area, and greater than 60% is abnormal.

3. What are the technical requirements of a chest radiograph for the cardiothoracic ratio to be considered accurate?

This measurement is accurate if the patient was radiographed in the upright position, in the posteroanterior projection, and with a standard 6-foot distance between the x-ray tube and the film. If the chest radiograph was taken in the anteroposterior projection or with a shorter distance between the x-ray tube and the film, the cardiac silhouette will be magnified. Semi-erect or supine positioning also makes the heart appear larger, as does expiration.

4. What can cause the heart to appear enlarged?

Chest wall deformity, such as pectus excavatum. Once such spurious causes have been eliminated, there are three major considerations to explain true cardiac enlargement:
- Pericardial disease, usually an effusion
- Valvular heart disease, which most often is due to mitral and aortic valvular disease
- Cardiomyopathy, usually due to ischemia

5. What cardiac chambers are enlarged in mitral stenosis?

The left atrium.

6. What cardiac chambers are enlarged in mitral insufficiency?

The left atrium and the left ventricle.

7. What happens to the heart in aortic stenosis?

A pressure load is imposed on the left ventricle, leading to hypertrophy rather than enlargement.

8. What happens to the heart in aortic insufficiency?

A volume load is imposed on the left ventricle, and the left ventricle dilates.

9. What is the best way to detect individual cardiac chamber enlargement?

Enlargement of a single cardiac chamber can be impossible to detect on a chest radiograph. Cross-sectional imaging techniques such as echocardiography, CT, and MRI are superior modalities for addressing this issue. If cardiomegaly is the result of valvular heart disease, the more obvious the cardiomegaly, the more likely that multiple valves are dysfunctional.

10. What are the radiographic findings in left ventricular failure?

The chest radiographic findings generally parallel the mean left atrial pressure, more conveniently measured as mean pulmonary capillary wedge pressure. Pressures up to approximately 15 mmHg are normal.

11. What happens when the mean left atrial pressure reaches 15–20 mmHg?

Pulmonary venous hypertension occurs. This may be visible on an upright chest radiograph as cephalization—enlargement of the upper lobe pulmonary blood vessels until they are equal or greater in caliber than the lower lobe vessels. There are two caveats: (1) in the semi-erect or supine positions, cephalization is very difficult to identify and (2) if pulmonary venous hypertension is chronic, compensatory mechanisms can restore the normal appearance of the upper lobe vessels.

12. At what mean left atrial pressure does pulmonary edema occur?

Above 20 mmHg, fluid begins to leak from the pulmonary capillaries into the interstitium of the lung.

13. What are the radiographic findings in pulmonary edema?

The chest radiographic findings corresponding to this event are:
- Blurring of the margins of the central pulmonary vessels, especially toward the lung bases
- The appearance of Kerley lines

    A lines are diagonally oriented markings in the upper lobes.

    B lines are short, linear markings perpendicular to the pleural surfaces of the lower lobes.

    C lines are polygonal markings, also in the lower lobes; they are the most common of the Kerley lines.
- Thickening of the walls of the bronchi, which is apparent when they are seen on-end
- If elevated pressures persist, the edema fluid eventually spills into the alveoli.

14. How can interstitial pulmonary edema be distinguished from other forms of interstitial lung disease?

Because acute interstitial lung disease is nearly always due to pulmonary edema, comparing the current radiographs to the prior films is important. In addition, interstitial edema involves both lungs symmetrically most of the time. Bizarre distributions of pulmonary edema are possible, however. One common cause is pre-existing lung disease. For example, edema cannot form in regions of lung destroyed by emphysema. Edema may be distributed asymmetrically because the fluid follows gravity and the patient has been positioned on one side. Also, one lung may be "protected" from forming edema by the presence of a large thromboembolus, or congenital hypoplasia, or absence of the pulmonary artery.

15. How can alveolar pulmonary edema be distinguished from other forms of alveolar lung disease?

Alveolar edema may have a characteristic "butterfly" or "bat's wing" distribution with symmetrical involvement of the central portions of both lungs. Unfortunately, this is unusual. More commonly, alveolar edema coexists with interstitial edema, differentiating it from most cases of pneumonia, aspiration, and pulmonary hemorrhage. While the alveolar and interstitial abnormalities in pulmonary edema often change rapidly, even in a matter of hours, pneumonia usually moves more slowly. It is worthwhile to consider a sequence of radiographs in a given patient.

16. What is the nature of the pleural effusions associated with pulmonary edema?

Pleural effusions are small, transudative fluid collections that may be unilateral or bilateral. It has been said that a right pleural effusion is more common than a left pleural effusion in cardiac failure, but the literature does not bear this out.

Pleural effusions resolve more slowly than pulmonary edema. If chest radiographs are obtained during the recovery phase of an episode of cardiac failure, the lungs may be clear and the pleural disease may be the only indication of what has transpired.

17. What are the imaging options for detecting coronary artery disease?

A significant coronary artery stenosis can be identified directly by arteriography as part of a cardiac catheterization or indirectly by observing physiologic alterations under stress. Stress usually means exercise on a treadmill, with ECG monitoring. In the face of a 70% or greater narrowing of the cross-sectional area of a coronary artery, the relative perfusion of the myocardium supplied by the artery will decrease, and the ischemic myocardium will lose contractility.

18. How do the thallium and technetium nuclear scans for myocardial ischemia work?

The decrease in perfusion of the ischemic region, relative to the remainder of the myocardium, is the basis for the radiotracer studies of myocardial ischemia. Thallium-201 is an analog of potassium that is extracted from the circulation by cardiac myocytes. Technetium-99m sestamibi, another radiopharmaceutical, behaves similarly. If cross-sectional images using SPECT technology are obtained after the injection of the tracer at peak exercise, areas of decreased myocardial perfusion will be revealed as areas of diminished uptake. This must be tempered by the realization that regions of previously scarred, infarcted myocardium will also fail to take up the radiopharmaceutical. It is necessary, then, to perform the same study with the patient at rest as well as with exercise, whereas ischemic but viable myocardium will take up the tracer at rest but suffer a relative loss of uptake with exercise.

19. What is the role of stress echocardiography in the work-up of myocardial ischemia?

Echocardiography performed at rest and immediately after exercise can demonstrate loss of myocardial contractility, also known as hypokinesis, in regions of ischemic myocardium. Images obtained with the patient in the resting state must be compared to the post-exercise images to distinguish ischemic from scarred myocardium. Nevertheless, stress echocardiography is both less time-consuming and less expensive than the nuclear medicine tests, and it appears to be equally accurate. Both types of indirect studies are noninvasive, as opposed to cardiac catheterization, and are less expensive. If a revascularization procedure is contemplated, however, the patient must undergo coronary arteriography.

20. What are the common causes of a pericardial effusion?

Fluid in the pericardial space may be the result of infection, immune reactions, and many other causes. Often the reason for the effusion cannot be identified. Among infectious agents, viruses are the most common. The possibility of tuberculosis should be kept in mind. Common immune-mediated causes include the collagen-vascular disorders, drug reactions, especially procainamide, and the post-cardiac injury effusions seen after myocardial infarction and pericardiotomy.

21. What are other causes of a pericardial effusion?

Traumatic hemopericardium, neoplastic involvement of the pericardium (especially metastatic), radiotherapy-induced pericarditis, and uremia.

22. What imaging studies assist in the detection of pericardial effusion?

Rarely, pericardial effusion can be identified on the lateral chest radiograph as a vertically oriented opaque stripe between the anterior heart border with its relatively less opaque epicardial fat and the pericardial fat, which is located superficial to the pericardium. This has been called the "oreo cookie" sign and is accentuated with the patient in the supine position.

Echocardiography provides an inexpensive, convenient, and reliable means of detecting pericardial effusion. It can also provide clues to the presence of cardiac tamponade. If further evaluation is desired, CT and MRI are better ways of getting an overview of the pericardium, surveying the mediastinum, and identifying co-existing pleural disease.

BIBLIOGRAPHY

1. Grossman ZD, Katz DS, Santelli ED, et al: Elective workup of myocardial ischemia/coronary artery disease. In Cost-Effective Diagnostic Imaging: The Clinician's Guide, 3rd ed. St. Louis, Mosby, 1995.
2. Grossman ZD, Katz DS, Santelli ED, et al: Pericardial effusion. In Cost-Effective Diagnostic Imaging: The Clinician's Guide, 3rd ed. St. Louis, Mosby, 1995.
3. Miller SW: Cardiac Radiology: The Requisites. St. Louis, Mosby, 1996.
4. Marcus ML, Schelbert HR, Skorton DJ, et al: Cardiac Imaging: A Companion to Braunwald's Heart Disease. Philadelphia, W.B. Saunders, 1991.

19. LUNG CANCER

Corey D. Eber, M.D.

1. What is a solitary pulmonary nodule?

An opacity seen on a chest radiograph must meet the following criteria to be considered a solitary pulmonary nodule:

- It must be solitary. Multiple nodules suggest an entirely different set of diagnostic possibilities (notably pulmonary metastases from an extrathoracic primary neoplasm).
- It must be pulmonary. Remember that artifacts and lesions arising from the skin, subcutaneous soft tissues, ribs, and pleura may all produce shadows on chest radiographs that mimic the appearance of a pulmonary nodule. A true pulmonary nodule usually can be seen on at least two different views of the chest, and should look roughly the same on both views. Occasionally, a CT scan is needed to confirm that a suspected nodule seen on a chest radiograph does indeed arise within the lung.
- It must be nodular or roughly spherical. Linear opacities do not count. Also, most authorities agree that a pulmonary nodule should be no larger than 3 cm in diameter. Spherical opacities larger than 3 cm are usually called pulmonary masses.

2. If a new solitary pulmonary nodule is discovered in an adult patient with known extrathoracic malignancy, is the pulmonary nodule more likely to be a metastasis from the tumor or is it more likely to represent a new primary lung cancer?

A solitary pulmonary nodule in a patient with an extrathoracic primary neoplasm usually represents a new primary lung cancer. However, if the patient has a primary melanoma or sarcoma, a solitary metastasis may be more likely.

3. What radiographic characteristics suggest that a solitary pulmonary nodule is probably benign?

Calcification, very fast or very slow growth rate, small size, and smooth external margins; however, while smooth external margins and a diameter of less than 2 cm favor a benign diagnosis, they are not specific enough characteristics to exclude malignancy.

4. Which patterns of calcification in a pulmonary nodule reliably indicate that the nodule is benign?

"Benign" calcifications in a pulmonary nodule have the following characteristics:
- Calcification that is diffusely present in the nodule
- Central calcification
- "Popcorn" calcification (multiple large areas of calcification)
- Laminar calcification (rings of calcification)

Eccentric or stippled internal calcifications can occur in both benign and malignant lesions and cannot be used to discriminate between them.

5. What is the typical growth pattern of lung cancer versus benign pulmonary nodules?

Lung cancers tend to grow over time. Nodules that have been radiographically stable for two or more years or that have doubled in volume in less than one month are, respectively, growing too slowly or too quickly and are very unlikely to be primary lung cancer.

6. What characteristics of a solitary pulmonary nodule suggest an increased likelihood of malignancy?

- Size. The larger the nodule, the greater the likelihood of malignancy.
- Margins. Spiculated margins or a lobulated contour increase the probability that a nodule is malignant.

• Age of patient. The older the patient, the higher the likelihood that a pulmonary nodule is malignant.
• Enhancement characteristics. It has been recently suggested that malignant pulmonary nodules enhance more intensely with intravenous contrast than do benign pulmonary nodules.

7. What role does computed tomography play in the evaluation of solitary pulmonary nodules?

CT may reveal additional pulmonary nodules, indicating that a whole new set of diagnoses must be considered. CT is much better than plain chest radiographs in demonstrating calcification in nodules. CT determination of enhancement characteristics may distinguish benign from malignant nodules. CT can demonstrate enlarged hilar and mediastinal lymph nodes, and adrenal and skeletal lesions, that may represent metastases. When these lesions are present, it may be easier and more expedient to biopsy them rather than the pulmonary nodule, since the tumor may be simultaneously diagnosed as well as staged.

8. How reliable is wall thickness in differentiating cavitary bronchogenic carcinomas from benign cavitary lesions (such as lung abscesses)?

Measurement of the thickest part of the cavity wall can be a very reliable way of distinguishing malignant from benign pulmonary cavities. Greater than 95% of cavities with a maximal wall thickness of 4 mm or less will be benign, and about 90% of cavities with a maximal wall thickness of 16 mm or more will be malignant. If the maximal wall thickness of a cavity is between 5 mm and 15 mm, it is considered indeterminate.

9. What type of bronchogenic carcinoma most commonly cavitates?

Squamous cell carcinoma. Small cell carcinoma rarely cavitates.

10. Which primary pulmonary neoplasm can produce extensive mediastinal adenopathy as its sole or most significant radiographic finding?

Small cell carcinoma of the lung (Fig. 1). Lymphoma, leukemia, and metastases from renal cell carcinoma, melanoma, and testicular cancer can also cause extensive mediastinal lymphadenopathy with few, if any, associated parenchymal abnormalities.

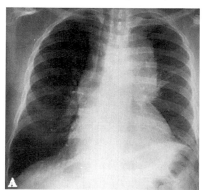 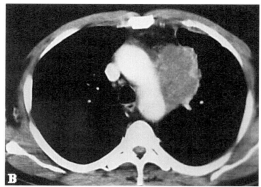

FIGURE 1.   Frontal chest radiograph *(A)* demonstrates a large mass in the left anterior mediastinum and elevation of the left hemidiaphragm (presumably secondary to phrenic nerve invasion). CT *(B)* confirms the presence of a mass in the left prevascular region (low density areas in the mass suggest necrosis). CT showed no pulmonary lesion.

11. What is a Pancoast tumor?

A Pancoast tumor is a bronchogenic carcinoma that arises at the apex of the lung, invades adjacent soft tissue and skeletal structures, and produces any or all of the following signs and symptoms:

Chest pain, back pain, or shoulder/hand pain
Horner's syndrome (miosis, ptosis, anhydrosis)
Atrophy of the muscles of the hand on the involved side

12. What types of bronchogenic carcinoma produce the Pancoast syndrome?

Any cell type of lung cancer can occur in this region and produce the Pancoast syndrome, but squamous cell carcinoma and adenocarcinoma are the most common.

13. What is the "reverse S sign of Golden"?

Also known as the "S" sign of Golden, this refers to a convex bulge in the medial aspect of the minor fissure, seen in some patients who have right upper lobe atelectasis. Normally when the right upper lobe collapses, the lateral portion of the minor fissure rises obliquely toward the apex of the chest, but the course of the minor fissure remains straight from its medial to its lateral end. If right upper lobe collapse is caused by a large central tumor which obstructs the right upper lobe bronchus, the medial portion of the minor fissure may bow inferiorly as it bends around the central obstructing lesion. The bowed appearance of the minor fissure is referred to as the "reverse S sign of Golden"; it implies the presence of a central mass (Fig. 2).

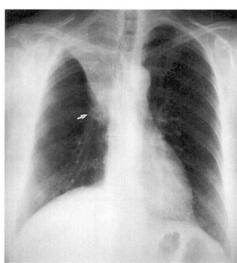

FIGURE 2. Frontal chest radiograph demonstrates partial atelectasis of the right upper lobe. Convexity of the medial aspect of the minor fissure (arrow) is caused by a large central mass. This contour is described as the "reverse S sign of Golden," and is a characteristic presentation of bronchogenic carcinoma.

14. Where do bronchogenic carcinomas usually occur?

Lesions occur most often in the upper lobes, especially in the anterior segment. They also occur more frequently in the right lung (3 to 2 ratio).

15. What are the four major types of bronchogenic carcinoma?

Squamous cell, small cell carcinoma, large cell carcinoma, and adenocarcinoma.

16. How does squamous cell carcinoma typically present radiographically?

As a central mass that may be associated with atelectasis or postobstructive pneumonia. Cavitation is common, occurring in up to 30% of cases.

17. How does adenocarcinoma present radiographically?

Adenocarcinoma often presents as a peripheral nodule or mass. Bronchoalveolar cell carcinoma, a variant of adenocarcinoma, can also present as a solitary pulmonary nodule but may produce multiple pulmonary nodules or area(s) of chronic air-space opacity. This tumor should always be considered as a possible cause for an apparent pneumonia that fails to resolve (Fig. 3).

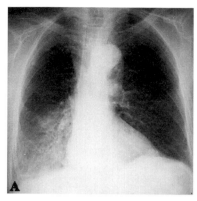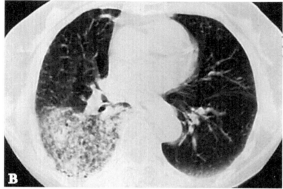

FIGURE 3. Consolidation in the right lower lobe seen on frontal chest radiograph *(A)* and CT *(B)*. This progressed despite antibiotic therapy. Biopsy proved bronchoalveolar carcinoma.

18. How does small cell carcinoma present radiographically?

Small cell carcinoma usually presents as a central mass (in 80% of cases), which is often associated with extensive mediastinal lymphadenopathy. Cavitation is extremely rare. Distant metastases are usually present at the time of diagnosis.

19. How does large cell carcinoma present radiographically?

Large cell carcinoma typically presents as a large, peripheral mass.

20. What is the TNM classification of the primary tumor (the "T") in lung cancer?

T1—A tumor that is 3 cm or less in greatest diameter, surrounded by lung or visceral pleural, and without evidence of invasion proximal to a lobar bronchus (except for superficial endobronchial tumors that may extend proximal to the main bronchus).

T2—A tumor that is more than 3 cm in greatest diameter, or a tumor of any size that either invades the visceral pleura or has associated atelectasis or obstructive pneumonitis extending to the hilar region. At bronchoscopy, the proximal extent of demonstrable tumor must be within a lobar bronchus, or at least 2 cm distal to the carina. Any associated atelectasis or obstructive pneumonitis must involve less than an entire lung.

T3—A tumor of any size which directly extends into the chest wall, diaphragm, mediastinal pleura, or pericardium, without involving the heart, great vessels, trachea, esophagus, or vertebral bodies; or a tumor in a bronchus that is within 2 cm of the carina without involving the carina.

T4—A tumor of any size with invasion of the mediastinum, involving the heart, great vessels, trachea, esophagus, vertebral body, or carina; or the presence of a malignant pleural effusion.

21. What is the TNM classification of nodal involvement (the "N") in lung cancer?

N1—Metastases to lymph nodes in the peribronchial region, the ipsilateral hilar region, or both, including direct extension.

N2—Metastases to ipsilateral mediastinal lymph nodes and subcarinal lymph nodes

N3—Metastases to contralateral mediastinal or hilar lymph nodes, ipsilateral or contralateral scalene, or supraclavicular nodes.

22. What is the importance of the distinction between Stage IIIa and Stage IIIb lung cancer?

Stage IIIa (T3 N0–1 M0, T1–3 N2 M0) lung cancer is potentially surgically resectable, while Stage IIIb (any T N3 M0, T4 any N M0) lung cancer involves invasion of vital mediastinal structures, metastases to non-resectable nodes, or a malignant pleural effusion. Stage IIIb lung cancers are not resectable.

23. What is the incidence of multiple pulmonary carcinomas?

Synchronous lesions are uncommon, with an incidence below 5%. The estimated incidence of metachronous lesions (second cancer appearing at a later time, usually > 1 year) in patients who have been treated for lung cancer (and presumably cured) is 10–15%. The average time interval is 4 to 5 years.

24. What is the role of CT in evaluating the mediastinal lymph nodes in patients with bronchogenic carcinoma?

This is controversial. The size of mediastinal lymph nodes is used to determine the likelihood that they harbor metastases; although tumor can be present in very small lymph nodes, generally the larger the nodes, the greater the chance that metastases are present (in patients with bronchogenic carcinoma). Clinically, the problem is where the size threshold should be set; if the threshold is too high, many patients who have nodal metastases may undergo extensive pulmonary surgery for disease that is already unresectable.

One working algorithm is as follows: patients with bronchogenic carcinoma who have mediastinal lymph nodes greater than one centimeter in short axis diameter should have these nodes biopsied before extensive resectional surgery to exclude the possibility of nodal metastases. If there are no nodes greater then one centimeter in short axis diameter, surgery can be performed, and the mediastinal lymph nodes can be biopsied at that time. The rationale for the latter step is that even if microscopic nodal metastases are present in normal size lymph nodes, surgery with adjuvant chemotherapy or radiation therapy may improve the patient's survival and may therefore be justified. This approach, however, is somewhat controversial.

25. What are carcinoid tumors?

Neuroendocrine neoplasms that are pathologically related to small cell carcinoma of the lung. Although they comprise only 1–2% of all pulmonary neoplasms, they account for 85% of all benign pulmonary tumors.

26. How are carcinoid tumors classified?

Carcinoid tumors are often classified as typical or atypical based on their histologic appearance. Typical carcinoid tumors have fewer mitoses, and are, in general, better organized than atypical carcinoids. Metastases are less common and survival rates are significantly better in patients who have typical carcinoid tumors when compared to patients with atypical carcinoids. Either type of carcinoid tumor may present as a peripheral pulmonary nodule or as a central mass. Central carcinoid tumors are often in part endobronchial, and may produce varying degrees of airways obstruction.

27. What are the radiographic findings of a central carcinoid?

A central mass, atelectasis, regional air-trapping, and post-obstructive pneumonia. Calcification may also be seen within carcinoid tumors, which is often easier to appreciate on CT scans (Fig. 4).

28. Is carcinoid syndrome common in patients who have pulmonary carcinoid tumors?

The carcinoid syndrome consists of paroxysmal episodes of facial flushing, tachycardia, and hypotension. Patients may also wheeze, have secretory diarrhea, and may develop cardiac valvular problems. Carcinoid syndrome is very uncommon in patients with pulmonary carcinoid tumors (0–3%). The reason for this is unknown but may be related to the small size of most pulmonary carcinoids.

29. What are the most common primary tumors of the trachea?

Primary tracheal tumors are uncommon, accounting for less than one percent of all pulmonary neoplasms. They are often initially misdiagnosed because:
- They are difficult to see on chest radiographs, and this area is often not examined closely when radiographs are reviewed.
- They are rare.
- Patients present with symptoms (wheezing, cough, dyspnea) that are nonspecific and that suggest the more common diagnoses of asthma, chronic bronchitis, or emphysema.

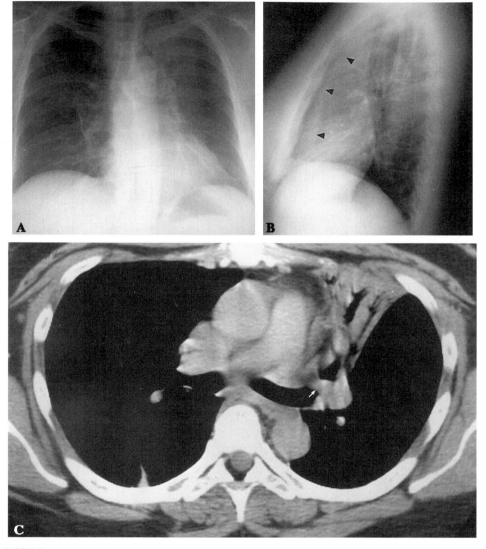

FIGURE 4.   Frontal chest radiograph *(A)* shows diffuse opacity in the left upper lobe, which obscures the left heart border. The lateral view *(B)* reveals marked anterior displacement of the major fissure (arrowheads) consistent with left upper lobe atelectasis. Thin-section CT *(C)* demonstrates a soft-tissue nodule (arrow) in the left upper lobe bronchus. Air-bronchograms suggest early or incomplete obstruction. At surgery, a carcinoid tumor was found.

Squamous cell carcinoma accounts for over 50% of all primary tracheal neoplasms. Adenoid cystic carcinoma and mucoepidermoid carcinoma are much less common.

30. What are pulmonary hamartomas, and how can they be diagnosed?

Pulmonary hamartomas are benign neoplasms composed of cartilage, fat, and fibrous tissue. They typically present radiographically as well-circumscribed pulmonary nodules. Plain chest radiographs rarely reveal the presence of calcification ("popcorn" calcification is uncommon, but should suggest this diagnosis when visible), but CT scans often demonstrate both calcium and fat in these lesions, confirming the diagnosis of hamartoma. In cases where the CT scan is nondiagnostic, percutaneous needle aspiration often allows the correct diagnosis to be made, and excisional biopsy can be avoided (Fig. 5).

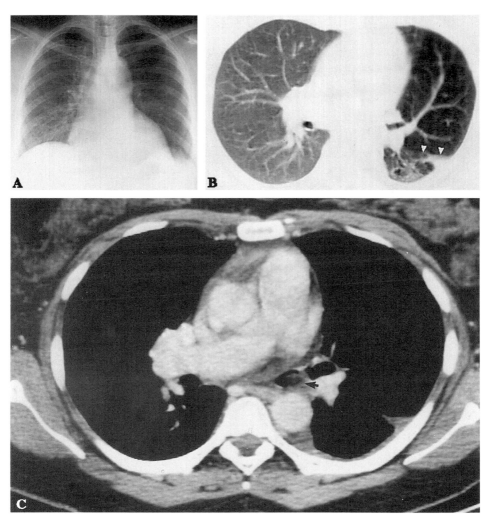

FIGURE 5. Frontal chest radiograph *(A)* demonstrates hyperlucency of the left lung in a patient with a chronic cough. Irregular opacity in the left base probably represents atelectasis. CT *(B)* shows low attenuation (density) in the left upper lobe, with posterior displacement of the major fissure (arrowheads), consistent with air-trapping. Mediastinal windows *(C)* reveal a fat-containing nodule (arrow) at the origin of the left upper lobe bronchus. At surgery, a hamartoma was found.

31. Where are pulmonary metastases usually located?

The most common pathway of metastatic disease to the lungs is via the pulmonary arteries. Since perfusion is gravity dependent metastases are usually more numerous at the lung bases. Pulmonary metastases also tend to be peripheral, with approximately 90% located in the outer third of the lung.

BIBLIOGRAPHY

1. Fraser RG, Pare JAP, Fraser RS, Pare PP: Synopsis of Diseases of the Chest, 2nd ed. Philadelphia, W.B. Saunders, 1994.
2. Groskin SA: Heitzman's The Lung—Radiologic-Pathologic Correlations, 3rd ed. St. Louis, Mosby, 1993.

III. Gastrointestinal Radiology

20. NORMAL RADIOGRAPHIC ANATOMY: GASTROINTESTINAL

Douglas S. Katz, M.D., and Burton M. Gold, M.D.

1. What are the parts of the stomach (Fig. 1)?
Gastroesophageal junction, cardia, fundus, body, antrum, and pylorus.

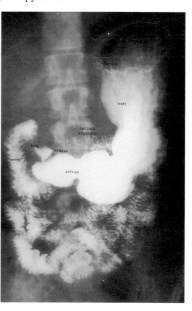

FIGURE 1. Single contrast upper GI series film shows the parts of the stomach.

2. What is the normal mucosal pattern of the stomach called?
The area gastricae, which is observed on double contrast studies.

3. What are the larger folds in the stomach called?
The rugae.

4. Where is the ligament of Treitz?
At the duodenal-jejunal junction.

5. What are the valvulae conniventes, also known as the plicae circularis?
The circumferential transverse folds of the small bowel.

6. Are there usually more transverse folds per unit length in the jejunum or in the ileum?
In the jejunum.

7. What are the parts of the colon (Figs. 2 and 3)?

Ileocecal valve, cecum, appendix, ascending colon, transverse colon, descending colon, sigmoid colon, and rectum.

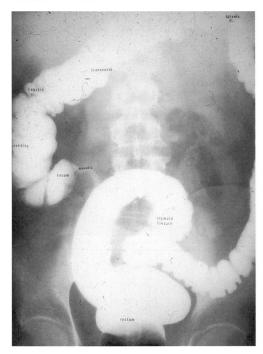
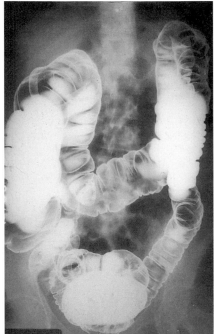

FIGURE 2 *(Left)*.   Single contrast barium enema film shows the various parts of the colon.
FIGURE 3 *(Right)*.   Double contrast barium enema.

8. What are the haustra?

The transverse folds of the colon. In contrast to the valvulae conniventes, they are incomplete, meaning that they are not circumferential.

9. On a plain film of the abdomen, what structures may normally contain gas?

The stomach and colon often contain gas. The small bowel may contain some gas, especially in the left upper quadrant.

10. What are the main reasons that fluoroscopy is performed during radiographic studies of the bowel?

It enables the radiologist to observe dynamic physiologic changes (such as peristalsis and gastroesophageal reflux), the pliability of the luminal gastrointestinal tract wall, fixation of structures, and to properly position the patient for fluoroscopic spot films.

11. What structures are normally seen when examining the pharynx (Fig. 4)?

- Valleculae (paired structures)
- Pyriform sinuses (also paired structures)
- Base of the tongue
- Epiglottis

12. What type of mucosal folds are seen in the thoracic esophagus?

Longitudinal thin folds, which are best seen on partially collapsed mucosal relief films. Rarely, distal, transiently seen, horizontal folds—the so-called "feline esophagus"—may be seen, often in association with gastroesophageal folds.

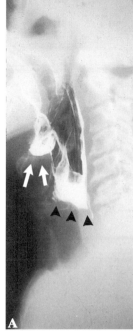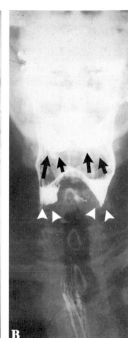

FIGURE 4. Lateral (*A*) and frontal (*B*) views of the pharynx, from a double contrast pharyngogram, shows the valleculae (arrows) and the pyriform sinuses (arrowheads).

13. Name the normal indentations on the thoracic esophagus (Fig. 5).

- Aortic knob
- Left mainstem bronchus
- Left atrium
- Diaphragmatic hiatus

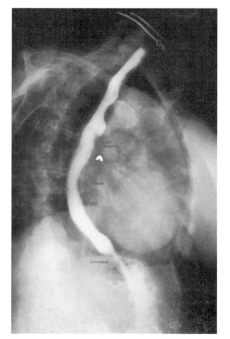

FIGURE 5. Oblique view of the thoracic esophagus from a single contrast barium swallow shows normal areas of indentation from adjacent structures.

14. Name the parts of the duodenum (Fig. 6).
  • Duodenal bulb (D1, or first portion of the duodenum)
  • Descending duodenum (D2)
  • Horizontal duodenum (D3)
  • Ascending duodenum (D4)

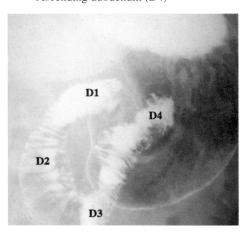

FIGURE 6. Oblique view from a double contrast upper GI series shows rugal folds of the stomach and the parts of the duodenum.

15. What are the parts of the biliary tree and pancreatic ducts that may be seen on an ERCP (endoscopic retrograde cholangiopancreatogram)? (Fig. 7)

Biliary tree	Pancreatic duct
Right and left hepatic ducts	Head
Common hepatic duct	Body
Cystic duct	Tail
Gallbladder	
Common bile duct	

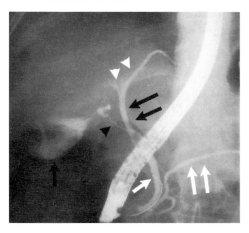

FIGURE 7. Image from an ERCP shows the endoscope in the descending duodenum and visualization of the biliary tree and pancreatic duct (gallbladder = arrow; cystic duct = arrowhead; common bile duct = white arrow; common hepatic duct = two arrows; right and left hepatic ducts = white arrowheads; pancreatic duct = two white arrows).

16. What structures are important to identify on a barium enema that signify that the entire colon has been filled with barium?
    The cecum, the ileocecal valve, the terminal ileum, and the appendix.

17. What abdominal organs are routinely seen on an abdominal ultrasound?
    Liver, gallbladder, spleen, pancreas (Fig. 8), and kidneys.

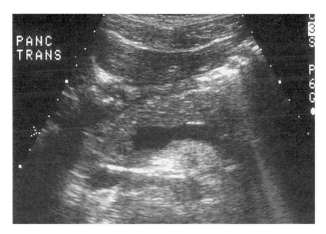

FIGURE 8.   Normal transverse sonographic view of the pancreas.

18. What structures can be identified in the liver on ultrasound (Fig. 9)?

The hepatic parenchyma is examined to evaluate its echotexture and to look for hepatic masses. The portal vein, the common bile duct, and the hepatic artery can all be seen in the porta hepatis. The diameter of the common bile duct should be measured routinely. The hepatic veins are seen as they enter the inferior vena cava.

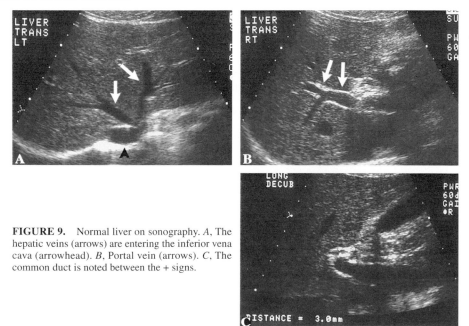

FIGURE 9.   Normal liver on sonography. *A*, The hepatic veins (arrows) are entering the inferior vena cava (arrowhead). *B*, Portal vein (arrows). *C*, The common duct is noted between the + signs.

19. What portions of the pancreas can be seen on ultrasound?

Sometimes the entire pancreas, including the head, the uncinate process, the body, and the tail, are visualized. Occasionally, the pancreatic duct can be seen, although it should measure no more than 2 mm in diameter. It may be difficult to see portions of the pancreas, especially the pancreatic tail, or the entire pancreas may not be seen; this is a common problem in obese patients or in patients with overlying bowel gas.

20. What is the normal gallbladder wall thickness on ultrasound?
Less than 3 mm (Fig. 10).

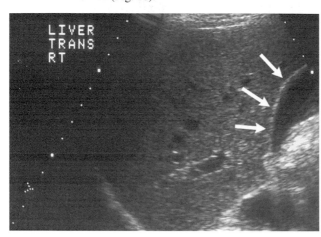

FIGURE 10.   Normal gallbladder on sonography. The wall (arrows) is less than 3 mm in diameter.

21. What is the basic lobar anatomy of the liver?
The liver is divided into left and right lobes by a plane that contains the gallbladder and the middle hepatic vein. The left hepatic lobe is divided into medial and lateral segments (relative to the liver, not the midline of the patient) by the fissure for the ligamentum teres and by the left hepatic vein. The right hepatic lobe is divided into anterior and posterior segments by a plane containing the right hepatic vein.

22. Where in the liver is the caudate lobe?
The caudate lobe extends off the medial aspect of the right hepatic lobe. It is separated from the left hepatic lobe, which is anterior to it, by the fissure for the ligamentum venosum.

23. What is the papillary process of the caudate lobe?
A small fingerlike projection of tissue that extends medially from the caudate lobe, between the portal vein, which is directly in front of it, and the inferior cava, which is directly behind it. This structure must not be confused with lymph nodes, which may occur in this region.

24. What vascular structure is found behind the pancreas?
The splenic vein.

25. What are the five major branches of the abdominal aorta (Fig. 11)?
1. Celiac artery
2. Superior mesenteric artery
3. Inferior mesenteric artery
4. Right renal artery
5. Left renal artery

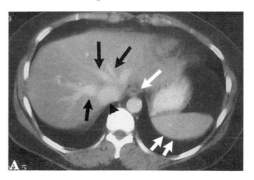

FIGURE 11.   Normal anatomy on CT. *A,* The hepatic veins (arrows) enter the inferior vena cava (arrowhead). The esophagus (white arrow), spleen (white double arrows), and aorta are noted.

Continued on following page.

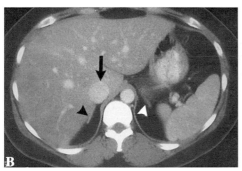
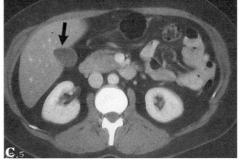

FIGURE 11 *(Cont.).* *B*, The inferior vena cava passes through the liver (arrow). The stomach is seen, as are portions of both adrenal glands (arrowheads). *C*, Gallbladder (arrow).

26. What two vascular structures join in front of the uncinate process of the pancreas to form the portal venous confluence?
The splenic and superior mesenteric veins.

BIBLIOGRAPHY

1. Ell SR: Handbook of Gastrointestinal and Genitourinary Radiology. St. Louis, Mosby, 1992.
2. Zeman RK, Fox SH, Silverman PM, et al: Helical (spiral) CT of the abdomen. AJR 160:719–725, 1995.

21. RADIOLOGY OF THE ESOPHAGUS

Jonathan Hartman, M.D.

1. What radiologic studies can be used to image the esophagus?
1. Barium esophagram
2. CT/MR
3. Endoscopic ultrasound

2. What is the value of these studies?
The barium study provides fine mucosal detail and permits fluoroscopic visualization of esophageal motility. CT does not permit detailed evaluation of the mucosa but does provide information about the tissues surrounding the esophagus: it evaluates extension of tumor and determines the presence or absence of lymph nodes. Endoscopic ultrasound is the noninvasive test of choice for determining the level of invasion of malignancy, although this modality is not as widely available as the other modalities.

3. What are the advantages of endoscopy over radiographic studies?
The esophagus is directly visualized, and abnormalities may be biopsied. However, this procedure is much more invasive and costly than an esophagram and should be reserved for cases in which there is uncertainty regarding a diagnosis or when tissue must be obtained.

4. What are the layers of the esophagus?
The esophagus is lined by squamous cell epithelium, the mucosa, throughout its course. Deep to the mucosa are the submucosa and the muscularis propria. Striated muscle is present in the upper third of the esophagus; smooth muscle is present throughout the esophagus. The esophagus has no adventitial layer.

5. **What types of disorders cause dysphagia?**
    • Mechanical causes
    • Motility disorders, including diffuse esophageal spasm, "nutcracker esophagus," and achalasia
    • Generalized muscular disorders, including muscular dystrophy and myasthenia gravis
    • Generalized neurologic disorders, including Parkinsonism, multiple sclerosis, and cerebrovascular disease
    • Connective tissue disorders, especially scleroderma

6. **What is the ideal position for studying a patient with dysphagia under fluoroscopy?**
    With the patient supine, to eliminate the effects of gravity on barium transit.

7. **What are some intrinsic mechanical causes of dysphagia?**
    1. Stricture   4. Esophageal carcinoma
    2. Schatzki's ring   5. Benign esophageal tumors
    3. Esophageal web

8. **What are some extrinsic mechanical causes of dysphagia?**
    1. Mediastinal neoplasms and/or lymphadenopathy
    2. Mediastinal benign masses such as duplication cysts/bronchogenic cysts
    3. Vascular abnormalities, such as an aberrant right subclavian artery
    4. Large anterior cervical spine osteophytes

9. **What are the esophagraphic findings of reflux?**
    The primary purpose of studying a patient with symptoms of reflux is not so much to prove that reflux exists as to exclude any morphologic or functional sequelae of the condition. Findings include thickened folds, a granular appearance of the mucosa, inflammatory polyp formation, ulceration, stricture, and abnormal motility. Specific findings will vary according to the chronicity and severity of the reflux.

10. **What is Barrett's esophagus?**
    Named for Norman Rupert Barrett, an English surgeon (1903–1979), Barrett's esophagus is progressive columnar metaplasia of the esophageal mucosa, secondary to chronic irritation, usually from gastroesophageal reflux. Barrett's esophagus may progress to carcinoma in situ and invasive adenocarcinoma. Patients may have symptoms of reflux or dysphagia, but up to half have no symptoms.

11. **What are the radiographic findings in Barrett's esophagus?**
    Esophageal stricture, hiatal hernia, reflux, thickened mucosal folds, ulceration, and a reticular mucosal pattern. While patients at high risk for Barrett's esophagus by radiographic criteria most often are confirmed with this diagnosis at biopsy, a barium esophagram is not as sensitive as endoscopy.

12. **A "beaked" distal esophagus indicates what disease?**
    Abrupt narrowing to a tight, symmetric stenosis, or "beaking" of the distal esophagus, is most consistent with achalasia. Abnormal innervation of the esophagus results in an absence of normal peristalsis, with subsequent esophageal dilatation, and abnormally elevated lower esophageal sphincter tone, which causes the distal beaking (Fig. 1). Other processes that result in distal esophageal stricture formation can mimic this appearance.

13. **What benign conditions should be considered when a mucosal mass is seen on an esophagram?**
    Papilloma, inflammatory polyp, and adenoma. Papillomas are by far the most common type of benign mucosal mass. However, benign tumors account for only a small percentage of esophageal tumors.

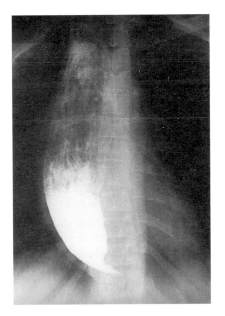

FIGURE 1. Anteroposterior radiograph from a barium esophagram, demonstrating marked esophageal dilatation with "beaked" narrowing distally, characteristic of achalasia. Note lucency within the barium column, representing undigested food. (Courtesy of Dr. Beth Wadler.)

14. What is the most common benign type of submucosal esophageal tumor?

Leiomyomas, which are tumors composed of bands or whorls of smooth muscle cells. About 60% occur in the distal third of the esophagus, 30% in the middle third, and 10% in the proximal third (because the proximal third is predominantly composed of striated muscle).

15. What is the appearance of an esophageal leiomyoma on an esophagram?

These lesions usually appear as a smooth, submucosal filling defect but may also have a significant exophytic or intraluminal component; although leiomyomas up to 20 cm in diameter occasionally exist, the tumors are usually between 3–5 cm when diagnosed. While they may cause dysphagia, they are not prone to bleeding, as are gastric leiomyomas; nor do they undergo malignant degeneration.

16. What are some uncommon or rare benign submucosal lesions of the esophagus?

Duplication cysts, fibrovascular polyps, lipomas, fibromas, granular cell tumors, and hemangiomas.

17. What is a Schatzki's ring?

Named for Richard Schatzki, a German-born American radiologist (1901–1992), this is a thin, ring-like constriction of the distal esophagus measuring 2–5 mm in height. The ring may vary in the degree of its constriction, producing the classic symptom of dysphagia for solids to a greater degree than liquids. Symptoms are particularly common when the diameter at the ring is less than 13 mm.

18. Which esophagram view best demonstrates a Schatzki's ring?

A view of the distal esophagus obtained with the patient prone and in a slight right anterior oblique position.

19. What is the most common infection affecting the esophagus?

Candida albicans. Most cases occur in immunocompromised patients, but about a fourth occur secondary to local stasis from disorders such as scleroderma or achalasia. The absence of thrush does not exclude esophageal candidiasis; only half of patients with esophageal disease have oral involvement.

20. What is the typical appearance of Candida on an esophagram?

Mucosal plaques and submucosal edema, often in a longitudinal linear pattern. In AIDS patients, aggressive infection may give the esophagus a "shaggy" appearance, often with ulcerations (Fig. 2).

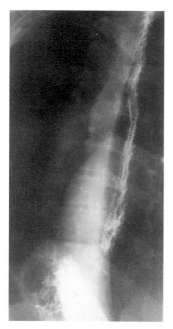

FIGURE 2.   Right anterior oblique radiograph from a barium esopha-gram, which shows marked, diffuse "shaggy" mucosal irregularity of severe Candida esophagitis in an immunocompromised patient. (Courtesy of Dr. Natalie Strutynsky.)

21. What viral organisms cause esophageal ulceration?

Herpes and cytomegalovirus, which occur in immunocompromised patients.

22. How does CMV esophagitis appear on an esophagram?

As one or a few giant ulcers, measuring 1–3 cm in diameter. Multiple small ulcers also may be seen, in which case the appearance is indistinguishable from herpes esophagitis. HIV itself can pro-duce large esophageal ulcers that are indistinguishable from those due to cytomegalovirus.

23. What medications are commonly implicated as causes of esophageal ulcers?

Tetracycline, aspirin, other NSAIDs, potassium chloride, iron sulfate, ascorbic acid, and quinidine.

24. What is the pathophysiology of drug-induced esophageal ulcers?

Taking medications with little or no fluid to aid in peristalsis and taking medications at bedtime result in stasis and mucosal irritation; the inherent acidity, alkalinity, or other irritative chemical properties of the medication by itself are not enough to produce ulceration. Disorders resulting in esophageal narrowing or dysmotility are predisposing factors for drug-induced ulceration. These ulcers are usually superficial and most commonly are seen in the midesophagus.

25. What are other causes of esophageal stricture?

- Corrosive ingestion
- Radiation
- Prolonged nasogastric intubation
- Crohn's disease
- Scleroderma
- Dermatologic disorders including pemphigoid and epidermolysis bullosa

26. What is the difference between uphill and downhill varices?

Uphill varices, or varices that form as a result of portal hypertension, are seen in the lower esophagus around the gastroesophageal junction. Downhill varices, which result from superior vena cava obstruction, are seen in the mid esophagus.

27. What is the radiographic appearance of varices?

Varices appear as serpentine submucosal filling defects on an esophagram, which are effaced when the esophagus is distended.

28. Can esophageal carcinoma mimic varices?

Yes, there are actually "varicoid" carcinomas that may superficially mimic varices on an esophagram. True varices will be effaced when the esophagus is distended with barium, while varicoid carcinoma will not be effaced due to the constrictive submucosal spread of the tumor.

29. If a patient presents with a soft-tissue mass extending up from the esophagus and prolapsing into the mouth, what is the diagnosis?

Fibrovascular polyp. This rare, benign tumor is thought to arise from loose submucosal tissue in the region of the pharyngoesophageal junction, to which chronic traction is applied due to peristalsis. A mass of redundant adipose, fibrous, and vascular tissue covered by normal squamous epithelium, fibroepithelial polyps causes dysphagia or wheezing. Sudden death due to airway obstruction also has been reported from these polyps.

30. What is the imaging appearance of a fibrovascular polyp?

A smoothly marginated intraluminal mass, often with a lobulated contour, which may displace the trachea anteriorly and can change in position during the course of an esophagram. If the margins of the polyp are more irregular or the pedicle is not identified, the polyp may be mistaken for a carcinoma. CT frequently shows a fatty component, which is diagnostic.

31. What is the appearance of an esophageal duplication cyst on imaging?

A mural mass, which if large enough, may appear as a middle mediastinal mass on chest radiographs. The cystic nature of the mass is usually revealed on CT, because the density of the cyst is close to that of water. However, if the cyst contains proteinaceous material, the CT density may be greater than that of water. Generally, esophageal duplication cysts do not communicate with the esophageal lumen.

32. What therapeutic maneuvers can be taken in the radiology department to manage acute impaction of food in the esophagus?

Intravenous injection of glucagon in combination with oral administration of water and an effervescent agent is effective in 70% of cases. However, if obstruction has been present for more than 24 hours, there is an increased risk of esophageal laceration or perforation.

33. Where does food get stuck in the esophagus?

At normal areas of narrowing, including at the level of the aortic arch, at the level of the left mainstem bronchus, at the gastroesophageal junction, and at areas of abnormal narrowing, including stricture and tumor.

34. What is the most common malignant tumor of the esophagus?

Squamous cell carcinoma, which accounts for 80% of esophageal malignancies, 7% of all GI malignancies, and 1% of all malignancy. Patients present with dysphagia, weight loss, and retrosternal chest pain (Fig. 3).

35. What is the appearance of esophageal cancer on esophagrams?

An irregular intraluminal mass, which may be sessile, polypoid, or ulcerated. Less common presentations include infiltrative and varicoid forms (Fig. 3).

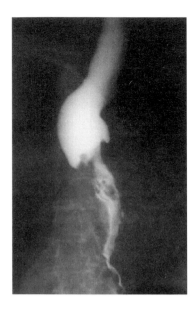

FIGURE 3. Right anterior oblique radiograph from a barium esophagram, in which barium outlines a large, fungating mass within the mid esophagus. Squamous cell carcinoma was diagnosed on biopsy. (Courtesy of Dr. Natalie Strutynsky.)

36. Why does CT understage esophageal cancer?

CT is used to evaluate direct tumor extension and metastases. CT cannot detect early tumor extension into adjacent tissues or lymphatic spread in nodes that are not enlarged.

37. How is esophageal tumor treated?

By total excision, if possible, with chemotherapy and radiation therapy for unresectable disease or as adjuvant therapy. Recently, there has been success using metallic stents to relieve obstructive symptoms in patients with unresectable tumor. Five-year survival is less than 10%.

38. What are some risk factors for squamous cell cancer of the esophagus?
- Tobacco and alcohol
- Achalasia (usually in the mid or distal esophagus, with a lag time of about 20 years, 5% prevalence)
- Stricture from lye ingestion (30–40 year lag time, 5% prevalence)
- Plummer-Vinson syndrome (controversial)
- Familial tylosis palmaris et plantaris (rare condition of hyperkeratosis of palms and soles and papillomatosis of the esophagus, carries a 70% risk; consider prophylactic esophagectomy)

39. If an esophageal cancer is not squamous cell, what type is it most likely?

An adenocarcinoma, which accounts for about 20% of esophageal cancer. Most of these cancers arise in Barrett's esophagus; about 10% of patients with Barrett's esophagus eventually develop adenocarcinoma.

40. Can esophageal adenocarcinoma be distinguished radiographically from squamous cell cancer?

No. Early lesions appear as a plaque-like mass, a stricture, or superficial mucosal irregularity, and more advanced lesions appear as an ulcerated mass, an extensive luminal narrowing, or a varicoid lesion. Extension into the gastric cardia is common, as these lesions generally arise in the lower esophagus. There is a 9:1 predominance in males over females.

41. What tumor may occur in the esophagus of AIDS patients?

Kaposi's sarcoma. The radiographic appearance is that of multiple polypoid lesions or submucosal masses, which may ulcerate, producing a target appearance.

42. What are some rare tumors of the esophagus?
- Small-cell carcinoma
- Spindle-cell carcinoma
- Leiomyosarcoma
- Melanoma
- Adenoid cystic carcinoma
- Mucoepidermoid carcinoma
- Lymphoma
- Secondary invasion by tumor*
- Metastases*

* More common than other entities.

43. What is a Zenker's diverticulum?

Named after Friedrich Albert von Zenker, a German pathologist (1825–1898), it is a true diverticulum of the upper esophagus located at the level of the upper esophageal sphincter. There is controversy over its etiology. While abnormal contraction and relaxation of the cricopharyngeus muscle probably contributes to its formation, some studies have shown abnormal muscle fiber configuration in some cases as well as a high association with hiatal hernia and gastroesophageal reflux, raising the possibility of an irritative or inflammatory cause.

44. How do patients present with a Zenker's diverticulum, and what is the appearance of the diverticulum on an esophagram?

Patients present with dysphagia, choking, halitosis, regurgitation of undigested food, or with a neck mass. The diverticulum is seen on esophagrams in the midline at the level of the pyriform sinuses, extending inferiorly and posterior to the cervical esophagus.

45. What other types of esophageal diverticula are there?
- Traction diverticula related to fibrosis from adjacent infected lymph nodes
- Pulsion diverticula from abnormal motility
- Epiphrenic diverticula, located just above the diaphragm (rare)

46. What are the plain film findings of Boerhaave's syndrome?

Named after the Dutch physician Herman Boerhaave (1668–1738), it is traumatic rupture of the distal esophagus, usually following forceful retching. Chest radiographic findings include pneumomediastinum, pleural effusion (usually left), and pneumothorax.

47. How can Boerhaave's syndrome be diagnosed at fluoroscopy?

Using a water-soluble contrast agent, extravasation of the contrast from the distal esophagus is seen. The tear usually originates just above the gastroesophageal junction on the left.

48. A patient with arthritis of her hands and dry skin presents with dysphagia. What disease does she have?

Scleroderma. She has developed esophageal dysmotility and fibrosis.

BIBLIOGRAPHY

1. Gore RM, Levine MS, Lauter I (eds): A Textbook of Gastrointestinal Radiology. Philadelphia, W.B. Saunders, 1994.
2. Levine MS: Radiology of the Esophagus. Philadelphia, W.B. Saunders, 1989.
3. Ott DJ, Gelfand DW (eds): Radiology of the upper gastrointestinal tract. Radiol Clin North Am 35(2):1994.

22. GASTROINTESTINAL HEMORRHAGE

Kenneth D. Murphy, M.D.

1. How is gastrointestinal hemorrhage classified?

According to location of the bleeding site. Lower GI hemorrhage is defined as bleeding within the alimentary tract distal to the ligament of Treitz. Upper GI hemorrhage is bleeding from a point proximal to the ligament of Treitz. Upper and lower GI bleeding can be further subdivided according to whether the source of hemorrhage is arterial or venous.

2. What are the causes of upper GI bleeding?

- Peptic ulcer disease
- Acute hemorrhagic gastritis
- Esophageal varices
- Mallory-Weiss syndrome
- Neoplasm
- Dieulafoy disease
- Vascular-enteric fistula
- Visceral artery aneurysm
- Vascular malformations

3. What are the most common causes of gastric bleeding?

Gastric varices, gastric ulcer disease, and acute hemorrhagic gastritis. Gastric varices are a complication of portal hypertension. Isolated gastric varices without esophageal varices suggest splenic vein thrombosis. Gastric ulcer disease is most commonly peptic in etiology. The majority of ulcers are benign. Bleeding from gastric varices and ulcer disease can be severe and life-threatening. Hemorrhagic gastritis, also known as erosive gastritis, is a common cause of mild upper GI hemorrhage. Hemorrhagic gastritis is often associated with alcohol use, emotional stress, or antiinflammatory medications.

4. What is Dieulafoy disease?

A rare cause of massive upper GI hemorrhage, due to erosion of an abnormally enlarged submucosal artery, typically in the proximal stomach. The diagnosis is frequently confirmed at surgery or autopsy. Inflammatory changes are noticeably absent when the artery is examined histologically. Endoscopy may show a bleeding artery centered in a shallow ulcer.

5. What are the angiographic findings in Dieulafoy disease? How is the disease treated?

Rapid extravasation of contrast from a slightly enlarged, otherwise normal artery in the gastric cardia or fundus. Treatment primarily has been surgical, or with transcatheter embolization. Critics question whether it is a real disease, based on the lack of pathologic and radiologic features.

6. What artery is responsible for gastric hemorrhage?

The left gastric artery, in 85% of cases. This is usually the first branch off the celiac artery. On rare occasions, the left gastric artery can originate off the splenic artery or off the aorta.

7. What is the Mallory-Weiss syndrome?

A cause of massive, painless hematemesis, the syndrome occurs after a violent episode of vomiting that results in a tear of the submucosal venous plexus of the distal esophagus. The syndrome is most common in male alcoholics (Fig. 1).

8. What are the angiographic findings in the Mallory-Weiss syndrome? How is the disorder treated?

Acute extravasation at the cardioesophageal junction, with contrast outlining the distal esophagus or the proximal stomach (Fig. 2). The differential diagnosis of this angiographic appearance includes ulcerative gastritis and a proximal gastric ulcer. The Mallory-Weiss tear is commonly self-limited, but transcatheter embolization of the left gastric artery is recommended for hemorrhage refractory to conservative management.

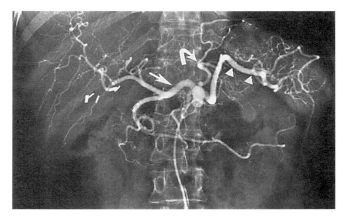

FIGURE 1. Celiac arteriogram demonstrates the three major branches: common hepatic artery (arrow), splenic artery (arrowheads), and left gastric artery (curved arrow).

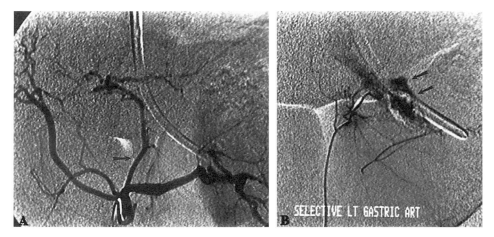

FIGURE 2. Mallory-Weiss syndrome. *A*, Celiac arteriogram demonstrates a common trunk of the left gastric and left hepatic arteries (arrow). *B*, Selective left gastric arteriogram demonstrates extravasation from a Mallory-Weiss tear (arrows).

9. What is the diagnostic work-up for upper GI bleeding?

Prior to the work-up, the patient is stabilized with IV fluids, blood transfusions, and correction of coagulopathy as needed. A nasogastric tube is usually placed for gastric decompression and documentation of upper tract blood loss. The initial diagnostic study is endoscopy, because arterial and venous hemorrhage can usually be distinguished, which is important for correct clinical management.

10. How is venous bleeding managed?

Venous bleeding, typically from gastroesophageal varices, is initially managed with endoscopic sclerotherapy. If variceal hemorrhage is recurrent or refractory to sclerotherapy, consideration of a transjugular intrahepatic portosystemic shunt (TIPS) or a surgical portosystemic shunt is warranted. Balloon tamponade of esophageal varices with a Blakemore tube can be performed as a temporizing measure.

11. How is arterial bleeding managed?

With endoscopic sclerotherapy, percutaneous transcatheter embolization, or surgery. After localization of the site and origin of upper GI hemorrhage, prompt treatment is critical for survival.

12. What is a TIPS?

A transjugular intrahepatic portosystemic shunt is a newly developed interventional procedure for treatment of variceal hemorrhage and ascites from portal hypertension. The procedure involves creation of an intrahepatic shunt from the portal vein to the hepatic vein (Fig. 3). Balloon angioplasty catheters are used to dilate the intrahepatic tract, which is subsequently supported with a metallic stent. The entire procedure is performed percutaneously via a jugular vein approach. The shunt allows variceal decompression with cessation of bleeding. In cases of persistent bleeding despite a TIPS, the shunt provides access to the varices for transcatheter embolization.

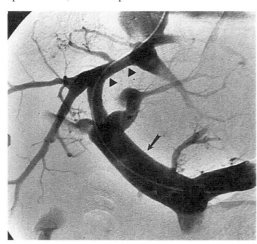

FIGURE 3. A TIPS shunt between the portal vein (arrow). and hepatic vein (arrowheads).

13. What are the indications for mesenteric arteriography for GI bleeding?

Severe, life-threatening hemorrhage or bleeding refractory to medical management. In select cases of chronic, intermittent GI blood loss where the endoscopic and diagnostic work-up is negative, arteriography may be beneficial in disclosing an occult lesion such as angiodysplasia.

14. What are the contraindications to mesenteric arteriography for GI bleeding?

The primary contraindication is hemodynamic instability. Patients with massive GI hemorrhage who are clinically unstable despite aggressive resuscitation may require surgical exploration. Residual barium in the bowel is a relative contraindication to mesenteric arteriography, because the barium may obscure detection of contrast extravasation.

15. What is the technique for angiographic evaluation of GI bleeding?

An arterial sheath is positioned in the common femoral artery, and a 5-French catheter with an angled tip is used to selectively catheterize the appropriate vessel(s). Images are obtained in the arterial, capillary, and venous phases of contrast injection. Glucagon should be administered intravenously prior to contrast injection, to reduce bowel peristaltic activity. The angiographic finding of acute hemorrhage is contrast extravasation into the bowel lumen. The contrast-filled bladder should be emptied to avoid obscuring contrast extravasation from bowel situated in the pelvis. Any medication with blood pressure lowering effects should be avoided, as hypotension may result in cessation of bleeding.

16. Where are the mesenteric arteries located?

To facilitate rapid selective catheterization and minimize procedural time, the origin of the mesenteric arteries with respect to bony landmarks is important. The celiac artery arises from the anterior aortic wall at the T12–L1 interspace. The superior mesenteric artery originates off the anterior aortic wall at the L1 vertebral body level. The inferior mesenteric artery originates off the anterolateral aortic wall at the L2–L3 interspace.

17. What are the causes of lower gastrointestinal bleeding?

- Diverticulosis
- Angiodysplasia
- Inflammatory bowel disease
- Ischemic colitis
- Neoplasm
- Vasculitis
- Aortoenteric fistula
- Aneurysm
- Mesenteric varices

18. Is lower GI bleeding always from a lower GI bleeding site?

No. In 10% of patients with severe rectal hemorrhage, the source is proximal to the ligament of Treitz.

19. What is diverticulosis?

An acquired condition in which overactivity of smooth muscle in the bowel wall results in herniation of mucosa and submucosa through the muscular layers, forming an outpouching known as a diverticulum. The diverticulum forms where colonic arterioles penetrate the mucosal wall of the bowel. Males and females are affected equally. One proposed cause of diverticular disease is a diet low in roughage and high in refined fiber. About 80% of diverticula occur in the descending colon, with a majority in the sigmoid colon.

20. What are complications of diverticular disease?

Infection and hemorrhage. Diverticulitis is an infectious complication that occurs when a diverticulum perforates and a localized, pericolic abscess results. Clinically significant hemorrhage is a rare complication of diverticulitis. Bleeding from diverticula usually results from trauma to the "exposed" arteriole that penetrates the mucosal wall at the neck of the diverticulum. Although diverticular disease is more common in the descending colon, approximately half of the bleeding occurs in the ascending colon. It is theorized that the wider neck of the right-sided diverticula exposes a longer segment of colonic arteriole to injury. In the elderly, bleeding from diverticula is the leading cause of severe blood loss, although the bleeding stops without intervention 80–90% of the time.

21. What is the incidence of severe bleeding after polypectomy?

As high as 2.2%. The bleeding can occur immediately after the procedure or can be delayed up to 2 weeks. Most post-polypectomy hemorrhages are self-limiting and respond to conservative management.

22. What is angiodysplasia?

Also known as vascular ectasia or arteriovenous malformation, angiodysplasia is a vascular lesion primarily localized to the colon that can result in severe bleeding. The lesion is a tuft of thin-walled vessels in the submucosa. The most common site is the cecum and ascending colon. At colonoscopy, angiodysplasia appears as a small reddish lesion that is sometimes ulcerated. Barium studies are usually unremarkable because the lesion is small and located in the submucosa. Bleeding tends to be low-grade and intermittent, but is occasionally massive. The hemorrhage stops spontaneously in 90% of cases, with an 85% risk of recurrent bleeding.

23. What are the angiographic features of angiodysplasia?

Selective superior mesenteric arteriography usually demonstrates a cluster or tuft of vessels in the right colon during the arterial phase of injection. There is early venous opacification, typically of the ileocolic vein (Fig. 4). In up to 25% of cases, multiple lesions can be identified.

24. What are the causes of gastrointestinal hemorrhage in AIDS?

AIDS is associated with infection and neoplasm of the gastrointestinal tract, which can occasionally result in hemorrhage. The neoplastic causes of GI hemorrhage in AIDS include Kaposi's sarcoma and lymphoma. The primary infectious etiology is cytomegalovirus colitis. In most cases, arteriography enables localization of the bleeding site and facilitates transcatheter treatment with embolic agents or vasoconstrictive drugs.

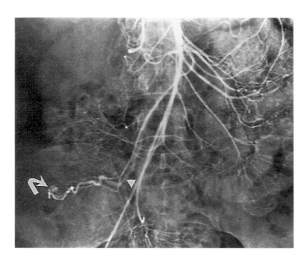

FIGURE 4. Selective superior mesenteric angiogram demonstrates angiodysplasia of the right colon. Note the "tuft" of vessels (curved arrow) and early draining vein (arrowhead).

25. What is the diagnostic work-up for lower GI hemorrhage?

Prior to the work-up, the patient is stabilized. The possibility of an anorectal source such as hemorrhoids or rectal fissure should be evaluated by physical examination supplemented by anoscopy or rigid sigmoidoscopy. Further endoscopic evaluation with colonoscopy may be performed. After clinical and endoscopic evaluation, scintigraphy is recommended. A positive nuclear medicine study warrants arteriography in the hemodynamically stable patient, and surgery should be considered if the patient is unstable. If the nuclear medicine study is negative, the bleeding rate is generally too slow to demonstrate by angiography.

26. What scintigraphic examinations are available for lower GI bleeding?

Technetium-99m labeled red blood cells and technetium sulfur colloid. For both studies, the respective agent is injected intravenously and scintigraphic images with digital interfacing are obtained every 30 seconds for about 60 minutes. Digital interfacing allows the images to be displayed in a "cine-loop" to enhance localization of the bleeding site. Extravasation of blood is represented by focal accumulation of tracer activity that moves within the bowel lumen.

27. Why is scintigraphy more sensitive for detecting GI hemorrhage than arteriography?

Because bleeding rates as low as 0.1 ml/min can be detected, while arteriography usually requires a bleeding rate of 0.5 to 1.0 ml/min for detection.

28. Why is a labeled red blood cell scan superior to sulfur colloid scan for detecting GI bleeding?

The labeled red blood cells have a longer intravascular half-life than sulfur colloid, which permits delayed images to be obtained, up to 24 hours after administration. Also, the liver and spleen background activity is significantly less with labeled red blood cells than with sulfur colloid. Detection of bleeding points in the colon or small bowel overlying the liver and spleen is therefore improved. The overall sensitivity for detection of hemorrhage is greater with labeled red blood cells than with sulfur colloid.

29. What mesenteric vessels are responsible for lower GI hemorrhage?

The superior and inferior mesenteric arteries are primarily responsible; the superior mesenteric artery (SMA) supplies the jejunum, ileum, cecum, appendix, ascending colon, and transverse colon, while the inferior mesenteric artery (IMA) supplies the descending colon, sigmoid colon, and rectum. The SMA and IMA should be catheterized first at mesenteric arteriography for lower GI hemorrhage. Complete arteriographic evaluation for lower GI bleeding necessitates a celiac arterial study, as middle colic branches to the transverse colon can originate from the dorsal pancreatic artery off the splenic artery.

30. What are the transcatheter treatment options for GI hemorrhage?

Embolization versus intraarterial infusion of a vasoconstrictive drug.

31. What is the role of embolotherapy in GI hemorrhage?

Transcatheter embolotherapy is temporary or permanent occlusion of the vessel supplying the bleeding lesion. Vessel occlusion decreases the pulsatile pressure head, allowing the patient's own coagulation factors to facilitate hemostasis. The technique involves transcatheter deployment of the embolic agent proximal to the bleeding point (Fig. 5). The tissue distal to the site of vessel occlusion is rendered ischemic. The upper GI tract is rich in collateral communications that minimize the impact of ischemia and the incidence of bowel infarction. For upper GI hemorrhage, embolotherapy is preferred over intraarterial infusion of vasoconstrictors. In contrast, embolization of the mesenteric circulation to the lower GI tract is associated with a higher incidence of ischemic complications such as bowel infarction. Therefore, intraarterial infusion of vasoconstrictive agents is preferred over embolotherapy for lower GI hemorrhage.

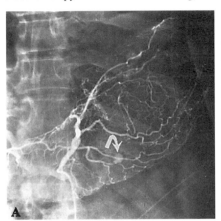 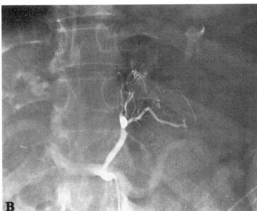

FIGURE 5. Gastric hemorrhage. *A*, Selective left gastric arteriogram demonstrates bleeding site (curved arrow). *B*, Left gastric arteriogram after embolization with gel foam demonstrates cessation of bleeding.

32. What are the indications for transcatheter embolization?

1. Acute arterial hemorrhage from an upper GI source.
2. Failure of vasoconstrictors to stop a lower or upper GI hemorrhage.

33. What are the contraindications to transcatheter embolotherapy?

A stenosis at the origin of the bleeding mesenteric artery. A catheter placed across a mesenteric arterial stenosis increases the risk of acute thrombosis and secondary ischemia.

34. What agents are used in embolotherapy?

The main embolic agents are gelatin (Gelfoam) and metallic oils. Other embolic agents not routinely used in the mesenteric circulation include polyvinyl alcohol foam (PVA), dehydrate ethanol, sodium tetradecyl sulfate, microfibrillar collagen, and acrylic tissue adhesives.

35. What is Gelfoam?

A gelatin product available in powder form or in sheets. The sheets can be cut into pledgets tailored in size for occlusion of the desired artery. The powder has a particulate size of 40–60µ, which primarily occludes capillaries. Gelfoam induces a panarteritis that promotes thrombosis. The embolic effect is temporary, lasting a few days to 2 weeks. Gelfoam is the preferred embolic material for gastric bleeding. In cases of peptic erosion the defect in the bleeding artery can allow pledgets of Gelfoam to pass into the bowel lumen. In such cases, a coil is placed proximal to the bleeding site.

36. What are metallic coils?

Permanent embolic agents composed of stainless steel or platinum. Some coils have Dacron fibers attached to promote thrombogenicity. The coils are available in a variety of lengths, diameters, and configurations. The coils are deployed via a catheter, with a guidewire or a coil pusher. Correct sizing of coils with respect to the target vessels is important to prevent coil migration into a nontarget vessel.

37. What is the technique for embolization of a bleeding duodenal ulcer?

The most common arterial source for a bleeding duodenal ulcer is the gastroduodenal artery (GDA). The GDA is usually the first major branch off the common hepatic artery. The GDA terminates at the right gastroepiploic artery and the anterior-superior pancreaticoduodenal artery. The anterior-superior pancreaticoduodenal artery communicates with the SMA via the inferior pancreaticoduodenal artery. As a result, occlusion of the GDA proximal to the bleeding site alone is insufficient, as the pancreaticoduodenal arteries will provide retrograde flow from the SMA to promote continued bleeding. Therefore, effective embolization of the GDA requires occlusion of the proximal and distal GDA, thus "trapping" the bleeding site (Fig. 6). Metallic coils are the preferred embolic agent for GDA occlusion.

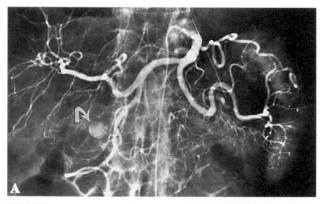

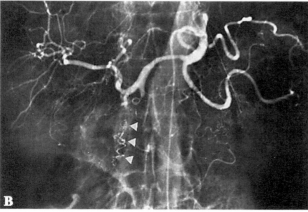

FIGURE 6.   Duodenal hemorrhage. *A*, Selective celiac angiogram demonstrates extravasation (curved arrow). *B*, Metallic coils (arrowheads) placed in the GDA proximal and distal to the bleeding site ensure occlusion.

38. What is vasopressin?

A drug that induces smooth muscle cell contraction in the GI tract and vascular bed. The drug has two mechanisms for promoting hemostasis in the GI tract. First, it induces contraction of the bowel wall to tamponade the exposed arterioles responsible for bleeding in diverticulosis. Secondly, the drug induces vasoconstriction in the mesenteric circulation to diminish flow and stop bleeding. Vasopressin is short acting and therefore requires continuous infusion.

39. What is the protocol for vasopressin infusion for GI hemorrhage?

Vasopressin can be administered for both upper and lower GI bleeding. It is delivered via a catheter selectively positioned in the proximal segment of the bleeding artery. Vasopressin is initially administered at 0.2 units/min for 20 minutes, and a repeat arteriogram is performed. If the bleeding has stopped, the catheter is secured into position and the infusion is continued at 0.2 units/min for 12–24 hours (Fig. 7). If there is no further bleeding, the infusion is tapered over 24 hours. If the bleeding persists after 20 minutes, the infusion rate is doubled to 0.4 units/min for an additional 20 minutes. If the double dose therapy stops bleeding after 20 minutes, the infusion is continued at 0.4 units/min for 6–12 hours. If the bleeding has subsided after 6–12 hours, the infusion dose is tapered over 24–48 hours. If the bleeding persists after a trial of 0.4 units/min, embolization or surgery is indicated.

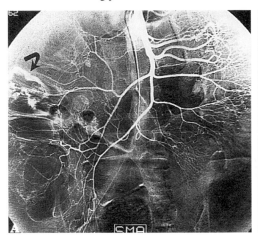 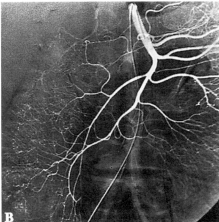

FIGURE 7. Lower gastrointestinal hemorrhage. *A*, Selective superior mesenteric arteriogram demonstrates bleeding in the right colon from diverticulosis (curved arrow). *B*, After vasopressin therapy, the bleeding has stopped.

BIBLIOGRAPHY

1. Durham JD, Kumpe DA, Rothbarth LJ, Van Stiegmann G: Dieulafoy disease: Arteriographic findings and treatment. Radiology 174:937–941, 1990.
2. McNally PR: GI/Liver Secrets. Philadelphia, Hanley & Belfus, 1996, pp 351–372.
3. Palmaz JC, Waltman AC: Dieulafoy disease: A real entity? Radiology 174:942, 1990.
4. Sharma VS, Valgi K, Bookstein JJ; Gastrointestinal hemorrhage in AIDS: Arteriographic diagnosis and transcatheter treatment. Radiology 185:447–451, 1992.

23. PEPTIC ULCER DISEASE

Douglas R. DeCorato, M.D., and Carolyn L. Raia, M.D.

1. Which cell produces gastric acid?

The parietal cell, which produces hydrochloric acid.

2. Which cell produces intrinsic factor?

The parietal cell.

3. What is the function of intrinsic factor?

Intrinsic factor is essential for the absorption of vitamin B_{12}, in the terminal ileum.

4. What cell secretes pepsinogen?
The chief cell.

5. Where do gastric contractions begin?
There are several types of gastric contractions; however, the constrictor wave, which propels food, begins in the body of the stomach and proceeds toward the antrum. This pushes the stomach contents to the pyloric channel.

6. What are some causes of thickened gastric folds?
1. Gastritis
2. Lymphoma
3. Adenocarcinoma
4. Varices
5. Ménétrier's disease

7. What are the radiologic findings in gastritis on an upper GI series (Fig. 1)?
Erosions, thickened folds, nodules, and polyps. Each of these findings may be found alone or in combination.

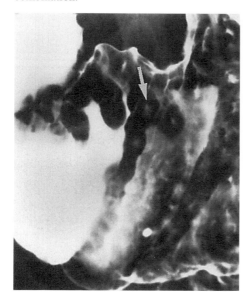

FIGURE 1. Gastritis. Note the thickened folds in the gastric antrum and the punctate erosions (arrow).

8. What is the typical appearance of gastric erosions?
Small linear collections of barium, which tend to line up with the gastric folds. These lesions are distinct from ulcers; they do not penetrate through to the submucosa.

9. What is the most common location for gastric erosions?
The antrum.

10. What are the symptoms of a gastric ulcer?
Abdominal pain is the most common presenting symptom. Symptoms suggestive of gastric ulcer include pain at night and pain exacerbated by food.

11. What is the differential diagnosis of gastric ulcers?
There are multiple benign and malignant causes. Benign causes include peptic ulcer disease (PUD), gastric erosions, and ulcers in benign masses such as leiomyoma. Malignant causes include carcinoma, lymphoma, leiomyosarcoma, and metastases.

12. Does location help in differentiating benign and malignant gastric ulcers?

Ulcers along the lesser curvature of the stomach are more likely to be benign. However, location by itself does not ensure that an ulcer is benign. Both benign and malignant ulcers can be found at any location in the stomach. An ulcer high in the gastric fundus must be considered suspicious by its location alone.

13. What are the radiologic signs of a benign gastric ulcer?
- Projection of the ulcer crater beyond the expected location of the gastric wall
- Hampton's line: a thin, sharply demarcated line with parallel, straight margins at the base of the ulcer crater
- Ulcer collar: a lucent ring that separates the ulcer crater from the gastric mucosa
- Ulcer mound, which is caused by mucosal edema

14. What are the radiologic signs of a malignant gastric ulcer (Fig. 2)?
- Gastric folds do not reach the edge of the ulcer crater
- Gastric folds are irregular, amputated, or clubbed
- Ulcer crater does not project beyond the expected location of the gastric wall
- Carman's meniscus sign, and the Kirkland complex (Fig. 3). Carman's meniscus refers to a finding described on a single contrast barium examination, where compression of the edges of a malignant ulcer causes the walls of the ulcer to touch and trap barium. The trapped barium is located in the ulcer bed, which has a meniscoid appearance (the inner margin is concave toward the lumen). The Kirkland complex refers to the heaped margins of the ulcer, which touch. This projects as a lucent rim around the ulcer on upper GI studies where the anterior abdominal wall is compressed by the radiologist.

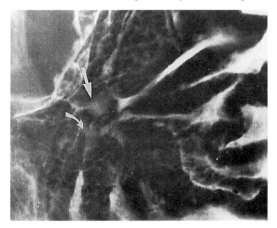 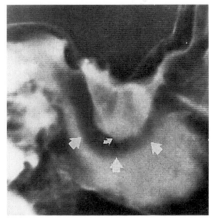

FIGURE 2 (Left). Malignant gastric ulcer. Demonstrated en face, this malignant ulcer (straight arrow) is associated with irregular mucosal folds, which unlike a benign ulcer do not radiate from the ulcer crater, but rather terminate at the ulcer mound or mass (curved arrow).

FIGURE 3 (Right). Carmen's meniscus sign: A malignant gastric ulcer which projects into the stomach. In addition, note Carmen's meniscus sign (curved arrow) where the compressed edges of the malignant ulcer trap barium. Kirkland complex: The heaped up margins of the ulcer, which touch to produce a lucent rim around the ulcer (arrowheads).

15. What are the complications of a gastric ulcer?

Bleeding, perforation, and fistula formation, which is rare.

16. What is the most common cell type in gastric cancer?

Adenocarcinoma, in 95% of all gastric cancer.

17. Is there an association between pernicious anemia and gastric neoplasms?
Yes, patients with pernicious anemia are at increased risk of developing gastric cancer.

18. What are the usual symptoms of a duodenal ulcer?
Abdominal pain is the most frequent complaint. Pain usually occurs 90–180 minutes after eating. Pain will often wake the patient at night and is usually relieved quickly by eating or ingesting antacids.

19. What is the differential diagnosis of duodenal ulcers?
Benign etiologies include peptic ulcer disease and Crohn's disease. Malignant causes include primary cancers and metastatic disease.

20. What organism is currently considered an important etiologic factor in peptic ulcer disease?
Helicobacter pylori.

21. What is the most common location of a duodenal ulcer (Fig. 4)?
About 95% of duodenal ulcers occur in the first portion of the duodenum.

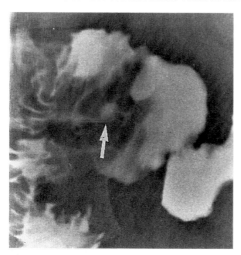

FIGURE 4.   Duodenal ulcer. Small collection of barium (arrow) which represents the ulcer crater projected en face. In addition, note the normal-appearing folds projecting to the ulcer crater.

22. What percentage of duodenal ulcers are found in the post-bulbar region?
About 3–5%.

23. What is Zollinger-Ellison syndrome?
A rare disorder caused by a gastrin-secreting non-beta islet cell tumor or tumors. Most of these tumors are found in the pancreas.

24. What is a major clue that Zollinger-Ellison syndrome is likely to be present?
When ulcers are found in a postbulbar location, especially when they are multiple.

25. What is a giant duodenal ulcer?
An ulcer of the duodenal bulb that is larger than 2 cm in size. They are sometimes difficult to diagnose despite their large size, because they can be confused with a deformed bulb, or they may coexist with a deformed bulb and also be missed.

26. What is the cloverleaf deformity?
Chronic deformity of the duodenal bulb due to scarring from peptic ulcer disease. It can be difficult to exclude a coexistent active ulcer in these patients.

27. What are the radiologic findings in duodenitis?
Thickening of the duodenal folds is the most sensitive but least specific sign. The folds are generally greater than 5 mm thick. Other signs include mucosal nodularity, erosions, and deformity of the folds.

28. Are duodenal bulb tumors malignant or benign?
Almost always benign, duodenal bulb tumors include adenomas, leiomyomas, and lipomas.

BIBLIOGRAPHY

1. Amberg JR, Juhl JH; The stomach and duodenum. In Juhl JH, Crummy AB (eds): Paul and Juhl's Essentials of Radiologic Imaging, 6th ed. Philadelphia, Lippincott-Raven, 1993.
2. Buck JL, Pantongrag-Brown L: Gastritides, gastropathies, and polyps unique to the stomach. Radiol Clin North Am 32:1215–1231, 1994.
3. Eisenberg RL: Gastrointestinal Radiology: A Pattern Approach, 3rd ed. Philadelphia, Lippincott-Raven, 1995.
4. Glick S: Duodenal ulcer. Radiol Clin North Am 32:1259–1274, 1994.
5. Guyton AC: Textbook of Medical Physiology, 9th ed. Philadelphia, W.B. Saunders, 1996, pp 846–847.
6. Maklansky D, Lindner AE, Kurzban JD: Gastric neoplasms. In Taveras JM, Ferrucci JT (eds): Radiology–Diagnosis–Imaging–Intervention, vol. 4. Philadelphia, J.B. Lippincott, (Looseleaf).
7. Maruyama M, Baba Y: Gastric carcinoma. Radiol Clin North Am 32:1233–1252, 1994.
8. Stevenson GW: Gastric ulcers. In Taveras JM, Ferrucci JT (eds): Radiology–Diagnosis–Imaging–Intervention, vol. 4. Philadelphia, J.B. Lippincott, (Looseleaf).
9. Thompson WM: Duodenal ulcers. In Taveras JM, Ferrucci JT (eds): Radiology–Diagnosis–Imaging–Intervention, vol. 4. Philadelphia, J.B. Lippincott, (Looseleaf).

24. INFLAMMATORY DISEASES OF THE LARGE BOWEL

Douglas S. Katz, M.D., and Burton M. Gold, M.D.

APPENDICITIS

1. What are some plain film signs of appendicitis? (Fig. 1)
- An appendicolith, a right lower quadrant calcification found in 10% of patients with acute appendicitis
- Abnormal bowel gas pattern, including focal ileus in the right lower quadrant
- Loss of the normal fat planes, including the right psoas shadow
- Extraluminal soft-tissue mass
- Free intraperitoneal gas (rare)
- Scoliosis of the lumbar spine, convex to the left

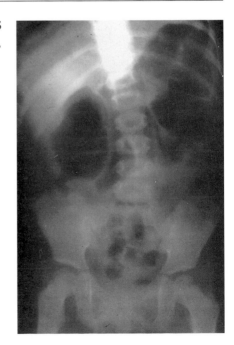

FIGURE 1. Supine film of the abdomen shows an appendicolith, a deformed spastic cecum, and scoliosis of the lumbar spine in a young child with appendicitis.

2. How specific are these signs?

Not very. The presence of an appendicolith in the correct clinical setting is highly suggestive of appendicitis and is the most specific plain film sign, although calcifications such as a phlebolith (a calcification in a vein) or a ureteral stone may simulate an appendicolith.

3. Why image patients with suspected appendicitis?

Many surgeons will go immediately to the operating room if a patient has classic signs and symptoms of appendicitis. However, a significant percentage of patients will present with atypical signs and symptoms. Many conditions will simulate appendicitis, especially gynecologic disorders. Also, since a negative exploration for appendicitis is much more expensive than an imaging study, patients, especially those with atypical or nonspecific presentations, probably would benefit from preoperative imaging.

4. What imaging studies can be used to diagnose appendicitis?

In children, an ultrasound is the best test since there is no ionizing radiation. Thin adults also can be imaged with sonography. Obese patients, patients who cannot tolerate sonography due to marked pain, and patients with equivocal ultrasound results should undergo a CT scan. Some institutions, with limited experience in right lower quadrant sonography, go directly to CT in all adults.

5. What are the sonographic findings of appendicitis? (Fig. 2)

An appendix dilated to greater than 6 mm in cross-section and that is non-compressible. During right lower quadrant sonography, the appendix is identified and the transducer is used to push directly on the appendix. A normal appendix can be compressed to a diameter less than 7 mm.

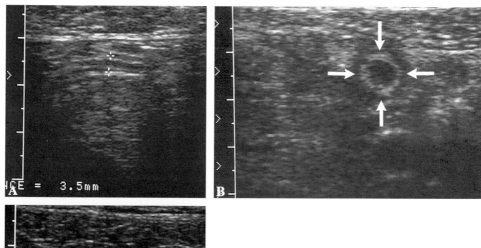

FIGURE 2. *A,* Normal appendix shown on sonography. The appendix measures less than 6 mm in diameter. *B* and *C,* Appendicitis demonstrated on sonography. *B,* The appendix, seen in cross-section, measures greater than 1 cm in diameter (arrows) and was noncompressible during the examination. *C,* Ultrasound image of a different patient. The appendix (between the + signs) is quite distended; the blind ending tip is seen, which proves that this structure is the appendix and not the cecum or ileum.

6. What are the findings of appendicitis on contrast-enhanced CT? (Fig. 3)

A dilated appendix (greater than 6 mm in cross-section) with an enhancing wall and inflammatory changes in the adjacent fat.

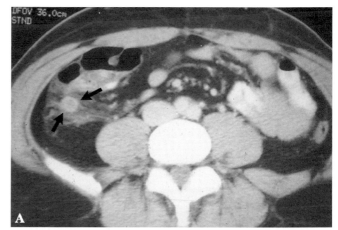

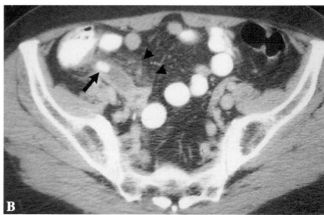

FIGURE 3. Two cases of acute appendicitis on CT. *A*, Contrast-enhanced CT. The appendix (seen in cross-section) is distended, its wall enhances (arrows), and there is periappendiceal inflammation. *B*, Contrast-enhanced CT of a different patient. The appendix (seen as a tubular structure) is dilated and contains an appendicolith (arrow); there is inflammation of the surrounding fat (arrowheads).

7. Which study, ultrasound or CT, is operator-dependent?

Ultrasound. Right lower quadrant sonography may be difficult, particularly in adults, and requires substantial experience.

8. What are some complications of appendicitis?
- Appendiceal perforation
- Phlegmon or abscess
- Subacute or chronic appendicitis

9. What is the best imaging test to diagnose the complications of appendicitis?

A contrast-enhanced CT (Fig. 4).

10. Is there a role for a barium enema in establishing the diagnosis of appendicitis?

While it was used in the past, the barium enema has no significant current role in the diagnosis of appendicitis. The diagnosis of appendicitis on a barium enema can be excluded only if the entire appendix, including the tip, filled with barium; unfortunately, the appendix does not completely fill with barium in up to a third of normal patients.

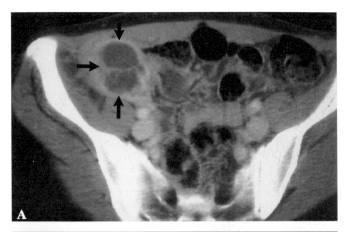

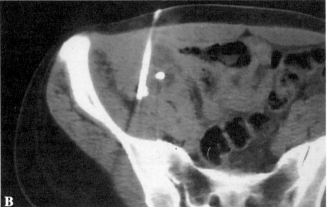

FIGURE 4. *A*, A 36-year-old woman with fever and right lower quadrant pain. There is an anterior right lower quadrant collection, which has low-density central areas, and peripheral enhancement (arrows) represents an abscess secondary to appendicitis. *B*, A percutaneous drainage catheter was placed into the collection by an interventional radiologist.

11. How can an appendiceal abscess be treated?

With antibiotics and percutaneous catheter drainage. After the patient's inflammatory process is allowed to "cool down," the appendix can be removed surgically.

DIVERTICULITIS

12. What is the difference between diverticulitis and diverticulosis?

Diverticulosis means that multiple diverticula (usually the term is used to refer to the colon) are present. Colonic diverticula are a common cause of lower gastrointestinal bleeding. Diverticulitis occurs in 10–20% of people with known diverticulosis. Diverticulitis is an inflammatory process caused by stagnation of inspissated feces within a diverticulum with subsequent perforation (usually localized) of the diverticulum. Both diverticulosis and diverticulitis affect older people. The sigmoid colon is the most commonly affected portion of bowel.

13. What is the best imaging test for diverticulitis?

CT, which allows the bowel wall and the adjacent fat to be directly visualized. Ultrasound has a limited role; a barium enema is minimally invasive, although it is useful in imaging patients with suspected diverticulitis.

14. What are some plain film signs seen in diverticulitis?

The findings usually are nonspecific, but there may be free intraperitoneal air, pelvic extraluminal air collection(s), localized ileus, pelvic fluid, and a pelvic soft-tissue mass.

15. What are the barium enema findings in diverticulitis? (Fig. 5)

• Diverticula
• Narrowed colonic lumen with spasm, muscular hypertrophy
• Extrinsic mass effect on the colonic lumen, e.g., by thickened bowel wall/abscess
• Colonic fixation
• Pointing and distortion of individual diverticula
• Perforation of barium outside the colonic lumen with sinus tracts or fistulas, or paracolic barium collections in abscesses, or free intraperitoneal spillage of barium

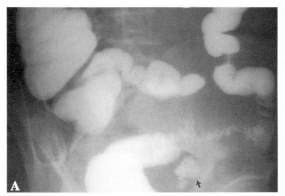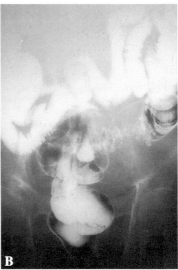

FIGURE 5. *A*, Oblique view from a single contrast barium enema shows spastic narrowing of the sigmoid colon, a deformed diverticulum, and a paracolic abscess collection (arrow). *B*, Angled view of the sigmoid colon on this single contrast barium enema film shows the spastic, narrowed sigmoid colon, with intramural fistulous tracts.

16. What are the CT findings in diverticulitis? (Fig. 6)

• Diverticula	• Inflammation of the adjacent fat
• Colonic wall thickening	• Fluid inflammation in the root of the sigmoid mesentery
• Abscess(es)	• Localized extraluminal air or occasionally free intraperitoneal air

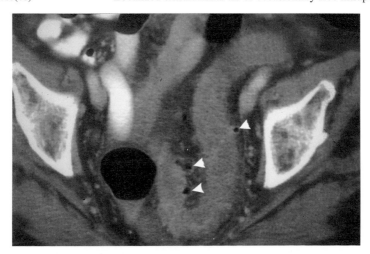

FIGURE 6. An 89-year-old man with left lower quadrant pain and fever from diverticulitis. CT image shows thickening of the wall of the sigmoid colon, diverticula (arrowheads), and inflammation of the adjacent fat.

17. Can a carcinoma simulate diverticulitis?

Yes, especially a carcinoma that has perforated. It can be difficult or impossible to distinguish the two radiographically. Long segments of involvement, with filling of diverticula in this region on a barium enema, more strongly points to diverticulitis. Likewise on CT, edema in the root of the sigmoid mesentery favors diverticulitis. However, there are exceptions to each of these rules, and follow-up imaging studies and/or endoscopy with biopsy may be indicated. Also, carcinoma and diverticulitis occasionally coexist.

18. Can a diverticular abscess be drained percutaneously?

Yes, and this step may convert a multiple-stage surgery into a single surgical procedure, following abscess drainage.

INFECTIOUS, INFLAMMATORY, AND ISCHEMIC COLITIS

19. What patients are affected by ischemic colitis?

Older patients.

20. What are the plain film and CT findings in ischemic colitis? (Fig. 7)

 • Thickening of the colonic wall, with luminal narrowing and transverse ridging
 • "Thumbprinting" of the bowel wall, due to edema
 • Fixed, rigid, tubular, ahaustral bowel loops
 • Pneumatosis (gas in the bowel wall)
 • Free gas in the peritoneal cavity (uncommon) or in the mesenteric veins and portal vein. The latter two signs are especially ominous and indicate progression of ischemia to infarction.

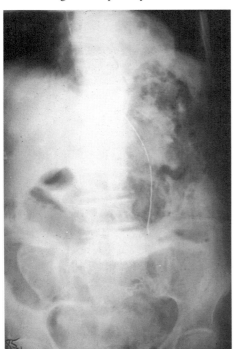

FIGURE 7.   Abdominal radiograph reveals extensive changes of linear and bubbly forms of pneumatosis intestinalis in a patient with chronic bowel ischemia.

21. What is the most common finding on plain films in ischemic colitis?

Most plain films are normal or show a nonspecific ileus pattern.

22. What are the classic barium enema findings in colonic ischemia?

1. Thumbprinting (in 75% of cases)
2. Transverse ridges
3. Ulcers
4. Spasm

5. Strictures
6. Intramural barium (due to sloughed necrotic bowel with intramural tracking)

23. Are there benign causes of pneumatosis? (Fig. 8)

Yes. There is a large differential diagnosis, including idiopathic causes, collagen vascular diseases, steroids, and chronic obstructive pulmonary disease.

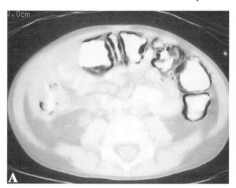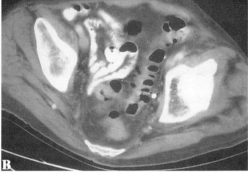

FIGURE 8. Two examples of "benign" colonic pneumatosis secondary to steroids, demonstrated on CT. *A*, Linear pneumatosis in a young child. *B*, Elderly man on steroids for idiopathic pulmonary fibrosis. Cystic pneumatosis of the sigmoid colon mimics diverticulosis. Free air (not shown) was also present in the peritoneal cavity. The patient remained asymptomatic and free air resolved over several days following conservative therapy.

24. What is a characteristic plain film appearance of pseudomembranous colitis?

The most characteristic finding in severe cases is the presence of thickened haustrae and thumbprinting, with a shaggy border to the colon. Megacolon occurs in some cases. Plain films may be normal.

25. What is the cause of pseudomembranous colitis?

Intestinal mucosal damage is produced by the cytotoxin produced by the enteric pathogen *Clostridium difficile*.

26. What is the appearance of pseudomembranous colitis on a barium enema or on a CT?

The actual pseudomembranes may be seen as irregular nodular or plaque-like filling defects. There may be poor mucosal coating, with blunted, thickened haustra. On CT, the bowel wall is thickened and edematous (Fig. 9).

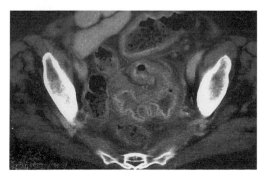

FIGURE 9. Marked thickening of the wall of the sigmoid colon, which enhances, in this patient with pseudomembranous colitis.

27. What is a complication of pseudomembranous colitis?
Toxic megacolon, which can lead to bowel perforation and death. For this reason, a barium enema is contraindicated when toxic megacolon is suspected. Plain films show significant dilatation of the colon (greater than 6 cm or more in diameter) and bowel wall edema.

28. What are some infectious causes of colitis?
Common causes include shigella and salmonella. Other infectious causes include gonococcus, cytomegalovirus, amebiasis, tuberculosis, and lymphogranuloma venereum.

29. What are some noninfectious, nonischemic causes of colitis?
1. Ulcerative colitis/Crohn's disease
2. Radiation therapy
3. Chronic laxative abuse

30. What is an early finding of ulcerative colitis on a barium enema?
The bowel mucosa has a granular pattern.

31. What are some later findings of ulcerative colitis on a barium enema?
Relatively deep ulcers, called collar button ulcers. Mucosal involvement is contiguous, beginning in the distal colon and extending to the proximal colon. The ileum may be involved; the ileocecal valve remains open, leading to "backwash" ileitis.

32. What are late findings of ulcerative colitis on a barium enema?
The colonic mucosa becomes featureless and rigid, having a "lead pipe" appearance. Areas of dysplasia and carcinoma may develop but may be difficult to detect.

33. What are early findings of Crohn's disease on a barium enema?
Superficial mucosal ulcers, which look like small bulls' eyes (aphthous ulcers).

34. What are some later findings of Crohn's disease on a barium enema?
Deeper ulcerations may occur. There are often "skip" areas of involvement. The entire GI tract may be involved—from the pharynx to the anus.

35. What is a serious complication of ulcerative colitis?
Toxic megacolon.

BIBLIOGRAPHY

1. Balthazar EJ, Birnbaum BA, Yee J, et al: Acute appendicitis: CT and US correlation in 100 patients. Radiology 190:31–35, 1994.
2. Balthazar EJ: Disorders of the appendix. In Gore RM, Levine MS, Laufer I (eds): Textbook of Gastrointestinal Radiology. Philadelphia, W.B. Saunders, 1994, pp 1310–1341.
3. Cho KC, Morehouse HT, Alterman D, Thornhill BA: Sigmoid diverticulitis: Diagnostic role of CT: Comparison with barium enema studies. Radiology 176:111–115, 1990.
4. Jeffrey RB Jr, Laing FC, Townsend RR: Acute appendicitis: Sonographic criteria based on 250 cases. Radiology 167:327, 1988.
5. Jeffrey RB Jr, Ralls PW: CT and Sonography of the Acute Abdomen, 2nd ed. Philadelphia, Lippincott-Raven, 1996.
6. Laufer I, Levine MS: Double Contrast Gastrointestinal Radiology, 2nd ed. Philadelphia, W.B. Saunders, 1992.
7. Taourel PG, Deneuville M, Pradel JA, et al: Acute mesenteric ischemia: Diagnosis with contrast-enhanced CT. Radiology 199:632–636, 1996.

25. BOWEL OBSTRUCTION

Sunah A. Kang Feng, M.D., and Natalie Strutynsky, M.D.

1. What is the initial radiologic examination for suspected small bowel obstruction?

An abdominal series of radiographs, consisting of a PA chest radiograph and flat and upright abdominal films. Although only 50–60% sensitive for obstruction, they are usually the first radiologic exam obtained for suspected small bowel obstruction.

2. What are some common signs of small bowel obstruction on plain radiographs?
- Multiple air-fluid levels
- Absence of colonic distention
- A "stepladder" appearance of small bowel loops/air-fluid levels with unequal heights in loops of small bowel
- "String of pearls," which refers to a small amount of residual air in the fluid-filled small bowel loops (Fig. 1)

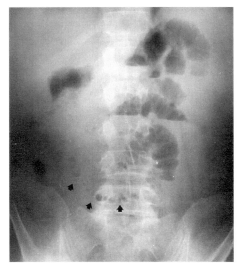

FIGURE 1. Upright radiograph shows multiple air-fluid levels in the dilated small bowel. The arrows demonstrate the string-of-pearls sign, which represents trapped air in the valvulae conniventes.

3. What is the "rule of threes" concerning the normal small bowel?
- Wall thickness less than 3 mm
- Valvulae conniventes (normal transverse small bowel folds) less than 3 mm thick
- Small bowel diameter less than 3 cm
- Less than 3 air-fluid levels per radiograph

4. Are multiple air-fluid levels at different heights on an upright film diagnostic of small bowel obstruction, and are multiple air-fluid levels at equal heights on an upright film diagnostic of a small bowel ileus?

Unfortunately not. These findings, while classic for their respective diagnosis, are neither sensitive nor specific, and air-fluid levels both at different heights and at equal heights on upright radiographs can be seen in either obstruction or ileus. The findings on radiographs in any patient must be correlated with the history and physical examination. Also, follow-up radiographs can be helpful in determining the correct diagnosis.

5. What are some other pitfalls of diagnosing small bowel obstruction based on plain films?
1. Proximal obstruction may be difficult to diagnose (air swallowing may mimic it).
2. The exact point of obstruction is difficult to determine based on plain films alone.
3. Dilated small bowel loops that are filled only with fluid may not be appreciated as obstruction.
4. A nasogastric tube removes air, which is the intrinsic "contrast" on plain films.
5. A "sentinel loop," or focal adynamic segment of small bowel, may simulate obstruction.
6. It is difficult to determine on postoperative films if actual obstruction is present, vs. ileus.

6. If an upright abdominal film cannot be obtained because a patient is too ill to sit up, what other views can be obtained?
A decubitus film, which is a frontal film obtained with the patient rolled over so that one side of the body is down and the other is up; the x-ray beam is parallel to the floor.

7. What are the most common causes of small bowel obstruction?
Adhesions, the most common cause, occur in up to 70% of all cases. Incarcerated hernias are responsible for 10% of cases and neoplasms about 5% (Fig. 2).

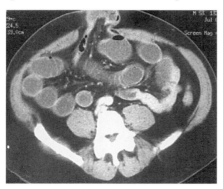

FIGURE 2. CT image shows a ventral hernia containing small bowel loops, which causes a small bowel obstruction. No evidence of strangulation is seen, as the bowel wall is not thickened.

8. What are some uncommon causes of small bowel obstruction, due to blockage of the lumen?
Gallstone ileus, bezoars and foreign bodies, and parasites, such as ascaris.

9. What is gallstone ileus, and what are the radiologic findings?
A large gallstone is impacted in the terminal ileum, a relatively narrow area, causing small bowel obstruction. Most commonly, the gallstone has eroded from the gallbladder wall into the duodenum, creating a duodenal-biliary fistula. Therefore, pneumobilia (air in the biliary tract) may be seen. The gallstone may or may not be visible in the abdomen (Fig. 3).

10. What are some uncommon causes of small bowel obstruction, due to a mural lesion?
- Inflammatory bowel disease
- Hematoma
- Stricture (e.g., from radiation therapy)
- Primary small bowel tumor (lymphoma, leiomyosarcoma)

11. What are some uncommon causes of small bowel obstruction, due to an extrinsic lesion?
Carcinomatosis and abscess.

12. If a large bowel lesion is suspected as the cause of a small bowel obstruction (and an associated proximal large bowel obstruction, e.g., due to a colon cancer), what radiologic exam should be performed? Should a small bowel series be performed first?
A single contrast barium enema (i.e., using barium or water-soluble contrast only, without air). Alternatively, a CT scan can be performed. Conventional wisdom states that, before a small

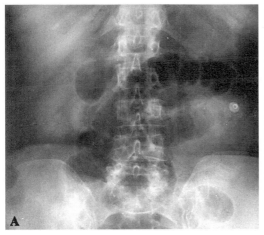
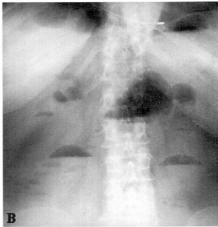
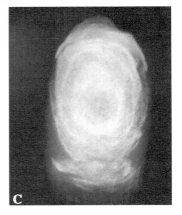

FIGURE 3. *A*, Dilated small bowel loops are seen, suggestive of a small bowel obstruction. However, small areas of gas are seen in the right upper quadrant overlying the liver silhouette. *B*, With the patient upright, pneumobilia in the porta hepatis is better demonstrated (tubular lucencies projecting just under the right breast.) Gallstone ileus is therefore the likely diagnosis. The stone is not visible. *C*, Radiograph of the laminated gallstone, which was found lodged in a distal small bowel loop at surgery.

bowel study is performed, if a colonic lesion is possibly responsible for the obstruction, a barium enema should be performed because barium in an obstructed colon, versus in the small bowel, may become hardened and form concretions as the colon resorbs the water from the barium suspension.

13. What are the relative advantages and disadvantages of using barium versus water-soluble contrast (gastrografin) during a small bowel study to evaluate a small bowel obstruction?

Water-soluble contrast progresses rapidly through the small bowel, but the influx of fluid caused by the hyperosmolar contrast dilutes the contrast, limiting visualization of the distal small bowel. Water-soluble contrast also causes cramping and vomiting in some patients with obstruction. Aspiration of gastrografin in the lungs is potentially dangerous, since the hyperosmolarity of the contrast can cause pulmonary edema, similar to salt water drowning. Barium provides better visualization of the small bowel, especially distally. If aspiration occurs, barium is inert and is therefore safer than gastrografin. However, if a CT, US, or nuclear medicine study of the abdomen is needed, the barium may significantly interfere with all of these procedures.

14. What is the role of CT in the work-up of bowel obstruction?

CT is valuable in confirming the diagnosis of bowel obstruction, determining the level of obstruction, establishing the cause, and diagnosing complications such as strangulation and perforation. CT is the imaging test of choice in patients with suspected bowel obstruction.

15. What is the role of enteroclysis in the evaluation of a small bowel obstruction?

Enteroclysis is superior to a routine small bowel series and to CT in the evaluation of low-grade or subacute/intermittent obstruction.

16. How is enteroclysis carried out?

An intestinal tube is placed nasally or orally into the duodenal-jejunal junction. Barium is infused at a rate of about 100 cc/min for a total volume of 300–400 cc. Methylcellulose or air is infused after barium is administered, which provides a double-contrast effect for visualization of the mucosal folds. Both fluoroscopy and spot films are used during the study.

17. What are contraindications to enteroclysis?

Complete (or high-grade/acute) small bowel obstruction; the presence of infarction/perforation.

18. What causes strangulation, and what are the radiographic findings on plain films?

Obstruction and strangulation of the venous drainage from the bowel or the segmental blood supply to the bowel causes strangulation. Initially there are thickened valvulae secondary to edema, and eventually featureless bowel ensues due to the effacement of the valvulae.

19. What is a closed-loop obstruction?

Closed-loop obstructions are caused by adhesions, volvulus, or internal hernias. They are seen as a U-shaped loop of distended bowel, because of the obstruction of the bowel at two points. The plain film findings are not specific but may show a gas-filled or fluid-filled and distended bowel loop. A closed-loop obstruction is a surgical emergency due to the high incidence of associated bowel infarction and perforation.

20. What are the CT findings in closed-loop obstruction?

A U-shaped loop of bowel may be identified. A "beak" sign is also found at both narrowed ends of the bowel loop. The mesentery may be seen converging toward the root of the obstruction (the "whorl" sign).

21. What are the CT findings in strangulation?

Strangulations may be seen in closed-loop obstruction, although the two terms are not synonymous. Other conditions that may lead to strangulation include an incarcerated hernia and a volvulus. In strangulation, a circumferentially thickened loop of bowel with an enhancing wall and submucosal edema (i.e., a "target sign") may be seen. Additional findings include pneumatosis, blunting of the valvulae conniventes, and congestive changes in the adjacent mesentery. The true accuracy of CT for determining the presence of strangulation is not known.

22. What is the risk of recurrence of small bowel obstruction?

After a laparotomy, the lifetime risk of small bowel obstruction is about 5%. After an operation for lysis of adhesions, the risk rises to around 12%.

23. What are the plain film findings of large bowel obstruction?
- Dilated colon, especially a dilated cecum
- Small bowel dilatation (in 25% of cases, due to reflux of gas through the ileocecal valve)
- Air-fluid levels in the colon, especially distal to the hepatic flexure (Fig. 4)

24. What are the common causes of large bowel obstruction?
1. Primary or metastatic carcinoma in 60–80% of cases
2. Diverticular disease in 10%
3. Sigmoid volvulus in 5%

25. What are less common causes of large bowel obstruction?

Cecal volvulus, hernias, intussusception, benign tumors, fecal impaction, and adhesions.

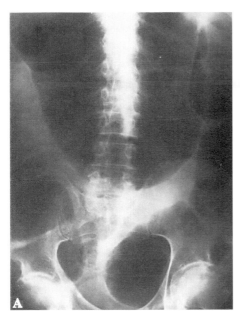 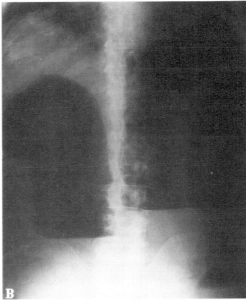

FIGURE 4. *A*, Supine radiograph shows dilated large bowel. *B*, Upright film shows several air-fluid levels. These findings are consistent with a large bowel obstruction.

26. When is the cecum considered significantly distended on plain films?

The normal caliber of the cecum is up to 9 cm, and the rest of the large bowel can be up to 6 cm without being considered dilated. There is little risk of perforation of the large bowel until the cecum is dilated by more than 12 cm and until the rest of the bowel is dilated by more than 9 cm.

27. How should an emergency barium enema for suspected large bowel obstruction be performed?

With a single contrast barium enema. Barium should be instilled up to but not beyond a tight stenosis; the proximal barium becomes concentrated as the bowel resorbs water, causing impaction. If perforation is suspected, water-soluble contrast should be given.

28. In what part of the bowel does volvulus commonly occur, and what are the risk factors?

Sigmoid volvulus is much more common than cecal volvulus, accounting for 75% of cases of large bowel volvulus. Large bowel volvulus is more common in older patients with chronic constipation, where the sigmoid colon becomes elongated and redundant. People with a high-residue or high-fiber diet are also at increased risk. Cecal volvulus is caused by a hypermobile cecum due to incomplete embryologic fixation of the ascending colon (Fig. 5). Volvulus of the transverse colon is rare.

29. What is the "coffee bean" sign?

In a patient with volvulus of the large bowel, the walls of the two limbs of the closed loop curve around and are adjacent to each other. Because the involved bowel walls are edematous, the adjacent walls form a dense white line on the radiograph. The line is surrounded by the curved and dilated gas-filled lumen, outlining a "coffee bean" shaped area (Fig. 6). If the dilated loop of bowel is filled with fluid, the volvulus becomes the "pseudotumor" sign.

30. What does the "beak sign" refer to?

In a patient with a volvulus, twisting of the mesenteric attachment around itself results in narrowing of the bowel lumen at both ends of the closed loop. This narrowing gives the sharp, pointed "bird's beak" appearance (Fig. 7).

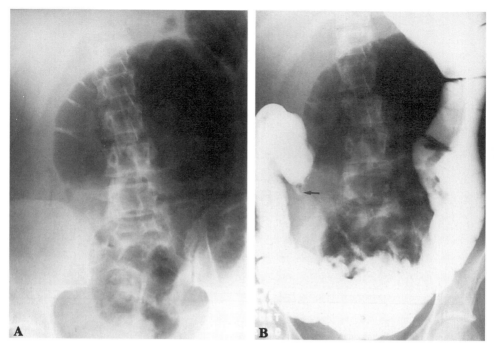

FIGURE 5. *A*, Supine scout film for a barium enema shows a dilated loop of large bowel in the left upper quadrant, which is suspicious for a cecal volvulus. *B*, Image from a barium enema demonstrates the "beak sign" leading up to the air-filled cecum, diagnostic of a cecal volvulus. The distended cecum is displaced into the left upper quadrant. This is a common finding in this condition.

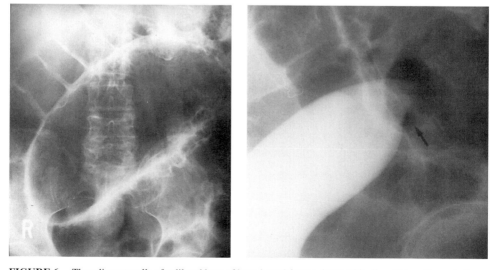

FIGURE 6. The adjacent walls of a dilated loop of large bowel form a dense white line. This radiograph shows the coffee bean sign, indicative of volvulus. The long axis of the "bean" usually points toward the right lower quadrant in cecal volvulus and the left lower quadrant in sigmoid volvulus. However, in this patient, the sigmoid was ectatic and the gas-filled transverse colon is the clue that this is a sigmoid volvulus.

FIGURE 7. Lateral view from an enema on this patient demonstrates the "beak sign," where the mesentery twists and narrows the lumen.

31. What are two nonmechanical causes of large bowel obstruction?

Toxic megacolon and paralytic ileus.

32. When is a barium enema contraindicated?

In the presence of perforated bowel, toxic megacolon, and portal venous gas.

33. What is Ogilvie's syndrome?

Pseudoobstruction, where the large bowel is markedly distended due to paralytic or adynamic ileus. The patient has a disproportionately small amount of pain relative to the amount of large bowel distention. Ogilvie's syndrome can be treated by colonoscopy, although a single contrast enema can be performed to rule out other causes of obstruction. The underlying cause is thought to be an imbalance in the sympathetic and parasympathetic innervation of the colon (Fig. 8).

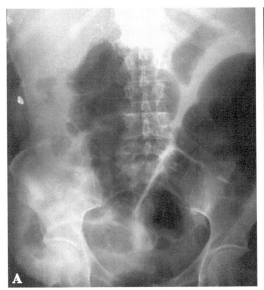 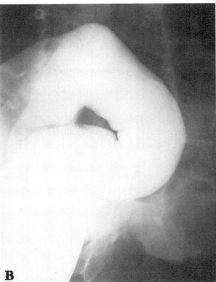

FIGURE 8. *A*, Dilated large bowel loops are seen on a supine film. *B*, On barium enema, no obstructing lesion is identified in the rectum or sigmoid. This patient had pseudoobstruction, which should be considered in the appropriate clinical setting.

34. What conditions cause pseudoobstruction?

- A variety of neurologic conditions
- Diabetes
- Hypothyroidism
- Scleroderma
- Amyloidosis
- Chronic renal failure
- Congestive heart failure
- Electrolyte imbalances

35. Is CT specific in demonstrating bowel ischemia and infarction?

The results of studies on the ability of CT to diagnose bowel infarction are mixed. Megibow found that 10 of 16 patients with strangulation had positive findings on CT indicative of ischemia, while Smerud's retrospective review found that in 23 cases of mesenteric ischemia, CT was not significantly better than plain radiography in detecting bowel infarction.

BIBLIOGRAPHY

1. Balthazar EJ, George W: Holmes lecture. CT of small bowel obstruction. AJR 162:255–261, 1994.
2. Gore RM, Eisenberg RL: Large bowel obstruction. In Gore RM, Levine MS, Laufer I (eds): Textbook of Gastrointestinal Radiology. Philadelphia, W.B. Saunders, 1994.

3. Herlinger H, Rubesin SE: Obstruction. In Gore RM, Levine MS, Laufer I (eds): Textbook of Gastrointestinal Radiology. Philadelphia, W.B. Saunders, 1994.
4. Jeffrey RB Jr: CT and Sonography of the Acute Abdomen. New York, Raven Press, 1988.
5. Megibow AJ: Bowel obstruction—evaluation with CT. Radiol Clin North Am 32:861–870, 1994.
6. Smerud MJ, Johnson CD, Stephens DS: Diagnosis of bowel infarction: A comparison of plain films and CT scans in 23 cases. AJR 154:99–103, 1990.

26. IMAGING OF PANCREATIC DISEASE

Douglas S. Katz, M.D.

1. What are some of the causes of pancreatitis?

Alcoholism and common duct stones, which together account for 80% or more of all cases of pancreatitis. Less common causes include hypercalcemia, various medications, hereditary pancreatitis, trauma, and viral infections.

2. How does an inflamed pancreas appear on ultrasound?

Enlarged and hypoechoic, which refers to decreased brightness. The pancreas is normally bright, or echogenic, on ultrasound and is usually brighter than the pancreas.

3. Does a normal-appearing pancreas on ultrasound exclude pancreatitis?

No. Pancreatitis is a clinical/laboratory diagnosis.

4. How does an inflamed pancreas appear on CT? (Fig. 1)

The pancreas may appear enlarged and edematous, with decreased density compared with normal. There may be fluid or inflammatory changes in the adjacent fat. Similar to ultrasound, a normal pancreas on CT does not exclude pancreatitis.

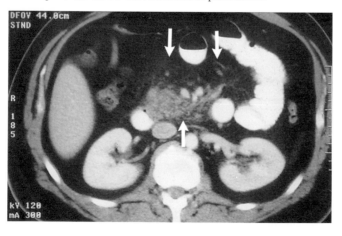

FIGURE 1. Pancreatitis. There is mild inflammation (arrows) of the fat around the pancreatic head, which is swollen on this CT image.

5. What is the colon cutoff sign in pancreatitis?

Inflammation can spread from the pancreas to the left upper quadrant, which induces a focal small bowel ileus in this region called a sentinel loop. On plain films, gas in the transverse colon appears "cut off" at the left upper quadrant (Fig. 2).

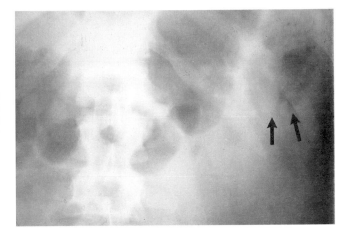

FIGURE 2. Close-up view of a supine abdominal radiograph shows the "cutoff sign" (arrows) of the descending colon, in pancreatitis.

6. **What are some other findings in pancreatitis on plain films and barium studies? (Fig. 3)**
   - Dilated duodenal "C loop" on an upper GI study, due to enlargement of the pancreatic head
   - Spiculation of the medial duodenal border due to inflammation
   - Swollen ampulla on an upper GI study
   - Pleural effusions, especially on the left
   - Calcifications of the pancreas in chronic pancreatitis

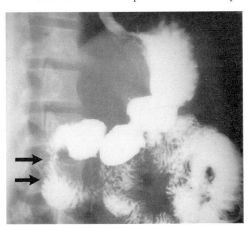

FIGURE 3. Upper GI series radiograph in a patient with pancreatitis. The inflammatory process has produced proximal descending duodenal spastic narrowing (arrows).

7. **What is the best imaging test for staging pancreatitis?**
   Contrast-enhanced CT. The pancreas can be difficult to visualize on ultrasound, especially in obese patients or in patients with overlying bowel gas. Also, patients with severe abdominal pain may not be able to tolerate sonography.

8. **Does the CT appearance of pancreatitis always correlate with a patient's clinical condition?**
   No, but CT provides valuable information about the status of the pancreas and about complications that may have developed. The severity of pancreatitis on CT does correlate with patient prognosis.

9. **What are some complications of pancreatitis that can be identified on CT?**
   Hemorrhage, pseudocyst formation (Fig. 4), pseudoaneurysm formation (Fig. 5), and development of pancreatic abscess or necrosis.

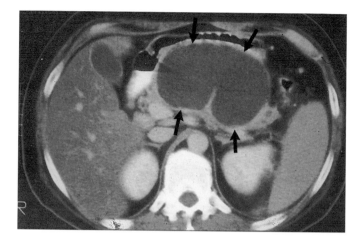

FIGURE 4. Large pancreatic pseudocyst demonstrated on CT (arrows).

FIGURE 5. Large pseudoaneurysm (arrows) of the gastroduodenal artery, which developed several weeks after this patient presented with pancreatitis.

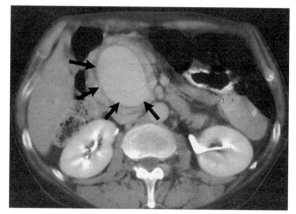

10. What is a pseudocyst, and where can it form?

A pseudocyst is a loculated fluid collection that is walled off by adjacent organs, structures, or fibrosis but does not have a true epithelialized wall. If they form in patients with pancreatitis, pseudocysts usually develop within a few weeks after an episode of pancreatitis begins. They are more common in patients with recurrent episodes of pancreatitis. A pseudocyst can form almost anywhere in the abdomen and pelvis but is most common in the pancreas or immediately adjacent to the pancreas. Pseudocysts are often connected to the pancreatic duct.

11. What are the interventions and the indications for intervention in a patient with a pseudocyst?

Interventions typically include percutaneous or endoscopic drainage. Indications include the following:

- A large pseudocyst, typically over 5 cm, especially if symptomatic. Larger cysts are at increased risk of rupture, which may lead to further complications, such as fistula formation and life-threatening hemorrhage.
- Suspected superinfection
- Pseudocyst that obstructs the biliary system or the bowel

12. How can ultrasound distinguish a pseudocyst from a pseudoaneurysm?

Color Doppler can be used to determine if a cystic structure is vascular. A pseudoaneurysm may develop as a complication of pancreatitis, and rupture of a pseudoaneurysm is usually fatal. It is especially important to determine that a pseudocyst is not an aneurysm prior to drainage.

13. How can a pseudoaneurysm be repaired?

A radiologist can perform an arteriogram to determine the vessel(s) feeding the pseudoaneurysm (e.g., the gastroduodenal artery, which is a branch of the celiac artery) and embolize its origin, typically with metal coils.

14. How can a pancreatic abscess be diagnosed and treated?

Untreated pancreatic abscess is almost uniformly fatal. The diagnosis can be difficult to establish; on CT only about 20% of fluid collections that prove to be abscesses contain gas, and most fluid collections on CT that are related to pancreatitis are not infected. The index of suspicion needs to be high, and patient with new fever or significant clinical deterioration should be promptly imaged with CT and suspicious fluid collections aspirated. The treatment of pancreatic abscess is controversial. Even with optimal therapy, mortality is 50% or more. Success with percutaneous drainage has been mixed, and some authorities favor open surgical drainage and debridement.

15. What is the differential diagnosis of diffuse pancreatic calcification? (Fig. 6)

Causes of chronic pancreatitis, which include alcoholic pancreatitis, cystic fibrosis, and hereditary pancreatitis.

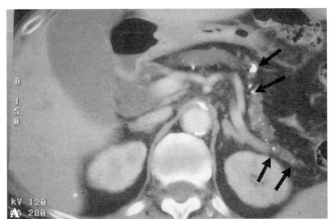

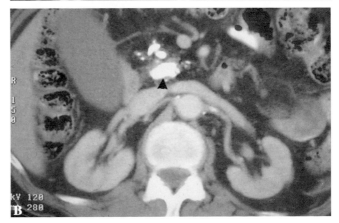

FIGURE 6. Chronic pancreatitis. Scattered calcifications (arrows) are seen in the pancreas. There is a large stone in the common duct (arrowhead, *B*), and the pancreas is atrophic.

16. What is the "chain-of-lakes"?

The appearance of the pancreatic duct as seen on an ERCP in patients with chronic pancreatitis (Fig. 7). Alternating areas of narrowing and dilatation give this appearance. Also, filling defects such as stones and sludge can be identified.

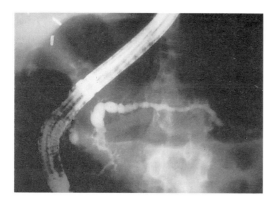

FIGURE 7. Spot radiograph from an ERCP shows a dilated ectatic main pancreatic duct, with a chain-of-lakes appearance, and ectasia of the secondary pancreatic ductal branches.

17. What is the most common tumor of the pancreas?
Adenocarcinoma.

18. What is the prognosis of patients with adenocarcinoma of the pancreas?
Only a small percentage of patients with pancreatic adenocarcinoma are candidates for surgical excision because local invasion or metastatic disease has already occurred. Pancreatic tail and body cancers are usually larger at detection than pancreatic head cancers, because cancers in the pancreatic head usually present with jaundice when they are relatively small. Overall, the prognosis remains dismal, with a mean survival after diagnosis of several months. The prognosis is slightly better if a small pancreatic head cancer is identified and resected (Fig. 8).

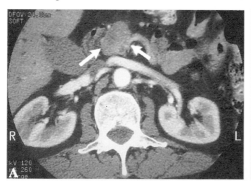
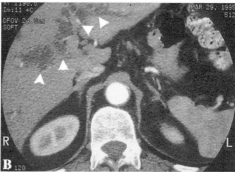

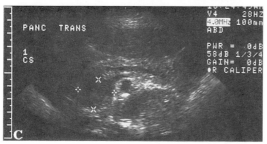

FIGURE 8. Small pancreatic head cancer (arrows, A) with resultant biliary dilatation (arrowheads, B). C, Different patient with a small pancreatic head mass (carcinoma). A 2.3 × 2.7 cm hypoechoic mass is visualized on sonography.

19. What is the best noninvasive test for staging pancreatic cancer?
Contrast-enhanced CT. The technique should be optimized with thin sections obtained using a helical CT scanner, through the region of the pancreas. Endoscopic ultrasound is playing an increasingly important role in local staging of pancreatic cancer.

20. How does a pancreatic cancer typically appear on CT?

As a mass that is relatively decreased in density compared with the normal pancreas. Pancreatic cancer often bulges the contour of the pancreas and may directly invade adjacent structures.

21. What are some CT findings that usually indicate that a pancreatic tumor is not resectable? (Fig. 9)

Specific criteria will vary depending on the institution and the aggressiveness of the surgeon, but CT findings include the following:

1. A tumor 3 cm or larger
2. Invasion/encasement of adjacent major arteries and veins, such as the celiac and superior mesenteric vessels
3. Invasion of adjacent organs, excluding the duodenum
4. Metastatic disease, typically to the liver and the peritoneum

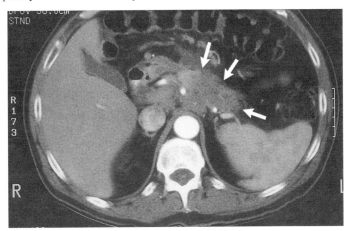

FIGURE 9. Unresectable pancreatic cancer. A mass (arrows) envelops the celiac artery and its branches.

22. What is the "double duct" sign?

A tumor of the pancreatic head often obstructs both the pancreatic duct and the common bile duct, dilating both of them. By itself, this sign is strongly suggestive of but not diagnostic of pancreatic cancer. The double duct sign is seen on CT, US, and ERCP (Fig. 10).

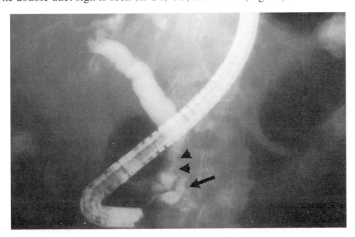

FIGURE 10. Spot radiograph from an ERCP of a patient with pancreatic cancer shows a double duct sign. There is obstruction of the pancreatic duct (arrow) and irregular narrowing of the common bile duct (arrowheads).

23. In a patient with pancreatic cancer and obstructive jaundice who is not a surgical candidate, what can be done to palliate the jaundice?

A stent may be placed into the common bile duct through the obstruction, preferably endoscopically. If this approach is not successful, a stent may be placed by an interventional radiologist using a percutaneous approach through the liver.

24. Are all low-density areas in the pancreas on CT cancer?

No. Occasionally cysts or focal areas of chronic pancreatitis can simulate a small pancreatic cancer. There is no reliable way to distinguish these findings on imaging studies.

25. Are there other types of pancreatic tumors?

Yes: islet cell tumors, cystic tumors, and metastases.

26. What are some types of islet cell tumors?

- Insulinomas—most commonly, they are benign tumors; all other types of islet cell tumors are most often malignant
- Gastrinomas—the cause of Zollinger-Ellison syndrome, they may be found in the pancreas or outside it (e.g., in the wall of the duodenum) and may be multiple
- Glucagonomas
- Somatostatinomas
- Nonfunctioning islet cell tumors

BIBLIOGRAPHY

1. Balthazar EJ, Freeny PC, van Sonnenberg E: Imaging and intervention in acute pancreatitis. Radiology 193: 297–306, 1994.
2. Balthazar EJ, Ranson JHC, Naidich DP, et al: Acute pancreatitis: Prognostic value of CT. Radiology 156:767, 1985.
3. Freeny PC: Radiologic diagnosis and staging of pancreatic ductal adenocarcinoma. Radiol Clin North Am 27:121–128, 1989.
4. Jeffrey RB Jr, Ralls PW: CT and Sonography of the Acute Abdomen, 2nd ed. Philadelphia, Lippincott-Raven, 1996, pp 160–204.
5. Kloppel G, Maillet B: Classification and staging of pancreatic nonendocrine tumors. Radiol Clin North Am 27:105–120, 1989.
6. Lu DSK, Verdantham S, Krasny RM, et al: Two-phase helical CT for pancreatic tumors: Pancreatic versus hepatic phase—enhancement of tumor, pancreas, and vascular structures. Radiology 199:697–701, 1996.
7. Thoeni RF, Blankenberg F: Pancreatic imaging: Computed tomography and magnetic resonance imaging. Radiol Clin North Am 31:1085–1113, 1993.

27. LIVER DISEASE

Douglas S. Katz, M.D.

1. What is meant by the "starry sky" appearance of the liver on ultrasound?

In some patients with acute hepatitis, the echogenicity of the liver decreases as the parenchyma becomes edematous, and the portal triads stand out as relatively bright areas, giving the appearance of a starry sky.

2. Is a diagnosis of hepatitis usually established by imaging?

No.

3. Can the liver have a completely normal sonographic appearance in acute hepatitis?

Yes, and it often does.

4. What can happen to the wall of the gallbladder in hepatitis?
It can become thickened.

5. What happens to the liver in cirrhosis, as demonstrated on cross-sectional imaging studies?
Over time, the liver becomes nodular and atrophic. The right hepatic lobe may atrophy more than the caudate lobe and the left hepatic lobe, although this finding is variable.

6. What does cirrhotic liver parenchyma look like on ultrasound, CT, and MR (Fig. 1)?
On ultrasound, the echotexture of the cirrhotic liver becomes heterogeneous and coarse; nodularity of the liver surface may be seen. Small nodules seen within the liver on CT and MR represent various types of regenerating nodules. The nodules may have a variable appearance but typically do not enhance significantly with intravenous contrast.

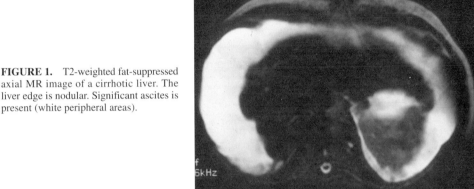

FIGURE 1. T2-weighted fat-suppressed axial MR image of a cirrhotic liver. The liver edge is nodular. Significant ascites is present (white peripheral areas).

7. What other findings may be present on cross-sectional imaging studies in patients with cirrhosis? (Fig. 2)

Ascites   Portal vein abnormalities (thrombosis, slow flow)
Varices   Development of hepatocellular cancer
Splenomegaly

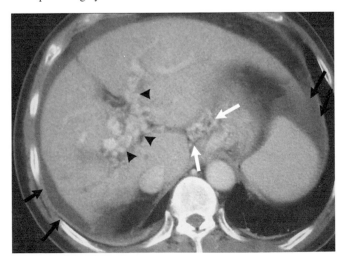

FIGURE 2. Cavernous transformation of the portal vein. CT image of a patient with cirrhosis shows ascites (arrows). Multiple vessels representing collateral venous channels are present instead of a normal portal vein (arrowheads). Varices are adjacent to the stomach (white arrows).

8. Does a normal cross-sectional imaging study exclude cirrhosis?
   No.

9. How does a hepatocellular cancer appear on cross-sectional imaging studies? (Fig. 3)
   It may appear as a focal lesion, which can invade the portal or hepatic veins. Hepatocellular cancer can also be multifocal or may be found diffusely in the liver. It usually has a heterogeneous appearance. On CT and MR, it typically enhances more than the adjacent liver after intravenous contrast is administered, especially if the liver is imaged within about 20 seconds after contrast is given (during the "hepatic arterial phase" of contrast enhancement of the liver, since hepatocellular cancer is hypervascular and is fed by the hepatic artery).

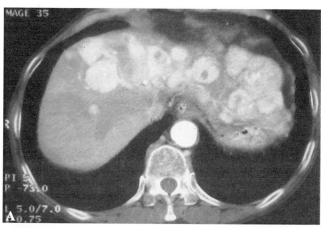

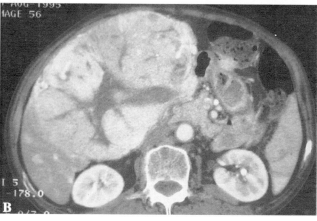

FIGURE 3.   This 74-year-old man with chronic viral hepatitis presented with abdominal pain and weight loss. There is massive replacement of the liver by hepatocellular cancer. *A,* Numerous foci of hypervascular tumor are seen in the liver. *B,* Inferiorly, there is a very large confluent area of tumor with central lower density areas consistent with necrosis.

10. When is a patient with cirrhosis and hepatocellular cancer usually not considered a candidate for liver transplantation?
   When metastases are present. Also, many authorities recommend against transplantation if a tumor greater than 3 cm in diameter is present or if there is strong evidence of portal or hepatic venous invasion.

11. What is the most common benign tumor of the liver?
   A hemangioma, which is a benign vascular tumor.

12. Where in the liver is a hemangioma most commonly found?
   In the posterior segment of the right hepatic lobe. Hemangiomas are more common in women.

13. How does a hemangioma appear on ultrasound?

Small hemangiomas are usually uniformly hyperechoic (bright) (Fig. 4).

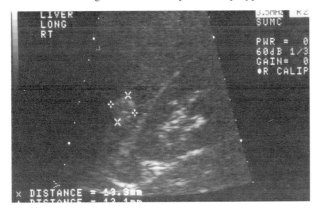

FIGURE 4. Echogenic, incidentally discovered 1.4-cm lesion in the posterior segment of the right hepatic lobe in this middle-aged woman is consistent with a hemangioma.

14. How does a hemangiomia appear on CT and MR? (Fig. 5)

On contrast-enhanced CT or MR, they usually have a very specific appearance. Initial images show peripheral discontinuous nodular contrast enhancement. Delayed images show more uniform contrast enhancement of the lesion. This appearance is so characteristic that usually no additional work-up is needed. On T2-weighted MR images, they are very bright.

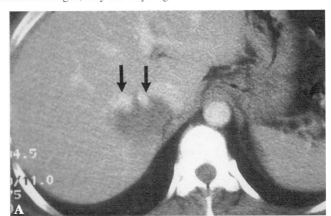

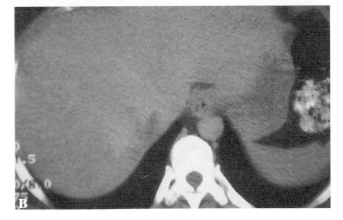

FIGURE 5. *A,* Early image of the liver after intravenous contrast administration. There is a hypodense lesion with peripheral nodular enhancement (arrows). *B,* Delayed image obtained several minutes after contrast enhancement shows contrast "filling in" the lesion.

15. What nuclear medicine study is diagnostic of a hemangioma?

A radiolabeled red blood cell scan. A portion of a patient's red blood cells are tagged to a radiopharmaceutical, Tc99m, and early and delayed (typically at 2 hours) images of the liver are obtained. Because hemangiomas are composed of venous spaces, take up red blood cells, and hold onto them, they appear as areas of activity in the liver on delayed images. This is diagnostic of a hemangioma.

16. Are there other benign liver tumors?

Yes; in particular, adenoma and focal nodular hyperplasia. Both are hypervascular lesions that occur most commonly in women. Adenomas may hemorrhage and are associated with the use of oral contraceptives. Focal nodular hyperplasia is usually an incidental lesion.

17. What tumors commonly metastasize to the liver?

Gastrointestinal tumors, especially colorectal cancer, breast cancer, and lung cancer. Virtually any tumor can metastasize to the liver.

18. What imaging test is most often used to look for liver metastases?

Usually a contrast-enhanced CT scan. MR can be used as the initial modality, but it is typically more expensive than CT; it is, however, particularly useful if a patient has a contraindication to receiving intravenous iodine-based contrast. Unenhanced CT is usually less sensitive than contrast-enhanced CT for detecting liver metastases. Alternatively, MR can be used as a problem-solving tool to further characterize an abnormality seen on another imaging modality. Ultrasound (Fig. 6) is usually less sensitive than CT or MR for detecting liver metastases.

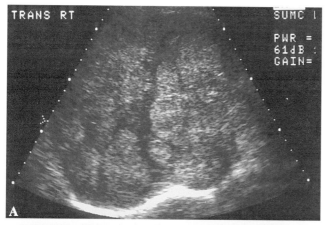

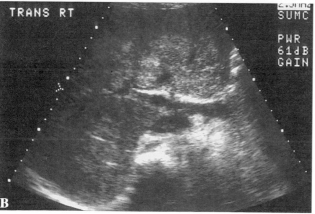

FIGURE 6. *A* and *B*, Diffuse liver metastases from colon carcinoma. The echogenicity of the liver is very heterogeneous; discrete lesions are difficult to discern.

19. How do metastases appear on CT?

Most metastases enhance less than normal liver and therefore are hypodense relative to the surrounding normal liver (Fig. 7). Some metastases can calcify, especially mucin-producing GI tract tumors. Some tumors are hypervascular relative to the normal liver and appear bright, especially if images are obtained immediately after intravenous contrast is given.

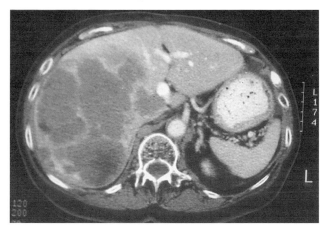

FIGURE 7. Large liver metastases from colon carcinoma. Contrast-enhanced CT shows replacement of the right hepatic lobe and a portion of the left hepatic lobe by hypodense lesions.

20. Which modalities can be used to guide a percutaneous liver biopsy?

CT and ultrasound.

21. What are the advantages and disadvantages of CT and US in providing guidance for liver biopsy?

Ultrasound provides real-time imaging guidance, and no radiation is involved. With CT, the needle may be easier to see than with ultrasound, but the imaging in not quite real-time and there is some minimal radiation exposure.

BIBLIOGRAPHY

1. Baron RL, Oliver JH III, Dodd GD III, et al: Hepatocellular carcinoma: Evaluation with biphasic, contrast-enhanced, helical CT. Radiology 199:505–511, 1996.
2. Hanafus K, Ohashi I, Himeno Y, et al: Hepatic hemangioma: Findings with two-phase CT. Radiology 196:465–469, 1995.
3. Hollett MD, Jeffrey RB Jr, Nino Murcia M, et al: Dual-phase helical CT of the liver: Value of arterial-phase scans in the detection of small malignant hepatic neoplasms. AJR 164:879–884, 1995.
4. Jeffrey RB Jr, Ralls PW: CT and Sonography of the Acute Abdomen, 2nd ed. Philadelphia, Lippincott-Raven, 1996, pp 30–73.
5. Miller WJ, Baron RL, Dodd GD III, et al: Malignancies in patients with cirrhosis: CT sensitivity and specificity in 200 consecutive transplant patients. Radiology 193:645–650, 1994.
6. Oliver JH III, Baron RL, Federle MP, Rochette HE Jr: Detecting hepatocellular carcinoma: Value of unenhanced or arterial phase CT imaging or both used in conjunction with conventional portal venous phase, contrast-enhanced CT imaging. AJR 167:71–77, 1996.
7. Runimeny E, Weissleder R, Stark DD, et al: Primary liver tumors: Diagnosis by MR imaging. AJR 152:63, 1989.

28. TUMORS OF THE STOMACH, SMALL INTESTINE, AND COLON

Burton M. Gold, M.D.

1. What is the most common type of mucosal polyp in the stomach?

Inflammatory or hyperplastic polyps (Fig. 1). They usually are multiple and well under 1 cm in size. They are most often found in the body and antrum of the stomach, do not ulcerate, and have no malignant potential.

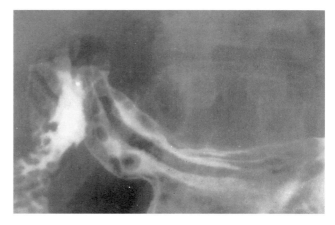

FIGURE 1. Image from a double contrast upper gastrointestinal series shows at least three distal antral polyps.

2. Are there any stomach polyps that do have malignant potential?

Yes, adenomatous polyps, which are usually isolated lesions that are significantly larger than inflammatory polyps. Adenomatous polyps may ulcerate and have a malignant potential that increases with their size.

3. What is the most common benign intramural gastric tumor?

Leiomyoma (Fig. 2). Two-thirds of leiomyomas in the gastrointestinal tract occur in the stomach. About 40% of all benign gastric tumors are leiomyomas. Most appear as submucosal masses of varying sizes that may ulcerate.

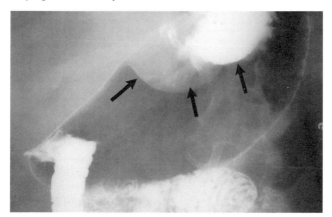

FIGURE 2. A large submucosal leiomyoma (arrows) in the body and fundus of the stomach is seen on this image from a double contrast UGI series.

4. What are some other benign intramural gastric tumors?
Neurofibromas, lipomas, hemangiomas, duplication cysts, and ectopic pancreatic rests.

5. What complication can occur two decades after partial gastrectomy for the treatment of peptic ulcer disease?
Gastric adenocarcinoma, a tumor that usually presents as a lobulated mass or stricture in the gastric remnant and often involves the anastomosis.

6. What are other predisposing factors for gastric carcinoma?
- High oral intake of nitrates
- Pernicious anemia
- Atrophic gastritis
- Gastric adenomatous polyps
- Ménétrier's disease

7. What percentage of gastric carcinomas occur in the fundus or cardia of the stomach?
About 30–40%. They are often difficult to detect and may be quite subtle on an upper GI series.

8. What are the radiologic appearances of gastric cancer on an upper GI series?
1. Polypoid mass with or without ulceration and with or without nodularity (Fig. 3)
2. Flat superficial spreading cancer, sometimes with very shallow ulcerations
3. Scirrhous submucosally infiltrating carcinomas (leather bottle stomach) (Fig. 4)

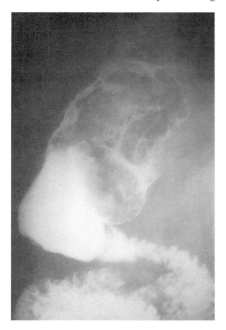

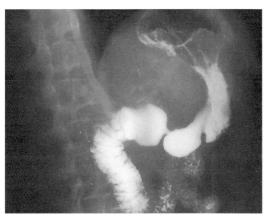

FIGURE 3 *(Left).*   Lateral view of the stomach from a single contrast UGI series shows a large polypoid mass in the fundus and body of the stomach.

FIGURE 4 *(Right).*   Single contrast UGI series image shows a diffusely infiltrating scirrhous carcinoma (linitis plastica) involving the body and most of the antrum of the stomach, with luminal narrowing.

9. What primary tumors most commonly metastasize to the stomach?
Melanoma, Kaposi's sarcoma (Fig. 5), breast cancer, pancreatic cancer, and colon cancer.

10. If a tumor extends from the antrum of the stomach across the pylorus to involve the duodenal bulb, is it more likely to be a carcinoma or a lymphoma?
Although lymphoma more commonly extends across the pylorus into the duodenum, gastric carcinomas are much more common than lymphoma (fewer than 2% of gastric malignancies are lymphoma). Therefore, carcinoma is the correct answer (Fig. 6).

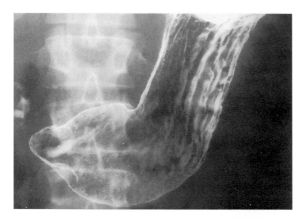

FIGURE 5. Image from a double contrast UGI series shows a submucosal nodule of Kaposi's sarcoma along the distal greater curvature of the stomach.

FIGURE 6. Gastric adenocarcinoma in the antrum, extending across the pyloric canal to involve the duodenal bulb.

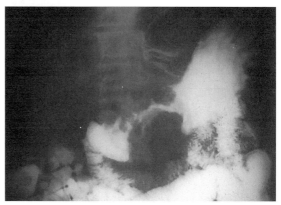

11. What are the radiologic and histologic forms of gastric lymphoma?
Radiologic
   Diffuse or focal fold thickening/infiltration (Fig. 7)
   Lobulated or ulcerated polypoid/nodular mass(es)
   Multiple nodules
Histologic
   About 90–95% of cases are histiocytic or lymphocytic lymphoma
   About 5–10% are Hodgkin's disease

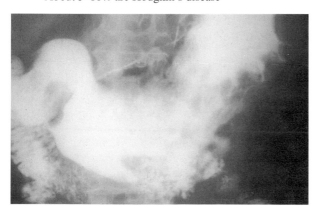

FIGURE 7. Histiocytic lymphoma of the stomach. There are markedly thickened folds in the fundus and body of the stomach.

12. Which polyposis syndromes may involve the stomach?
• Familial polyposis coli (adenomatous polyps)
• Gardner's syndrome (adenomatous polyps)
• Peutz-Jegher's syndrome (hamartomatous polyps) (Fig. 8)
• Cronkhite-Canada syndrome (inflammatory or juvenile-type hamartomatous polyps)
• Juvenile polyposis (hamartomatous polyps)
• Cowden's disease (hamartomatous polyps)

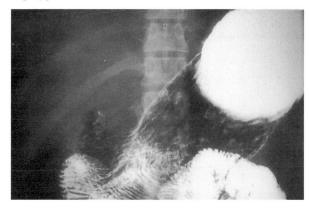

FIGURE 8. Image from a double-contrast UGI series reveals multiple gastric polyps in a patient with Peutz-Jeghers syndrome.

13. What are the mechanisms of tumor spread to the bowel?
Direct extension or invasion, peritoneal seeding, and hematogenous metastases.

14. In what conditions do patients have an increased incidence of duodenal carcinoma (usually at or below the ampulla of Vater)?
Gardner's syndrome and celiac disease (nontropical sprue). These tumors may be polypoid, ulcerated, or annular.

15. What is the primary small bowel tumor that produces a characteristic syndrome of flushing and diarrhea?
Carcinoid (Fig. 9), which arises from argentaffin cells and initially grows as an intramural nodule in the distal ileum. The tumor invades the serosa and mesentery; it incites a desmoplastic reaction, which leads to kinking, fixation, tethering, and obstruction of adjacent small bowel loops. The carcinoid syndrome of flushing, diarrhea, and occasionally bronchospasm is a late finding that is infrequent.

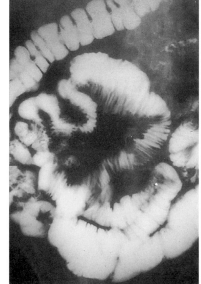

FIGURE 9. A carcinoid tumor separates loops of small bowel. There is spiculation and tethering of the folds of the small bowel in the right lower quadrant.

16. What percentage of small bowel adenocarcinomas are found in the duodenum, the jejunum, and the ileum?
- Duodenum, 40% (Fig. 10)
- Jejunum, 35%
- Ileum, 25%

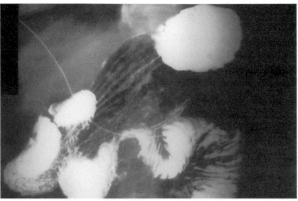

FIGURE 10. Adenocarcinoma producing marked luminal narrowing and mucosal destruction in the fourth portion of the duodenum.

17. What is the typical appearance of small bowel adenocarcinoma on barium studies?
An infiltrating circumferential mass with mucosal destruction and ulceration, with or without proximal dilatation. Duodenal tumors are sometimes polypoid.

18. What polyposis syndromes most commonly involve the small bowel?
1. Peutz-Jegher's syndrome
2. Cowden's disease
3. Cronkhite-Canada syndrome
4. Gardner's syndrome (desmoid tumor in the mesentery)

19. What two tumors are the most common causes of hematogenous metastases to the small bowel?
Melanoma and bronchogenic carcinoma

20. What is the distribution of lymphoma in the small bowel?
Small bowel lymphoma is more common distally than proximally, paralleling the distribution of lymphoid tissue in the small bowel.

21. What are the usual radiographic appearances of small bowel lymphoma?
- Mucosal effacement with segmental narrowing; infiltrative form
- A mass with an amorphous collection of barium communicating with the lumen of an abnormal small bowel loop; endoexoenteric form
- Diffuse nodules, with or without ulcers (Fig. 11)
- Aneurysmal dilatation

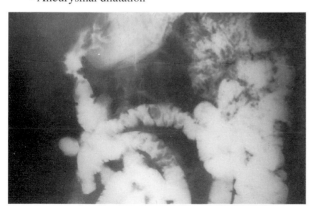

FIGURE 11. Multiple nodules in the midabdominal small bowel in a patient with lymphoma.

22. Name two tumors found in the appendix.
Mucocele and carcinoid.

23. Do colorectal cancers usually have a precursor lesion?
Yes, most colorectal carcinomas arise from pre-existing adenomas. This is known as the "adenoma-carcinoma sequence." Thus, the incidence and mortality of colorectal carcinoma can be reduced by interrupting this sequence by diagnosing polyps on double contrast barium enemas (Fig. 12) or colonoscopy, followed by endoscopic polypectomy. Although most adenomas probably will never evolve into carcinoma, approximately 5% of endoscopically resected adenomas contain invasive carcinoma. The time required for an adenoma to evolve into a carcinoma is quite variable but usually averages 10–15 years.

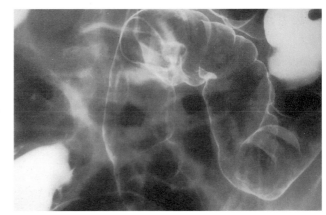

FIGURE 12.   Midsigmoid colonic pedunculated polyp seen on a double contrast barium enema.

24. What are the histologic types of colonic adenoma?
• Tubular, 75%
• Tubulovillous, 15%
• Villous, 10%. These have the highest incidence of malignancy.

25. What factors determine the risk of malignancy in an adenomatous polyp?
Size, histologic type, and degree of epithelial dysplasia. The incidence of invasive malignancy is less than 1% in adenomas smaller than 1 cm, 10% in adenomas measuring 1–2 cm, and more than 30% in adenomatous polyps larger than 2 cm.

26. What two major types of polyposis syndromes involve the colon?
    1. Familial adenomatous polyposes syndromes, which include familial polyposis coli and Gardner's syndrome
    2. Hamartomatous polyposis syndrome, including Peutz-Jegher's syndrome, Cowden's syndrome, Cronkhite-Canada syndrome, and juvenile polyposis

27. Other than prior adenomatous polyps, what conditions are associated with an increased incidence of colon cancer?
    1. Personal or family history of colorectal polyps or cancer
    2. Chronic ulcerative colitis. In patients with pancolitis, the incidence usually starts to increase after the patient has ulcerative colitis for 10 years, and then about 10% of patients develop cancer every decade.

28. What are the two commonly used classifications of colon cancer?
    1. Modified Duke's classification
    2. The TNM (tumor, node, metastases) classification

29. What are the different radiographic appearances of colon cancer on barium enemas?
- Polyps
- Polypoid mass (Fig. 13)
- Circumferential narrowing—apple core or napkin ring lesion (Fig. 14)
- Flat plaque-like lesions, producing abnormal lines or a reticular/villous surface pattern
- Linitis plastica form, with a long area of narrowing with tapered margins

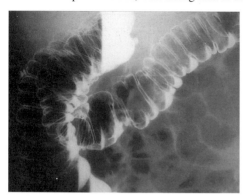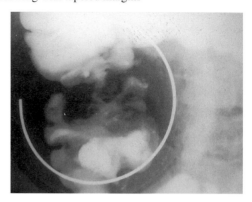

FIGURE 13.   Lobulated polypoid mass in the transverse colon, produced by adenocarcinoma.

FIGURE 14.   "Apple core" narrowing of the proximal ascending colon due to adenocarcinoma.

30. What percentage of patients with colorectal cancer have synchronous cancers?

5%. Also, about one-third to one-quarter have at least one synchronous adenomatous polyp. Thus, the entire colon must be studied carefully for the presence of multiple lesions.

31. What metastases from other organs most commonly involve the colon, and how do they get there?

Spread to the colon occurs by direct invasion from cancers of the ovary (Fig. 15), uterus, kidney, prostate, cervix, and gallbladder; by intraperitoneal seeding from cancers of the ovary, stomach, pancreas, and colon; and by embolic metastases from melanoma and cancers of the lung and breast.

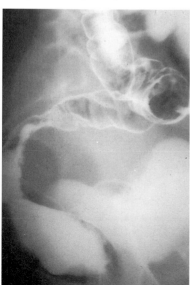

FIGURE 15.   Lateral view of the rectum shows metastases to the anterior wall of the rectosigmoid, from endometrioid cancer of the ovary.

32. What are the most frequent sites and forms of colonic lymphoma?

The cecum and the rectum are the most frequent sites. Small nodules are seen in 45% of cases, but other manifestations include large intramural (Fig. 16) or intraluminal masses, focal strictures, and large extrinsic masses.

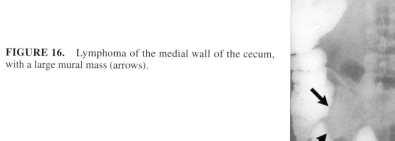

FIGURE 16.   Lymphoma of the medial wall of the cecum, with a large mural mass (arrows).

BIBLIOGRAPHY

1. Freeny PC, Stevenson GW: Margulis and Burhenne's Alimentary Tract Radiology, 5th ed. St. Louis, Mosby-Year Book, 1994.
2. Gore RM, Levine MS, Laufer I: Textbook of Gastrointestinal Radiology. Philadelphia, W.B. Saunders, 1994.

---

29. GALLBLADDER AND BILIARY DISEASE

Douglas S. Katz, M.D.

---

1. What is the best way to diagnose gallstones?

Gallstones are common in the general population and are often found incidentally on plain films, ultrasound, and, less commonly, on CT scans (Fig. 1). The best test for gallstones is ultrasound, which is noninvasive and very accurate. A gallstone on ultrasound is echogenic: it appears as a white structure that casts a dark shadow behind it. Gallstones are usually mobile unless they are fixed to the gallbladder wall. Occasionally, a large anterior gallstone may obscure the entire gallbladder, making the diagnosis difficult.

2. What percentage of gallstones are visible on plain radiographs?

Only about 20%.

3. What are the ultrasound findings of cholecystitis? (Fig. 2)

The two most specific signs of cholecystitis are gallstone(s) and a sonographic Murphy's sign, which is pain corresponding directly to the gallbladder, as demonstrated by sonography. Additional supportive signs are fluid around the gallbladder and thickening of the gallbladder wall to greater than 3 mm. Occasionally, a stone may be impacted in the neck of the gallbladder.

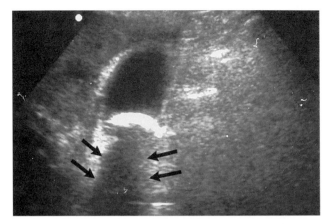

FIGURE 1.   A large stone is demonstrated in the gallbladder. There is posterior acoustic shadowing (arrows) from the stone.

FIGURE 2.   Acute cholecystitis on sonography. The gallbladder wall is significantly thickened (between the + signs) and there is sludge in the gallbladder. Stones were seen (not shown), and a sonographic Murphy's sign was present at the time of the examination.

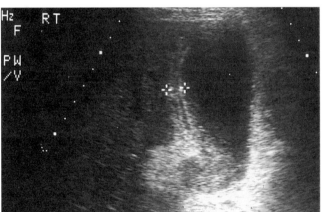

4. What other imaging test can establish the diagnosis of cholecystitis?

A nuclear medicine test called a HIDA scan, named for the first version of the radiopharmaceutical used in this exam. Like ultrasound, it is very accurate in establishing or excluding the diagnosis of acute cholecystitis.

5. Which test is preferable, a HIDA or an ultrasound?

The choice may depend on institutional preference, the relative costs of the procedures, and the ease of obtaining the study, particularly after regular working hours. In some circumstances, such as when the ultrasound is performed first and it is equivocal, the studies may be complementary. Ultrasound shows the anatomy better, and alternative diagnoses may be established if the gallbladder is normal. The HIDA scan shows the physiology better.

6. How does a HIDA scan work (Fig. 3)?

The radiopharmaceutical is injected intravenously and is selectively taken up by the liver and the biliary system. Images of the right upper quadrant are obtained serially over time. Patients should be NPO for at least 4 hours prior to the study. Normally, the gallbladder fills with HIDA; this effectively excludes acute cholecystitis, because cystic duct obstruction is the hallmark of acute cholecystitis. If the gallbladder does not fill with HIDA and the small bowel does, morphine can be given intravenously, which contracts the sphincter of Oddi; a normal gallbladder will then fill with HIDA. If the gallbladder does not fill with the radiopharmaceutical, the cystic duct is obstructed, and acute cholecystitis is diagnosed.

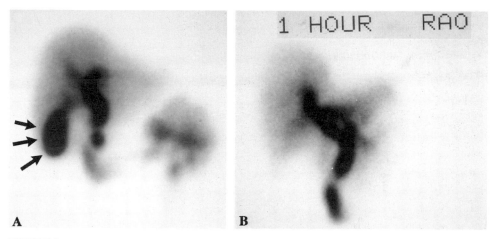

FIGURE 3. *A*, Normal HIDA scan. The gallbladder has filled with radionuclide (arrows). *B*, Acute cholecystitis. The common duct and a portion of the duodenum have filled with radionuclide, but the gallbladder does not fill despite the administration of morphine. (Courtesy of Dr. Zachary Grossman.)

7. What are some causes of false negative and false positive HIDA scans?

If a patient has just eaten, the gallbladder will be contracted and may not fill with HIDA, giving a false positive study for acute cholecystitis. If a patient has not eaten for many hours, the gallbladder may be full of bile or sludge and may not fill with HIDA, also giving a false positive study. If a patient has chronic cholecystitis, the gallbladder may not fill on the initial images but may fill on later images. A small percentage of patients with acute cholecystitis will have false negative HIDA scans, because the cystic duct is not obstructed. In these cases, particularly if the index of suspicion is high, it may be useful to perform ultrasound or, if ultrasound was performed and was negative, follow-up ultrasound.

8. How is acalculous cholecystitis diagnosed and treated?

Cholecystitis can develop in patients without gallstones. Hospitalized patients, such as those in cardiac intensive care units, are most likely to develop this condition, which may be due to ischemia. Acalculous cholecystitis may be diagnosed with ultrasound or a HIDA scan, but the accuracy of both of these examinations is lower than with acute calculous cholecystitis. If a patient with known or suspected acalculous cholecystitis is too ill to undergo cholecystectomy, as is often the case, a drain can be placed—at the bedside, if necessary—into the gallbladder under imaging guidance (e.g., ultrasound).

9. What are some complications of cholecystitis that can be seen or suggested on sonography?

1. Gangrenous cholecystitis
2. Emphysematous cholecystitis
3. Gallbladder perforation
4. Liver or pericholecystic abscess

10. Is CT a good test for diagnosing acute cholecystitis?

No, because the exam occasionally may be negative in the face of acute cholecystitis. However, not uncommonly, when CT is performed for nonspecific fever or abdominal pain, the diagnosis may be established or suspected on CT. CT is a good test for clarifying or diagnosing suspected complications of acute cholecystitis such as liver or pericholecystic abscess (Fig. 4).

11. What are some causes of gallbladder wall thickening other than cholecystitis?

Cirrhosis, ascites, hypoproteinemia, hepatitis, adenomyomatosis, and gallbladder cancer.

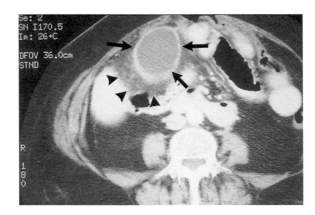

FIGURE 4. Acute cholecystitis on CT. The gallbladder is distended, its wall is thickened and enhances with intravenous contrast (arrows), and there is significant inflammation in the pericholecystic fat (arrowheads).

12. **A soft tissue mass is seen in the gallbladder on ultrasound and does not move when the patient's position is changed. What is the differential diagnosis?**

If the mass is 5 mm or smaller and does not cast a shadow, it is most likely a small adherent stone, a small polyp, or adherent ("tumefactive") sludge. Masses larger than 1 cm should be considered malignant until proven otherwise (Fig. 5).

FIGURE 5. Sonographic image of the gallbladder shows two polyps in the gallbladder. There is no posterior acoustic shadowing, and the polyps are much less echogenic than stones.

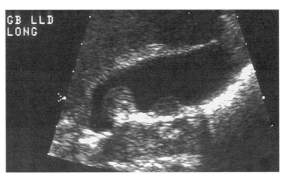

13. **What are the other imaging presentations of gallbladder cancer?**

In addition to a focal soft tissue mass, gallbladder cancer may present with focal or diffuse thickening of the gallbladder wall. There may be direct invasion of adjacent organs, especially of the liver, and metastases. Associated gallstones are common. The diagnosis is often made by pathologic examination of a cholecystectomy specimen.

14. **What is the prognosis of a patient with gallbladder cancer?**

Dismal.

15. **Calcification is seen throughout the gallbladder wall on plain films or CT. What is the diagnosis, and what should be done (Fig. 6)?**

This condition is known as porcelain gallbladder and is strongly associated with the development of gallbladder cancer. Most authorities advocate removal of the gallbladder.

16. **Air is seen in the gallbladder wall on plain films or CT. What is the diagnosis?**

Emphysematous cholecystitis (Fig. 7).

17. **What is the most common cause of emphysematous cholecystitis?**

Clostridium perfringens, in about a third of cases. Elderly diabetics have a predisposition for developing this condition. Patients may be ill at the time of diagnosis or may become ill shortly after plain films are obtained.

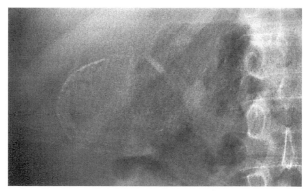

FIGURE 6.   Plain film of the right upper quadrant reveals calcification of the wall of the gallbladder (porcelain gallbladder).

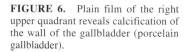

FIGURE 7.   Upright abdominal film shows emphysematous cholecystitis, with gas in the gallbladder wall and a gas-fluid level in the lumen of the gallbladder.

18. What is the best way to diagnose a common duct stone?

The best initial test is ultrasound, although it is not highly accurate. Dilated bile ducts are usually seen if the stone is obstructing the common duct, although it may be difficult to visualize the stone directly in many patients. At endoscopy, a retrograde cholangiogram (ERCP) can be performed. While accurate, ERCP is relatively invasive. A stone is seen at ERCP as a persistent filling defect. Also, at ERCP therapeutic maneuvers can be attempted (e.g., stone extraction after sphincterotomy). Alternatively, a less invasive new examination that has shown excellent results in diagnosing common duct stones is magnetic resonance cholangiography. Using heavily-weighted T2 images, without administering any contrast, the bile acts as an intrinsic contrast agent against which common duct stones appear as filling defects. MR cholangiography can be performed without any special preparation and on most commercially available MR scanners. CT, performed without contrast, may also be useful for detecting a common duct stone.

19. What is the best test to visualize dilated bile ducts, and what is the differential diagnosis for this finding?

Ultrasound is the best initial test. In addition to a common duct stone, causes for dilated bile ducts include biliary stricture and pancreatic, primary biliary, and metastatic tumors.

20. What other tests can be used to work up biliary obstruction?

CT can be used to look for an obstructing tumor or to further stage a mass identified on sonography. MR cholangiography may have a role in looking for a common duct stone or characterizing a duct stricture. For further diagnosis and therapy, ERCP is usually the next step (Fig. 8); if an ERCP cannot be performed, a percutaneous transhepatic cholangiogram (PTC) is an alternative exam, but it is more invasive than ERCP because the liver is traversed by a needle. At endoscopy, ultrasound may be used to examine the local anatomy near the stomach and duodenum (an ultrasound transducer is mounted in a special endoscope). The radiologist and gastroenterologist involved in the care of such a patient need to tailor the imaging work-up to the individual patient with biliary obstruction.

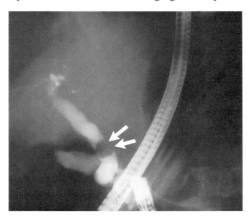

FIGURE 8. ERCP reveals a single common bile duct stone (arrows).

21. How can a primary biliary tract tumor—a cholangiocarcinoma—present on imaging studies?

Cholangiocarcinoma is often difficult to diagnose because its presentation may be insidious. Cholangiocarcinoma may take a variety of forms, from a polypoid mass or an irregular stricture in the common bile duct, to an obstructing mass at the junction of the right and left hepatic ducts (a Klatskin tumor), or a peripheral liver mass that is difficult to distinguish from a primary liver tumor. The prognosis is usually quite poor, and the only hope for cure is early resection (Fig. 9).

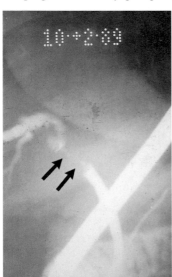

FIGURE 9. Cholangiocarcinoma produces irregular narrowing (arrows) of the proximal hepatic duct on an ERCP.

22. What are some of the complications of laparoscopic cholecystectomy, and how can they be diagnosed with imaging?

Laparoscopic cholecystectomy is now the surgical method of choice for removing the gallbladder, but a variety of complications can occur. The common duct may be accidentally tied off; biliary ductal dilatation will be seen on ultrasound, the differential being a retained common duct stone. ERCP or HIDA scan may be appropriate in this setting. A bile leak may be suspected, and HIDA is appropriate in these circumstances. Other complications include abscess, hematoma, dropped gallstone (into the peritoneal cavity, which serves as as source of infection), and, rarely, liver infarction. These can be assessed using a variety of imaging studies, especially CT, ultrasound, and ERCP (Fig. 10).

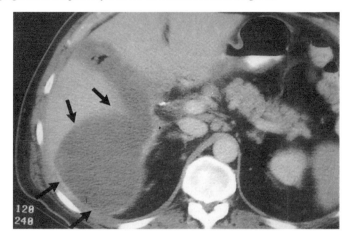

FIGURE 10. A 54-year-old man after laparoscopic cholecystectomy, with continued right upper quadrant pain. There is a collection of fluid (arrows) contiguous with the cholecystectomy site. A HIDA scan (not shown) confirmed a bile leak.

BIBLIOGRAPHY

1. Choledocholithiasis: Evaluation with MR cholangiography. AJR 167:1441–1445, 1996.
2. Datz FL: Handbook of Nuclear Medicine, 2nd ed. St. Louis, Mosby, 1993.
3. Glenn F, Becker CG: Acute acalculous cholecystitis. Ann Surg 195:131–136, 1982.
4. Jeffrey RB Jr, Ralls PW: CT and Sonography of the Acute Abdomen, 2nd ed. Philadelphia, Lippincott-Raven, 1996, pp 74–121.
5. Krishnamurthy GT, Turner FE: Pharmacokinetics and clinical application of technetium-99m-labeled hepatobiliary agents. Semin Nucl Med 20:130–149, 1990.
6. Ralls PW, Colletti PM, Lapin SE, et al: Real-time sonography in suspected acute cholecystitis. Radiology 155:767–771, 1985.

30. INFLAMMATORY BOWEL DISEASE

Robert J. Botash, M.D., and Douglas S. Katz, M.D.

1. Figure 1 shows a frontal radiograph from a small bowel follow-through of a 29-year-old woman with chronic right lower quadrant pain, diarrhea, and weight loss. Note the tubular narrowing of the terminal ileum with loss of the normal mucosal pattern. What is the likely diagnosis?

Crohn's disease (regional enteritis).

2. What are the two primary diagnostic considerations in inflammatory bowel disease?

Crohn's disease and ulcerative colitis. Not uncommonly, elements of both disorders may be present, both clinically and histologically.

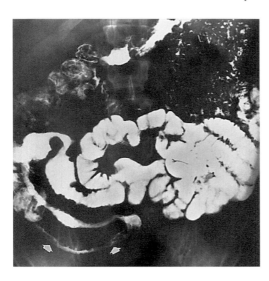

FIGURE 1.   String sign. Fibrosis of the terminal ileum results in stricture formation (arrows).

3. What part of the bowel is most commonly affected by Crohn's disease?

The terminal ileum, although any part of the gastrointestinal tract may be involved. Crohn's disease is a chronic, inflammatory disorder of unknown etiology that presents most commonly in the second and third decades of life.

4. What is meant by "skip lesions" in Crohn's disease?

Crohn's disease is characterized by a discontinuous or segmental granulomatous process, with diffuse transmural inflammation of the bowel. Involved areas may be separated by radiographically normal segments.

5. What produces the "cobblestone" appearance of the bowel in Crohn's disease?

Longitudinal and transverse linear ulcers produce a cobblestone appearance of the mucosa (Fig. 2).

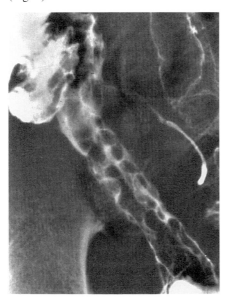

FIGURE 2.   Criss-crossing ulcerations in the terminal ileum produces a cobblestone appearance.

6. What is the "string sign"?

Progressive inflammation and fibrosis result in rigidity and stricture formation, which are referred to as the string sign (see Fig. 1). In addition, fistulas may occur between adjacent bowel loops (Fig. 3) or end blindly, resulting in the formation of abscess cavities.

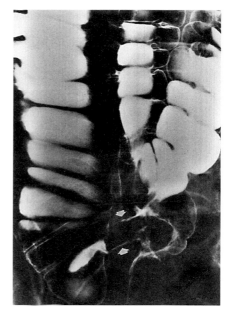

FIGURE 3. Transmural inflammation has resulted in fistula formation (arrows) between the small bowel and colon.

7. Where does bowel inflammation occur in ulcerative colitis?

Inflammation is limited to the mucosa. Disease begins in the rectum and may spread proximally in the colon to varying degrees.

8. Are skip lesions seen in ulcerative colitis?

No. Involvement of the colon is continuous and symmetrical.

9. What is "backwash" ileitis?

Reactive inflammatory changes in the terminal ileum due to "backwash" from the inflamed colon. The ileocecal valve may become fixed in an open position. In contrast, patients with Crohn's disease often have stricture or spasm of the terminal ileum, which produces the string sign.

10. Is the rest of the small bowel involved in ulcerative colitis?

No. Only the most distal portion of the terminal ileum is involved, as described above.

11. What other typical locations of the gastrointestinal tract are involved by Crohn's disease?

Usually, in addition to the terminal ileum, the proximal large bowel (cecal region) is involved. Less commonly, other areas of the small bowel are affected. Rarely, the stomach and esophagus are affected; if they are involved, almost always there is or has been disease in the more typical locations as well.

12. What are the typical superficial ulcers seen in early Crohn's disease called?

Aphthous ulcers. They may be found anywhere from the pharynx to the rectum.

13. What are the typical early ulcerations in ulcerative colitis called?

"Collar-button" ulcers (Fig. 4). They are deeper than the aphthous ulcers because the submucosa is involved.

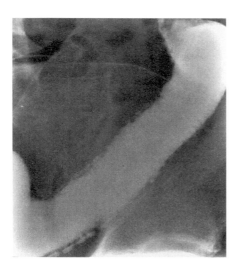

FIGURE 4.   Collar button ulcers.

14. What is toxic megacolon? In what inflammatory bowel disease is it usually found?

Toxic megacolon is significant gaseous distention of the colon (Fig. 5), which may progress to perforation. This condition, which is occasionally seen in ulcerative colitis, may be suggested on plain films. Suspected toxic megacolon is a contraindication to barium enema examination.

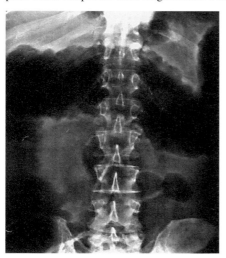

FIGURE 5.   Toxic megacolon. Dilatation of the colon is seen in this patient with fulminant ulcerative colitis.

15. What are pseudopolyps?

Hyperplastic, inflamed regenerating mucosa results in pseudopolyp formation, which is typical of relatively late ulcerative colitis (Fig. 6).

16. What is meant by the "lead-pipe" colon?

Progressive fibrosis in ulcerative colitis causes shortening and rigidity of the colon with loss of the haustral pattern (Fig. 7).

17. Are patients with inflammatory bowel disease at increased risk for developing colon cancer?

Yes, especially in ulcerative colitis, but the risk is also increased with Crohn's disease. Such cancers can be difficult to detect, both endoscopically and radiographically.

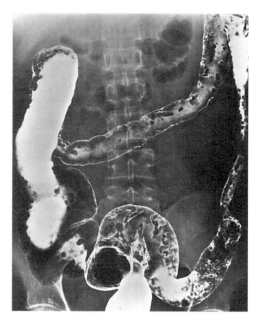 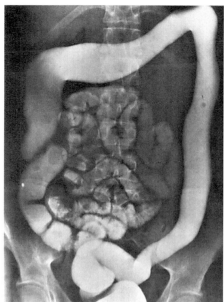

FIGURE 6 *(Left)*.   Pseudopolyps appear as filling defects in the colon.

FIGURE 7 *(Right)*.   Shortening and loss of haustral markings in the fibrotic phase of ulcerative colitis.

18. What biliary condition are patients with inflammatory bowel disease predisposed to develop?
    Sclerosing cholangitis, which is most typically associated with ulcerative colitis and is also a risk factor for the development of cholangiocarcinoma.

19. What stone-forming conditions are patients with inflammatory bowel disease at risk of developing (especially in Crohn's disease)?
    Gallstones and urinary tract stones.

20. Which radiographic examinations are useful in evaluating inflammatory bowel disease?
    Barium enema (to be used cautiously during active disease; contraindicated with toxic megacolon)—for evaluating the extent of colonic disease and complications such as cancer
    Small bowel follow-through—for evaluating the small bowel, especially the ileum
    CT—for detecting complications such as fistula and abscess formation
    Endoscopic retrograde cholangiopancreatography (ERCP)—for evaluating suspected sclerosing cholangitis

21. What conditions outside the gastrointestinal tract can be seen in inflammatory bowel disease?
    Sacroiliitis
    Iritis or uveitis
    Skin findings, such as erythema nodosum

BIBLIOGRAPHY

1. Bartram CI, Laufer I: Inflammatory bowel disease. In Laufer I, Levine MS (eds): Double Contrast Gastrointestinal Radiology, 2nd ed. Philadelphia, W.B. Saunders, 1992, pp 579–645.
2. McNally PR: GI/Liver Secrets. Philadelphia, Hanley & Belfus, 1996, pp 383–385.

31. ABDOMINAL CALCIFICATIONS

Robert J. Botash, M.D., and Douglas S. Katz, M.D.

1. Describe the findings in the abdominal radiograph (Fig. 1) of a 43-year-old obese woman with right upper quadrant pain radiating to the back.

Two round, laminated calcifications can be seen in the right upper quadrant.

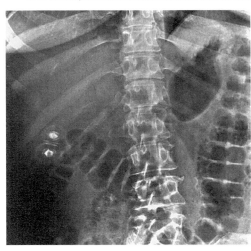

FIGURE 1. Laminated calcifications are present in the right upper quadrant.

2. A film from a subsequent endoscopic retrograde cholangiogram (ERC), which is an injection of water-soluble, iodine-based contrast into the common duct after it is cannulated endoscopically, confirms that the calcifications are within the gallbladder. What is the definitive diagnosis?

Cholelithiasis. The cause of calcifications on abdominal radiographs usually can be determined from their size, shape, and position (Fig. 2). When the site of the calcification corresponds to the location of the patient's symptoms, additional imaging studies may be required to confirm the location and to evaluate the secondary effects.

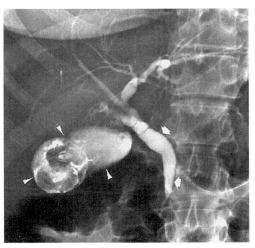

FIGURE 2. Spot image from an ERC demonstrates contrast in the gallbladder surrounding the structures seen on plain films (arrowheads) (Arrows = common bile duct.)

3. What percentage of gallstones are radiolucent (i.e., cannot be seen on plain radiographs)?

About 80%. Up to 20% of gallstones contain enough calcium that they can be seen on radiographs. Gallstones are usually rounded if solitary. Multiple gallstones are usually faceted.

4. What is a porcelain gallbladder?

This term refers to extensive calcification of the gallbladder wall (Fig. 3).

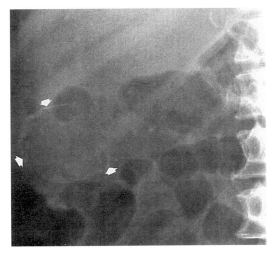

FIGURE 3.   Diffuse peripheral calcification of the gallbladder wall.

5. Porcelain gallbladders are usually resected. Why?

There is a high incidence of gallbladder carcinoma (either existing at the time of diagnosis or occurring in the future) in patients with porcelain gallbladders.

6. What is your radiographic diagnosis for Figure 4?

Chronic pancreatitis. Pancreatic calcifications are pathognomonic of chronic pancreatitis. Calcifications are most often present in the head of the pancreas but may extend to involve the body and tail as well.

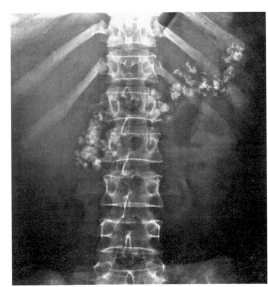

FIGURE 4.   Calcifications in the mid abdomen, from chronic pancreatitis.

7. What structures are seen in Figure 5?

Arterial calcifications are present in the splenic artery (arrowheads), iliac arteries (arrows), and renal arteries (open arrows). The splenic artery usually follows a serpentine course in the left upper quadrant. Venous calcifications (phleboliths) are commonly seen in the pelvis and are of no consequence.

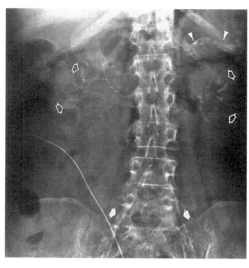

FIGURE 5. Diffuse calcification of several structures. A dialysis catheter is present in the right lower quadrant.

8. What percentage of urinary tract calculi are visible on plain films?

About 80%. They may be identified in the kidneys, ureters, or bladder.

9. What is the most sensitive imaging test for abdominal calcification?

CT, which is far more sensitive than plain radiographs.

10. A CT scan shows a few, small, punctate calcifications in the liver and the spleen. What is the diagnosis?

This common finding on CT usually relates to previous (and usually asymptomatic) infection from histoplasmosis. It is usually of no clinical significance.

11. A focal area of "sunburst" calcification (i.e., spicules of calcification radiating from a central point) is seen in the liver on plain films or CT. What is the diagnosis?

Hemangioma. Although hemangioma, a benign lesion of the liver, is common (and almost always asymptomatic), on rare occasions it may calcify in a "sunburst" pattern. This pattern of calcification is diagnostic of a hemangioma.

12. List other causes of calcification in the liver.
- Previous infection other than granulomatous disease (e.g., bacterial)
- Other, more unusual infections (e.g., atypical mycobacterial, *Pneumocystis carinii* [in patients with AIDS], or echinococcus)
- Old trauma
- Metastatic disease (typically from mucin-producing tumors, such as colorectal cancer)
- Primary malignancies of the liver

13. List other causes of calcification in the spleen.

The differential diagnosis is similar to that for liver calcification: old trauma or infection, metastatic tumor, benign primary lesions such as hemangioma, and benign cysts (whether primary or, more commonly, secondary to old trauma).

14. Do pancreatic malignancies calcify?

Adenocarcinoma of the pancreas almost never calcifies. Other unusual tumors of the pancreas, both benign and malignant (e.g., various cystic tumors of the pancreas), may contain calcification.

15. An area of rim calcification is seen adjacent to the lumbar spine, just off the midline on a frontal radiograph of the abdomen. What is the likely diagnosis? What should be done?

The diagnosis may be calcification in the aorta, which may or may not be dilated. If both walls of the aorta are closely seen and the vessel does not appear dilated, an aneurysm is unlikely. However, if only one wall is seen, an aneurysm may or may not be present. If the patient is asymptomatic, the most effective (and inexpensive) exam to perform is ultrasound, which rapidly excludes or diagnoses an abdominal aneurysm.

16. List the most common causes of adrenal calcification.
   • Old hematoma (e.g., from hemorrhage in a newborn or hemorrhage due to trauma or anticoagulation)
   • Old infection, typically tuberculosis or other granulomatous infections
   • Calcification is unusual in adrenal tumors

17. Diffuse foci of calcification are seen throughout the abdominal wall. What are the diagnostic possibilities?
   • Systemic condition in which calcium is deposited (i.e., various hypercalcemic states)
   • Abdominal wall infarction, such as from nematodes
   • Disorders of muscle such as dermatomyositis

BIBLIOGRAPHY

1. Eisenberg RL: Diagnostic Imaging in Internal Medicine. New York, McGraw-Hill, 1985, pp 726–736.
2. Freedman M: Calcium deposits in the abdomen. In Freedman M (ed): Clinical Imaging: An Introduction to the Role of Imaging in Clinical Practice. New York, Churchill Livingstone, 1988.

IV. Genitourinary Radiology

32. GENITOURINARY TRACT: NORMAL ANATOMY, NORMAL VARIATIONS, AND BASIC RADIOGRAPHIC PROCEDURES

Douglas S. Katz, M.D., and Steven Perlmutter, M.D.

1. What is the most basic radiographic study of the urinary tract?

Intravenous pyelography (IVP), also known as intravenous urography (IVU) or excretory pyelography.

2. How is an IVP performed?

An initial scout radiograph of the abdomen and pelvis is obtained. A catheter or butterfly needle is then placed into a peripheral vein (e.g., antecubital), and iodine-containing contrast is hand-injected. Immediately after the contrast is injected, a repeat radiograph is obtained, followed by additional films over the next 30 minutes or so.

3. Why is the IVP customized by the radiologist?

To solve the particular clinical problem. For example, if the history is hematuria in an older patient, tomograms of the kidneys are obtained. These blur the anatomy in front of and behind a particular depth in the patient, allowing the selected plane of tissue to be seen better. In this clinical setting, the bladder should be radiographed both full and empty to look for a bladder tumor. If a child is examined with an IVP, there is no need for tomograms; it is best to obtain as few radiographs as possible to limit the radiation dose.

4. What is purpose of the scout radiograph on an IVP?

The scout is used to examine the bones, bowel gas pattern, and soft tissues. In particular, the presence of any calcifications within the urinary tract should be noted, because they may be subsequently obscured by the contrast material. If a possible renal calcification is suspected, it may be useful to obtain an oblique film (e.g., angled 45° off the frontal midline) to determine whether the calcification is truly within the kidney. A renal calcification overlies the kidney on all projections, whereas a calcification outside the kidney will project off the kidney on the oblique view.

5. What is the purpose of the compression device that may be used during an IVP?

The compression device usually consists of a belt with two inflatable balloons that are placed on the anterior abdominal wall, overlying the ureters, during an IVP. It is usually applied after the ureters are visualized, to distend the proximal ureters and collecting systems for optimal visualization.

6. List the contraindications to applying a compression device during an IVP.

Urinary tract obstruction
Abdominal aneurysm
Recent abdominal surgery
In addition, the device is not needed in children.

7. Identify the following structures on the normal urograms (Fig. 1): kidney, ureter, bladder, minor calyx, major calyx, and renal pelvis.

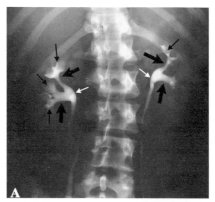
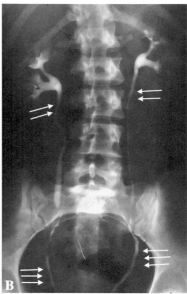
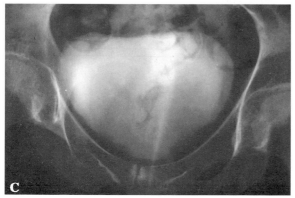

FIGURE 1. Normal intravenous pyelography. The kidneys, minor calyces (small black arrows), major calyces (large arrows), renal pelvis (white arrows), proximal ureters (double white arrows), distal ureters (triple white arrows), and bladder (*C*) are shown.

8. What is the normal orientation of the kidneys in the body?

Normally, the kidneys parallel the psoas muscles so that the lower poles of the kidneys lie anterior and lateral to the upper poles.

9. So what?

Many normal variants exist. Deviation from the normal axis suggests that a mass may be displacing the kidney or ureter. The normal variants include nonrotation or malrotation during the embryologic ascent of the kidney. Masses that shift the renal axis may arise from the kidney or adjacent structures.

10. A single kidney is seen in the abdomen on a CT scan (Fig. 2A). What are the diagnostic possibilities?

- Congenital single kidney (other associated genitourinary anomalies are common)
- A second kidney may be present in an ectopic location, such as the pelvis (Fig. 2B) or, rarely, the thorax
- Prior resection of a kidney
- Renal hypoplasia or atrophy
- Nonfunctioning kidney (secondary to obstruction, trauma, or renal artery or vein occlusion)

11. What is a horseshoe kidney?

A horseshoe kidney is a fusion anomaly in which the lower poles of the kidneys fuse across the midline. The connecting tissue may be functioning or nonfunctioning (e.g., fibrous tissue). Horseshoe kidneys are recognized by a change in the orientation of the kidneys—the lower poles are located closer to the midline than the upper poles, which is the reverse of normal (Fig. 3).

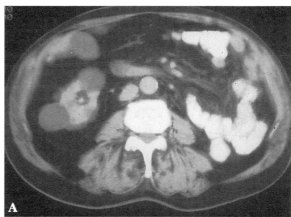

FIGURE 2. In the abdomen, a right kidney is present, but there is no left kidney (*A*). A left pelvic kidney is identified on lower images of the same patient. (*B*). Note the multiple simple renal cysts.

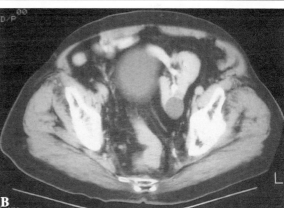

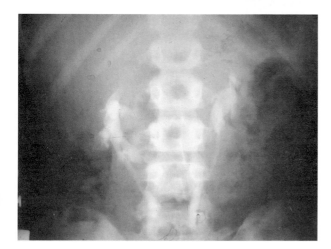

FIGURE 3. Horseshoe kidney in an 8-year-old. The lower poles are medially located; the ureters project anteriorly and are bowed around the bridge of tissue connecting the kidneys.

12. What is the significance of a horseshoe kidney since it is a normal variation?

Horseshoe kidneys are more susceptible to traumatic injury. Because the proximal ureters must pass over the connecting tissue between the lower renal poles, there often is poor drainage. The stasis of urine predisposes the kidney to infection and stones.

13. What is a retrocaval ureter (Fig. 4)?

In some patients the proximal ureter follows an abnormal course, hooking behind and then medial to the inferior vena cava. There may be obstruction of the ureter, which generally involves the right ureter and is caused by anomalous development of the inferior vena cava.

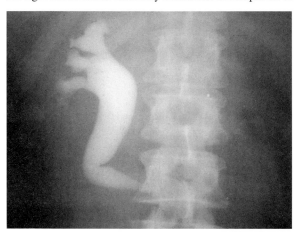

FIGURE 4. Retrograde right ureterogram reveals a retrocaval ureter. Notice narrowing of the ureter at the approximate point where it crosses the psoas muscle. The proximal ureter is dilated.

14. What is meant by a dromedary hump?

Sometimes the spleen causes an impression on the upper lateral aspect of the left kidney, which is referred to as the dromedary hump (Fig. 5). It should be recognized as a normal variation of no significance.

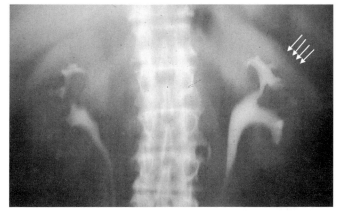
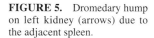

FIGURE 5. Dromedary hump on left kidney (arrows) due to the adjacent spleen.

15. What is meant by duplication of the collecting system?

A portion or all of the collecting system and ureter of one or both kidneys may be duplicated. Partial duplications commonly involve the proximal ureter and are rarely significant. Complete duplications may have clinical consequences. Separate ureters drain the upper and lower poles of the kidney. The upper pole ureter frequently inserts in an ectopic location in the bladder inferior and medial to the usual ureteral orifice, and may become obstructed. Although the ureter from the lower pole inserts into a normal location in the bladder, it often is incompetent, allowing urine to reflux into the ureter and kidney.

16. The term *cobra head* refers to what normal variation?

Some people have a ureterocele, which is an outpouching of the distal ureter into the bladder. This finding, which may be unilateral or bilateral, is usually not significant. On an IVP the thin walls of the distal ureter are outlined by contrast. The ureterocele resembles a cobra head (Fig. 6).

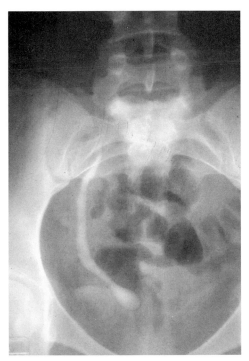 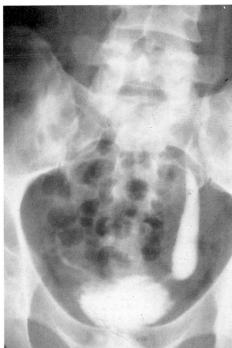

FIGURE 6 *(Left)*. A 37-year-old man with a simple ureterocele on intravenous pyelography. The distal right ureter has a "cobra head" appearance.

FIGURE 7 *(Right)*. A 33-year-old man with primary megaureter. The distal left ureter is dilated but there is a short segment of narrowing just before the ureterovesical junction; the latter area is the adynamic (abnormal) segment responsible for the ureteral dilatation.

17. What congenital condition causes dilatation of the ureter, except for the lowest portion of the ureter?

Primary megaureter (Fig. 7). The nondilated distal portion is called the adynamic segment, which lacks peristalsis, causing functional rather than mechanical obstruction. This entity must be distinguished from other causes of ureteral dilatation such as mechanical obstruction (e.g., by a stone or tumor), reflux, previous obstruction, etc.

18. What anatomy can be identified on a renal ultrasound?

Ultrasound is an inexpensive, safe, and relatively easy method of determining renal size. The parenchyma is evaluated for cysts and masses, and for echogenicity, and the collecting system is examined for dilatation, which usually signifies hydronephrosis. The bladder is easily examined when it is full. The ureters are not usually seen unless they are dilated. Doppler can be used to evaluate the renal vasculature.

19. What is the best way to visualize the uterus and ovaries?

Ultrasound is the mainstay of female reproductive tract imaging. It is safe and relatively inexpensive, and no radiation is involved. Ultrasound may be used in numerous situations to scan the uterus and the ovaries—for example, to evaluate a suspected pelvic mass, to look for an ectopic pregnancy, and to evaluate the uterus for possible fibroids.

20. Which ultrasound techniques can be used to scan the female pelvis?

Ultrasound of the female pelvis may be performed using a transabdominal probe, which is placed on the skin. The bladder should be full if this approach is used. Alternatively, or in addition to transabdominal scanning, a specialized ultrasound probe is placed transvaginally. It provides better detail because the probe is much closer to the uterus and the ovaries than with transabdominal scanning. During the pelvic ultrasound, the uterine size and shape are assessed, the endometrial stripe is measured, and the ovaries are identified and examined. The presence or absence of free fluid and masses is noted.

21. Are there any supplemental examinations other than ultrasound for examining the female reproductive tract?

There are several, and they are used in specific situations. CT is used to evaluate the pelvis for possible tumors or abscesses and may be used in conjunction with ultrasound or as a primary modality. MR has multiple uses, including confirming pelvic developmental abnormalities, staging pelvic tumors (e.g., cervical and uterine cancer), and evaluating uterine fibroids. The advantages of MR include multiplanar imaging, the ability to characterize tissue better than ultrasound, and the absence of radiation. Hysterosalpingography (HSG) is usually performed by cannulating the cervical os and injecting iodinated contrast into the uterus and fallopian tubes. One purpose of this procedure is to determine whether the fallopian tubes are open—if the contrast spills into the peritoneal cavity, they are. For selected patients, the HSG may be combined with a transvaginal sonogram—hysterosonography. This technique is useful in evaluating abnormalities of the endometrial cavity (e.g., differentiating an endometrial polyp from a submucosal fibroid).

22. Identify the following structures on the CT images in Figure 8*A–C*.

Kidneys, renal cortex, renal medulla, main renal artery, main renal vein, and bladder.

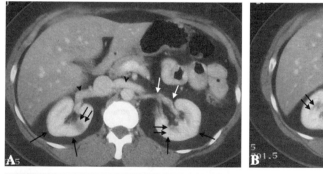
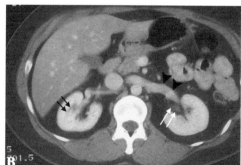
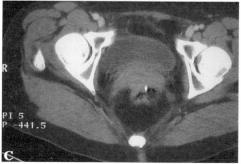

FIGURE 8. Normal anatomy of the urinary tract on CT. *A* and *B*, Renal cortex (arrows), medulla (double arrows), renal veins (arrowheads), and left renal artery (white arrows). Left renal collecting system/ureteropelvic junction (double white arrows, *B*). *C*, Bladder.

23. What is the advantage of CT compared with IVP?

With CT, cross-sections of the body are obtained; thus overlying structures, such as bowel gas, do not obscure urinary tract anatomy. CT shows subtle density differences, which an IVP cannot do, and the renal vessels can be evaluated. Masses can be characterized—for example, simple cysts can usually be distinguished from renal tumors.

24. What is the purpose of a renal nuclear scan?

DTPA, an agent which is filtered by the kidneys, is tagged to the radionuclide technetium-99m. The radiopharmaceutical agent is injected intravenously, and images of the urinary tract are obtained with a gamma camera. This procedure is performed in the nuclear medicine department. Although the resolution of a nuclear scan is inferior to that of a IVP or CT, functional information is easily obtained. The glomerular filtration rate of each kidney can easily be estimated. A renal nuclear scan may be used in many different situations, including for following patients in renal failure, and for determination of whether hypertension is due to a renovascular cause (i.e., a captopril renal scan to exclude renal artery stenosis).

25. When should MR be used to evaluate the kidneys?

When a CT scan is warranted (e.g., when a renal mass or abscess is suspected) but intravenous contrast cannot be administered, because of either contrast allergy or abnormal renal function, MR can be performed. Gadolinium, the contrast agent used for MR, can be safely administered in such circumstances.

26. What is the current role of renal angiography?

Renal angiography is currently used only for selected indications, such as evaluation and possible treatment (by balloon angioplasty) of renal artery stenosis, or for the treatment of renal hemorrhage by embolic occlusion of the bleeding renal artery branches.

27. How is the male urethra best evaluated?

It depends on the clinical situation. If the patient is a young male, with a possible anomaly (e.g., valves in the posterior urethra), the best test is a voiding cystourethrogram (VCUG), in which the bladder is catheterized through the urethra and images are obtained while the child urinates. If the patient is an adult with a possible stricture, a retrograde urethrogram is obtained (Fig. 9).

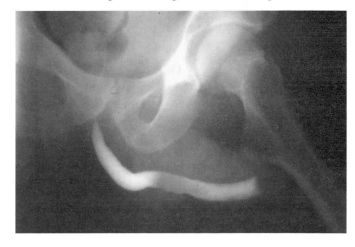

FIGURE 9.   Normal image from a retrograde (male) urethrogram.

28. What is the basic anatomy of the male urethra?

On a normal male urethrogram, the following structures are evaluated: the prostatic urethra, membranous urethra, bulbous urethra, and penile urethra. The anterior urethra is composed of the penile and bulbous segments, and the posterior urethra is composed of the membranous and prostatic segments.

29. Is there such a thing as a female urethrogram?

Yes. Because the female urethra is short, it is rarely injured in trauma. However, a woman may present with symptoms suggesting a diverticulum of the urethra (believed to be postinfectious in origin). Such a patient may present with a history of immediate postvoid dribbling, recurrent urinary tract infections, and pain on intercourse. A VCUG or a urethrogram performed with a catheter designed to evaluate the female urethra will usually demonstrate the diverticulum.

30. What is a cystogram?
A catheter is placed from the urethra into the bladder, and iodinated contrast is injected into the bladder under fluoroscopic control. Two situations for which this study is indicated are possible traumatic rupture of the bladder and urinary incontinence in a woman.

31. Which normal structures are identified on a scrotal ultrasound?
The testicles should be seen as uniformly echogenic structures. The epididymal heads are also seen routinely. Doppler is used to look at the vascular flow within the testes. This is useful in excluding testicular torsion.

BIBLIOGRAPHY

1. Davidson AJ, Hartman DS: Radiology of the Kidney and Urinary Tract, 2nd ed. Philadelphia, W.B. Saunders, 1994.
2. Ell SR: Handbook of Gastrointestinal and Genitourinary Radiology. St. Louis, Mosby, 1992.

33. URINARY TRACT CALCULI

Douglas S. Katz, M.D.

1. What initial imaging test is usually ordered to find urinary tract stones?
Plain radiographs. The majority of urinary tract stones, particularly if they are relatively large (e.g., > several mm) are detectable on a plain radiograph. However, other calcifications may be confused with urinary tract stones (e.g., a phlebolith in the pelvis, which is a venous calcification, often with a lucent center, that is of no clinical significance) and vice versa. In addition, overlying structures such as bones and bowel gas may obscure a urinary tract calcification.

2. What does a urinary tract calcification look like on a plain radiograph?
A calcification blocks the transmission of the x-ray beam; thus it appears as a white area on the radiograph.

3. What other modalities can detect urinary tract calcifications?
Ultrasound and computed tomography. On ultrasound, a calcification appears as a white area (echogenic) with shadowing behind it. On CT, a calcification appears as a very white (dense) area.

4. What is the most sensitive radiologic test for urinary tract stones?
CT, performed without contrast, is highly sensitive for detecting urinary tract stones (Fig. 1).

5. Urinary tract stones composed primarily of calcium are often visible on plain films. What types of stones are less visible or not visible at all on plain films?
Stones composed primarily of cystine are minimally dense on plain films. Stones composed of urate are invisible (radiolucent) on plain films.

6. Are any urinary tract stones radiolucent on CT?
No. Virtually all urinary tract stones, regardless of their composition, are visible on CT.

7. What is meant by the term *renal colic*?
Renal colic refers to the presence of crampy flank pain, which may radiate to the groin; the pain is due to the passage of a stone through the ureter.

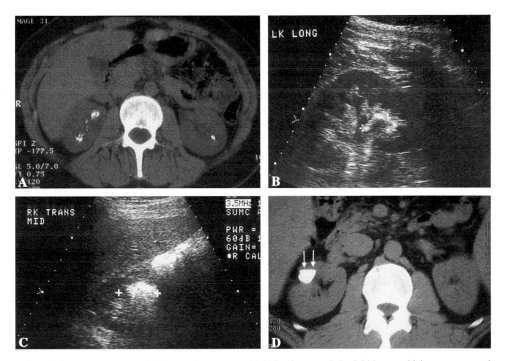

FIGURE 1. *A*, Unenhanced CT image demonstrates high density areas in both kidneys, which represent renal calculi. *B*, Sagittal ultrasound image of the left kidney of a patient with a lower pole collecting system stone (between the + signs; note posterior acoustic shadowing). There is mild dilatation of the collecting system. *C* and *D*, Echogenic area is noted between + signs, in the upper pole of the right kidney of this man (*C*). Unenhanced helical CT image shows this area represents "milk of calcium" layering posteriorly in a calyceal diverticulum or in a renal cyst (arrows).

8. What are the options for imaging a patient with a possible ureteral stone?

Traditionally, a frontal film of the abdomen and pelvis (called a KUB for kidneys, ureters, and bladder) is obtained, and an intravenous pyelogram (IVP, also known as an intravenous urogram) is performed. Typically, 50 to 100 ml of iodine-based contrast is injected intravenously, and a series of radiographs of the abdomen and pelvis is obtained.

9. What are the imaging findings of a ureteral stone on an IVP (Fig. 2)?

Acute ureteral stones often obstruct (completely or incompletely) the portion of the urinary tract that is above it. The kidney that is obstructed enhances with contrast later than the unobstructed kidney. This finding may be subtle in low-grade obstruction or obvious in high-grade obstruction, in which the obstructed kidney may not be seen at all on the initial images. The collecting system of the obstructed kidney is usually dilated; when contrast finally fills it, the ureter may demonstrate a standing column of contrast that ends at the ureteral stone. Often the stone is small and cannot be seen directly on the radiographs. On occasion, because of the diuretic effect of the intravenous contrast, the IVP may actually help the patient to pass a small stone out of the ureter.

10. Are there alternative ways of diagnosing an acute ureteral stone?

Some authorities advocate the use of ultrasound (Fig. 3). Usually, the ureteral stone cannot be seen, but it is inferred by the clinical context and the presence of obstruction on the symptomatic side (i.e., the collecting system and/or ureter is dilated). Problems with ultrasound include false-negative diagnoses in early obstruction and a low yield in visualizing the stone itself.

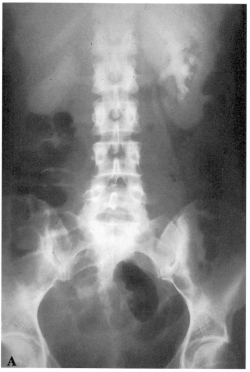

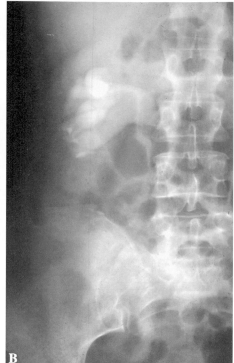

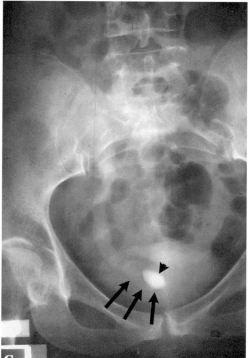

FIGURE 2.   *A*, A 40-year-old man with left renal colic. There is persistent opacification of the obstructed left kidney, while contrast has cleared from the right kidney. Note vicarious excretion of contrast by the gallbladder. *B* and *C*, A 59-year-old woman with right flank pain. There is hydroureteronephrosis due to a stone (arrowhead) in a right ureterocele (arrows). (Courtesy of Steven Perlmutter, M.D.)

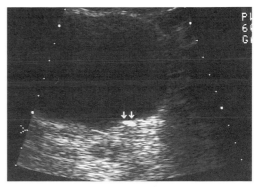

FIGURE 3. Transverse image from a bladder sonogram of a patient with left flank pain. A small calcification is present in the left ureterovesical junction (arrows).

11. Is there any role for CT in this situation?

Yes. In the experience of the author as well as physicians at several institutions, spiral (helical) CT of the abdomen and pelvis performed without contrast is a good test for diagnosing acute renal colic (Fig. 4). The stone is seen directly in the ureter, and associated findings such as dilatation of the collecting system and ureter, swelling of the affected kidney, and edema around the kidney and ureter are commonly seen. Other advantages include the speed of the examination (minutes compared with hours for some IVPs), avoidance of any risk of a contrast reaction, and possibly decreased radiation dose (which adds up as film after film is obtained during an IVP). An alternative diagnosis also may be established on an unenhanced spiral CT, such as appendicitis or diverticulitis. Finally, CT often avoids the common problem of distinguishing residual edema at the ureterovesical junction, which causes some obstruction although the stone has already passed through the ureter, from a retained small stone at the ureterovesical junction, which may not be seen easily on plain films or IVP.

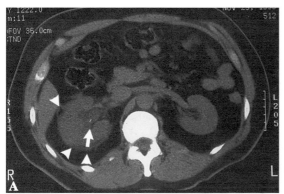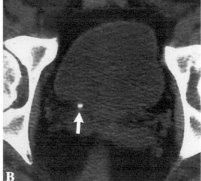

FIGURE 4. Unenhanced helical CT of a patient with right flank pain. There is swelling of the right kidney, hydronephrosis (arrow), and perinephric edema (arrowheads) (*A*), due to a stone at the right ureterovesical junction (*B*, arrow).

12. Are there any disadvantages of unenhanced spiral CT?

Yes. It may be more expensive than an IVP, and occasionally it is difficult to distinguish a true ureteral stone from a phlebolith.

13. A patient has multiple calcifications in both kidneys, corresponding to the renal medulla (medullary nephrocalcinosis). What is the differential diagnosis?

The three major causes of this finding are hyperparathyroidism (with hypercalcemia), medullary sponge kidney, and renal tubular acidosis (Fig. 5).

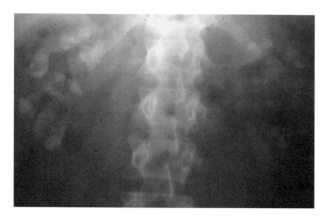

FIGURE 5. A 39-year-old man with microscopic hematuria following a motor vehicle accident. There is bilateral medullary nephrocalcinosis, presumably secondary to medullary sponge kidney. (Courtesy of Steven Perlmutter, M.D.)

14. What is medullary sponge kidney?

Patients affected by medullary sponge kidney have dilatation of the collecting tubules in the medulla and are often asymptomatic. However, some may have problems relating to stones and/or infection. The presence of dilated tubules alone is a common finding on IVP that is usually of no significance; for a diagnosis of medullary sponge kidney, both the tubular ectasia and the medullary stones should be present. The appearance of the tubules on IVP has been likened to a bouquet of flowers. Medullary sponge kidney is associated with several other conditions, including hepatic fibrosis and Caroli's disease.

15. What imaging modalities are used to guide lithotripsy and to follow patients after the procedure?

Plain films and ultrasound. Many lithotripsy devices have an ultrasound transducer (for diagnosis only, somewhat different from the device used to produce ultrasound waves that break up the stones) that is used to image a stone and to localize it for lithotripsy. Follow-up radiographs are usually used to image patients after lithotripsy.

16. What is meant by *Steinstrasse*?

The term (from the German, meaning stone street) refers to the stream of tiny stone fragments that may fill the ureter after lithotripsy—and may obstruct it (Fig. 6). A ureteral stent is often placed by the urologist cystoscopically before lithotripsy to prevent this complication.

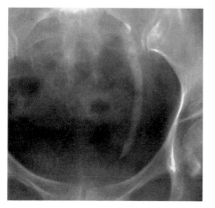

FIGURE 6. Radiograph of the pelvis of a 70-year-old man following lithotripsy. There are diffuse calcifications in the distal left ureter, representing stone fragments (Steinstrasse). (Courtesy of Steven Perlmutter, M.D.)

17. What is a staghorn calculus?

A large stone that fills most or all of the renal collecting system. Staghorn stones are usually visible on plain films (Fig. 7); they form a cast of the calyces and the renal pelvis and are difficult to treat.

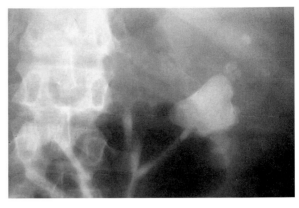

FIGURE 7. Radiograph of a 43-year-old man with cystine stones. There is a staghorn calculus, which fills the left renal pelvis. Satellite stones are also seen in the calyces. (Courtesy of Steven Perlmutter, M.D.)

18. What are the potential complications of a ureteral stone?

An obstructing stone may lead to urinary infection. In addition, because of the increased pressure in the urinary system, a portion of the collecting system may "blow out." This condition usually resolves spontaneously but occasionally leads to a significant amount of extravasation of urine into surrounding soft tissues.

19. If a ureteral or renal pelvic stone does not resolve after conservative treatment (fluids, pain medication, lithotripsy), what are other therapeutic options?

The urologist may attempt to extract the stone through a scope placed through the urethra and the bladder into the ureter. Alternatively, an interventional radiologist may place a relatively small-diameter catheter into the renal collecting system percutaneously. This catheter can be converted into a larger tract in the operating room so that the urologist can extract the stone(s). Contact lithotripsy also may be performed at that time.

20. What chronic infectious or inflammatory condition is associated with a staghorn calculus?

Xanthogranulomatous pyelonephritis is a condition in which a staghorn calculus (usually composed of triple phosphate crystals—magnesium ammonium phosphate) forms in association with infection from urease-splitting organisms. Chronic obstruction and infection result. Central cystic spaces form, usually involving all, but occasionally only part, of the kidney. Spread of this process to the adjacent perinephric tissues is common. Cure usually requires nephrectomy.

21. Which patients develop bladder stones? (Fig. 8)

Usually patients with bladder outlet obstruction (e.g., from prostatic hypertrophy or functional obstruction, as in a quadriplegic).

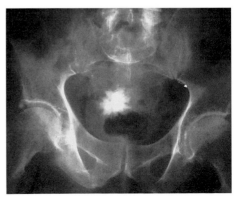

FIGURE 8. Elderly man with prostatic enlargement who fell and has a right subcapital femoral fracture and urinary retention. There is a "Jackstone" calculus in the bladder. (Courtesy of Steven Perlmutter, M.D.)

BIBLIOGRAPHY

1. Dunnick NR, McCallum RW, Sandler CM: Textbook of Uroradiology, 2nd ed. Baltimore, Williams & Wilkins, 1997.
2. Katz DS, Lane MJ, Sommer FG: Unenhanced helical CT of ureteral stones: Incidence of associated urinary tract findings. AJR 166:1319–1322, 1996.
3. LeRoy AJ: Diagnosis and treatment of nephrolithiasis: Current perspectives. AJR 163:1309, 1994.
4. Smith RC, Rosenfield AT, Choe KA, et al: Acute flank pain: Comparison of non-contrast-enhanced CT and intravenous urography. Radiology 194:789–794, 1995.
5. Van Arsdalen KN, Banner MP, Pollack HM: Radiographic imaging and urologic decision making in the management of renal and ureteral calculi. Urol Clin North Am 17:171–190, 1990.

34. URINARY OBSTRUCTION

Douglas S. Katz, M.D.

1. Why is it important to recognize renal obstruction?
Over time, obstructed kidneys may lose function permanently.

2. A patient presents with suspected renal obstruction. What is the best initial imaging test for renal obstruction?
Ultrasound. It is relatively inexpensive, safe, and effective. The presence of hydronephrosis usually correlates with obstruction. The cause of obstruction also may be identified.

3. Hydronephrosis and/or hydroureter is identified on ultrasound, but the cause is unclear. What should be done next?
A CT scan (Fig. 1) or an intravenous pyelogram may identify the cause of obstruction (e.g., unilateral obstruction from a ureteral stone or metastatic disease obstructing the ureters). If the BUN and creatinine are elevated, an MR may be performed or an unenhanced CT of the abdomen and pelvis. Finally, direct injection of contrast into the urinary tract may be performed.

4. List the other common causes of urinary tract obstruction.
Prostatic hypertrophy or cancer, urinary tract stricture, primary urinary tract tumor.

5. How do patients with obstructing urinary tract stones usually present?
With acute flank pain and hematuria.

6. List the common causes of ureteral strictures.
Previous stones, prior instrumentation, prior infections, and intrinsic narrowing (ureterovesical or ureteropelvic junction obstruction).

7. What are three common causes of urethral stricture?
Prior infection (e.g., gonococcal), prior trauma, and prior instrumentation or catheterization (Fig. 2).

8. Does a dilated ureter or collecting system always mean that obstruction is present?
No. Dilatation usually equates with obstruction, but there are exceptions. If previous obstruction has been relieved, there may be residual dilatation without obstruction. States of increased urine production—for example, in pregnancy—may lead to dilatation without obstruction.

9. Does a normal renal ultrasound exclude obstruction?
No. In very early obstruction, the collecting system and ureter may not have had a chance to dilate. In addition, unusual conditions (e.g., tuberculosis, retroperitoneal fibrosis) may fibrose the collecting system and ureter, leading to obstruction without dilatation.

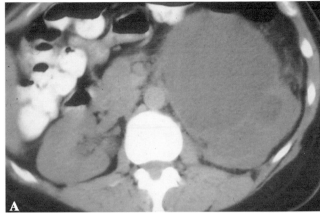

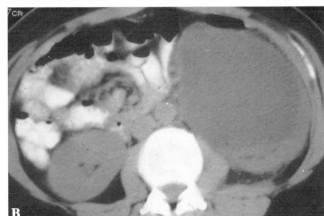

FIGURE 1. *A* and *B*, A 41-year-old woman with left abdominal pain and a palpable mass. CT (performed with oral but no intravenous contrast) reveals marked dilatation of the left renal collecting system. The ureter was normal, and there was no evidence of a mass at the ureteropelvic junction. Diagnosis: chronic left ureteropelvic junction obstruction.

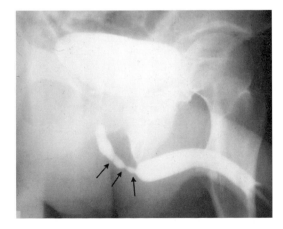

FIGURE 2. Retrograde urethrogram performed on a 27-year-old man shows a beaded area of narrowing of the bulbous urethra (arrows) from prior infection. (Courtesy of Steven Perlmutter, M.D.)

10. What does an acutely obstructed kidney look like on an IVP or contrast-enhanced CT?

There is a delay in the normal excretion of contrast by an obstructed kidney, and the collecting system, when it is visualized, is usually dilated. On an IVP, it may be difficult to see any significant renal excretion in high-grade obstruction on early images. Occasionally, the increased pressure causes a calyx to rupture, and urine (and contrast in the urine) extravasates from the urinary tract.

11. A patient with a known abdominal aortic aneurysm develops bilateral renal obstruction. What may have happened?

Retroperitoneal fibrosis, incited by the aneurysm, may have occurred. The ureters may be deviated (typically medially) and become obstructed by fibrous tissue that envelops them (Fig. 3).

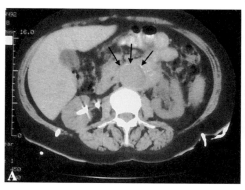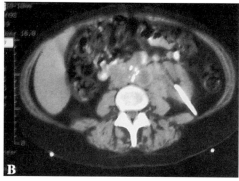

FIGURE 3. Bilateral ureteral obstruction from retroperitoneal fibrosis related to an abdominal aortic aneurysm (arrows). Note the nephrostomy tubes which were placed to relieve the obstruction which had developed due to encasement of the ureters by the fibrotic process.

12. List the other common causes of retroperitoneal fibrosis.

Drugs, such as methysergide

Tumors, both primary and metastatic

Idiopathic (most common)

13. What is a good way to exclude urinary tract obstruction if it is still strongly suspected, despite a negative or equivocal ultrasound, when the BUN and creatinine are elevated and intravenous contrast cannot be given?

A nuclear renal scan is a good test in this setting. Normal bilateral renal excretion of the radiopharmaceutical agent excludes significant obstruction.

14. What if the collecting system(s) and/or ureter(s) are dilated on ultrasound, yet obstruction is doubted. What can be done?

Several noninvasive examinations can exclude obstruction. The presence of bilateral jets of contrast from the ureters into the bladder when the bladder is examined by color Doppler shows that the ureters are not completely obstructed and are passing urine. This study is relatively easy to do. Alternatively, if this does not solve the problem, and if intravenous contrast can be given, an IVP may be performed or a nuclear scan may be obtained. Furosemide may be given during the scan to distinguish a dilated collecting system and/or ureter that is not obstructed from one that is—the radiopharmaceutical washes out of a non-obstructed system rapidly.

15. Once obstruction is identified, what are the options for treatment?

A urologist can place a stent from a transurethral approach into the bladder and ureter. Such a stent is typically a plastic tube coiled at each end (called a "double J" ureteral stent). One end is placed in the renal pelvis and the other end in the bladder. Contrast injected during the procedure may identify the cause of the obstruction.

16. What if this approach is unsuccessful?

A radiologist can place a catheter into the ureter through the kidney, using a percutaneous approach. Ultrasound may be helpful in guiding a needle into the renal collecting system, through which contrast is injected under fluoroscopic guidance to confirm its correct placement. A series of wires and dilators is used to create a path for the catheter, which is then placed with one end coiled in the renal collecting system and the other end outside the patient to drain urine.

17. What are the potential complications of percutaneous nephrostomy tube placement?
    Infection and bleeding, although uncommon, are the most common complications. Rarely, a structure such as bowel may be transgressed.

18. Why do ureteral stents (whether placed transurethrally or percutaneously) need to be changed relatively frequently?
    They often become clogged with debris if left in place for a significant period of time.

BIBLIOGRAPHY

1. Davidson AJ, Hartman DS: Radiology of the Kidney and Urinary Tract, 2nd ed. Philadelphia, W.B. Saunders, 1994.
2. Ritchie WW, Vick CW, Glocheski SK, et al: Evaluation of azotemic patients: Diagnostic yield of initial US examination. Radiology 167:245–247, 1988.

35. RENAL FAILURE

Douglas S. Katz, M.D.

1. A patient presents with newly diagnosed renal failure. What is the best initial test to exclude urinary obstruction, which is usually the most easily reversible cause of renal failure?
    Ultrasound. Although only about 10% or less of all cases of renal failure are due to obstruction of the urinary tract, these patients are important to identify so that the urinary tract can be decompressed and further deterioration of renal function be prevented. When obstruction is present, dilatation of the renal collecting system is usually present. However, early obstruction may not be evident on ultrasound.

2. What radiologic test can estimate the glomerular filtration rate (GFR) of each kidney?
    A nuclear renal scan. Technetium-99m, a radioactive isotope, is tagged to a compound that is filtered by the kidney, typically either diethylene triamene pentaacetic acid (DTPA) or mercaptoacetyltriglycine (MAG3), and is injected intravenously. Because the amount of injected radioactive isotope is known and the amount of radioactive compound excreted by each kidney can be calculated by drawing a region of interest on a computer, the GFR of each kidney can be estimated by relatively straightforward calculations. The nuclear renal scan is useful for monitoring the function of each kidney in patients with renal failure. It is accurate, relatively inexpensive, and noninvasive.

3. If both kidneys appear bright (hyperechoic) on a renal ultrasound in a patient with renal failure, what is the differential diagnosis?
    Numerous diseases such as diabetes and hypertension cause the echogenicity of the kidneys to increase over time. The term *medical renal disease* is usually applied because the differential diagnosis is broad and a specific cause usually cannot be determined based on ultrasound or other imaging modalities. Over time, the kidneys atrophy. To establish a specific diagnosis, a renal biopsy is often indicated.

4. What is the best imaging modality for guiding renal biopsy?
    Ultrasound. With real-time ultrasound guidance, the lower pole of the kidney can be biopsied, and the main renal vessels (and other structures) can be avoided (Fig. 1).

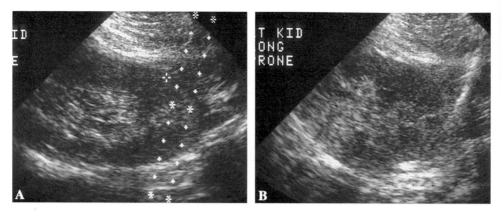

FIGURE 1. *A*, Renal biopsy. Initial sonographic image of the lower pole of the left kidney in a patient who has acute renal failure shows the planned course of the biopsy needle. *B*, Bright area is the needle entering the lower pole of the left kidney.

5. List the most common complications of renal biopsy.

Perinephric and intraparenchymal hemorrhage (very common, at least to some extent, but usually not clinically significant)

Introduction of infection (very uncommon with sterile technique)

Development of an arteriovenous fistula or pseudoaneurysm (uncommon and usually of no clinical significance, if small)

Puncture of an adjacent structure (e.g., the bowel—rare if direct sonographic visualization is used)

6. Intravenous contrast is usually contraindicated when the creatinine becomes significantly elevated (e.g., > 2). If a contrast study of a patient in renal failure is required, what are the options?

Perform the study without contrast (e.g., CT)

Use another imaging modality (e.g., ultrasound or MR)

If angiography is required, use nonionic contrast; limit the dose given; or use alternative methods (e.g., CO_2 angiography, if available).

7. Is intravenous gadolinium, the contrast agent used for MR, contraindicated in renal failure?

No. There is no known upper limit for creatinine above which it is unsafe to use gadolinium. MR is helpful for imaging a patient in renal failure when other imaging modalities (e.g., unenhanced CT) cannot answer the clinical question.

8. A patient presents with untreated renal failure and multiple large cysts in both kidneys on ultrasound. One of his parents had a similar condition. What is the diagnosis?

Autosomal dominant polycystic kidney disease (Fig. 2). This diagnosis can be established by ultrasound or CT. Patients may develop cysts in other organs, such as the liver and pancreas; over time they develop renal insufficiency.

9. What central nervous problem may occur in patients with polycystic kidney disease?

About 15% develop intracranial aneurysms, which may be clinically silent or may bleed. MR angiography is an ideal examination for screening patients with polycystic kidney disease for such aneurysms.

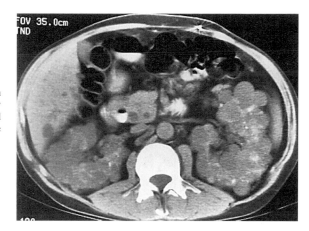

FIGURE 2. CT image of a patient with autosomal dominant polycystic kidney disease. Both kidneys are enlarged and contain numerous cysts. Several cysts are also present in the liver.

10. A patient with chronic renal failure (e.g., from chronic glomerulonephritis) develops multiple cysts in both kidneys. What has happened?

Patients with chronic renal failure, especially those kept alive on dialysis, commonly develop multiple bilateral renal cysts (Fig. 3). The cysts are usually small but may become large and resemble those seen in autosomal dominant polycystic kidney disease. The exact etiology of this condition is unknown. Patients are at increased risk for developing renal cell cancer. It is controversial whether (and if so, how) to screen these patients for renal cell cancer.

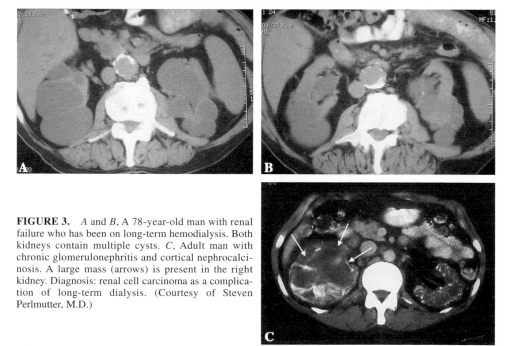

FIGURE 3. *A* and *B*, A 78-year-old man with renal failure who has been on long-term hemodialysis. Both kidneys contain multiple cysts. *C*, Adult man with chronic glomerulonephritis and cortical nephrocalcinosis. A large mass (arrows) is present in the right kidney. Diagnosis: renal cell carcinoma as a complication of long-term dialysis. (Courtesy of Steven Perlmutter, M.D.)

11. Why not remove the native kidneys in all patients with chronic renal failure?

There is no proven benefit to this approach. In addition, the native kidneys may still be functioning to some extent; they also produce substances, such as erythropoeitin, that are of value to the patient.

12. A 25-year-old man presents with slightly enlarged, echogenic kidneys and renal failure. He also has pneumonia and white plaques in his mouth. What is the diagnosis?

AIDS. HIV-related nephropathy (which occurs through a variety of mechanisms) has a tendency to preserve or slightly increase renal size (Fig. 4).

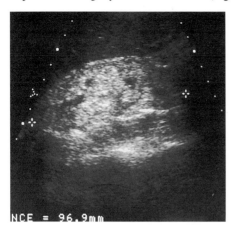

FIGURE 4. Sagittal image of the right kidney demonstrates markedly increased echogenicity of the parenchyma (compare with the liver, which is anterior to the kidney). Note that the renal size is normal (almost 10 cm in length), which is unusual in this patient who has relatively long-standing renal failure.

13. A radiograph of the abdomen of a patient shows diffuse calcifications of the cortex of both kidneys. What is the differential diagnosis?

This unusual finding suggests a few diagnoses, all of which are rare:

Cortical necrosis, usually due to a serious hypotensive episode (classically a crisis related to bleeding in pregnancy)

Oxalosis, a rare hereditary disorder

Alport's disease, which is associated with high-frequency hearing loss and renal failure

BIBLIOGRAPHY

1. Davidson AJ, Hartman DS: Radiology of the Kidney and Urinary Tract, 2nd ed. Philadelphia, W.B. Saunders, 1994.
2. Dunnick NR, McCallum RW, Sandler CM: Textbook of Uroradiology, 2nd ed. Baltimore, Williams & Wilkins, 1997.

36. RENOVASCULAR HYPERTENSION

Kenneth D. Murphy, M.D.

1. What is renovascular hypertension (RVH)?

A clinical condition characterized by elevated systemic blood pressure that results from abnormal renal arterial vasculature and impaired nephron perfusion. The abnormal arterial vasculature is typically a stenosis that can occur anywhere from the origin of the renal artery off the aorta, to the distal end of an intrarenal afferent arteriole.

2. What is the prevalence of RVH?

Hypertension affects 10–15% of the U.S. population. The prevalence of RVH within the hypertensive population has been estimated at 5%.

3. What is the pathophysiology of RVH?

Renal artery stenosis results in a reduced blood flow and glomerular filtration rate (GFR). The GFR is regulated by the juxtaglomerular complex. As a response to a diminished GFR secondary to RAS, the juxtaglomerular cells release renin. Increased renin results in increased conversion of angiotensinogen to angiotensin I. Angiotensin I is rapidly converted to angiotensin II in the lung, by angiotensin-converting enzyme (ACE). Angiotensin II is a potent vasoconstrictor that results in hypertension. Angiotensin II also stimulates the secretion of aldosterone, which results in sodium retention that further exacerbates the hypertension.

4. What clinical characteristics of hypertension suggest a renovascular origin?

1. Continuous flank bruit
2. Recent onset
3. Onset after age 50
4. Accelerated hypertension within 6 months
5. Uncontrollable hypertension
6. Sudden rise in serum creatinine
7. Worsening renal function in response to ACE inhibitors
8. Presence of other vascular disease

5. What causes renal artery stenosis?

The most common cause is atherosclerosis, followed by renal artery dysplasia. Uncommon causes include aortic dissection, neurofibromatosis, Takayasu's disease, radiation, polyarteritis nodosa, renal artery aneurysm, and aortic coarctation.

6. What are the clinical features of atherosclerotic RAS?

Patients tend to be older (mean 50–60 years) than those with essential hypertension. Atherosclerotic RAS has a slight male predominance. Acceleration of previously mild hypertension is also suggestive of atherosclerotic RVH. Patients with atherosclerotic RVH tend to have mild chronic renal insufficiency due to RAS-induced ischemic nephropathy or hypertension-induced nephrosclerosis.

7. What is the angiographic appearance of atherosclerotic RAS?

Atherosclerotic RAS results from atheromatous plaques compromising the lumen of the renal artery. The lesions can be single, multiple, unilateral, or bilateral. The stenosis is typically located within the proximal renal artery; however, lesions within smaller intrarenal branches can occur. An ostial lesion is a stenosis of the proximal renal artery located within 5 mm of the aorta (Fig. 1). The narrowing may range from a small plaque to complete occlusion. The configuration of the stenosis ranges from circumferential to eccentric.

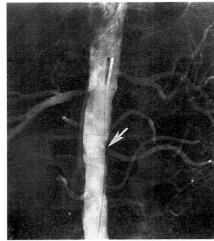

FIGURE 1. Abdominal aortogram demonstrates an ostial stenosis of an accessory left renal artery (arrow).

8. What is renal artery dysplasia?

A condition affecting medium-size arteries, where the various layers of the arterial wall proliferate, resulting in a stenosis. Renal artery dysplasia can be classified into six types: intimal hyperplasia, medial dissection, medial hyperplasia, medial fibroplasia, perimedial fibroplasia, and adventitial fibroplasia.

9. What is the most common type of renal artery dysplasia?

Medial fibroplasia, also referred to as fibromuscular dysplasia (FMD).

10. What are the clinical features of fibromuscular dysplasia?

FMD is the second most common cause of RAS in adults and the most common cause of RVH in children. FMD accounts for one-third of all cases of RAS. FMD typically occurs in young adults in their third and fourth decades, with a strong female prevalence of 3:1. The renal lesions can be associated with an abdominal bruit and with renin-mediated hypertension. FMD can involve other medium-size arteries, including the carotid, iliac, and mesenteric vessels. FMD of the carotid circulation is associated with intracranial aneurysms.

11. What are the angiographic features of FMD?

The findings reflect the underlying pathology. In FMD, there are alternating bands of thickened, fibrotic media with thinned areas devoid of smooth muscle and internal elastic lamina. These pathologic changes in the vessel wall create a characteristic string-of-beads appearance on angiography (Fig. 2). FMD is typically located in the middle or distal third of the renal artery. In up to two-thirds of cases, FMD is bilateral. When unilateral, FMD more commonly involves the right artery. Although the string-of-beads configuration is typical of FMD, renal artery dysplasia has a spectrum of appearances. Stenoses can be focal, diffuse, tapered, abrupt, irregular, circumferential, or eccentric (Fig. 3).

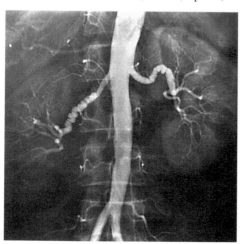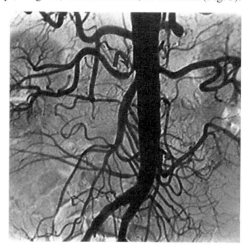

FIGURE 2 *(Left)*. Bilateral fibromuscular dysplasia in a young woman.

FIGURE 3 *(Right)*. Tapered stenosis in proximal right renal artery (curved arrow) proved to be an atypical renal artery dysplasia.

12. What are the causes of pediatric renovascular hypertension?

The most common cause is FMD. Others include neurofibromatosis (Fig. 4), the middle aortic syndrome, arteritis, and Williams' syndrome.

13. What hypertensive patients should be screened for RVH?

Patients that have a flank bruit, accelerated hypertension, uncontrollable hypertension, one small kidney, worsening of renal function in response to ACE inhibitors, onset of hypertension in a child or young adult, and severe vascular disease elsewhere.

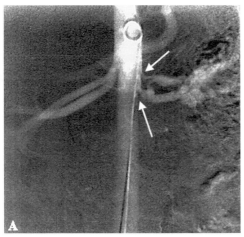
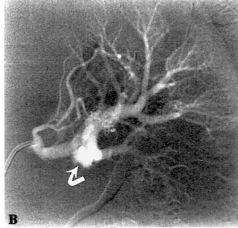

FIGURE 4. Neurofibromatosis. *A*, Abdominal aortogram demonstrates duplicated left renal arteries with high grade stenoses proximally (arrows). *B*, Selective left renal arteriogram demonstrates an intrarenal artery aneurysm (curved arrow), another finding typical of neurofibromatosis.

14. What diagnostic tests are available for the evaluation of suspected RVH?

- Plasma renin activity
- Renal vein renin activity
- Ultrasound
- Computed tomography
- Magnetic resonance imaging
- Scintigraphy
- Intravenous urography
- Angiography

15. What is the plasma renin activity test?

An inexpensive simple blood test that measures renin activity in the peripheral venous system. The exam may be performed with or without captopril stimulation. It is considered positive if the captopril-stimulated plasma renin activity is ≥ 12 ng/ml/hr, the plasma renin activity is increased by at least 10 ng/ml/hr above baseline, and the captopril-stimulated plasma renin activity is at least 150% of the baseline activity. The sensitivity and specificity when performed with captopril stimulation is 79% and 70%, respectively.

16. What is renal vein renin analysis?

A procedure used to determine the physiologic significance of RAS that is difficult to grade. The procedure is performed by selective catheterization of the renal veins and aspiration of a blood sample. The left renal vein catheter must be positioned beyond the origin of the left gonadal vein to avoid sample dilution. The right renal vein can be sampled closer to the inferior vena cava (IVC) because the right gonadal vein empties directly into the IVC. Ideally, patients should be off all ACE inhibitors and beta-blockers several days prior to the procedure. Chronic administration of ACE inhibitors and beta-blockers stimulates plasma renin secretion. A study is considered positive if the ratio of renal vein renin activity in one kidney to the other is greater than 1.5:1.0. The usefulness of renal vein renin analysis to predict the benefit from revascularization remains controversial; the sensitivity is only 65%. Also, the examination is invasive.

17. What is the role of duplex ultrasound in evaluating suspected RVH?

Duplex ultrasonography is a noninvasive imaging modality that can detect RAS. The use of potentially nephrotoxic contrast is omitted, an obvious benefit in patients with underlying renal disease. The study is performed by localizing the renal arteries with color flow Doppler. Overlying bowel gas is minimized by having the patient fast 12 hours prior to the procedure. Several renal artery parameters are measured. Limitations of this technique include overlying bowel gas that obscures the renal arteries, tortuous renal arteries that can falsely increase the velocities, and difficulty in detecting accessory or multiple arteries. The examination is highly operator- and time-dependent.

The role of renal ultrasound is controversial in this setting; some authorities do not recommend it for suspected RVH.

18. What is the role of CT?

Modern CT imaging with helical scanners has enhanced the potential for RAS detection by CT. Thin slices are acquired through the renal arteries, with image acquisition timed in concert with optimal contrast opacification from an intravenous injection. The images can be reformatted into coronal and sagittal planes to facilitate interpretation. The limitations include the need for a large volume of contrast and diminished sensitivity for visualizing small vessels compared with conventional angiography.

19. What is the role of MR?

The advances of MR technology and the development of magnetic resonance angiography (MRA) have created a novel imaging ideal for RAS, in that iodinated contrast can be avoided. Phase contrast and time-of-flight MRA enable the flow of blood to be evaluated. MRA is ideal for evaluating the proximal 4–5 cm of the renal arteries (Fig. 5). The resolution of distal and small accessory branches is limited; however, this is improving with the development of new MR software. There is excellent correlation between a normal MRA and absence of RAS. The correlation between an abnormal MRA and the presence of a stenosis also has been established.

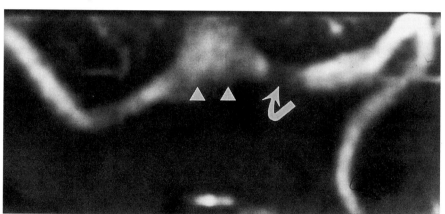

FIGURE 5.   Magnetic resonance angiography demonstrates a left renal artery stenosis (curved arrow) and infrarenal aortic occlusion (arrowheads).

20. How are nuclear renal studies performed in suspected RVH?

Renal scintigraphy is performed by administering a radioactive labeled compound that is cleared by the kidney. The most commonly used radionuclide agents for renal imaging are Tc99m DTPA and Tc99m MAG3. The radioactivity of the kidney is measured as a function of time, enabling estimation of the GFR and the estimated renal plasma flow (ERPF). The evaluation for RAS by radionuclide examination can be enhanced by administering an ACE inhibitor such as captopril. The ACE inhibitors block efferent arteriolar vasoconstriction, which results in a decrease in GFR and ERPF. A unilateral drop in GFR in excess of 30% with respect to the opposite side, after captopril administration, is suggestive of RAS. Another finding suggestive of RAS is asymmetric renal uptake and size (Fig. 6).

21. What are the advantages and disadvantages of a nuclear renal study? What is its role in suspected RVH?

The advantages are that it is noninvasive, omits the need for iodinated contrast, and may be performed in patients with renal insufficiency. Disadvantages include the diminished sensitivity and specificity in patients with bilateral RAS or a stenosis affecting one of multiple renal arteries. Many authorities believe that a captopril nuclear renal study is a fairly good screening examination for

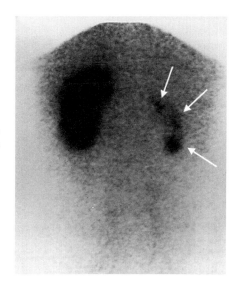

FIGURE 6. Posterior view from a Tc99mDTPA study demonstrates diminished right renal uptake and size (arrows) in a patient with right renal artery stenosis.

suspected RVH, especially because the negative predictive value of a normal study is high. Patients with positive or equivocal examinations should undergo further testing, either with additional noninvasive studies such as MRA or with renal angiography, for definitive diagnosis and therapy.

22. What are the IVP findings suggestive of RAS?

Delayed and increasingly dense nephrogram, prolonged urine transit time, ureteral notching from arterial collaterals, and asymmetric nephrogram size; however, for a variety of reasons, including poor sensitivity, IVP is not recommended in the workup of suspected RVH.

23. What is the role of angiography in suspected RVH?

Conventional angiographic examination for RAS remains the "gold standard." The invasiveness of the procedure limits its application to patients with a high clinical suspicion for RVH. The advantages are that it enables accurate detection, localization, and quantification of RAS in the main and distal branches, and multiple/accessory renal arteries can be effectively evaluated. The arteriogram also facilitates planning of revascularization procedures. Angiography is indicated if a patient has an abnormal renal vein renin study, nuclear scan, MRA, or other studies.

24. How is a renal angiogram performed?

An initial abdominal aortogram is performed with a "pigtail" type catheter placed in the aorta, usually via the transfemoral approach. If the femoral approach cannot be used, i.e., if iliac occlusive disease is present, an axillary or brachial approach is warranted. The catheter is positioned at the upper border of the L2 vertebral body, the anticipated site of the renal arteries. An aortogram is performed in the frontal projection. An additional view in the left anterior oblique position is sometimes necessary to profile the left renal artery origin. Digital subtraction angiography is favored because it requires smaller contrast volumes. If a stenosis is detected, selective renal artery catheterization is generally avoided to minimize the risk of a dissection or occlusion. If no main artery stenosis is detected, selective catheterization is mandatory to evaluate for distal or small branch stenoses. Multiple or accessory renal arteries should be carefully scrutinized for a stenosis.

25. What are the angiographic findings in RAS?

- Diameter of the aorta decreased by 50%
- Poststenotic dilatation
- Diminished ipsilateral renal size
- Diminished velocity of flow
- Collateral vessels
- Pressure gradient greater than 20% of peak systolic pressure (Fig. 7)

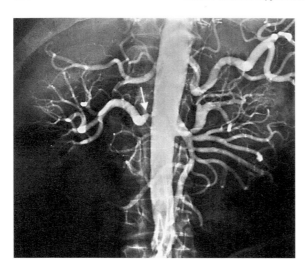

FIGURE 7. High-grade right renal artery
stenosis (arrow) with post-stenotic dilatation.

26. What is a reasonable screening algorithm for the evaluation and treatment of RVH?

Patients with hypertension should be initially evaluated by history and physical examination. If the clinical suspicion for RVH is low, standard medical therapy without further work-up is sufficient. If there is clinical suspicion for RVH, the plasma renin activity before and after ACE inhibitor administration should be measured. If this is normal, medical therapy is indicated without further diagnostic tests; if it is elevated, further work-up with a captopril-stimulated nuclear scan, MR/MRA, helical CT is justified. If one or more of these diagnostic studies is positive, angiography is indicated. An angiographically detected stenosis can be treated percutaneously with angioplasty or stent placement. Surgery or further therapy can be reserved for angioplasty or stent failures.

27. What are the treatment options for RAS?

The natural history of atherosclerotic lesions in the renal artery is progression over time to complete occlusion and secondary renal failure. The natural history of FMD is less clear; these patients are typically symptomatic and undergo treatment. The main therapeutic options for RAS are:

1. Conservative medical management
2. Percutaneous transluminal angioplasty (PTA)
3. Percutaneous intravascular stent placement
4. Surgery

Medical management of RVH is less desirable due to side effects of drugs and the failure to inhibit further progression of disease. Surgical revascularization with endarterectomy, reimplantation, or bypass graft is well established but is limited by the associated morbidity and mortality in high-risk patients. Percutaneous techniques including angioplasty and stent placement continue to gain acceptance in the treatment of RAS.

28. What are the indications for renal artery PTA?

1. Refractory hypertension
2. Noncompliance with or intolerance of antihypertensive medications
3. Loss of renal mass
4. Worsening renal function while on antihypertensive medications

29. What are the techniques for renal artery PTA?

The stenotic renal artery is carefully catheterized (Fig. 8), and the stenosis is crossed with a guidewire. A balloon oversized by 15% of the vessel diameter is inflated at the stenosis. A typical renal artery balloon diameter is 5–7 mm. Heparin and antispasmodics such as nitroglycerin are administered. After balloon dilatation, the vessel is evaluated with a repeat contrast injection.

Angioplasty is considered successful if there is less than 30% residual stenosis, there is no dissection, and there is no persistent pressure gradient.

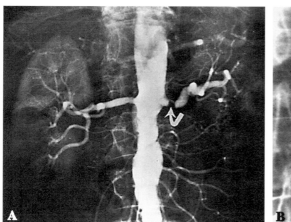
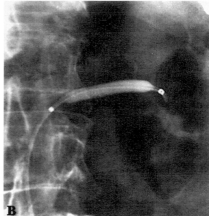
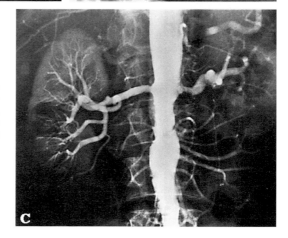

FIGURE 8.   Renal angioplasty. *A*, Abdominal aortogram demonstrates high-grade, proximal, left renal artery stenosis (curved arrow). *B*, Balloon dilatation of stenosis. *C*, Post-angioplasty demonstrates satisfactory result with less than 30% residual stenosis and no dissection.

30. How is the outcome of renal PTA for RVH classified?

A cure is a diastolic blood pressure ≤ 90 mm Hg with at least a 10 mm Hg decrease from pre-PTA levels. An improvement is a 15% decrease in diastolic pressure to a value < 110 mg Hg but > 90 mm Hg. A failure is defined as a less than 15% decrease in diastolic pressure with the diastolic pressure > 90 mm Hg, or a diastolic pressure > 110 mm Hg.

31. What is the success of renal artery PTA?

The technical success is 85–95%. The immediate benefit from hypertension is 90–100% for FMD and 80% for atherosclerotic disease. In one study, long-term follow-up 3 years after renal PTA demonstrated 80% of patients with cured or improved hypertension. FMD lesions respond more favorably to PTA than atherosclerotic lesions. Factors that predispose to PTA restenosis include atherosclerotic etiology, ostial location, and a residual post-PTA stenosis greater than 30%. Due to the high PTA restenosis rate of ostial lesions, alternative treatment such as surgery or stent placement should be considered.

32. What are the complications of renal PTA?

The overall complication rate is 5–10%. Complications include arterial rupture, thrombosis, dissection, peripheral renal embolus, renal failure, renal infarction, perinephric hematoma, and puncture-site hematoma.

33. When is renal intravascular stent placement indicated?

Stent placement is reserved for a suboptimal or failed angioplasty. Elastic recoil, residual stenosis > 30%, or dissection all constitute a suboptimal PTA result. The largest clinical experience worldwide in renal stent placement has been with the balloon-expandable Palmaz stent (Cordis-Johnson and Johnson Interventional Systems, Miami, FL). The stent is placed via a guiding catheter and is deployed with balloon inflation (Fig. 9). The short-term results of stent placement are encouraging, but ongoing clinical trials will define long-term patency rates, restenosis rates, and clinical benefit.

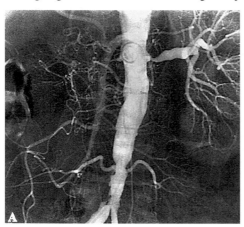 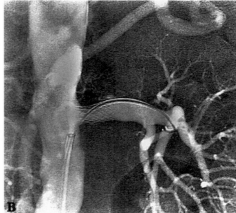

FIGURE 9. Solitary left kidney. A, Aortogram demonstrates proximal left renal artery stenosis. B, Post-stent angiogram demonstrates restored patency without dissection.

BIBLIOGRAPHY

1. Laragh JH, Brenner BM (eds): Hypertension: Pathophysiology, Diagnosis, and Management, 2nd ed. Philadelphia, Lippincott-Raven, 1995.
2. Muller FB, Sealey JE, Case DB, et al: The captopril test for identifying renovascular disease in hypertensive patients. Am J Med 80:633–644, 1986.
3. National Heart, Lung, and Blood Institute: Working Group on Renovascular Hypertension: Detection, evaluation, and treatment of renovascular hypertension. Final report. Arch Intern Med 147:820–829, 1987.
4. Roubidoux MA, Dunnick NR, Klotman PE, et al: Renal vein renins: Inability to predict response to revascularization in patients with hypertension. Radiology 178:819–822, 1991.

37. URINARY TRACT INFECTION

Douglas S. Katz, M.D.

1. Does a single, uncomplicated urinary tract infection in an adult need a radiologic workup?

No, especially if it occurs in a woman.

2. When should adult patients with urinary tract infections be imaged?

When conservative therapy (e.g., oral antibiotics) fails, when complications (e.g., abscess) are suspected, or when episodes of infection recur.

3. Which patients are predisposed to developing urinary tract infections?

Diabetics, patients with indwelling urinary catheters (e.g., Foley catheter, nephrostomy tube), and patients with structural abnormalities (e.g., ectopic ureter, duplication of the renal collecting system and ureter).

4. Is urinary tract infection spread hematogenously or by ascending in the urine?

Almost always by ascending in the urine (Fig. 1), although occasionally it may occur by hematogenous spread or by direct spread from adjacent structures (e.g., diverticulitis).

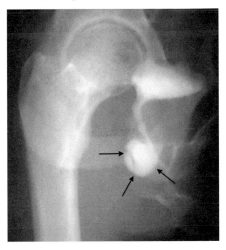

FIGURE 1. Oblique image from a voiding cystourethrogram shows a large diverticulum (arrows), which communicates with the urethra in this woman with recurrent urinary tract infections. The urethral diverticulum developed in the periurethral glands as a consequence of recurrent ascending infection.

5. What does uncomplicated pyelonephritis look like on ultrasound? On CT?

Patients with pyelonephritis often have completely normal imaging studies. However, wedge-shaped areas of decreased echogenicity may be seen on ultrasound in the kidneys. CT shows triangular areas of relatively decreased enhancement (Fig. 2).

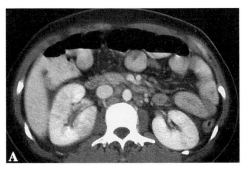 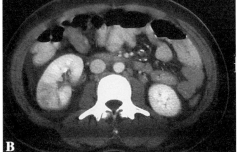

FIGURE 2. *A* and *B*, Acute pyelonephritis. The right kidney is swollen, and there are multiple wedge-shaped areas of decreased parenchymal enhancement.

6. What happens if renal infection progresses?

More pronounced areas of focal infection may occur and progress to form abscess(es).

7. What is the CT appearance of a renal abscess?

A mass-like area containing a central area that does not enhance with intravenous contrast. There is usually an enhancing wall, which may be associated with inflammatory changes in the adjacent tissue (inside or outside the kidney), and there may be direct spread of the abscess to the perinephric space.

8. How should a renal abscess be treated?

Small abscesses can be treated successfully with high-dose intravenous antibiotic therapy and possibly by simple needle aspiration. Large abscesses can be treated with a combination of intravenous antibiotics and percutaneous catheter drainage. Catheter drainage may be done with ultrasound or CT guidance.

9. **Cystitis is usually due to bacterial organisms ascending through the urethra. List some common noninfectious causes of cystitis.**
   Radiation
   Chemotherapy (especially cyclophosphamide)
   Eosinophilic cystitis

10. **What does cystitis look like on contrast studies? On ultrasound?**
    The bladder may be completely normal on imaging studies. Alternatively, the bladder mucosa may appear irregular on contrast studies (e.g., an IVP), and on ultrasound the bladder wall may be thickened and hypoechoic. This appearance may simulate a diffuse bladder tumor (Fig. 3).

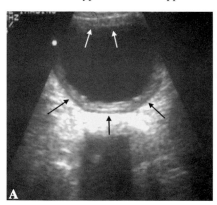 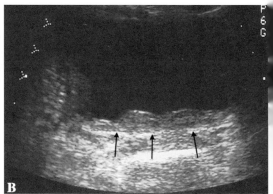

FIGURE 3. An 8-year-old boy with gross hematuria from cystitis secondary to adenovirus (*A*). (Case courtesy of Steven Perlmutter, M.D.) A different patient being treated with cyclophosphamide (B). Note the irregularly thickened bladder wall (arrows) in both patients.

11. **What is meant by the term *chronic pyelonephritis*?**
    The term is used to refer to patients who have suffered from chronic reflux of urine (from the bladder into the ureter and kidneys), usually with associated infection. The renal cortex may become atrophied in such patients, especially immediately opposite the upper and lower pole calyces.

12. **Which organisms cause gas-forming urinary tract infections?**
    Emphysematous pyelonephritis or cystitis is very uncommon and is associated with *Escherichia coli* infections, especially in diabetics. Patients are usually quite ill, and the infectious process may be life-threatening. Traditionally, emphysematous pyelonephritis, the most serious gas-forming infection in the urinary tract, was treated with nephrectomy, although some recent success has been reported with percutaneous drainage.

13. **What is the best study for suspected gas-forming infection in the urinary tract?**
    CT, although the diagnosis may be suspected or established on the basis of abnormal gas collections on plain films or ultrasound (Fig. 4).

14. **Which organisms cause both tiny abscesses in the kidneys and masses in the renal collecting system?**
    Fungal infections, especially with *Candida* sp. They are especially a problem in immunosuppressed patients. Fungal microabscesses can be seen on ultrasound or CT. Fungus balls may form in the renal collecting systems and ureters.

15. **Which infection causes calcifications to form in the wall of the bladder?**
    Schistosomiasis. The ureters may be involved, especially distally.

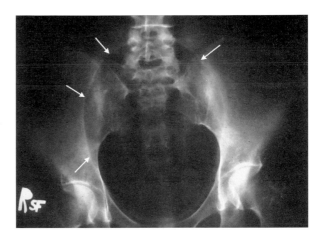

FIGURE 4. Emphysematous cystitis. The bladder is markedly distended and is filled with gas (arrows).

16. What are the imaging findings of urinary tract infection with tuberculosis?

Findings are usually unilateral/asymmetric:

Renal abscess, often with involvement of the perinephric space and the psoas muscle (acute phase)

Papillary necrosis

Strictures of the collecting system

Strictures of the ureter, which may have skip areas ("corkscrew ureter") or be continuous ("pipestem ureter") (Fig. 5)

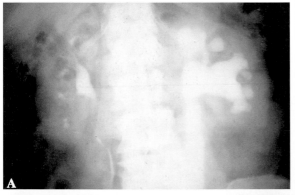

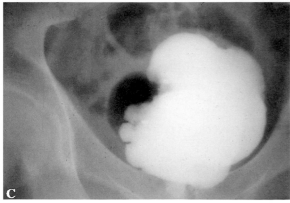

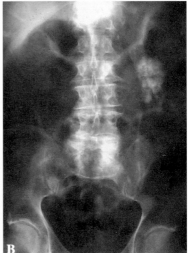

FIGURE 5. *A*, Intravenous pyelography shows strictures of the upper pole collecting system, dilatation of the collecting system and proximal ureter. *B*, Chronic tuberculosis. A "putty kidney," a small, calcified (autoinfarcted) left kidney is seen on this plain film. The left ureter is calcified. *C*, Cystography of a patient with tuberculosis of the bladder. The bladder contour is lobulated; there are pseudodiverticula secondary to fibrosis of the bladder wall. (Courtesy of Steven Perlmutter, M.D.)

Calcifications in the kidney and proximal ureter
Calcifications in the perinephric space and psoas muscle
Shrunken, heavily calcified, nonfunctioning kidney (autonephrectomy)

BIBLIOGRAPHY

1. Davidson AJ, Hartman DS (eds): Radiology of the Urinary Tract, 2nd ed. Philadelphia, W.B. Saunders, 1994.
2. Dunnick NR, McCallum RW, Sandler CM: Textbook of Uroradiology, 2nd ed. Baltimore, Williams & Wilkins, 1997.
3. Soulen MC, Fishman EK, Goldman SM, et al: Bacterial renal infections: Role of CT. Radiology 171:703, 1989.

38. URINARY TRACT TUMORS

Douglas S. Katz, M.D., and Steven Perlmutter, M.D.

1. What is the most common renal mass?

The most common renal mass is a simple cyst. They are more common in older patients and are found in approximately half the population over 50 years of age. Renal cysts are rarely clinically significant.

2. What is the best way to confirm that a renal mass is a simple cyst?

Ultrasound. The ultrasound appearance of a simple cyst is that of a round or oval mass with a paper thin wall, smooth margins, no internal echoes, and good through transmission, which means that more sound waves reach the tissues behind the cyst because they are not stopped by the fluid in the cyst.

3. Renal cysts are often detected incidentally on CT. What are the CT criteria for a simple cyst (Fig. 1)?

Analogous to the ultrasound criteria, a simple cyst should have an imperceptible or barely perceptible wall, and its contents should have a uniform low-density appearance, with Hounsfield unit measurements of 20 or less (i.e., close to water density). There should be no septations in the cyst, no associated calcification or soft-tissue mass, and no enhancement of the cyst.

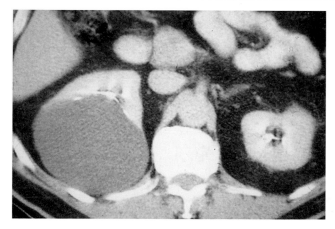

FIGURE 1. Large simple right renal cyst on contrast-enhanced CT. Note that the cyst wall is barely perceptible and that the density of the cyst is uniformly low compared with the normal adjacent renal parenchyma.

4. If a known or suspected renal mass is evaluated by CT, what should be done?

The CT should be performed using thin sections (e.g., 5 mm), and images should be obtained both before and after intravenous contrast. A renal cyst will not enhance after contrast administration;

thus Hounsfield unit measurements of the cyst's contents should be the same before and after contrast is given.

5. What if a mass fulfills all the criteria for a simple cyst but is denser than 20 Hounsfield units?

The cyst is most likely a hyperdense cyst. It either contains blood or proteinaceous (also called milk of calcium). Ultrasound should be performed to confirm that it is a simple cyst; hyperdense cysts on CT often appear as simple cysts on ultrasound. Alternatively, if Hounsfield unit measurements of the cyst's contents do not change before and after contrast, a hyperdense cyst is confirmed.

6. Can a renal cancer contain cystic areas (Fig. 2)?

Yes. There may be significant overlap in the appearance of a renal cell carcinoma and benign processes, (e.g., a complex cyst). The best way to analyze a renal mass (regardless of how it is initially detected) is to perform thin CT sections through the mass before and after intravenous contrast administration. The more complex the lesion (e.g., a mass with multiple septations that are thick and enhancing or the presence of enhancing soft-tissue elements) the more likely it is malignant. Depending on the CT appearance, a decision can be made whether to remove the lesion. Unfortunately, despite the best radiologic workup, there will be renal masses that are indeterminate for malignancy and have to be removed.

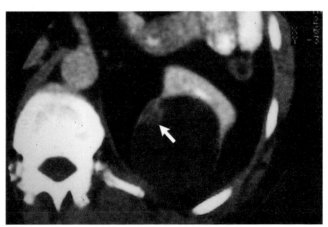

FIGURE 2. In contrast to the image shown in question 3, note the enhancing mural nodule (arrow) in this cystic renal cell carcinoma discovered in a 49-year-old man with microscopic hematuria.

7. A 60-year-old patient presents with hematuria (microscopic or macroscopic). Which radiologic test should be performed to exclude malignancy (Fig. 3)?

This seems like a simple question, but it is not. Some institutions perform intravenous pyelography (IVP) on all such patients; others go directly to a CT scan of the abdomen and pelvis. The CT scan should be performed with and without intravenous contrast; ideally, the bladder should be distended with urine to optimize detection of a bladder tumor; and delayed images should be obtained where appropriate (e.g., of the ureters and bladder). Unfortunately, even the best performed CT scan does not exclude a small bladder tumor, and cystoscopy is mandatory with persistent hematuria of unknown origin. Small carcinomas arising from the pelvocalyceal systems and the ureters (usually transitional cell carcinomas) may be better detected on an IVP than on CT.

8. Do any chronic or inherited conditions predispose a patient to developing a renal cell carcinoma?

Yes. Patients on long term dialysis are at risk for developing renal cell carcinoma. Individuals with the rare von Hippel Lindau syndrome often develop multiple renal cancers. A small percentage of other patients are afflicted by an inherited form of renal cell carcinoma in the absence of a syndrome; however, most renal cell cancers are sporadic.

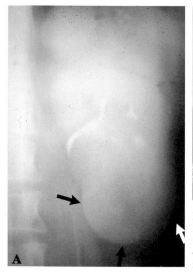

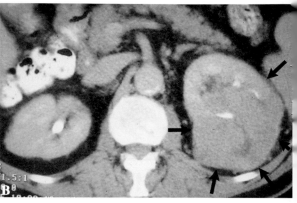

FIGURE 3. *A*, Tomogram from an intravenous pyelography in a 52-year-old man shows a mass in the lower pole of the left kidney (arrows), with lucent central areas. This renal cell cancer was subsequently resected. *B*, CT image shows a left renal cell cancer (arrows) in a different patient. Note the deformity of the collecting system.

9. Why is renal cell cancer called the internist's tumor?

Because the tumor may present with a variety of vague signs and symptoms, which may be systemic, such as fever, gastrointestinal symptoms, weight loss. Occasionally, it may present with erythrocytosis. Only in a relatively small percentage of cases is the classic triad of hematuria, flank pain, and a palpable renal mass present.

10. What is the basic staging system for renal cell cancer?

Stage I	Tumor confined to the renal capsule.
Stage II	Tumor extends through the renal capsule but is contained by the perinephric fascia.
Stage III	Tumor invades the main renal vein (and may extend into the inferior vena cava) and/or has metastasized to local lymph nodes, but is otherwise contained by the perinephric fascia.
Stage IV	Tumor has extended through the perinephric fascia to invade adjacent organs and/or metastasized to distant organs.

11. To which organs does renal cell cancer typically metastasize (Fig. 4)?

The lungs and bones. Lung lesions usually consist of multiple nodules (a miliary pattern), or less often a solitary nodule or lymphangitic infiltrates. A single pulmonary metastasis can be resected. Bone metastases from renal cell carcinoma are typically lytic and may expand the bone. Because renal cell cancer is highly vascular, metastases have a tendency to bleed.

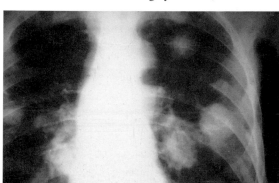

FIGURE 4. Large metastases are seen on the chest radiograph of this 69-year-old man with renal cell carcinoma.

12. What imaging test, other than CT, helps to stage renal cancer?

MR. A renal mass may be imaged in multiple planes, and vascular invasion can be assessed. MR can be used as a problem-solving tool after initial CT staging or as an alternative to CT in patients who cannot receive intravenous contrast.

13. CT shows multiple solid renal masses. What are the diagnostic possibilities (Fig. 5)?

Although unusual, multiple primary renal cancers may occur. More likely, this finding may represent metastatic disease. If multiple, relatively low-density masses are present, lymphoma is a likely diagnosis; usually, the CT shows other evidence of lymphoma on the CT.

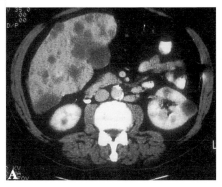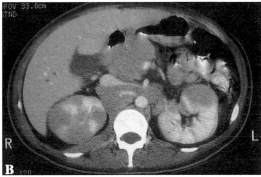

FIGURE 5. *A,* A 58-year-old man with metastatic lung cancer. Numerous liver lesions are demonstrated on this CT image, as well as metastases to both kidneys. *B,* Multiple relatively low-density lesions are seen in the kidneys in a different patient with lymphoma. There is also tumor surrounding the aorta and in the peripancreatic region.

14. A small (e.g., 2 cm) enhancing renal mass is discovered incidentally on a CT scan in an elderly patient. What should be done (Fig. 6)?

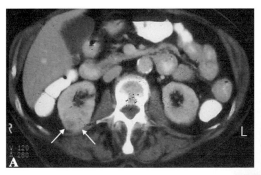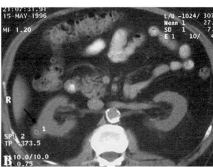

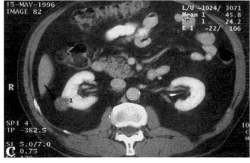

FIGURE 6. *A,* Elderly woman with a small mass in the right kidney, consistent with renal cell cancer (arrows). Note that the mass enhances heterogeneously. *B* and *C,* CT evaluation of a small exophytic right renal mass in a different patient, detected incidentally on abdominal sonography. Pre-contrast image (*B*) reveals the mass (arrows), which has a density of 27 Hounsfield units. After contrast administration (*C*), the mass enhances to 46 Hounsfield units, consistent with renal cell carcinoma.

Another seemingly straightforward question that is the source of a fair amount of controversy. Some authors advocate surgery for such lesions, unless the patient is very elderly or is a poor surgical risk. In these situations, a watchful approach is recommended because small renal cancers that do not grow significantly on follow-up studies tend to be low grade and are unlikely to become a subsequent clinical problem.

15. How does a transitional cell cancer appear on imaging studies (Fig. 7)?

On cross-sectional imaging studies or on an IVP, transitional cell cancer usually appears as a filling defect in the renal collecting system, ureter, or bladder. The filling defect may be polypoid, more sessile, or irregular. A relatively small percentage of transitional cell cancers contain calcifications. Transitional cell cancer in the renal pelvis may invade the renal parenchyma; it tends to infiltrate the kidney rather than form the focal renal mass seen with renal cell carcinomas.

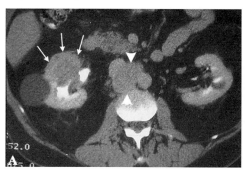 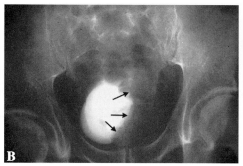

FIGURE 7. *A*, Elderly man with gross hematuria and a history of transitional cell carcinoma of the bladder. CT image shows a central mass in the right kidney, representing a metachronous transitional cell carcinoma (arrows) and an adjacent simple cyst. Metastatic lymphadenopathy is noted between the aorta and inferior vena cava (arrowheads). *B*, A different 57-year-old man with a nonfunctioning left kidney on intravenous pyelography (not shown) due to obstruction of the left ureter from a left bladder transitional cell cancer (arrows).

16. What are the major risk factors for transitional cell cancer (TCC)?

Smoking and occupational exposure to some chemicals (certain dyes). TCC has a strong tendency to be multifocal and to recur. TCC is, therefore, often treated by resection of the kidney, ureter, and a cuff of bladder from the involved side. It is much more common in men than in women.

17. What determines the resectability of a bladder TCC?

Superficial tumors are usually resectable either cystoscopically or by partial cystsectomy. Once the tumor extends deeply into the muscular wall of the bladder, a total cystectomy, irradiation, and/or chemotherapy is usually required. Cystectomy is generally not performed if there is an extension beyond the bladder (Fig. 8).

18. Which radiographic studies are useful in staging bladder cancer (Fig. 9)?

Unfortunately, although CT is fairly accurate in detecting bladder cancers that are not small (e.g., > 1 cm), it is inaccurate in determining the degree of local invasion. MR has also been disappointing. CT is useful in detecting extension of bladder tumor to local structures, determining whether pelvic lymphadenopathy is present, and for discovering metastatic disease. When there is bone pain or elevated alkaline phosphatase, bone scans are useful in detecting body metastases.

19. How can TCC in the bladder be distinguished from clot on ultrasound (Fig. 10)?

Blood clots tend to be more echogenic than bladder tumors and unlike tumors they can move when the patient changes position. Color Doppler may show blood flow in a bladder tumor but not in a blood clot. Also, blood clots in the urinary tract tend to lyse over a few days because of naturally occurring urokinase.

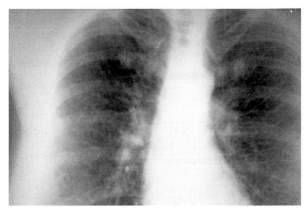

FIGURE 8. A 55-year-old woman with lymphangitic spread of transitional cell cancer in the lungs. Note the fine reticular interstitial pattern present throughout the lungs on this chest radiograph.

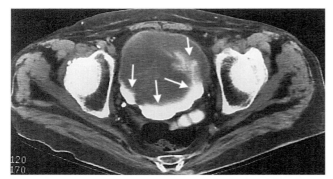

FIGURE 9. CT image shows a large transitional cancer almost completely filling the bladder. Brighter areas (arrows) represent the residual bladder lumen.

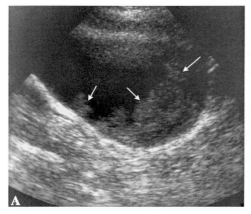
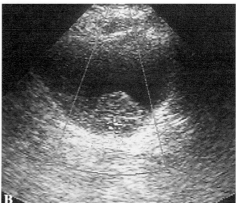

FIGURE 10. A 53-year-old man with hematuria following a recent renal transplant. Ultrasound reveals irregular tissue in the bladder (arrows, *A*). Doppler interrogation reveals flow in tissue (*B*, brighter areas correspond to flow that was present on original color image) consistent with tumor as opposed to clot.

20. Are there any other bladder tumors besides TCC (Fig. 11)?

There are a variety of unusual tumors of the bladder, both benign and malignant. The benign tumors include papillomas, smooth muscle tumors, and granulomas (such as from BCG instillation in the bladder as a treatment for superficial bladder cancer). Adenocarcinoma of the bladder is associated with congenital abnormalities including bladder extrophy and urachal diverticula. Sarcoma, lymphoma, and metastases may also involve the bladder.

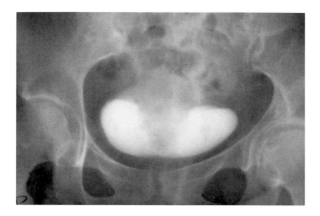

FIGURE 11. Delayed image of the bladder from an intravenous pyelogram demonstrates a large, irregular filling defect in the bladder of this 39-year-old woman. Pathologic examination of the mass revealed the lesion to be a nephrogenic adenoma, an unusual benign bladder tumor.

21. An Egyptian male presents with hematuria and a bladder mass. Calcification is seen on plain films and CT in the bladder wall. What is the likely diagnosis?

Squamous cell cancer of the bladder, due to chronic schistosomiasis.

22. A patient presents with mucus in the urine. What is a likely diagnosis (Fig. 12)?

Carcinoma of the urachus. The finding of mucinous cells in the urine is highly suggestive of this unusual diagnosis. Urachal tumors sit on the anterosuperior aspect of the bladder. The urachus is the remnant of the obliterated allantois, which runs from the bladder roof to the umbilicus. Urachal cancers are usually highly malignant adenocarcinomas that are often calcified on CT.

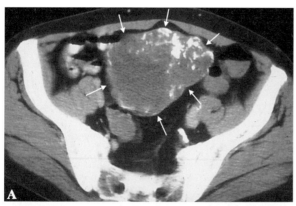

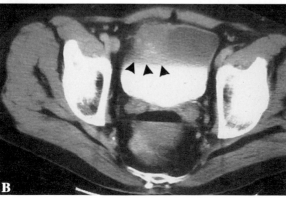

FIGURE 12. Complex, relatively low-density mass contains multiple areas of calcification (a, arrows) in a 60-year-old man with recurrent urinary tract infections. The mass is located at the anterosuperior aspect of the bladder (bladder is shown filled with contrast on the delayed image in B; bottom of mass: arrowheads). Diagnosis: urachal carcinoma.

23. A patient presents with repeated episodes of flushing, hypertension, and syncope while voiding. What is the likely diagnosis?

Pheochromocytoma of the bladder. This unusual location for a pheochromocytoma has a characteristic presentation—micturition syncope. Usually pheochromocytomas arise from the adrenal medulla. When they ensue from the sympathetic chain outside the adrenal gland they are more correctly called paragangliomas.

24. An echogenic mass is found incidentally on sonography in a middle-aged woman. CT performed to evaluate the mass shows that the majority of the lesion is composed of fat. What is the diagnosis (Fig. 13)?

Angiomyolipoma. These benign, uncommon tumors are usually found as solitary lesions in middle-aged women. They are composed of smooth muscle, fat, and blood vessels with thick walls. The presence of fat on CT (e.g., minus 30 Hounsfield unit measurement obtained in the mass) is diagnostic of an angiomyolipoma. Angiomyolipomas are usually asymptomatic, but when they become large they may present with flank pain and retroperitoneal bleeding. For this reason, large angiomyolipomas are often resected.

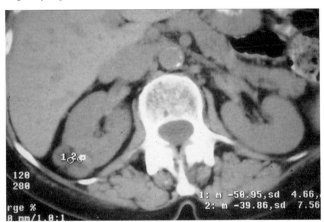

FIGURE 13. Unenhanced CT image reveals a mass in the right kidney in this asymptomatic middle-aged woman (CT was performed to confirm nature of mass, which was detected as an echogenic lesion on a sonogram performed to evaluate the right upper quadrant of the abdomen). Density measurements of the mass confirm the presence of fat (–40 to –60 Hounsfield units), consistent with an angiomyolipoma.

25. A 15-year-old has mental retardation, skin lesions, and multiple fatty masses in the kidneys on CT. What is the diagnosis (Fig. 14)?

Multiple renal angiomyolipomas due to tuberous sclerosis, an inherited disease characterized by mental retardation and skin lesions. Patients with this disease have hamartomas in various organs.

FIGURE 14. Multiple bilateral angiomyolipomas in this patient with tuberous sclerosis.

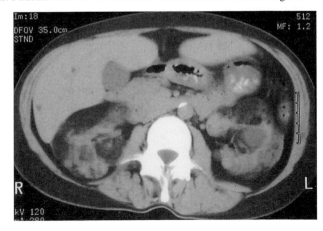

26. A 23-year-old woman has an incidentally detected left renal upper pole mass, which on T1-weighted MR images is relatively low in signal intensity. What benign mass has this appearance (Fig. 15)?

Oncocytoma. Unfortunately, there is too much overlap on cross-sectional imaging studies to distinguish them from renal cell carcinomas, and resection is necessary. If this benign neoplasm is suspected, the surgeon may opt to resect the tumor only and not remove the entire kidney, as is generally done for renal cell cancer.

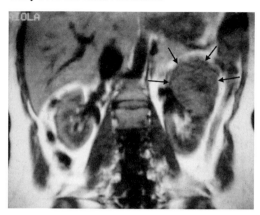

FIGURE 15. Sagittal T1-weighted MR image in this 23-year-old pregnant woman shows a mass in the upper pole of the left kidney (arrows). The lesion was later proven to be an oncocytoma.

27. What is the most common sarcoma of the kidney?

Leiomyosarcoma. Although sarcomas comprise only a few percent of renal tumors, leiomyosarcomas are most frequent. They may arise from the renal capsule at the periphery of the kidney or from the smooth muscle of vessels within the renal parenchyma.

28. What is the most common renal malignancy of childhood?

Wilms' tumor. This tumor is rare in adults. They have a poorer prognosis than in children. Children with Wilms' tumors may have sporadic hypoplasia of the iris, enlargement of the organs on one side of the body (hemihypertrophy), and various genitourinary developmental disorders.

29. What rare retroperitoneal developmental malformation tends to cross tissue boundaries and may involve the kidneys? (Hint: when this entity occurs in the neck of a fetus, it may be associated with Turner's syndrome.)

Lymphangioma. Its radiographic appearance is that of an elongated mass that tend to cross compartments of the retroperitoneum and may have a single cystic compartment or be multiseptated.

BIBLIOGRAPHY

1. Birnbaum BA, Jacobs JA, Ramchandi P: Multiphasic renal CT: Comparison of renal mass enhancement during the corticomedullary and nephrographic phases. Radiology 200:753–758, 1996.
2. Cohan RH, et al: Renal masses: Assessment of corticomedullary-phase and nephrographic-phase CT scans. Radiology 196:445–451, 1995.
3. Davidson AJ, Hartman DS (eds): Radiology of the Urinary Tract, 2nd ed. Philadelphia, W.B. Saunders, 1994.
4. Davidson AJ, Hartman DS, Choyke PL, et al: Radiologic assessment of renal masses: Implications for patient care. Radiology 202:297–305, 1997.
5. Dunnick NR, McCallum RW, Sandler CM: Textbook of Uroradiology, 2nd ed. Baltimore, Williams & Wilkins, 1997.
6. Johnson CD, Dunnick NR, Cohan RH, et al: Renal adenocarcinoma: CT staging of 100 tumors. AJR 148:59–63, 1987.
7. McClennan BL, Deyoe LA: Imaging evaluation of renal cell carcinoma: Diagnosis and staging. Radiol Clin North Am 32:55, 1994.
8. Silverman SG, et al: Small renal masses: Correlation of spiral CT features and pathologic findings. AJR 163:597–605, 1994.

39. RENAL TRANSPLANT IMAGING

Douglas S. Katz, M.D.

1. Which radiologic tests are useful in working up a patient who wants to donate a kidney for transplantation?

Traditionally, intravenous urography (also called intravenous pyelography) and renal angiography are performed on a potential living renal donor.

2. What information do these tests provide?

The transplant surgeon wants to know the anatomy of the kidney before the donor is brought to the operating room. Many surgeons prefer to transplant the left kidney; the left renal vein is easier to anastomose than the right renal vein because the left renal vein is longer. However, if a significant variation of the left kidney is discovered, such as a duplicated renal collecting system, the right kidney is transplanted.

3. What normal variations in renal vascular anatomy are important to discover preoperatively?

Variations in renal vascular anatomy are common. It is important for the surgeon to know in advance whether a normal variation of renal venous anatomy is present—for example, a left renal vein that goes behind the aorta or a circumaortic renal vein (that encircles the aorta). Otherwise the surgeon may inadvertently transect the vein.

4. How common are accessory renal arteries?

Very common. One or more may be present. The renal artery also may bifurcate early after its origin (prehilar branching), or it may be duplicated. The surgeon needs to know this in advance; otherwise, the arterial supply to a portion of the kidney may be disrupted.

5. What findings on an intravenous urogram preclude a potential renal donor from further consideration?

Discovery of an asymptomatic urinary tract tumor, such as a renal or a bladder cancer, or demonstration of a significant renal anomaly such as absence of one kidney or a horseshoe kidney (both kidneys are fused across the midline along their lower poles). The presence of significant stone disease also may exclude someone as a renal donor.

6. Angiography is a relatively invasive examination. Is there an alternative to performing renal angiography on potential living renal donors?

Yes. Recently, computed tomographic angiography has shown promise as an alternative examination to both renal angiography and intravenous urography. Thin cross-sectional images of the kidneys are obtained with a spiral (helical) CT scanner, as intravenous contrast is rapidly administered through a large-gauge peripheral intravenous catheter. The CT images show the renal vascular anatomy, including normal variations such as accessory renal arteries. Additional images of the kidneys, ureters, and bladder are also obtained as contrast passes through the urinary tract.

7. Which imaging tests are routinely performed immediately after a renal transplantation is completed?

Depending on the preference of the surgeon and/or the institution, nuclear imaging (renal scan) or ultrasound is performed (in selected instances, both may be performed). Both studies serve as a baseline for comparison with future examinations, especially if a problem develops. In addition, immediate posttransplantation complications are identified. A renal scan gives more physiologic information than an ultrasound, but the ultrasound demonstrates the anatomy more effectively. To perform a renal scan, a radiopharmaceutical agent is injected intravenously (usually DTPA tagged with technetium), and multiple images of the transplant are obtained. Initially, the perfusion to the transplant is evaluated as the agent reaches the transplant. Images are then obtained as the kidney excretes the agent into the collecting system and bladder.

8. Why is the gamma camera (nuclear medicine camera) placed over the patient's Foley catheter bag at the end of a renal transplant scan?
To check for radioactivity in the urine, which is expected if urine is excreted by the transplant.

9. What information does the radiologist need to know before scanning a patient in the immediate posttransplant period?
The radiologist needs to know basic information about the transplant—where the transplant is located and whether it was obtained from a cadaver or a living person. Some surgeons now transplant both kidneys from a cadaveric donor; obviously it is important to know this information before scanning a patient.

10. What group of patients may receive both renal and pancreatic transplants?
Diabetics. This type of transplant surgery is performed at selected centers. The combined transplant comes from a cadaver. Typically, the pancreas and a short segment of small bowel are anastomosed to the bladder. The pancreatic transplant can be imaged by both nuclear medicine and ultrasound techniques.

11. Which complications of renal transplantation occur in the immediate postoperative period?

Acute tubular necrosis (ATN)	Renal vein thrombosis
Rejection	Urine leak
Renal arterial thrombosis	

12. What is the classic finding on a nuclear renal scan in acute tubular necrosis?
The classic finding of ATN (which typically affects cadaveric kidney transplants) is a discrepancy between flow and function. Flow is relatively preserved (as is seen on the early images), but poor function is seen on the later images.

13. On follow-up renal nuclear scans, how can acute tubular necrosis and problems such as rejection be distinguished?
ATN typically improves, whereas with other problems, such as rejection, both flow and function may be decreased.

14. What are other potential causes of decreased flow and function on nuclear renal scans?
Renal arterial or venous thrombosis. If these diagnoses are suspected, urgent additional evaluation is indicated, because viability of the transplant is threatened.

15. How does a large active urine leak appear on a nuclear renal scan?
A photopenic defect adjacent to the kidney or bladder may initially be seen; it then fills in with activity.

16. How is a renal transplant ultrasound performed (Fig. 1)? How does a normal transplant appear on ultrasound?
The kidney is identified and measured, and the flow within the kidney is examined with color and power Doppler. Then the main renal artery and vein are identified and flow within them is evaluated. When the bladder is examined with color Doppler, a jet of color coming from the transplanted ureter shows that urine is passing normally out of the ureter. Small fluid collections around the transplanted kidney are expected immediately after surgery.

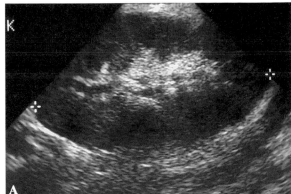

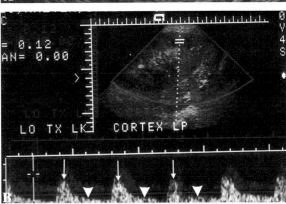

FIGURE 1. Normal sonographic appearance of a renal transplant (*A*). There is normal flow, with both a systolic (arrows) and a diastolic (arrowheads) component, in the segmental renal artery which is being sampled with Doppler in *B*.

17. An ultrasound performed on a patient who received a renal transplant several weeks ago reveals a large collection surrounding the kidney (Fig. 2). What is the differential diagnosis?

The collection may represent a hematoma, abscess, urinoma, or lymphocele. Depending on the clinical context, aspiration of the collection may be indicated to determine its nature, especially if infection is suspected. Aspiration can be performed easily by the radiologist under ultrasound guidance.

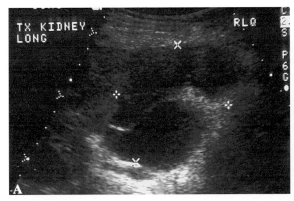

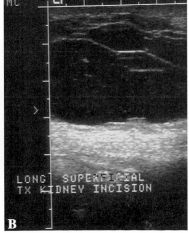

FIGURE 2. Complex collection adjacent to the transplanted kidney both inferiorly (*A*) and anteriorly (*B*). Patient complained of fever and pain. Diagnosis: lymphocele.

18. What ultrasound findings may indicate rejection (Fig. 3)?

Loss of the normal corticomedullary differentiation

Prominence of the renal pyramids

Decreased diastolic flow

Swelling of the mucosa of the collecting system and ureter

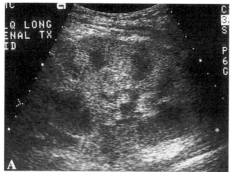
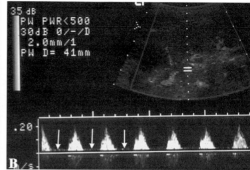

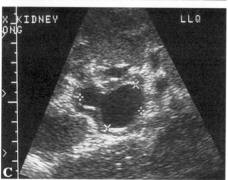

FIGURE 3.   Manifestations of acute rejection on sonography. In contrast to the appearance of the transplant in question 16, note the prominent renal pyramids, loss of corticomedullary differentiation, increased echogenicity, and abnormal appearing central renal sinus fat (*A*). Segmental renal arterial waveform has lost normal diastolic component (arrows, *B*). In a different patient (*C*), note thickening of the renal sinus mucosa due to edema (noted by x signs).

19. Are these findings specific for rejection?

Unfortunately not. Many of these signs may be due to one or more other causes, such as cyclosporine toxicity.

20. How is the diagnosis of rejection made more conclusively?

By renal biopsy. Clinical and laboratory evidence pointing to rejection, along with ultrasound findings, usually prompt an urgent biopsy.

21. What are the advantages of performing a renal transplant biopsy under ultrasound guidance?

The transplanted kidney is visualized under real-time guidance. The exact biopsy site—usually the cortex of the lower pole—can be targeted precisely, and the needle can be kept away from major vascular structures.

22. Obstruction of the transplanted kidney is suspected. What are the ultrasound findings of obstruction?

Mild dilatation of the renal collecting system is often seen in normal transplants. However, significant dilatation of the collecting system may represent obstruction (e.g., from a blood clot or ureteral stenosis).

23. A renal transplant patient develops hypertension, and stenosis of the transplanted renal artery is suspected. What ultrasound finding suggests the diagnosis?

The velocity in the renal artery should be measured with Doppler ultrasound near its anastomosis. A velocity significantly above 2 meters/sec suggests the diagnosis. Other techniques for evaluating suspected renal artery stenosis include MR angiography and CT angiography. For definitive diagnosis and therapy, conventional angiography should be performed. If significant stenosis is identified, angioplasty can be attempted.

24. What sign of chronic renal transplant rejection may be seen on plain films or CT (Fig. 4)?
Occasionally, calcifications in a chronically rejected renal transplant can be seen.

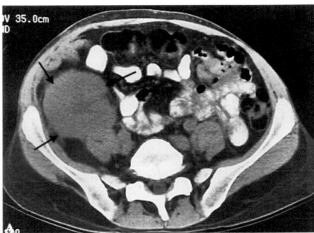

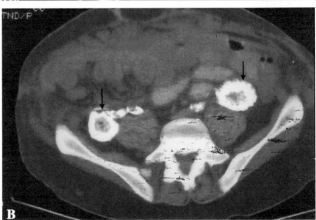

FIGURE 4. *A*, CT performed with oral contrast only shows a normal-appearing renal transplant in the right lower quadrant (arrows). *B*, CT image in a different patient with chronic transplant rejection, shows calcified, small bilateral renal transplants (arrows).

BIBLIOGRAPHY

1. Dubovsky EV, Russel CD, Erbas B: Radionuclide evaluation of renal transplants. Semin Nucl Med 25:49, 1995.
2. Genkins SM, Sanfillipo FP, Carroll BA: Duplex Doppler sonography of renal transplants: Lack of sensitivity and specificity in establishing pathologic diagnosis. AJR 152:535–539, 1989.
3. Grenier N, Douws C, Morel D, et al: Detection of vascular complications in renal allografts with color Doppler flow imaging. Radiology 178:217–223, 1991.
4. Orons PD, Zajko AB: Angiography and interventional aspects of renal transplantation. Radiol Clin North Am 33:461, 1995.
5. Rubin GD, Alfrey EA, Dake MD, et al: Assessment of living renal donors with spiral CT. Radiology 195:457–462, 1995.
6. Spring DB, Salvatierro O Jr, Palubinskas AJ, et al: Results and significance of angiography in potential kidney donors. Radiology 133:45–47, 1979.
7. Tublin ME, Dodd GD III: Sonography of renal transplantation. Radiol Clin North Am 33:447, 1995.

40. IMAGING OF THE ADRENAL GLANDS

Ali M. Gharagozloo, M.D., and Douglas S. Katz, M.D.

1. What clinical situations warrant imaging of the adrenal glands?
• Detection of metastases to the adrenal glands in patients with known primary neoplasms
• Assessment of patients with clinical and biochemical evidence suspicious for a hormone-producing mass
• Further characterization of an incidentally discovered adrenal mass.

2. Which imaging modalities are most often used in the evaluation of the adrenals?
CT, MRI, and, in neonates, ultrasound.

3. What is the best initial radiologic test for evaluating the adrenals?
CT. Although most adrenal masses are detectable on 10-mm contiguous axial images, for optimal evaluation thinner images (e.g., 5 mm) are obtained. Ultrasound is used mainly for evaluation of the adrenal glands in infants (e.g., rule out hemorrhage, neuroblastoma), because the paucity of retroperitoneal fat and the large size of the glands relative to the surrounding structures make them much more visible than in older children or adults.

4. What role does MRI play in the work-up of adrenal masses?
Although rarely used in the initial evaluation of the adrenal glands, MRI may help to characterize adrenal masses in more detail if CT is equivocal.

5. What other radiologic studies can be used to evaluate the adrenal glands?
Adrenal venous sampling, arteriography, and nuclear medicine are reserved for specific problem cases. Adrenal biopsy, usually performed under CT guidance, may be required in certain cases for definitive diagnosis.

6. What is the normal appearance of the adrenal glands on CT?
The adrenal glands may assume various shapes, including linear, triangular, H, or inverted Y, V, or L configurations. Each adrenal limb has straight or convex borders, may measure up to 4 cm in length, and normally should measure < 10 mm in thickness.

7. In which anatomic compartment of the retroperitoneum do the adrenal glands reside? What is their relationship to the surrounding structures?
The adrenal glands lie within the perirenal space (Fig. 1) near the upper pole of each kidney. The right adrenal gland is posterior to the right lobe of the liver and adjacent to the inferior vena cava. The left adrenal gland is anteromedial to the left kidney and lateral to the aorta and left crus of the diaphragm. Each adrenal gland is fixed to Gerota's fascia.

8. How can large adrenal masses be distinguished from upper pole renal masses?
It is difficult on axial CT images to distinguish a large adrenal mass from a large upper pole renal mass. It may be easier to make this distinction on MRI, because such a mass can be scanned in multiple planes (e.g., coronal and axial), although reformations in multiple planes can be performed on a spiral (helical) CT scanner. The location of the center of the mass and the displacement of nearby structures are helpful clues. For instance, a mass that displaces the inferior vena cava and the retroperitoneal fat anteriorly and the right kidney inferolaterally is more likely of adrenal than renal or hepatic origin.

9. What adjacent structures can simulate adrenal pathology?
Any nearby normal (or pathologic) structure can produce an adrenal pseudotumor. On the left, an accessory spleen, a tortuous splenic vessel, tumors of the pancreatic tail or left kidney, and a

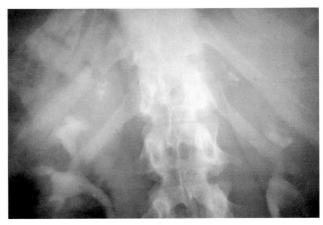

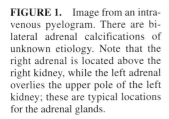

FIGURE 1. Image from an intravenous pyelogram. There are bilateral adrenal calcifications of unknown etiology. Note that the right adrenal is located above the right kidney, while the left adrenal overlies the upper pole of the left kidney; these are typical locations for the adrenal glands.

nearby unopacified loop of bowel are among the structures that can simulate adrenal pathology. Causes of right adrenal pseudotumors include renal and hepatic neoplasms and tortuous renal vessels.

10. How can adrenal pseudotumors be distinguished from true adrenal masses?

In most cases, careful inspection of the slices above and below the region in question reveals the contiguity of a pseudotumor with its site of origin. Liberal use of oral contrast to opacify the lumen of any nearby viscus and intravenous contrast to evaluate the enhancement pattern of the pseudotumor helps to clarify most problem cases.

11. How is the diagnosis of Cushing's syndrome initially established?

The diagnosis is initially made by clinical presentation, low-dose dexamethasone suppression test, and 24-hour urine cortisol levels.

12. What is the most common cause of Cushing's syndrome?

Eighty percent of cases are caused by bilateral adrenal hyperplasia due to an adrenocorticotropic hormone (ACTH)-producing pituitary adenoma (Cushing's disease), which is diagnosed clinically by virtue of its suppression with high-dose dexamethasone administration. Patients usually do not require imaging of the adrenal glands but should receive an MRI of the pituitary gland to localize the adenoma before surgical resection.

13. What are less common causes of Cushing's syndrome?

Fifteen percent of cases are due to an autonomous (but benign) adenoma of the adrenal. This diagnosis is suspected from the lack of suppression of ACTH even with high doses of dexamethasone. CT, using thin sections, is performed to localize the adenoma. Ectopic production of ACTH by a nonpituitary tumor such as a small cell lung cancer is rare; adrenal cortical carcinoma accounts for most of the remaining cases of Cushing's syndrome.

14. How does an adrenal adenoma appear on CT? What about adrenal hyperplasia?

Adrenal adenomas whether functional or not, appear as a focal low-density mass with biconvex margins (Fig. 2). The contralateral gland is either normal or atrophic (from suppression by a contralateral functioning adenoma). Aldosteronomas are typically smaller than cortisol-producing adrenal adenomas, but they cannot be reliably distinguished by CT alone. **Adrenal hyperplasia** may present as smooth or nodular thickening of the adrenal limbs. Because adrenal hyperplasia is often secondary to a systemic process, these findings are bilateral, and, in contrast with an adenoma, the overall configuration of the gland is maintained. Nearly 50% of hyperplastic adrenal glands have a normal CT appearance, because marked thickening must occur before it is detectable by imaging.

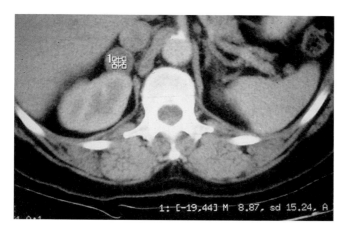

FIGURE 2. Image from a CT scan of a 62-year-old with lung cancer. There is a small incidental right adrenal lesion, the density of which is less than 10, consistent with an adenoma.

15. What is Conn's syndrome?

In 1955 Conn described a syndrome of primary hyperaldosteronism with hypokalemia, hypertension, elevated serum aldosterone, and low serum renin levels. Low serum renin levels distinguish primary hyperaldosteronism from renovascular or secondary hyperaldosteronism.

16. What are the two main causes of Conn's syndrome? Why is it important to distinguish the two?

Eighty percent of primary aldosteronism is caused by an adrenal adenoma. The remaining 20% is caused by adrenal hyperplasia. Adrenal carcinomas rarely produce enough aldosterone to cause Conn's syndrome. Imaging is critical, because aldosteronomas are managed surgically; whereas hyperplasia is managed medically. If thin-section CT does not reveal a mass, an aldosteronoma is still not excluded and adrenal venous sampling should be considered.

17. What are the clinical features of adrenal carcinoma?

Adrenal carcinoma is rare but highly malignant, with a zero percent 5-year survival rate. The tumor typically presents in the fifth decade of life. Because of inefficient hormone production by malignant cells, adrenal carcinomas are typically large (> 6 cm), and only 50% have clinical evidence of hyperfunction at presentation.

18. What are the major hormonal manifestations of adrenal carcinoma?

Cushing's syndrome, virilization, and feminization.

19. What is the CT appearance of an adrenal carcinoma?

The tumor appears as a large, suprarenal mass with areas of central low density representing necrosis. The margins are often irregular, and up to 30% may have calcifications. Enhancement with intravenous contrast is heterogeneous.

20. Does MRI have anything to add?

The inferior vena cava and (in the case of a left tumor) the left renal vein may contain tumor thrombus. The multiplanar capability of MRI and the ease of evaluating these vessels make MRI valuable in evaluating adrenal carcinoma.

21. From which part of the adrenal glands do pheochromocytomas arise?

From the adrenal medulla, which shares the same ectodermal embryonic origin as the paraspinal parasympathetic chain (Fig. 3). Therefore, although 90% arise from the adrenal medulla, they may occur anywhere from the skull base to the sacrum. Furthermore, unlike the adrenal cortex, which is derived from the primitive mesoderm, adrenal medullary tumors such as pheochromocytoma produce catecholamines.

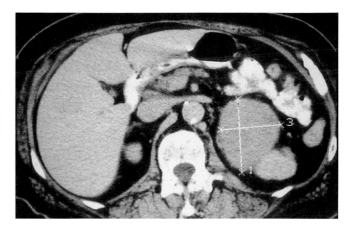

FIGURE 3. A 71-year-old woman with a left adrenal pheochromocytoma (between the x signs). (Courtesy of Dr. Steven Perlmutter.)

22. Of all patients with hypertension, how many have a pheochromocytoma?

Only 0.1%. A clinical diagnosis is based on a history of paroxysmal sweating and palpitations; urinary catecholamines (i.e., metanephrine, vanillylmandelic acid) are elevated.

23. What is the rule of tens?

Pheochromocytomas are bilateral in 10%, extraadrenal in 10% (Fig. 4), and malignant in 10% of cases; in addition, 10% occur in families. Associated syndromes are easily remembered by the mnemonic **VEIN**: **v**on-Hippel Lindau syndrome, **E**ndocrine neoplasms (in multiple endocrine neoplasia type II), **I**nherited, and **N**eurofibromatosis.

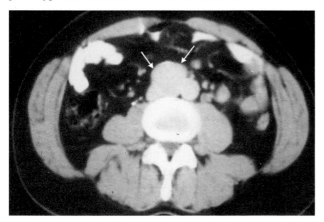

FIGURE 4. Mass between the aorta and inferior vena cava (arrows) is a pheochromocytoma of the organ of Zuckerkandl. This is the most common site of origin of an extraadrenal pheochromocytoma. (Courtesy of Dr. Steven Perlmutter.)

24. What is the most practical imaging approach for detecting pheochromocytomas before surgery?

Because 90% of pheochromocytomas arise from the adrenal glands, CT is the initial imaging test of choice. If no adrenal mass is detected, the entire abdomen and pelvis must be examined for the presence of an extraadrenal pheochromocytoma. If no mass is detected, the chest should be evaluated. Because CT has a sensitivity of only 60% in detecting extraadrenal pheochromocytomas, many radiologists prefer to continue the work-up with MRI.

25. What is the role of nuclear medicine examination with I[131]-MIBG?

Iodine[131]-labeled metaiodobenzyl guanidine (I[131]-MIBG) is the nuclear agent of choice for detecting or confirming the presence of a pheochromocytoma. I[131]-MIBG is taken up by adrenergic tissue and can detect pheochromocytomas with an accuracy comparable to other cross-sectional imaging tests. The entire body should be scanned after a single injection of I^{131}-MIBG; the test is most useful in detecting multifocal disease, metastases, and an extraadrenal primary tumor and also for confirmation of equivocal findings on CT and MRI.

26. What is the main disadvantage of MIBG?

Poor spatial resolution. MIBG should be correlated with other cross-sectional imaging tests (CT and MR).

27. What are the radiologic features of pheochromocytoma on CT? On MR?

On CT pheochromocytomas appear as well-circumscribed masses that often measure > 3 cm. Large masses may contain calcium and display central inhomogeneity due to hemorrhage and necrosis. On T2-weighted MR sequences, pheochromocytomas are usually exceptionally bright—and are referred to as light bulb lesions. However, adrenal carcinomas and cysts may have a similar appearance.

28. What is the danger in performing a percutaneous biopsy of a pheochromocytoma?

A hypertensive crisis, which can be life threatening, may be precipitated. Patients should be adequately blocked before biopsy with antiadrenergics against both alpha- and beta-catecholamines if a pheochromocytoma is suspected.

29. In what age group are neuroblastomas found?

Neuroblastomas occur in children (especially very young children). They arise from the sympathetic nervous system and are most commonly found in the adrenal glands. Neuroblastomas are malignant tumors (Fig. 5).

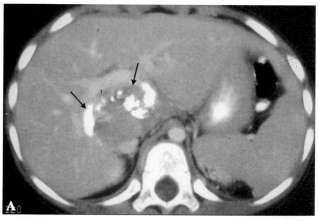

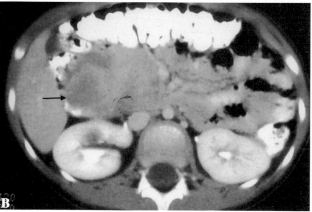

FIGURE 5. A 6-year-old boy with neuroblastoma of the right adrenal. Note the large, calcified mass adjacent to the right kidney and the liver (arrows).

30. What is the CT and MR appearance of adrenal neuroblastomas?

Neuroblastomas are typically large at presentation and may be palpable. On CT they may have irregular or lobulated margins and often cross the midline. Up to 40% have stippled calcification. On T2-weighted MR images, they are brighter than the liver. MR is especially valuable in evaluating extension of tumor into the spinal canal and is more sensitive than a bone scan in detecting metastases to the bone marrow. Cortical metastases have a graver prognosis and are best evaluated by bone scan.

31. What is an adrenal myelolipoma? Which CT feature establishes its radiologic diagnosis?

A relatively unusual hamartomatous lesion, myelolipomas contain erythroid, myeloid, and fatty elements (Fig. 6). A Hounsfield unit measurement of less than zero on CT indicates the presence of fat and helps establish the diagnosis, especially if the lesion is relatively large (vs. a nonfunctioning adenoma, which is also benign) and if gross fat is evident. Only in the presence of pain should surgical removal be considered.

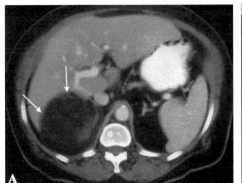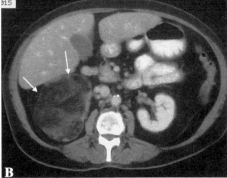

FIGURE 6.   Large fatty mass of the right adrenal (arrows), which is a myelolipoma. (Courtesy of Luann Teschmacher, M.D.)

32. What is an incidentaloma?

Incidentalomas are nonfunctioning adrenal adenomas that are discovered on imaging performed for other indications. They are seen in up to 8% of the population and have a higher incidence in the elderly and in patients with obesity, diabetes, and hypertension. Incidentalomas must be distinguished from metastases in patients with a known or suspected primary neoplasm, especially if it would change the management plan (i.e., a lung cancer that is otherwise resectable unless the adrenal lesion proves to be a metastasis).

33. Which primary neoplasms metastasize most commonly to the adrenal glands?

Lung, breast, thyroid, colon, and melanoma. Adrenals are the fourth most common site of metastases, and adrenal metastases are found in up to 25% of patients with a known primary. Even in the presence of a known primary cancer, an adrenal mass (especially if it is small) is more likely to be a nonfunctioning adenoma than a metastasis (Fig. 7).

34. Which radiologic tests can be used to distinguish a metastasis from a nonfunctioning adrenal adenoma?

Adenomas may be distinguished by the presence of some fat within them. If an adrenal mass contains fat on CT (initial images should be obtained with thin sections and no intravenous contrast in this context), or is of relatively low density on CT, or contains fat on MR (using in-phase and out-of-phase chemical shift images), the possibility of a metastasis can be reliably discarded. The radiologist should be consulted, because the correct use of cross-sectional imaging may avoid an adrenal biopsy in many cases (Fig. 8).

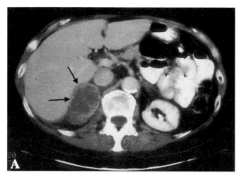 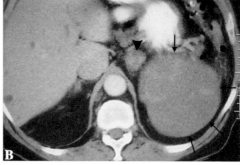

FIGURE 7. *A*, Metastatic right adrenal lesion (arrows) from lung cancer. *B*, In a different patient with a large left renal cancer (arrows), there is a metastasis to the left adrenal (arrowhead).

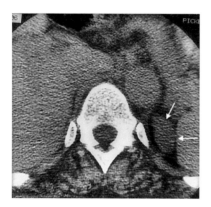

FIGURE 8. Unenhanced CT to evaluate a left adrenal lesion (arrows). Density was −7 Hounsfield units, consistent with an adenoma.

35. What are the advantages and disadvantages of performing an adrenal biopsy?

If cross-sectional imaging cannot resolve the question of whether an adrenal mass is benign or malignant, biopsy should be considered, especially if patient management will change depending on the result. Satisfactory specimens are obtained in about 85% of biopsies. Complications such as hematoma and pneumothorax may occur, although they are rare (about 2% of cases).

36. What are the most common causes of adrenal hemorrhage? What role does imaging play?

In neonates, adrenal hemorrhage is a relatively common problem and may be due to birth trauma, hypoxia, or sepsis. As in the evaluation of other adrenal masses in neonates, ultrasound is the initial imaging test of choice. In adults, anticoagulation, sepsis (e.g., from meningococci), and trauma are the most common causes. Adrenal hemorrhage due to trauma involves only the right adrenal gland in 80% of cases. It is postulated that the direct drainage of the right adrenal vein into the inferior vena cava allows the unimpeded transfer of force from a blow to the abdomen.

37. How does adrenal hemorrhage appear on ultrasound?

Initially, adrenal hemorrhage appears echogenic; within a short time, it becomes more hypoechoic and smaller. The most important differential diagnosis is congenital neuroblastoma, which is less common and, unlike hemorrhage, is vascular on color Doppler ultrasound. The distinction between adrenal hemorrhage and neonatal neuroblastoma can be made on follow-up ultrasound (e.g., 1 week or so later).

38. How does adrenal hemorrhage appear on CT?

CT should initially be performed without intravenous contrast (Fig. 9). Hemorrhage appears hyperdense during the acute and subacute phases and becomes progressively hypodense with time.

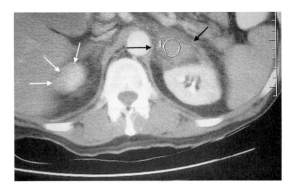

FIGURE 9. A 68-year-old man with back pain after cardiac surgery and anticoagulation. There is enlargement of the left adrenal (arrows), and to a lesser extent of the right adrenal (white arrows). The density of the left adrenal is 48, consistent with hemorrhage. Note the hazy borders of the adrenals.

39. What are the clinical features of Addison's disease?

Patients with primary adrenal insufficiency, or Addison's disease, present with hypotension, fatigue, anorexia, and weight loss. Due to loss of negative feedback from the adrenal cortex, the pituitary secretes more ACTH, which includes the melanocyte stimulating hormone fragment. Patients with Addison's disease can therefore be clinically differentiated from patients with pituitary or hypothalamic pathology by their characteristic hyperpigmentation of exposed skin surfaces.

40. What are the CT features of Addison's disease?

In the United States, an autoimmune process accounts for 80% of cases, and the adrenal glands may appear atrophied on CT. Tuberculosis accounts for the remaining 20% of cases as well as most cases worldwide. Tuberculosis and other granulomatous infections have a nonspecific masslike appearance on CT and in the chronic stage may show calcification.

BIBLIOGRAPHY

1. Dunnick NR: Adrenal imaging: Current status. AJR 154:927, 1990.
2. Korobkin M, Dunnick NR: Characterization of adrenal masses. AJR 164:643–644, 1995.
3. Korobkin M, Brodeur FJ, Yutzky GG, et al: Differentiation of adrenal adenomas from nonadenomas using CT attenuation values. AJR 166:531–536, 1996.
4. Lee MJ, Mayo-Smith WW, Hahn PF, et al: State-of-the-art MR imaging of the adrenal gland. RadioGraphics 14:1015, 1994.
5. Outwater EK, Mitchell DG: Differentiation of adrenal masses with chemical shift MR imaging. Radiology 193:877, 1994.
6. Szolar DH, Kammerhuber F: Quantitative CT evaluation of adrenal gland masses: A step forward in the differentiation between adenomas and nonadenomas? Radiology 202:517–521, 1997.
7. Welch TJ, Sheedy PF II, Davis HS, et al: Percutaneous adrenal biopsy: Review of a 10-year experience. Radiology 193:341–344, 1994.

41. SCROTAL IMAGING

Michael M. Abiri, M.D.

1. What are the common imaging modalities used for evaluation of scrotal diseases?

Sonography, nuclear scintigraphy, and MRI.

2. What are the indications for these modalities?

Sonography is the modality of choice for assessing known or suspected scrotal pathology. Nuclear scintigraphy is extremely helpful in evaluating suspected testicular torsion. MRI can be used when ultrasound is not conclusive or does not demonstrate a clinically suspected lesion.

3. How large is the normal testis?

The normal testis measures approximately 3 cm in transverse diameter by 5 cm in length.

4. What is the tunica albuginea? The tunica vaginalis?

Each testicle is encased in a dense membrane called the tunica albuginea. The tunica vaginalis is a membrane that covers the epididymis and almost the entire testis except for a small area posteriorly called the bare area. This area anchors the testis to the posterior wall of the scrotum, where the blood vessels, lymphatics, epididymal ducts, and nerves enter the testicle.

5. Where is the epididymis in relationship to the testis?

The epididymis surrounds the testicle. It is located superior and posterolateral to the testis and has three parts: head, body, and tail (Fig. 1).

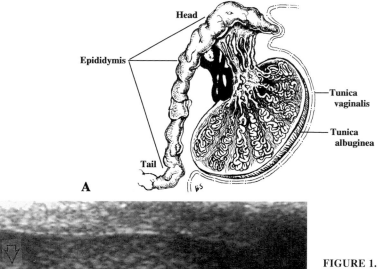

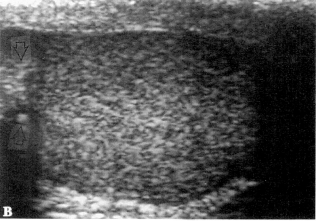

FIGURE 1. *A*, Normal testicular anatomy. *B*, Longitudinal section through the testicle. Note the homogeneous uniform gray scale appearance of the testes. The hypoechoic nodule demarcated by the arrowheads, superior to the testicle, represents the epididymal head.

6. What is the clinical significance of the bare area of the testis?

The size of the bare area is variable. Sometimes it is so small that it only leaves a short stalk attaching the testis to the scrotum. This is called the bell-clapper deformity, which is strongly associated with intravaginal testicular torsion. The bell-clapper deformity is bilateral in 40% of cases.

7. What are the five major indications for scrotal imaging?

Acute pain   Occult neoplasm
Palpable mass   Trauma
Scrotal enlargement

8. Which clinical conditions result in acute scrotal pain?

The most important possible diagnoses are torsion (either of the testes or, less commonly, of the appendages of the testes), epididymitis, and epididymo-orchitis. It is particularly important to diagnose testicular torsion in an expeditious fashion, because delay in surgical repair results in testicular infarction. The salvage rate after 12 hours is 20%. After 24 hours the torsed testis is usually not salvageable.

9. Which type of testicular torsion is more common?

There are two types of testicular torsion: intravaginal and extravaginal. Extravaginal torsion occurs in neonates and is less common. It involves the testes, its supporting structures, and the processus vaginalis in the inguinal canal. Extravaginal torsion clinically mimics the appearance of a strangulated hernia. Intravaginal torsion is more common; it occurs in young men in their teens and early twenties. Intravaginal torsion results from the bell-clapper deformity, as described above.

10. What causes epididymitis and orchitis?

Epididymitis and orchitis usually result from bacterial infection due to retrograde spread of organisms from the bladder and urethra. The organism(s) is variable, depending on the age of the patient. Infection usually begins in the tail and then extends to the body and head of the epididymis.

11. Which imaging modalities can be used to differentiate the main causes of acute scrotal pain?

Sonography and nuclear scintigraphy.

12. What are the sonographic findings of early and late testicular torsion?

An early torsion may be normal on gray-scale imaging, but absence of flow to the affected side is seen with color Doppler imaging. By 24 hours (the so-called missed torsion) the testicle has an abnormal appearance on gray-scale imaging as well, although the findings (including swelling of the testicle and epididymis and abnormal echotexture of the testicle) are not specific for torsion. Again, absence of flow is seen with color Doppler.

13. What are the scintigraphic findings of early and late torsion?

In early torsion, there is no flow to the affected side. In late torsion, there is "luxury flow" to the surrounding scrotal tissues, with no flow to the affected testis.

14. What are the sonographic and scintigraphic findings in epididymitis?

If there is no associated orchitis, the testicle has a normal gray-scale appearance, whereas the epididymis is engorged and hypervascular (Fig. 2). Nuclear imaging demonstrates increased flow to the epididymis.

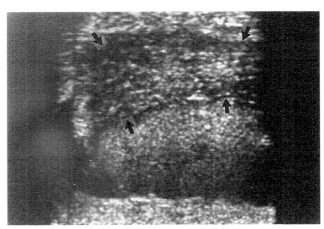

FIGURE 2. Note the normal gray scale appearance of the testes and the very enlarged hypervascular epididymis, demarcated by arrows.

15. What are the causes of gross scrotal enlargement?

A hydrocele is the most common etiology (Fig. 3). A hydrocele represents a benign collection of serous fluid that has accumulated between the two layers of the tunica vaginalis. Other collections that may form within the scrotal sac include a hematocele (after trauma), and a lymphocele (after surgery). Another common cause of scrotal enlargement is an inguinal hernia. The imaging findings depend on the contents of the hernia. Although an inguinal hernia is often clinically obvious, at times it may be necessary to perform an imaging test to distinguish between a hernia and a large hydrocele.

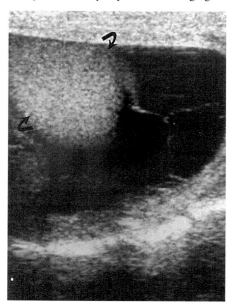

FIGURE 3. The testicle, defined by arrows, appears normal in its texture and has a uniform gray scale appearance. The testicle is surrounded by a large, septated hydrocele.

16. What is a varicocele? What is its clinical significance?

A varicocele is usually due to dilatation of the veins of the pampiniform plexus, which is located posterior to the testicle. A varicocele, however, may occur in any part of the scrotum, even within the testicle. There may be venous engorgement of the left gonadal vein, as it drains into the left renal vein. The right gonadal vein drains into the inferior vena cava. Infertility is associated with the presence of a varicocele. Varicoceles are seen in 15% of the normal population and in up to 35% of infertile men.

17. What is the main consideration in dealing with a palpable scrotal mass?

In general, palpable scrotal masses are divided into two categories: intratesticular and extratesticular. Extratesticular masses are rare and are generally benign. The only malignant extratesticular mass to consider is the paratesticular rhabdomyosarcoma, which occurs almost exclusively in children.

18. Why are intratesticular masses important to diagnose?

The majority of intratesticular masses are malignant. Although both primary and secondary malignancies of the testicle occur, the majority of testicular neoplasms are primary. Primary malignancies are most frequent in boys younger than 10 years, in men aged 20–40, and in men older than 60.

19. What primary tumors are found in the testes?

Primary tumors originate from germ cells or from the stromal cells of the testes. Germ cell tumors are more common and include seminomas, embryonal cell tumors, teratomas, choriocarcinomas, and mixed germ cell tumors.

20. What is the most common type of testicular germ cell tumor?

Seminoma (Fig. 4).

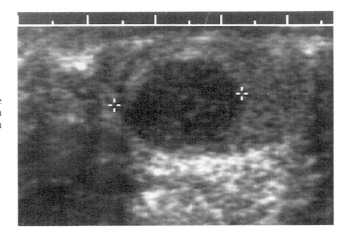

FIGURE 4. Cursors demarcate a focal hypoechoic mass within the testicle. This is a seminoma in this 54-year-old patient.

21. What is the most aggressive type of testicular germ cell tumor?
Embryonal cell carcinoma.

22. How often are stromal cell tumors benign?
Ninety percent are benign. Stromal cell tumors arise from either Sertoli cells or interstitial cells of Leydig and may present with feminizing signs.

23. What is the imaging test of choice in dealing with a palpable scrotal mass?
Sonography is both sensitive and cost-effective. Sonography clearly differentiates an intratesticular from an extratesticular mass.

24. What is the most common metastatic testicular tumor?
Lymphoma accounts for 1–8% of all testicular tumors. Leukemia is the second most common testicular metastatic tumor. In a patient over 60 years of age, the most common cause of a focal intratesticular mass is lymphoma.

25. What is the role of imaging in scrotal trauma?
After acute scrotal trauma, a hematoma may develop either within the layers of the tunica vaginalis (termed a hematocele) or within the testicle or epididymis. It is important to determine whether the testicle is intact or whether there is testicular rupture; surgical intervention may be necessary to treat testicular rupture. An isolated testicular hematoma may be observed without surgery. Again, ultrasound is the most cost-effective method of determining the integrity of the testicle. If sonography is nondiagnostic (findings of rupture may be subtle or indeterminate), MRI is helpful.

BIBLIOGRAPHY

1. Collings C, Cronan JJ, Grusmark J: Diffuse echoes within a simple hydrocele: Imaging caveat. J Ultrasound Med 13:439–442, 1994.
2. Doherty FJ: Ultrasound of the nonacute scrotum. Semin US CT MR 12:131–156, 1991.
3. Gersovich EO: High-resolution ultrasonography in the diagnosis of scrotal pathology. II: Tumors. J Clin Ultrasound 21:375–386, 1993.
4. Langer JE: Ultrasound of the scrotum. Semin Roentgenol 28:5–18, 1993.
5. Patel MD, Olcott EW, Kerschmann RL, et al: Sonographically detected testicular microlithiasis and testicular carcinoma. J Clin Ultrasound 21:444–452, 1993.
6. Ralls PW, Larsen D, Johnson MB, Lee KP: Color Doppler sonography of the scrotum. Semin US CT MR 12:109–114, 1991.
7. Rumack CM, Wilson SR, Charboneau JW: Diagnostic Ultrasound, 2nd ed. St. Louis, Mosby, 1998.
8. Tumeh SS, Benson CB, Richie JP: Acute diseases of the scrotum. Semin US CT MR 12:115–130, 1991.

42. IMAGING OF THE PROSTATE

Robert B. Poster, M.D.

1. What is the normal weight of the prostate in an adult?

Approximately 20 grams.

2. Which modalities are useful in estimating the weight of the prostate?

CT, MR, transabdominal ultrasound, and transrectal ultrasound. The volume can be estimated by multiplying the length times the width times the thickness times 0.52. This calculation gives an estimated volume, which is approximately equal to the weight of the prostate in grams.

3. What is the shape of the prostate?

The shape of the prostate is best described as a flattened cone. The tip of the cone represents the apex of the gland and is situated more caudally. The flattened portion of the cone is analogous to the base of the prostate and is situated more cranially.

4. What is the lymphatic drainage of the prostate?

Drainage of lymph from the prostate is to the internal and external iliac lymph nodes, including the obturator nodes.

5. What are the zones of the prostate?

The peripheral zone, central zone, and transitional zone. In young men, the peripheral zone occupies approximately 70% of the total volume of the prostate. The central zone occupies approximately 25%, and the transitional zone 5%. These percentages may change with age.

6. Can the zonal anatomy of the prostate be seen on contrast-enhanced CT?

No. Although zonal anatomy may be seen on occasion, it is not usually discernible (Fig. 1).

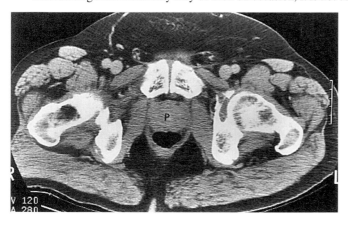

FIGURE 1. Axial CT image shows the prostate (P) as homogeneous in density. The zonal anatomy is not seen.

7. What information do T1- and T2-weighted MR images provide about the prostate?

The T2-weighted images best demonstrate the zonal anatomy of the prostate. The peripheral zone has high signal intensity, whereas the transitional zone has low signal intensity. The T2-weighted images are best for demonstrating lesions within the prostate. The T1-weighted images are useful for demonstrating areas of postbiopsy hemorrhage and the status of the neurovascular bundles and for determining whether there is gross invasion into the periprostatic fat (Fig. 2).

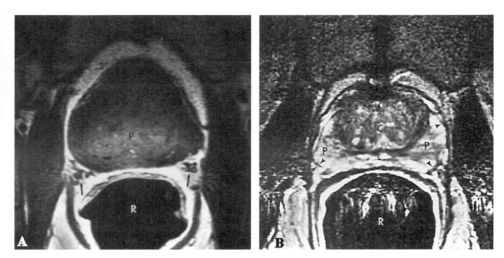

FIGURE 2. *A*, Normal prostate, T1-weighted images. The prostate (P) is homogeneous in signal intensity and is surrounded by bright periprostatic fat. The neurovascular bundles (dark arrows) are shown, as is the endorectal surface coil (ERSC) in the rectum (R). *B*, Normal prostate, T2-weighted image. The high signal intensity peripheral zone (P) is well demarcated from the inhomogeneous central gland. The prostatic capsule is seen as a dark area around the prostate (arrowheads) (R = endorectal surface coil in the rectum.)

8. What is the typical appearance of the seminal vesicles on the T1- and T2-weighted images?

On T1-weighted images, the seminal vesicles are usually low in signal, whereas on T2-weighted images they are high in signal (Fig. 3).

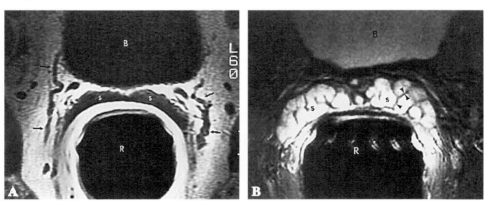

FIGURE 3. *A*, T1-weighted axial image. Seminal vesicles (S) are homogeneous in signal intensity. B = bladder. R = rectum with endorectal surface coil. Vessels are seen in the region (black arrows). *B*, Normal seminal vesicles on T2-weighted axial image. The seminal vesicles (S) are high in signal intensity. The walls of the seminal vesicles are well seen (arrowheads). B = bladder, R = endorectal surface coil in rectum.

9. The prostatic capsule is best seen on what modality?

MR imaging, performed with an endorectal coil, is the only modality that consistently demonstrates the prostatic capsule. The surgical capsule separates the peripheral and central zones from the transition zone and represents condensed connective tissue. On T2-weighted images, the prostatic capsule appears as a low signal intensity area (see Fig. 2).

10. What is the most common cause of prostatic calcification seen on plain radiographs and CT?
Primary prostatic calcification, which is due to calcium deposition in the corpora amylacea (Fig. 4).

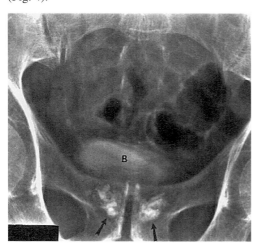

FIGURE 4. Calcification of the prostate is seen (arrows). Contrast is noted in the bladder (B) from a previous intravenous pyelogram.

11. What is the best way to visualize the prostate with ultrasound?
Transrectal ultrasound, which is typically performed with a high frequency transducer (7 Mega Hz or higher) (Fig. 5). The examination, like all ultrasound studies, is operator-dependent.

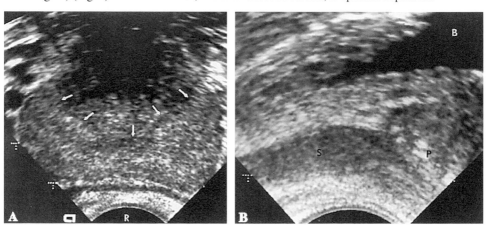

FIGURE 5. *A*, Transrectal axial sonogram demonstrates the peripheral zone (arrows) demarcated from the remainder of the prostate. R = rectum containing the endorectal ultrasound probe. *B*, Longitudinal transrectal sonogram demonstrates the seminal vesicle (S) and prostate (P). B = bladder.

12. Which zone of the prostate is the site of origin of the vast majority of benign prostatic hypertrophy?
The transitional zone is the site of origin of > 95% of benign prostatic hypertrophy (BPH).

13. Can prostatic hypertrophy be identified on plain radiographs?
No. Occasionally, prostatic calcifications or a large soft tissue mass may be seen, but for the most part there are no plain film findings of prostatic enlargement.

14. There is a debate over when an intravenous urogram should be performed in patients with benign prostatic hypertrophy. What circumstances warrant an intravenous urogram?
History of hematuria
Suspected renal or ureteral stones seen on plain film
Patients with an atypical history or BPH

15. List the major findings on an intravenous urogram of an enlarged prostate that causes bladder outlet obstruction.
Smooth or irregular impression on the bladder base from the enlarged prostate (Fig. 6)
Trabeculated, thick-walled bladder
Hydroureteronephrosis
Tortuosity and decreased peristalsis of the ureters
Bladder diverticula
"Fishhook" configuration to the distal ureter
Postvoid residual (although this finding is not always present, even in the presence of significant obstruction)

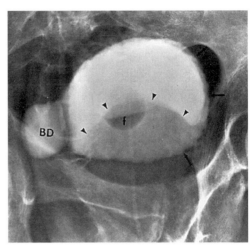

FIGURE 6.   A film of the contrast-filled bladder demonstrates the smooth impression on the bladder base, from an enlarged prostate (arrowheads). Also noted is a trabeculated bladder (arrows) as well as a bladder diverticulum (BD). f = Foley catheter balloon.

16. What are the major uses of transabdominal ultrasound of the pelvis in evaluating a patient with an enlarged prostate?
• The size and weight of the prostate can be estimated.
• Pre- and postvoid bladder volume measurements can be made noninvasively.
• Bladder wall thickening can be identified.
• Bladder diverticula may be seen.

17. Which patients with enlarged prostates undergo renal ultrasound?
Patients with renal insufficiency or obstructive symptoms.

18. What amount of urine is considered a significant postvoid residual?
About 200 cc of urine or greater.

19. What is the appearance of benign prostatic hypertrophy on T2-weighted MR images?
Stromal BPH appears dark on T2-weighted images. Nonstromal (glandular) BPH appears bright. A low signal intensity rim may be seen surrounding the nodules. A combination of these findings may be seen (Fig. 7).

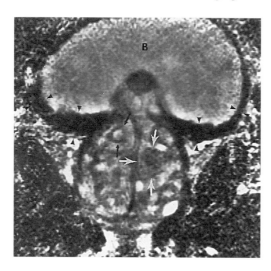

FIGURE 7. Coronal T2-weighted MR of the prostate demonstrates both stromal (white arrows) and glandular nodules of benign prostatic hypertrophy. The thickened bladder wall is nicely demonstrated (arrowheads).

20. What are the most commonly used screening tests for prostate cancer?
Digital rectal examination and monitoring of prostate specific antigen.

21. How is the diagnosis of prostate cancer usually made?
By biopsy of the prostate, which is often accomplished transrectally with ultrasound guidance (Fig. 8). Biopsies are generally performed in patients with an elevated prostate specific antigen or a suspicious digital rectal examination.

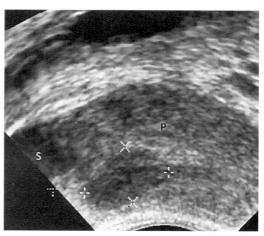

FIGURE 8. Longitudinal transrectal sonogram demonstrates a hypoechoic lesion (cursors) that on biopsy proved to be adenocarcinoma of the prostate (P). S = seminal vesicle.

22. What is the percentage of prostate cancer arising within each of the three zones?
Peripheral zone—70%
Central zone—10%
Transitional zone—20%

23. What is a simplified staging system for prostate cancer?
Stage A: Occult cancer (focal or diffuse)
Stage B: Cancer confined to the prostatic capsule
Stage C: Extracapsular spread
Stage D: Distant metastases

24. What findings are consistent with an advanced stage of prostate cancer?
Seminal vesicle invasion
Bony metastases
Bladder invasion
Lymphadenopathy

25. Why is it important to differentiate stage B from stage C prostate cancer?
In general, patients with stage B disease may undergo radical prostatectomy, whereas patients with stage C or D are often not considered candidates for radical prostatectomy because of the increased frequency of spread to the regional lymph nodes.

26. How is the possibility of recurrent prostate cancer best monitored?
By monitoring the level of prostatic specific antigen. Any rise in the level above that obtained after radical prostatectomy is worrisome for recurrent tumor.

27. What are two common causes of an elevated prostate specific antigen other than prostate cancer?
Prostatitis
Benign prostatic hypertrophy

28. What is the most common site of hematogenous metastases from the prostate?
Bone is involved in 85% of patients dying of prostate cancer. The most common sites (from most frequent to least frequent) are the pelvic bones, lumbar spine, femur, thoracic spine, and ribs.

29. What is the most commonly used radiologic test for detecting skeletal metastases from prostate cancer?
The radionuclide bone scan is more sensitive than plain films. Plain films of the skeleton may be used to clarify equivocal areas on the bone scan.

30. What is the most common plain film appearance of a bony metastasis from prostate cancer?
Eighty percent of bony lesions are osteoblastic; 5% may be osteolytic; 10–15% are mixed osteoblastic and osteolytic.

31. What other conditions may cause osteoblastic lesions in bone?
Metastases from other primary cancers
Lymphoma
Myelofibrosis
Many other lesions, benign and malignant

32. Which radiologic signs of prostate cancer may be seen on an intravenous urogram?
Defect at the bladder base that is irregular in outline
Edema of the bladder neck or trigone
Distal ureteral narrowing
Hydronephrosis
Bony metastases

33. Can transabdominal ultrasound of the prostate be used for detecting prostate cancer?
No. It does not have the spatial resolution necessary to detect small lesions within the prostate. Transrectal ultrasound is much more sensitive for detecting small lesions. However, transrectal ultrasound should not be used as a screening test for prostate cancer; it should be reserved for patients who have an abnormally elevated prostate specific antigen or a suspicious digital rectal examination.

34. How does transrectal ultrasound aid in the diagnosis of prostate cancer?

Transrectal ultrasound is useful for detecting suspicious lesions, guiding biopsies, and staging cancer locally. Unfortunately, there is a large degree of overlap in the sonographic appearance of benign and malignant lesions; thus sonography is not highly specific for diagnosing malignant prostate lesions.

35. What is the most common sonographic appearance of prostate cancer on transrectal sonography?

A hypoechoic lesion within the peripheral zone (see Fig. 8). The larger the lesion, the more likely it is cancerous.

36. On transrectal sonography, what lesions other than prostatic cancer may appear as a hypoechoic lesion in the peripheral zone?

Areas of fibrosis   Acute or chronic prostatitis
Benign prostatic hyperplastic nodules   Dilated prostatic ducts or cysts

37. Are stage A lesions easily detected by transrectal sonography?

No. Because of the inhomogeneous echogenicity of the central gland and the difficulty in identifying anteriorly located lesions, transrectal ultrasound is not highly accurate in detecting stage A lesions (Fig. 9).

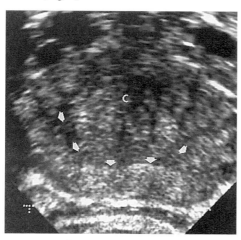

FIGURE 9.   Inhomogeneous central gland (C) is demarcated from the peripheral zone by arrows.

38. List three advantages of transrectal sonography-guided biopsy of the prostate vs. transperitoneal biopsy.

Improved patient tolerance
Fewer inadequate specimens
Decreased need for anesthesia

39. List three possible complications associated with transrectal ultrasound-guided biopsy.

Bleeding into urine, rectum, or semen
Infection
Acute urinary retention

40. What two precautionary measures minimize the risks of complications from a transrectal sonographically guided biopsy?

Ascertain that the patient takes no medications that may interfere with clotting of the blood (especially aspirin-containing products)
Prophylactic antibiotic coverage

41. Can CT differentiate between benign and malignant diseases of the prostate?

No. For the most part, CT cannot differentiate between benign and malignant lesions of the prostate in the absence of frank invasion outside the prostate.

42. Is CT an accurate examination for differentiating between stages B and C?

No. It is, however, useful in detecting distant metastases.

43. What is the most reliable sign of invasion of the seminal vesicles by prostate cancer on CT?

Asymmetric enlargement of the seminal vesicles.

44. What is the criterion for an enlarged lymph node?

A lymph node > 1 cm in largest dimension is suspicious for metastatic disease. MR and CT are about equally accurate in detecting abnormal lymph nodes. Unfortunately, signal characteristics of lymph nodes on MR are not useful in determining whether lymph nodes are enlarged because of tumor invasion.

45. List two advantages of MR over CT for evaluating the prostate.

Visualizing the gland in multiple planes
Differentiating zonal anatomy

46. What are the advantages of using an endorectal surface coil rather than the body surface coil (which is external to the patient) for imaging the prostate with MR?

The spatial resolution is greater with a transrectal surface coil than with a body coil. The transrectal surface coil demonstrates the prostatic capsule, whereas imaging with the body coil usually does not.

47. Should MR imaging of the prostate with an endorectal surface coil be used for screening and diagnosing prostate cancer?

No. MR imaging is used to help stage prostate cancer. It is not used for screening or diagnosing prostate cancer, because it is too expensive and not specific enough.

48. How do the majority of prostate cancers appear on T2-weighted images?

The majority of prostate cancers arise within the peripheral zone. They appear as a dark lesion against the background of the high signal intensity peripheral zone (Fig. 10).

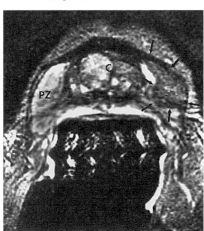

FIGURE 10. T2-weighted axial MR image shows a hypointense cancer nodule (arrows) within the peripheral zone. Compare this with the normal high signal peripheral zone (PZ). The central gland (C) shows adenomas secondary to benign prostatic hypertrophy.

49. Other than cancer, what may cause low signal intensity areas within the peripheral zone on T2-weighted images?

Prostatitis   Stromal disease within the peripheral zone
Granulomatous disease   Postbiopsy blood

50. How useful is MR in evaluating prostate cancers within the central portion of the gland?

Not very useful. The central gland appears inhomogeneous, and prostate cancer cannot be diagnosed within it.

51. What does invasion of the seminal vesicles from prostate cancer look like on MR imaging?

On the T2-weighted images, low signal intensity areas within the seminal vesicles and asymmetry in size may indicate tumor invasion. However, blood, changes secondary to radiation therapy, and other benign processes may appear as low signal intensity areas in the seminal vesicles (Fig. 11).

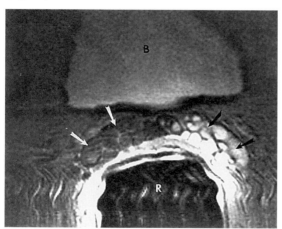

FIGURE 11. T2-weighted axial MR image shows low signal intensity of the right seminal vesicle (white arrows), consistent with tumor invasion from the prostate (pathologically proven). Normal left seminal vesicle is of high signal intensity (black arrows). B = bladder, R = rectum.

52. Can biopsy of the prostate affect the MR examination?

Yes. Postbiopsy hemorrhage may make the MR examination difficult to interpret. Hemorrhage may appear as low signal intensity areas on T2-weighted images, and thus mimic tumor in the peripheral zone or invasion of the seminal vesicles. There is also disruption of the capsule, which may mimic invasion into the periprostatic fat.

53. How useful is the intravenous contrast agent gadolinium in staging prostate cancer on MR?

At present, gadolinium has no value in assessing the prostate. In equivocal cases of seminal vesicle invasion, it may have some use.

54. What are the major limitations of endorectal surface coil MR in staging prostate cancer?

Inability to detect microscopic invasion
Inability to evaluate adenocarcinoma contained within the central or transitional zones
Inability to differentiate benign from malignant disease
In addition, the volume of large tumors is underestimated, and the volume of small tumors is overestimated by MR.

BIBLIOGRAPHY

1. Hamper UM, Sheth S: Prostate ultrasonography. Semin Roentgenol 28:57, 1993.
2. Langlotz C, Schnall M, Pollack H: Staging of prostate cancer: Accuracy of MR imaging. Radiology 194:645–646, 1995.

3. Hricak H, Thoeni R: Neoplasms of the prostate gland. In Pollack HM (ed): Clinical Urography. Philadelphia, W.B. Saunders, 1990, pp 1381–1403.
4. Talner LB: Specific causes of obstruction. In Pollack HM (ed): Clinical Urography. Philadelphia, W.B. Saunders, 1990, pp 1629–1751.
5. McCallum RW, Banner MP: Lower urinary tract calculi and calcifications. In Pollack HM (ed): Clinical Urography. Philadelphia, W.B. Saunders, 1990, pp 1889–1925.
6. Fair WR: Urinary Tract Inflammation: An Overview. Philadelphia, W.B. Saunders, 1990, pp 788–798.
7. Ramchandani P, Schnall MD: Magnetic resonance imaging of the prostate. Semin Roentgenol 28:74, 1993.
8. Shiebler ML, Schnall MD, Pollack HM, et al: Current role of MR imaging in staging adenocarcinoma of the prostate. Radiology 189:339, 1993.

V. Obstetrics and Gynecology

43. OBSTETRIC ULTRASOUND

Rhonda P. Osborne, M.D.

FIRST-TRIMESTER IMAGING

1. What are the advantages of transvaginal ultrasound in imaging patients in the first trimester of pregnancy or patients suspected of having an early pregnancy?

Transvaginal ultrasound allows the radiologist (or obstetrician) to place a high-frequency transducer nearer to the region of interest than transabdominal ultrasound. This position permits optimal visualization of the uterus, cervix, ovaries, and cul-de-sac. Subcutaneous fat and other overlying tissue degrade transabdominal ultrasound images.

2. Should both transvaginal and transabdominal sonography be performed in this setting?

Many authorities believe that a combination of techniques is best, and ideally both should be performed. One of the disadvantages of transvaginal sonography is that, although the resolution is far superior to transabdominal sonography, the higher portions of the pelvis may not be seen. Therefore, if transabdominal sonography is performed, it complements transvaginal sonography and prevents a mass or other abnormality from being missed.

3. What is the major disadvantage of transabdominal sonography?

Transabdominal sonography requires a full bladder and therefore is much more uncomfortable than transvaginal sonography. It also may take some time for the patient to fill her bladder.

4. Is it acceptable to perform either transvaginal or transabdominal sonography alone?

It depends. Some institutions or practices go directly to transvaginal sonography (no patient preparation is required) and only scan the pelvis transabdominally to clarify selected abnormalities (e.g., if an adnexal mass is seen, to identify its cranial extent). However, as stated above, the transabdominal sonogram provides a better survey of the pelvis and is helpful in orienting the transvaginal study; lesions outside the relatively short field of view of the intravaginal probe may be missed if the transabdominal scan is omitted. This approach, however, is more labor- and time-intensive. Alternatively, if a normal-appearing intrauterine gestation is seen transabdominally and both adnexal regions are unremarkable, it may be acceptable to stop at this point.

5. In which suspected condition is it especially critical to perform transvaginal ultrasound on a pregnant patient in her first trimester?

When an ectopic pregnancy is detected, especially if the β-HCG level is significantly elevated and no intrauterine pregnancy is detected by transabdominal sonography.

6. What is an anembryonic pregnancy?

Also known as a blighted ovum, an anembryonic pregnancy is a fertilized egg in which embryonic development has become arrested. Because early gestational sac growth parallels embryonic growth, a living embryo should be identified in all normal pregnancies when the gestational sac exceeds a certain critical size, defined as the discriminatory sac size.

7. What exactly is meant by the discriminatory sac size?

This concept is independent of the menstrual history, which may be inaccurate. There are discriminatory sac sizes for visualizing the embryo and yolk sac.

8. When should the gestational sac be visible?

Normally the gestational sac should be visible in the uterus at 5 weeks' menstrual age. The gestational sac should be 17 mm (mean sac diameter) by 6 weeks' menstrual age and should grow at approximately 1.13 mm/day. If the level of beta-human chorionic gonadotropin (β-HCG) is $\geq$ 1000 mIU/ml (second international standard), an intrauterine gestational sac should be seen on transvaginal sonography. If it is not visible, an ectopic pregnancy should be assumed until proved otherwise (by careful clinical, sonographic, and β-HCG follow-up).

9. When should the yolk sac be visible?

Using transabdominal sonography, the yolk sac should be visible when the mean diameter of the gestational sac exceeds 20 mm. Various transvaginal studies suggest that a yolk sac should be consistently visible when the gestational sac exceeds 8 mm.

10. When should the fetal pole be visible?

With transabdominal sonography, a fetal pole should be detected when the mean sac diameter is 25 mm. With transvaginal sonography, a fetal pole should be seen when the mean sac diameter reaches 16 mm.

11. When should the fetal heart beat be visible?

Using transabdominal sonography, cardiac activity should be noted by 7 weeks and 1–2 weeks earlier with transvaginal sonography. A heart beat should be seen when the embryo is $\geq$ 9 mm crown–rump length with transabdominal sonography and $\geq$ 5 mm crown–rump length with transvaginal scanning.

12. How is the appearance of the yolk sac used to determine the outcome of the pregnancy?

The upper limit of normal for yolk sac diameter between 5 and 10 weeks' menstrual age is 5.6 mm. Larger yolk sacs, abnormally shaped yolk sacs, or nonvisualized yolk sacs in the presence of an embryo are associated with fetal loss.

13. When is the amnion expected to fuse with the chorion?

The fetus grows within the amniotic sac, which is defined by the amniotic membrane. The amniotic sac grows to fill the chorionic cavity of the uterus by 14–16 weeks. Before this point, the amnion can be seen as a separate membrane or sac within the chorionic cavity.

14. When is the best time to measure fetal age accurately?

The accuracy of first-trimester fetal measurements (early with mean sac diameter, somewhat later in the first trimester with crown–rump length) in predicting fetal age has been well documented. During the third trimester, the individual genetic expression in fetal size results in a diverse population. Once fetal age has been established during early pregnancy, it should not be changed because of measurements made later in pregnancy.

15. What exactly is an ectopic pregnancy?

An ectopic pregnancy is a pregnancy that occurs outside the endometrial cavity. Ninety-five to 97% of ectopic pregnancies occur in the fallopian tube, most commonly in the ampulla and isthmus.

16. What are uncommon sites of ectopic pregnancies?

Two to 5% occur in the cornual region of the fallopian tube (the region of the opening of the tube into the uterus). Less than 1% occur in the ovary and about one-tenth of 1% occur in the cervix.

17. What is the classic triad of ectopic pregnancy? How often does it occur?

Abnormal vaginal bleeding, pelvic pain, and a palpable adnexal mass are present in < 50% of patients with ectopic pregnancy.

18. What are risk factors for ectopic pregnancy?

A history of pelvic inflammatory disease, endometriosis, intrauterine device, and prior ectopic pregnancy.

19. Describe the sonographic findings of an ectopic pregnancy.

The only diagnostic finding is the presence of a live embryo outside the uterus, but this is seen in <20% of patients. The spectrum of findings on sonography includes an adnexal mass, free fluid in the pelvis and/or abdomen, and, most importantly, the absence of an intrauterine pregnancy, especially when the β-HCG level in the serum has reached a certain critical value.

20. What is meant by a heterotopic pregnancy?

A heterotopic pregnancy is the coexistence of an intrauterine pregnancy and an ectopic pregnancy. The incidence of heterotopic pregnancy is approximately 1 in 30,000 pregnancies. The risk increases in patients with pelvic inflammatory disease and/or a history of previous ectopic pregnancy and in patients undergoing therapy for infertility.

SECOND- AND THIRD-TRIMESTER IMAGING

21. What is the most common abnormality of the fetal neural axis?

Open neural tube defects. Of these, anencephaly is the most common, occurring in 1 in 1000 pregnancies. Anencephaly is characterized by the absence of the brain and cranial vault; facial structures and orbits are present. The condition is uniformly fatal after birth. On sonography no brain or skull is seen, and the orbits have a bulging appearance. The fetus often has a frog-like appearance (Fig. 1).

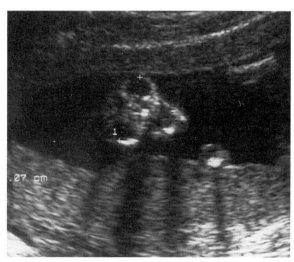

FIGURE 1. Anencephalic fetus with frog-like appearance.

22. Which neural axis abnormality is associated with a small cisterna magna?

The Chiari II malformation. In these fetuses, the contents of the posterior fossa are displaced caudally. Because the cerebellum abuts the occiput, it effaces the cisterna magna. This cerebellar deformity has been termed the banana sign (Fig. 2).

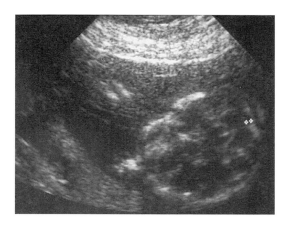

FIGURE 2. Banana sign. The cisterna magna (between calipers) is effaced and the cerebellum has lost its normal central concavity.

23. What associated abnormality is found in virtually all fetuses with the Chiari II malformation?
Meningomyelocele. Therefore, careful evaluation of the fetal spinal column is mandatory (although it should always be carefully examined at sonography in any case).

24. What is the lemon sign?
An additional feature associated with the Chiari II malformation is the lemon sign, which is an infolding of the frontal bones (Fig. 3).

FIGURE 3. Lemon sign. Infolding of the frontal bones is demonstrated (arrows). This fetus also has ventriculomegaly, and the "dangling choroid sign." The enlarged choroid plexus has assumed a gravitationally dependent position (arrowheads), with the enlarged atrium of the lateral ventricle.

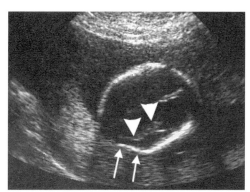

25. Is the lemon sign diagnostic of a Chiari II malformation?
No. The lemon sign may be an isolated finding of no significance in a small percentage of fetuses.

26. What are the causes of an enlarged cisterna magna?
Mega cisterna magna (usually a normal variation)
Dandy-Walker Syndrome (either the full blown malformation or its variant, in which the vermis is either completely or partially absent)
Arachnoid cyst of the posterior fossa (the vermis is intact, but is displaced)

27. What are the most common types of abdominal wall defect?
Omphalocele and gastroschisis.

28. Which is more common?
Omphalocele occurs more frequently than gastroschisis, with an incidence of 1:4000 live births as opposed to 1:12,000 for gastroschisis.

29. What is an omphalocele?

It is an abdominal wall defect that occurs in the midline, usually in the mid abdomen, with the umbilical cord inserting centrally into the defect. Although various contents protrude anteriorly from the abdominal wall, they are covered by a membrane.

30. What may the omphalocele contain?

Usually the liver and a portion of bowel (Fig. 4).

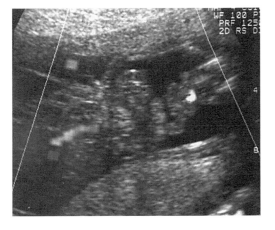

FIGURE 4.   Large omphalocele with herniation of the liver and other abdominal organs. The umbilical vein is seen centrally within the defect.

31. What is a gastroschisis?

It is an abdominal wall defect that occurs to the side of the midline, usually to the right of the umbilicus.

32. How else is gastroschisis different from an omphalocele?

Gastroschisis does not have a covering membrane. A portion of small bowel always herniates through the defect. Because there is no covering, the bowel is directly exposed to the amniotic fluid, and irreversible damage may occur to this portion of bowel. Ischemia may result from constriction at the defect, and subsequent bowel resection may be necessary.

33. Why is the prognosis better with gastroschisis than with an omphalocele?

Fetuses with an omphalocele have coexistent anomalies in 50–70% of cases and chromosomal anomalies in 40–60% of cases, whereas fetuses with gastroschisis rarely have associated anomalies or chromosomal abnormalities.

34. What is the pentalogy of Cantrell?

A rare condition that includes sternal, pericardial, diaphragmatic, and abdominal wall defects. Cardiac exstrophy and omphalocele are present.

35. What is the hallmark of an incompetent cervix?

Protrusion of the amniotic membranes through the internal cervical os. Sonography can detect early herniation of the membranes, especially in association with an intact external cervical os when physical changes in the cervix are not yet detectable by speculum and digital examination (Fig. 5). When a dilated cervical canal is detected, conservative management, surgical intervention (cerclage), or both may be instituted to prevent premature delivery. However, if the bulging membranes contain products of conception, early delivery is usually not preventable.

36. What is placenta previa? Who is at risk?

Placenta previa occurs when implantation of the fertilized ovum is abnormally low and the developing placenta covers all or part of the internal cervical os. Risk factors include previous Cesarean section, advanced maternal age, and increasing parity.

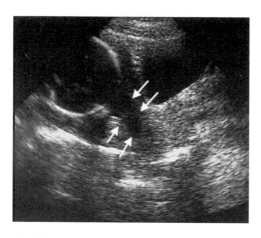

FIGURE 5. Dilated endocervical canal with anechoic bulging membranes (arrows).

37. What is the difference between partial previa and complete previa? What is a marginal previa?

In complete previa, the placenta has implanted on both sides of the cervix, completely bridging the internal os. In partial previa, the placenta implants on one side of the uterus and partially covers the internal os, whereas in marginal previa the placenta ends at the margin of the internal cervical os without covering it. Marginal and partial previa are often grouped together because ultrasound often cannot differentiate them.

38. What is the most common presentation of placenta previa?

Painless vaginal bleeding, which usually occurs in the third trimester, although it may occur as early as 20 weeks.

39. What is a low-lying placenta?

A placenta that extends within 2 cm of the internal os but does not abut it. While not technically a placenta previa, it still warrants evaluation.

40. What causes false-positive and false-negative results of evaluation for placenta previa?

False-positives may occur with lower uterine segment myometrial contractions. Evaluation should be repeated in 45 minutes or so to allow for muscular relaxation. Overdistention of the bladder may lead to apposition of the anterior and posterior walls of the lower uterine segment, simulating placenta previa. False-negatives may occur if the fetal head is low in the uterus and obscures the internal os.

41. Can transvaginal sonography be performed to evaluate placenta previa?

This issue is controversial, although standard transvaginal sonographic technique does not require direct contact between the external cervical os and the transducer face. Transperineal (translabial) ultrasound provides a good alternative for evaluating the relationship of the internal cervical os to the placenta.

42. What are the most severe complications of placenta previa?

Maternal hemorrhage secondary to premature detachment of the placenta, premature delivery, and perinatal death.

43. How are polyhydramnios and oligohydramnios diagnosed?

Although it is usually sufficient to note whether the amount of amniotic fluid is normal, increased, or decreased (Fig. 6), the volume of amniotic fluid can be assessed by several methods. In the first trimester, the volume of amniotic fluid is greater than the volume of embryonic mass. In the second trimester, fetal mass and amniotic fluid are relatively equal in volume. In the third trimester, the amount of amniotic fluid decreases relative to fetal mass.

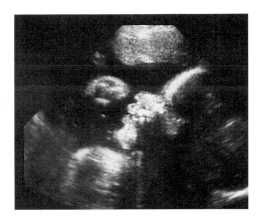

FIGURE 6.   Fetal profile with a normal amount of amniotic fluid around the fetal face.

With the single-pocket method, oligohydramnios can be diagnosed when the largest pocket of fluid is < 2 cm; polyhydramnios is diagnosed when a pocket of fluid > 8 cm is detected. If all four quadrants are examined, oligohydramnios is diagnosed when the sum of the four deepest pockets (one picked for each quadrant) is < 5 cm; polyhydramnios is diagnosed when the sum of the four deepest pockets is > 24 cm. Perinatal morbidity and mortality are increased with extremes of amniotic fluid volume.

44. What are the landmarks for measuring the biparietal diameter and the abdominal circumference?
The biparietal diameter (BPD) should be measured from the transverse axial plane of the fetal head, which includes the falx, cavum septi pellucidi, thalamic nuclei, and choroid plexus in the atria of the lateral ventricles. The critical landmarks for measurement of the abdominal circumference include the left portal vein (in the liver) and fetal stomach.

45. What structures should be routinely examined at sonography (Fig. 7)?
Cerebral ventricles, cerebellum, and cisterna magna
Diaphragm, heart (four-chamber view), umbilical cord insertion on the abdomen, stomach, kidneys, and bladder
Spine
Each examination should be tailored as needed, depending on the individual patient and history.

46. List the three basic types of twins.
Dichorionic diamniotic
Monochorionic diamniotic
Monochorionic monoamniotic

57. What do these terms mean?
Dichorionic diamniotic twins have two separate placentas, chorions, and amnions. The placentas may be fused or on separate sides of the uterus. All dizygotic twins are dichorionic diamniotic (but not all dichorionic diamniotic twins are dizygotic; some are monozygotic). Monochorionic diamniotic twins share a single placenta, but each has its own amnion. All monochorionic twins are monozygotic; this is the most common type of twinning. Monochorionic monoamniotic twins share a single placenta and a single amnion.

48. In the United States, what percentage of twins are dichorionic diamniotic and what percentage are monochorionic?
Eighty percent are dichorionic diamniotic and 20% are monochorionic. Of all monochorionic twins, only 2–3% are monoamniotic; these twins have a mortality rate as high as 50%. With ultrasound, the presence of twinning can be established at six weeks' gestational age by using endovaginal sonography. Dichorionic twins have a thicker membrane between them (Fig. 8), because it is

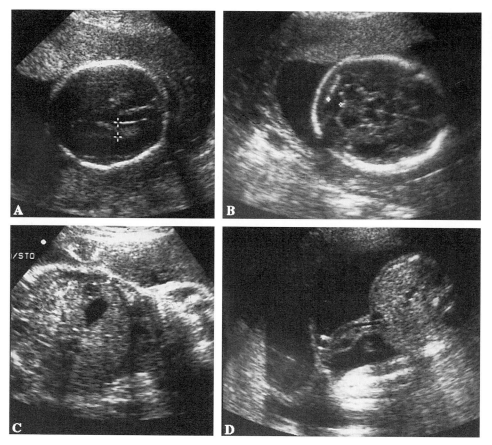

FIGURE 7.   *A*, Normal appearing fetal ventricle, with appropriate placement of calipers at the atrium for measurement. *B*, Calipers outline a normal appearing cisterna magna, with the adjacent cerebellum located anteriorly (on the right on the image). *C*, Intact fetal diaphragm with fluid-filled stomach just inferior (on the left on the image). *D*, Cord insertion.

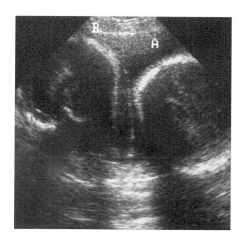

FIGURE 8.   Membrane separating diamniotic twins.

composed of two layers of chorion and two layers of amnion instead of amnion alone, as in a mono-chorionic diamniotic pregnancy. In monochorionic monoamniotic pregnancy, there is no separating membrane.

49. How many vessels are normally present in the umbilical cord?

Two arteries and one vein (Fig. 9). The spiral configuration of the cord is seen on a longitudinal view, in which the cord takes on the appearance of a braid. When an image is obtained perpendicular to the long axis of the cord, the two smaller, thicker-walled arteries can be seen flanking the slightly larger and thinner-walled vein.

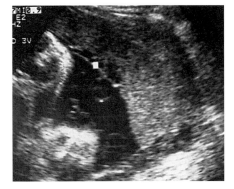

FIGURE 9.   Three vessel umbilical cord, in cross-section.

50. What is the most commonly detected anomaly of the umbilical cord?

A single umbilical artery. The single artery is usually larger than normal and approaches the size of the vein. When a single umbilical artery is detected, a more thorough search for associated fetal anomalies should be initiated. Associated anomalies occur in up to 50% of fetuses with a single umbilical artery. Although chromosomal abnormalities may be associated with a single umbilical artery, such fetuses usually have additional findings on sonography; the presence of a single artery with no other abnormalities is not an indication for amniocentesis.

51. What is the normal appearance of the cervix during the second trimester?

The cervix usually measures 3 cm long; the lower limit of normal is 2.5 cm (Fig. 10). The cervical canal width should not exceed 8 mm. If these criteria are not met, an incompetent cervix should be considered.

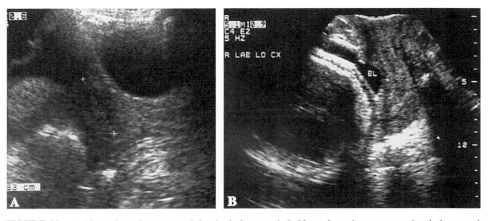

FIGURE 10.   *A*, Normal cervix on transabdominal ultrasound. *B*, Normal cervix on transperineal ultrasound. The fetal head is seen inferior to the nondistended urinary bladder (BL) and against the internal cervical os.

BIBLIOGRAPHY
1. Callen PW: Ultrasonography in Obstetrics and Gynecology, 3rd ed. Philadelphia, W.B. Saunders, 1994.
2. Kurtz AB, Middleton WB: Ultrasonography: The Requisites. St. Louis, Mosby, 1996.
3. Nyberg DA: Diagnostic Ultrasound of Fetal Anomalies. Text and Atlas. St. Louis, Mosby, 1990.

44. OVARIAN AND ADNEXAL IMAGING

Robert B. Poster, M.D.

1. Which imaging modality should be used first to evaluate the ovaries?
Ultrasound (Fig. 1).

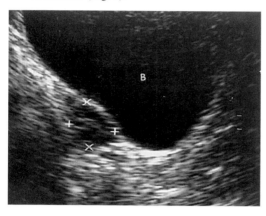

FIGURE 1. Normal ovary on transabdominal sonography (cursors) seen through the distended bladder (B).

2. When performing pelvic sonography in the nulliparous female, what structure is often a landmark for finding the ovaries?
The ovary is often anterior to the internal iliac artery.

3. What are three groups of patients in whom the ovaries may be difficult to visualize with ultrasound?
Patients on hormonal contraception, postmenopausal patients, and prepubertal patients.

4. Is transvaginal, or endovaginal, sonography more sensitive than transabdominal pelvic sonography for evaluating the adnexal structures (Fig. 2)?
Yes. With transvaginal sonography, the ultrasound probe is usually in closer proximity to the adnexae. This allows a higher frequency transducer to be used, which provides better resolution.

5. What is a potential disadvantage of transvaginal sonography to visualize the ovaries?
The field of view is less than with transabdominal sonography, and ovaries that are not within the field of view cannot be evaluated.

6. What are some contraindications to endovaginal sonography?
1. Prepubertal patients
2. Patients who are not and have never been sexually active
3. Recent instrumentation of the vagina, cervix, or endometrium
4. Patient with reluctance to have the exam

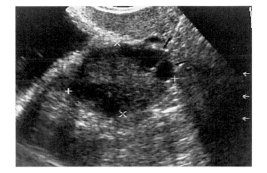

FIGURE 2. Normal ovary on transvaginal sonography (cursors), which contains several small follicles.

7. Which of the following modalities is least useful in evaluating the female reproductive organs: transabdominal sonography, transvaginal sonography, CT, or MR?
    CT.

8. Is free fluid in the cul-de-sac always an abnormal finding on sonography?
    No. While fluid in the cul-de-sac may be due to blood or pus, a small amount of physiologic fluid is normal in premenopausal women (Fig. 3).

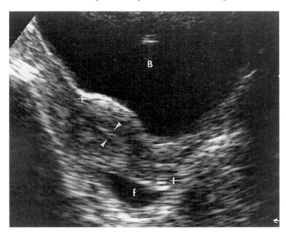

FIGURE 3. Physiologic free fluid (f) in the cul-de-sac, behind the uterus (cursors). B = bladder, arrowheads = endometrium.

9. What is the normal appearance of the ovaries on MR?
    The ovaries are seen as adnexal structures containing multiple follicles of high signal intensity on T2-weighted images (Fig. 4).

10. When sonography is equivocal, can MR determine whether an adnexal mass is arising from the ovary or the uterus?
    Yes.

11. What are the parts of the fallopian tube?
    Starting from the intramural (intrauterine) portion of the fallopian tube, there are the intramural, isthmic, and ampullary sections, with fibria extending off the distal ampullary section.

12. Is the normal fallopian tube routinely visible on transvaginal sonography?
    No, unless the fallopian tube is surrounded by fluid or contains fluid.

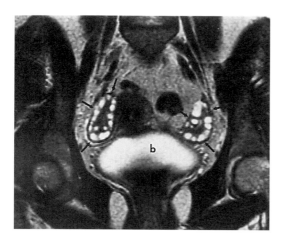

FIGURE 4. Normal ovaries (arrows) on T2-weighted coronal MR image, which contain multiple high signal intensity follicles.

13. What imaging modality best demonstrates the fallopian tubes?

A hysterosalpingogram (HSG). Patency of the fallopian tubes is demonstrated by showing free spillage of contrast from the tubes (Fig. 5).

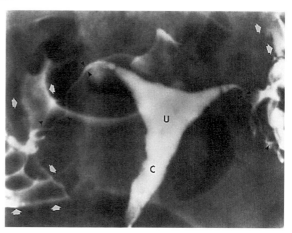

FIGURE 5. Normal hysterosalpingogram; the endocervical canal (C), the uterine cavity (U), and both fallopian tubes (black arrowheads) are demonstrated. Bilateral free spillage of contrast (white arrows) confirms that the fallopian tubes are patent.

14. What is the most common reason for performing a hysterosalpingogram?

To evaluate a patient with infertility.

15. What are some causes of infertility that may be demonstrated on a HSG?

- Blocked fallopian tubes
- Adhesions around the fallopian tube
- Salpingitis isthmica nodosa
- Adhesions within the uterine cavity
- Congenital anomalies
- Submucosal fibroids

16. What is the most common cause of hydrosalpinx?

Hydrosalpinx, a dilated, fluid-filled fallopian tube, is most commonly caused by obstruction of the distal tube secondary to pelvic inflammatory disease (Fig. 6).

17. What is salpingitis isthmica nodosa (SIN), and how may it affect fertility?

SIN is the presence of multiple diverticula extending from the isthmic portion of the fallopian tubes, usually secondary to pelvic inflammatory disease. SIN often can be associated with tubal pregnancy (Fig. 7).

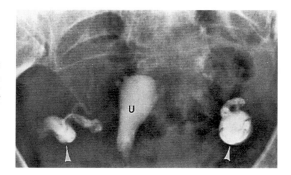

FIGURE 6. Hysterosalpingogram shows contrast collecting in both fallopian tubes, which are obstructed, representing bilateral hydrosalpinx (arrowheads). No free spillage of contrast is seen. U = uterine cavity.

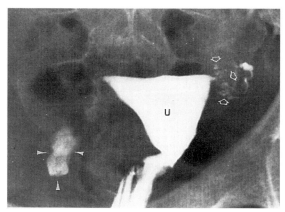

FIGURE 7. Salpingitis isthmica nodosa demonstrated on hysterosalpingogram. Multiple small diverticula (open arrows) extend from the isthmic portion of the left fallopian tube. U = uterine cavity. Arrowheads = calcified dermoid.

18. What are five postoperative fluid collections that may be seen within the pelvis, and what are their sonographic characteristics?

Urinoma, seroma, lymphocele, hematoma, and abscess. While the first three tend to be cystic and not contain internal echoes, hematoma and abscess often contain internal echoes within the fluid.

19. What are sonographic characteristics of a unilocular ovarian cyst?

The cyst contains no internal echoes, there is good through transmission of the sound waves, posterior wall enhancement is noted, and the walls of the cyst are smooth (Fig. 8).

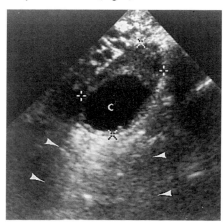

FIGURE 8. A cyst (C) is seen in the ovary (cursors) on transvaginal sonography. The cyst contains no internal echoes, has no perceptible wall, and has good through transmission (arrowheads).

20. Is a unilocular ovarian cyst in a woman of reproductive age almost always benign?
Yes, especially when the cyst measures less than 5 cm.

21. At what point in the menstrual cycle can a mature graafian follicle be seen?
At midcycle, prior to ovulation.

22. At what size is a unilocular ovarian cyst considered within normal limits in a premenopausal woman who is not taking oral contraceptives?
2.5 cm or less.

23. What is the most common cause of ovarian enlargement in young women?
Functional cysts.

24. What are three types of functional cysts in the ovary?
1. Follicular cysts
2. Corpus luteal cysts
3. Theca-luteum cysts

25. If an ovarian cyst is visible sonographically, what additional imaging study could be performed to confirm that it is a functional cyst?
A repeat examination at a different point in the menstrual cycle should show a decrease in size or resolution of the cyst.

26. What is a complicated cyst?
A cyst that contains internal echoes (Fig. 9).

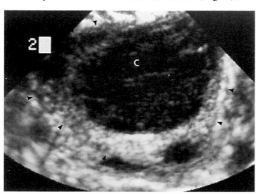

FIGURE 9. A complicated cyst (c) containing internal echoes is identified within the ovary (arrowheads).

27. What are the three most likely diagnoses for a small, complicated ovarian cyst seen by transvaginal sonography in a premenopausal woman?
1. Involuting follicle
2. Hemorrhagic cyst
3. Endometrioma

28. Of the functional cysts, which is related to hyperstimulation of the ovary?
Theca-luteum cysts.

29. What is ovarian hyperstimulation syndrome?
A potential complication of exogenous administration of hormones to assist in follicular development and ovulation in patients having difficulty conceiving. The ovaries may become very enlarged with multiple theca-luteum cysts. When accompanied by pleural effusions or ascites, there is a risk of electrolyte imbalance, hypotension, and oliguria (Fig. 10).

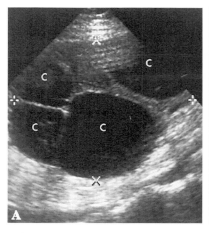
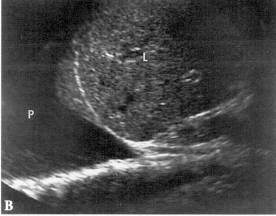

FIGURE 10. *A*, Ovarian hyperstimulation. A markedly enlarged ovary is seen on transvaginal sonography (cursors), containing multiple large cysts (c). *B*, Longitudinal image of the upper abdomen shows a pleural effusion (P) above the liver (L)

30. What ovarian lesions in postmenopausal women are worrisome for malignancy?

Solid lesions or complicated cysts. A unilocular cyst smaller than 5 cm in the ovary is not uncommon in postmenopausal women and can be followed sonographically.

31. What sonographic findings are associated with torsion of the ovary?

A unilaterally enlarged ovary, with multiple peripheral cortical follicles. Color Doppler may demonstrate absence of flow within the ovary.

32. What are some of the sonographic findings associated with pelvic inflammatory disease?

1. The endometrium may be thickened, secondary to endometritis.
2. Echogenic fluid, which represents pus, may be seen in the cul-de-sac.
3. A fluid-filled fallopian tube may be identified.
4. Masses within the ovaries may be seen secondary to ovarian abscesses.

33. What is the classic appearance of the ovaries in patients with polycystic ovaries?

The ovaries are enlarged and contain multiple small peripheral follicles. The stromal echogenicity is increased (Fig. 11).

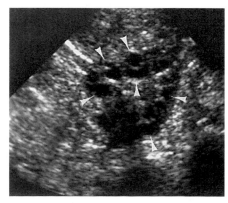

FIGURE 11. Multiple small cysts (arrowheads) line the periphery of an enlarged ovary on transvaginal sonography.

34. What is a sonographically complex mass?

A mass containing both solid and cystic components (Fig. 12).

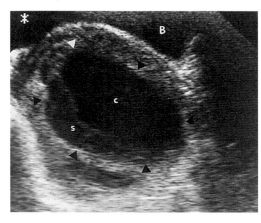

FIGURE 12. A complex mass (arrowheads) containing both solid (s) and cystic (c) components is demonstrated on pelvic sonography. B = bladder.

35. What are some causes of a complex adnexal mass in a nonpregnant patient?
Benign or malignant tumor, abscess, endometrioma, and hematoma.

36. What is endometriosis?
The presence of secretory endometrium in an ectopic location.

37. In what group of women is endometriosis most commonly found?
Infertile women of childbearing age.

38. Which test is considered the "gold standard" for diagnosing endometriosis?
Laparoscopy.

39. What is the most common site of endometriosis?
The ovaries.

40. What is the typical sonographic appearance of endometriomas?
These structures appear as cysts with diffuse low amplitude internal echoes, a visible wall, and enhanced through sound transmission (Fig. 13).

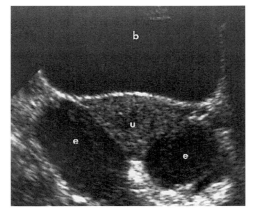

FIGURE 13. Bilateral endometriomas (e) exhibiting internal echoes and through transmission are seen on sonography. u = uterus, b = bladder.

41. What are some clinical situations in which MR may be useful in the evaluation of endometriosis?
- Screening young women who do not want to undergo surgery
- Documenting the extent of disease when adhesions limit laparoscopy
- Monitoring the response to treatment noninvasively

42. What are some MR characteristics of endometriomas?
1. Lesions exhibit high signal intensity on both T1- and T2-weighted images.
2. There are areas of decreased signal intensity within the lesions on T2-weighted images.
3. Multilocular high signal intensity cysts on T1-weighted images.
4. No fat is observed in the lesions.

43. What two lesions may mimic an endometrioma on MR?
Hemorrhagic cysts and ovarian cancer with hemorrhage.

44. What is the most common childhood ovarian tumor?
Dermoids (teratomas).

45. Should dermoid cysts be removed, since they are benign?
Due to the possible complications of rupture or torsion of the ovary, standard practice is to remove them.

46. What plain film findings may be seen with a dermoid cyst?
There is increased lucency representing fat. Radiopaque densities resembling teeth may be seen on plain films and should suggest the diagnosis (Fig. 14).

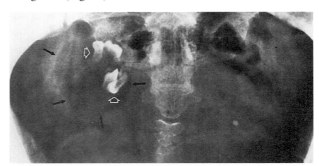

FIGURE 14. Structures resembling teeth (open arrows) are surrounded by an area of increased lucency consistent with fat (black arrows) in this patient with a dermoid.

47. Regarding dermoid cysts, what is the "tip of the iceberg" sign on sonography?
A highly echogenic mass with posterior shadowing is noted; the echogenic area hides the structures posterior to it (Fig. 15).

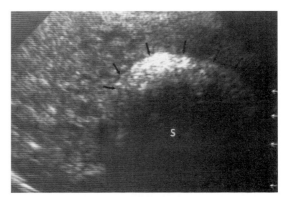

FIGURE 15. Echogenic mass on sonography (arrows) shadows out (s) structures posterior to it. This is the "tip of the iceberg sign" from a dermoid.

48. What is a dermoid plug?
An echogenic mural nodule in a predominately cystic mass (Fig. 16).

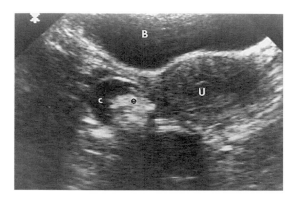

FIGURE 16. A right adnexal mass containing an echogenic nodule (e) and a cystic component (c) is seen on sonography in this patient with a dermoid.

49. What exam should be ordered when a dermoid cyst is suspected clinically but is not confirmed sonographically?

CT, which detects small amounts of fat as well as bony fragments or teeth.

50. On T1- and T2-weighted MR images, a dermoid may appear similar to an endometrioma. What additional MR sequence can help differentiate between these two lesions?

Fat-suppression imaging, because a dermoid contains fat but an endometrioma does not. On a fat-suppression image, therefore, areas of fat in a dermoid will become dark, while the hemorrhage in an endometrioma will remain bright despite fat suppression.

51. What are some of the MR characteristics of dermoid cysts?

- Signal intensity on T1- and T2-weighted images similar to fat elsewhere in the body
- Dermoid plugs
- Floating debris or fat within the lesion
- Chemical shift artifact
- Fat seen within the lesion as demonstrated by fat suppression

52. What are the most common primary neoplasms that metastasize to the ovary?

Breast, colon, and gastric neoplasms.

53. What characteristics of an ovarian lesion suggest that it is malignant?

- A solid ovarian mass
- Irregular solid areas
- Irregular margins
- Thick septae
- Size greater than 10 cm
- Ascites
- Matted loops of bowel

54. What are some benign ovarian neoplasms that are solid on sonography?

Ovarian fibromas, Brenner tumors, and thecomas.

55. What nongynecologic pelvic masses may simulate ovarian masses at sonography?

- Pseudomass from fecal material in the rectum
- Bowel neoplasm
- Abscess from appendicitis, Crohn's disease, or diverticulitis
- Bladder diverticula

56. Do low-resistance waveforms in an ovarian mass as measured by Doppler definitely indicate that a lesion is malignant?

No. While malignant lesions do demonstrate low resistance to flow (i.e., relatively high flow in diastole relative to systole in the arteries within a lesion), other lesions such as corpus luteal cysts and inflammatory masses also may show low resistance to flow.

BIBLIOGRAPHY

 1. Coleman BG: Transvaginal sonography of adnexal masses. Radiol Clin North Am 30:677, 1992.
 2. Coleman BG: Transvaginal sonography of normal pelvic anatomy. Radiol Clin North Am 30:663, 1992.
 3. Filly RA: Ovarian masses . . . what to look for . . . what to do. In Callen PW (ed): Ultrasonography in
    Obstetrics and Gynecology, 3rd ed. Philadelphia, W.B. Saunders, 1994, pp. 625–640.
 4. Laing FC: US analysis of adnexal masses: Art of making the correct diagnosis. Radiology 191:21, 1994.
 5. Jain KA, Friedman DL, Pettinger TW, et al: Adnexal masses: Comparison of specificity of endovaginal US
    and pelvic MR imaging. Radiology 186:697, 1993.
 6. McCarthy S: Magnetic resonance imaging of the normal female pelvis. Radiol Clin North Am 30:769, 1992.
 7. Mitchell DG: Benign disease of the uterus and ovaries: Applications of magnetic resonance imaging. Radiol
    Clin North Am 30:777, 1992.
 8. Occhipinti KA, Frankel SD, Hricak H: Ovary: Computed tomography and magnetic resonance imaging.
    Radiol Clin North Am 31:1115, 1993.
 9. Outwater EK, Dunton CJ: Imaging of the ovary and adnexa: Clinical issues and applications of MR imaging.
    Radiology 194:1–18, 1993.
10. Salem S: The uterus and adnexa. In Rumack CM (ed): Diagnostic Ultrasound. St. Louis, Mosby, 1994, pp
    383–412.
11. Stein SM, et al: Differentiation of benign and malignant adnexal masses: Relative value of gray-scale, color
    Doppler, and spectral Doppler sonography. AJR 164:381, 1995.

45. UTERINE AND CERVICAL IMAGING

Robert B. Poster, M.D.

1. What is the initial imaging study that should be used to evaluate the pelvis when a woman is suspected of having a problem related to the uterus or the cervix?

Ultrasound, given its relative ease of performance, its safety, and its relatively low cost. For transabdominal sonography, the bladder should be full enough to cover the uterine fundus (Fig. 1).

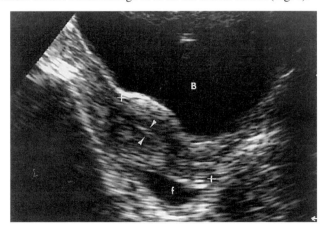

FIGURE 1. Transabdominal pelvic sonogram, sagittal view; the uterus (between +s) is visualized through the distended bladder (B). The endometrium is seen (arrowheads). Physiologic fluid is seen in the cul-de-sac.

2. What conditions limit the performance of a transabdominal pelvic sonogram?

Patients who cannot fill their bladder adequately, obese patients in whom the pelvic organs may not be visualized well, and a retroverted uterus, in which case the uterine fundus may not be seen well.

3. What are some advantages of transvaginal sonography over transabdominal sonography?

The major advantage is the ability to use higher frequency transducers, which provide better resolution. Also, the bladder does not need to be distended during transvaginal sonography.

4. What is the main disadvantage of transvaginal sonography?
The field of view is limited.

5. Which structure is more echogenic, the myometrium or the endometrium?
The endometrium (Fig. 2).

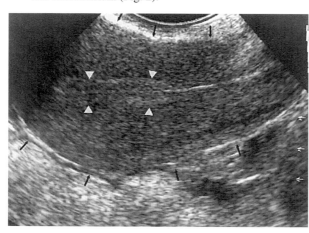

FIGURE 2. Transvaginal sonogram, longitudinal view; the endometrium (arrowheads) is identified as a linear echogenic structure within the uterus (arrows).

6. Is fluid in the cul-de-sac always an abnormal finding?
No, a small amount of fluid can be seen normally in the cul-de-sac in women in their reproductive years.

7. How is a hysterosalpingogram performed?
The cervical os is cannulated, and contrast is injected into the uterine cavity in a retrograde fashion (Fig. 3).

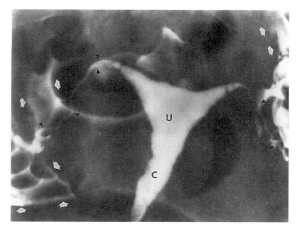

FIGURE 3. Hysterosalpingogram. Contrast is seen filling the endocervical canal (c) and the uterine cavity (U). The fallopian tubes (black arrowheads) and bilateral free spillage of contrast (white arrows) are demonstrated.

8. What is the most common reason for performing a hysterosalpingogram?
As part of the work-up of patients with infertility.

9. What are some uses of MR for imaging the pelvis?
• Diagnosis of müllerian duct anomalies noninvasively
• Preoperative evaluation of uterine fibroids, especially prior to planned myomectomy
• Differentiation of fibroids from adenomyosis

• Determination of whether a pelvic mass originates from the uterus or from the adnexa
• Characterization of some adnexal masses (e.g., teratoma vs. endometrioma)
• Monitoring of endometriosis noninvasively

10. What are some advantages of pelvic MR over CT?
Structures can be imaged in many different planes using MR. There is no ionizing radiation in MR, and the zonal anatomy of the uterus, cervix, and vagina can be identified.

11. T-2 weighted images show the zonal anatomy of the uterus. What are the different zones shown in the uterus on T2-weighted MR images?
The endometrial canal has high signal intensity. Surrounding the endometrial canal is the junctional zone, which is of low signal intensity and represents the compact muscle fibers of the inner myometrium. The outer myometrium is of intermediate signal intensity (Fig. 4).

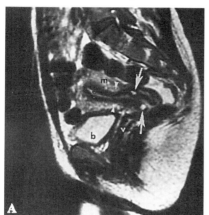 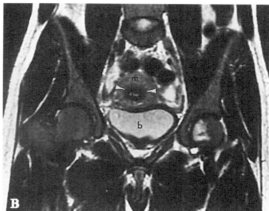

FIGURE 4. *A,* Sagittal T2-weighted MR image demonstrates zonal anatomy of the uterus. The high signal intensity endometrium (e) is surrounded by the dark signal intensity junctional zone. The myometrium (m) is of medium signal intensity. The cervix extends from the internal os (arrowheads) to the external os, which protrudes into the vagina (V). Nabothian cysts (arrows) are seen within the dark cervical stroma. *B,* Coronal T2-weighted MR image shows the high signal intensity endometrium (e) surrounded by the dark junctional zone (arrowheads) and the medium signal intensity myometrium (m). Bladder = b.

12. Why are T1-weighted images obtained when imaging the uterus with MR?
T1-weighted images help to characterize tissue and fluid, permit lymph nodes to be detected, and offer excellent contrast between the pelvic organs and the adjacent fat.

13. During what phase of the menstrual cycle is the endometrium widest?
In the midsecretory phase.

14. In the appropriate clinical setting, is thickening of the endometrium and echogenic material in the endometrial cavity diagnostic of retained products of conception?
No, because a large blood clot may have a similar appearance.

15. What is considered an abnormally thickened endometrial stripe in a postmenopausal woman?
The thickness of the endometrial stripe depends on whether the patient is receiving estrogen replacement therapy. Most authors agree that an endometrial stripe less than 5 mm is normal and greater than 10 mm is abnormal.

16. Which women are most at risk for developing endometrial cancer?
Postmenopausal women.

17. What are some etiologic factors associated with endometrial cancer?
Obesity, diabetes, hypertension, nulliparity, and excess estrogen (either endogenous or exogenous, particularly when unopposed by progesterone).

18. What is the most common presenting symptom of patients with endometrial carcinoma?
Vaginal bleeding—in postmenopausal women.

19. The diagnosis of endometrial cancer is made using which of the following modalities: transvaginal sonography, MR, contrast-enhanced CT, or endometrial biopsy?
Microscopic examination of an endometrial biopsy or curettage specimen. The other modalities may be helpful in staging endometrial cancer.

20. What ultrasound finding is suggestive of endometrial cancer?
Thickening of the endometrium (greater than 6 mm) in a postmenopausal patient with vaginal bleeding (Fig. 5).

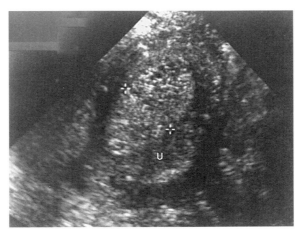

FIGURE 5.   Transvaginal sonogram, longitudinal view. Markedly thickened endometrium (between +s) is seen in a patient with endometrial cancer. Myometrium of the uterus = U.

21. What other conditions can give a thickened endometrium in a postmenopausal woman?
Endometrial hyperplasia, an endometrial polyp, endometritis, and blood in the endometrial cavity.

22. Is an irregular filling defect in the uterine cavity, as seen on a hysterosalpingogram (HSG), most likely due to endometrial cancer?
No. The most likely diagnosis is uterine synechiae (scar tissue). The filling defect(s) in this condition persists even when large amounts of contrast are introduced into the uterine cavity. Endometrial cancer or an early intrauterine pregnancy may give a similar appearance. However, these findings are rare in the patient who usually undergoes an HSG. Also, with these entities, the filling defect will become less apparent or obliterated with increasing amounts of contrast (Fig. 6).

23. Is MR a useful screening test for endometrial cancer?
No. While MR may be useful for staging endometrial cancer, it has no role in detecting the disease. The cancer, which is usually bright on T2-weighted images, is often difficult to distinguish from normal endometrium.

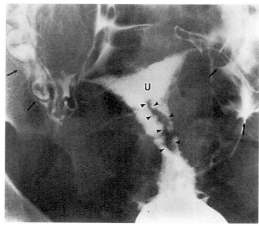

FIGURE 6. Uterine synechiae shown on a hysterosalpingogram as an irregular filling defect in the lower uterine cavity (arrowheads) (U). Bilateral free spillage of contrast (arrows) confirms patency of the fallopian tubes.

24. Is MR the most accurate method of staging endometrial cancer?

No, surgical staging is. However, MR is the most useful noninvasive imaging method. MR can demonstrate the depth of invasion of the myometrium as well as abnormal regional lymph nodes (Fig. 7).

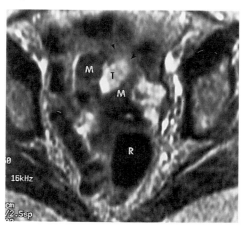

FIGURE 7. Endometrial cancer shown on an axial T2-weighted MR image. High signal intensity endometrial cancer extends through the full width of the myometrium (M). Arrowheads = tumor extending through the wall of the myometrium. R = rectum.

25. What finding on MR is highly suggestive that endometrial cancer is confined to the endometrium?

The junctional zone is intact.

26. MR may depict the degree of invasion of endometrial cancer into the myometrium. Why is this important?

There is a direct correlation between the depth of myometrial invasion and the incidence of lymph node metastases in endometrial cancer.

27. What is one limitation of MR in staging endometrial cancer in postmenopausal women?

The presence or absence of invasion of tumor through the junctional zone is important in staging endometrial cancer, but the junctional zone is often not seen well in postmenopausal women.

28. What is the most common neoplasm of the uterus?

Leiomyomas, or fibroids, which occur in 20–30% of women older than 30.

29. How can a leiomyoma be characterized by location?
- An intramural leiomyoma is confined to the myometrium.
- A submucosal leiomyoma projects into the uterine cavity.
- A subserosal leiomyoma projects from the peritoneal surface of the uterus.

30. In which location are leiomyomas most likely to cause symptoms?
In a submucosal location. They can cause infertility as well as irregular or heavy bleeding.

31. What symptoms can subserosal leiomyomas cause?
While most subserosal leiomyomas are asymptomatic, large subserosal leiomyomas may cause symptoms by pressing on adjacent organs, ligaments, and nerves.

32. Are uterine leiomyomas the most commonly calcified lesions of the female genital tract?
Yes. Calcifications within a fibroid are typically stippled or whorled (Fig. 8).

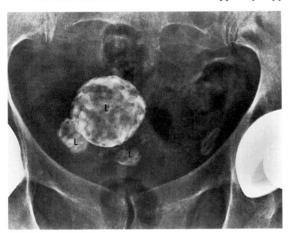

FIGURE 8.   Plain film of the pelvis shows typical calcifications within three separate uterine leiomyomas (L).

33. Is a smooth filling defect in the uterine cavity on HSG diagnostic of a submucosal fibroid?
No. An endometrial polyp or an air bubble may also appear as a smooth filling defect on an HSG (Fig. 9).

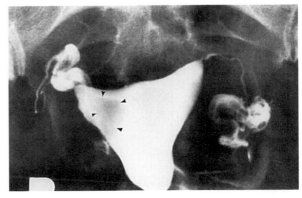

FIGURE 9. A submucosal fibroid shown on a hysterosalpingogram. A smooth filling defect (arrowheads) within the uterine cavity represents the fibroid.

34. What pathologic condition may a retroverted uterus simulate at transabdominal sonography?
The fundus of a retroverted uterus may simulate a fibroid. At transvaginal sonography, it should be easy to distinguish a retroverted fundus from a fibroid (Fig. 10).

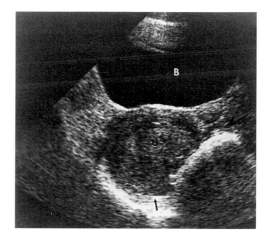

FIGURE 10. A retroverted uterus (u) shown on a transabdominal pelvic sonogram. Bladder = B. Fundus = arrow).

35. What is the typical sonographic appearance of a uterine fibroid?

Fibroids most commonly appear as discrete hypoechoic masses within the uterus (Fig. 11). However, the spectrum of appearances of fibroids is varied. Fibroids may cause diffuse enlargement of the uterus or may be multiple discrete masses. Fibroids may contain calcification or cystic areas and occasionally may be hyperechoic.

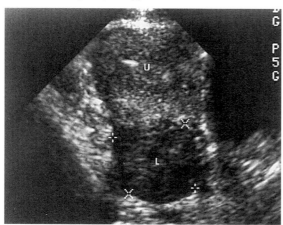

FIGURE 11. Longitudinal view from a pelvic sonogram shows a leiomyoma (L) in the posterior aspect of the uterus (U), which is well circumscribed, round, and hypoechoic.

36. Are leiomyosarcomas easily differentiated on sonography from fibroids?

No. A leiomyosarcoma may appear identical to a rapidly growing or degenerating fibroid. Leiomyosarcomas are rare and account for less than 2% of uterine malignancies.

37. What is the typical appearance of a fibroid on MR?

Typical fibroids, or leiomyomas, appear as sharply defined, round masses with uniform low signal intensity on T1- and T2-weighted images (Fig. 12).

38. What is the most accurate imaging modality for assessing the size, number, and location of fibroids?

MR.

39. Should MR be performed in all patients suspected of having fibroids?

No; ultrasound is easier to perform and less expensive than MR.

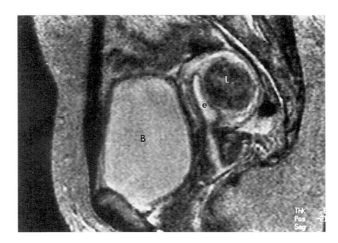

FIGURE 12. Leiomyoma on a T2-weighted sagittal image. A round, low signal intensity intramural leiomyoma (L) is seen in the posterior aspect of the uterus. Endometrium = e; bladder = b.

40. Name five uses for MR in the evaluation of fibroids.
  1. Prior to a myomectomy, MR accurately localizes individual fibroids.
  2. Assessing the response of fibroids to hormone treatment.
  3. Evaluating adnexal masses when ultrasound is inconclusive as to whether they are uterine in origin.
  4. When sonography is technically limited or indeterminate.
  5. To differentiate a leiomyoma from adenomyosis.

41. Is it easy to distinguish a leiomyoma from a leiomyosarcoma on MR?
  While marked enlargement or degenerative changes within a fibroid may be suggestive of a leiomyosarcoma, in most cases it is not possible to distinguish a leiomyoma from a leiomyosarcoma.

42. What is adenomyosis?
  Invasion of the basal layer of the endometrium into the myometrium. Unlike endometriosis, no cyclic changes are observed.

43. What is the treatment for adenomyosis?
  Hysterectomy.

44. Which imaging modality is best for establishing the diagnosis of adenomyosis: sonography, CT, HSG, or MR?
  MR.

45. What are the MR findings of adenomyosis?
  The most specific finding is widening of the junctional zone (greater than 5 mm), which is seen on the T2-weighted images. The widened area may be diffuse or focal. When focal, they are oval. They have irregular and indistinct boundaries with the myometrium. Occasional foci of high signal intensity may also be noted on the T2-weighted images (Fig. 13).

46. What are some distinguishing features on MR between an adenomyoma (a focal area of adenomyosis) and a leiomyoma?
  Leiomyomas tend to be rounder, with smooth margins. Adenomyomas are more irregular in shape and have ill-defined margins.

47. Is the diagnosis of adenomyosis easy to establish at sonography?
  No. Sonographically, the uterus may appear diffusely enlarged. This finding is difficult to distinguish from an enlarged fibroid uterus. MR is useful in distinguishing these two possibilities.

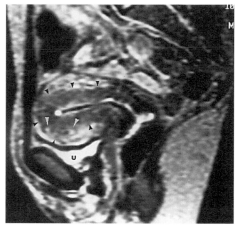

FIGURE 13.   Diffuse adenomyosis. A T2-weighted sagittal image shows diffuse widening of the junctional zone, with indistinct margins (black arrowheads). Punctate areas of high signal intensity are noted (white arrowheads).

48. What is a müllerian duct anomaly?
A congenital anomaly that results from nondevelopment or nonfusion of the müllerian ducts, which can occur to varying degrees.

49. What disorders are associated with müllerian duct anomalies?
- Menstrual disorders
- Infertility, including spontaneous abortions
- Premature labor
- Dystocia
- Abnormal fetal presentation

50. Abnormalities relating to what nongynecologic organ are associated with müllerian duct anomalies?
In up to 50% of patients with müllerian duct anomalies, there are associated abnormalities of the kidney(s), particularly agenesis or ectopia.

51. What is the primary imaging modality for diagnosing müllerian duct abnormalities?
Hysterosalpingography.

52. An HSG in combination with the physical examination is usually adequate to assess which müllerian duct anomaly? In what instances would MR imaging of the pelvis be useful in further diagnosing müllerian duct anomalies?
MR is useful in distinguishing a septate from a bicornuate uterus. It is also useful in identifying an obstructed rudimentary uterine horn in patients who have a unicornuate uterus.

53. Why is it important to distinguish a septate from a bicornuate uterus?
A septate uterus may be repaired by hysteroscopic metroplasty. A bicornuate uterus requires transabdominal surgery if repair is necessary.

54. Can HSG reliably distinguish between a septate and a bicornuate uterus?
No. If the angle of the uterine cavity is 75° or less, the diagnosis is usually a septated uterus. With angles greater than 75°, it is difficult to distinguish a septated from a bicornuate uterus (Fig. 14).

55. What is the major criterion for distinguishing a bicornuate from a septated uterus on MR?
A fundal notch or indentation greater than 1 cm is diagnostic of a bicornuate uterus. A bicornuate uterus will usually show a septum that is of higher signal intensity, often similar to the myometrium. With a septate uterus, the septum is usually of lower signal intensity. However, this finding is not always reliable in distinguishing the two entities (Fig. 15).

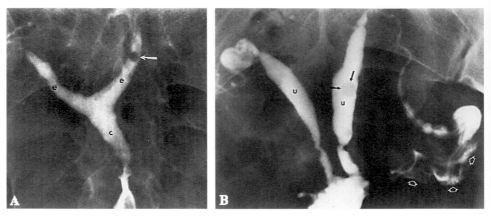

FIGURE 14. *A*, Hysterosalpingogram demonstrates a bicornuate uterus. Two endometrial cavities (e) are separated by a wide angle. C = endocervical canal. Arrow = air bubble. *B*, Septate uterus on HSG. Two endometrial cavities (u) are separated by an angle of less than 75°. The septum extends into the cervix. Free spillage is seen on the left (open arrows). An air bubble (black arrows) moved in the left endometrial cavity.

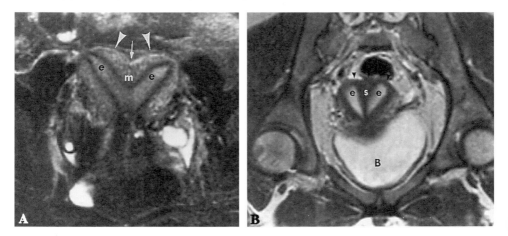

FIGURE 15. A, Bicornuate uterus shown on a coronal T2-weighted MR image. The two endometrial cavities (e) within two uterine horns (arrowheads) are separated by myometrial tissues (m). A fundal notch is demonstrated (arrow). B, Septate uterus shown on a coronal T2-weighted image. The two endometrial cavities (e) are separated by a low signal intensity septum (s). The fundal contour is smooth (arrowheads). B = bladder.

56. Which müllerian duct anomaly will have a typical "banana-shape" uterine cavity on MR?
The unicornuate uterus.

57. What do cystic structures within the cervix on sonography usually indicate?
The presence of nabothian cysts, which are secondary to obstructed and dilated endocervical glands.

58. What is the most common gynecologic malignancy in women of menstrual age?
Cervical cancer.

59. Is transvaginal sonography a good screening exam for carcinoma of the cervix?
No. Screening for cervical cancer is done with a Pap test. Sonography may play a role in the staging of cervical cancer.

60. Which imaging modality is most useful in staging cervical cancer?

MR is useful in estimating tumor size, depth of stromal invasion, parametrial extension, and lymph node involvement.

61. What is the appearance of cervical cancer on T2-weighted images?

Cervical cancer appears as a high signal intensity area; cervical stroma is of low signal intensity.

62. What does an intact cervical stroma on MR indicate?

The chances that the tumor has spread outside the endocervical canal are less than 10% (Fig. 16).

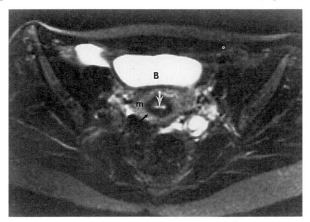

FIGURE 16. A T2-weighted axial MR image shows an intact dark cervical stroma (black arrow) surrounding the endocervical canal (white arrow). Smooth muscle (m) is seen as medium signal intensity around the periphery of the cervix. B = bladder.

63. What is the first imaging modality that should be used to confirm the location of an intrauterine device?

Ultrasound. An intrauterine device appears as an echogenic structure that often has distal acoustic shadowing. If the location cannot be determined at sonography, a plain film of the pelvis could be performed to determine whether the device is present or is lying in the peritoneal cavity. A CT scan can also demonstrate the position of an intrauterine device (Fig. 17).

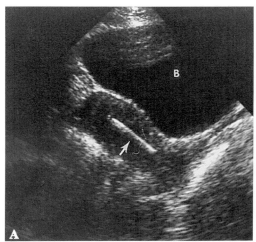
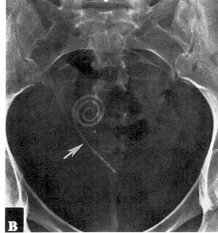

FIGURE 17.   *A*, A sonographic image demonstrates an intrauterine device (arrow) as a linear echogenic structure in the endometrial canal. Bladder = B. *B*, Plain film of the pelvis shows the IUD (arrow).

(Continued on following page.)

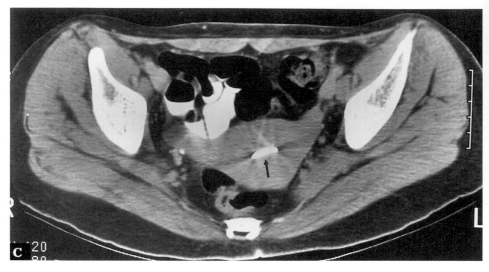

FIGURE 17 *(Cont.).* C, CT shows the IUD (arrow) in the uterus.

BIBLIOGRAPHY

1. Hall DA, Yoder IC: Ultrasound evaluation of the uterus. In Callen PW (ed): Ultrasonography in Obstetrics and Gynecology, 3rd ed. Philadelphia, W.B. Saunders, 1994.
2. Holt SC, Levi CS, Lyons EA, et al: Normal anatomy of the female pelvis. In Callen PW (ed): Ultrasonography in Obstetrics and Gynecology, 3rd ed. Philadelphia, W.B. Saunders, 1994.
3. Karasick S: Hysterosalpingography. Urol Radiol 13:67, 1991.
4. McCarthy S: Magnetic resonance imaging of the normal female pelvis. Radiol Clin North Am 30:769, 1992.
5. Mogavero G, Sheth S, Hamper UM: Endovaginal sonography of the nongravid uterus. Radiographics 12:969, 1993.
6. Salem S: The uterus and adnexa. In Rumack CM (ed): Diagnostic Ultrasound, 2nd ed. St. Louis, Mosby, 1998.
7. Schnall MD: Magnetic resonance evaluation of acquired benign uterine disorders. Semin Ultrasound CT MR 15:4, 1994.
8. Schnall MD: Magnetic resonance evaluation of uterine malignancies. Semin Ultrasound CT MR 15:27, 1994.
9. Wagner BJ, Woodward PJ: Magnetic resonance evaluation of congenital uterine anomalies. Semin Ultrasound CT MR 15:4, 1994.
10. Wagner BJ, Woodward PJ, Farley TE: MR imaging in the evaluation of female infertility. Radiographics 13:293, 1993.
11. Yoder IC: Diagnosis of uterine anomalies: Relative accuracy of MR imaging, endovaginal sonography, and hysterosalpingography. Radiology 185:343, 1992.

VI. Musculoskeletal Radiology

46. OSTEOPOROSIS

Zachary D. Grossman, M.D., and Kevin R. Math, M.D.

1. What is osteoporosis, and how does it differ from osteomalacia and osteopenia?

Osteoporosis is a generalized decrease in overall bone mass, with the bone that is present remaining normally mineralized. It is caused by insufficient formation or increased resorption of bone matrix. *Osteomalacia* is characterized by poor mineralization of normal, or sometimes increased, volumes of osteoid. It can be thought of as a qualitative deficiency in the bone, while osteoporosis is a quantitative abnormality. *Osteopenia* ("poverty of bone") is a general, nonspecific term that encompasses both of the above diseases. This term is used to describe a pathologically decreased quantity of bone when the exact cause of the radiographically decreased bone density is unknown.

2. In what demographic groups is osteoporosis most prevalent?

Females, light hair and eyes, Northern European or Asian ancestry, slender body habitus, and the elderly (senile osteoporosis).

3. Name some dietary, environmental, and pharmacologic causes of osteoporosis.

Deficiency states such as poor calcium and/or vitamin D intake, scurvy, malnutrition/anorexia nervosa; excess caffeine and/or alcohol intake; smoking; weightlessness; immobilization/disuse; medications such as steroids, heparin, and phenytoin.

4. What systemic and congenital/genetic diseases have an increased incidence of osteoporosis?

Endocrine states: hyperparathyroidism (primary and secondary), Cushing's syndrome, estrogen deficiency (postmenopausal women), hypogonadism (e.g., Turner's syndrome), hyperthyroidism, and acromegaly.

Congenital/genetic: osteogenesis imperfecta, homocystinuria, mucopolysaccharidoses, sickle cell disease, thalassemia, and neuromuscular diseases.

Other: intestinal malabsorption syndromes, neoplastic (e.g., multiple myeloma, metastasis, infiltrative marrow diseases, rheumatoid arthritis, amyloidosis, and liver disease).

5. Are conventional radiographs sensitive enough to diagnose osteoporosis?

No. About 20–40% of bone mineral mass must be lost before radiographic findings are evident.

6. What radiographic features are useful in diagnosing osteoporosis?

Decreased bony density, cortical thinning, accentuation of trabecular stress lines due to resorption of secondary trabeculae (best seen at femoral neck), and prominence of vertebral body endplates.

7. How is the third metacarpal bone useful in diagnosing osteoporosis?

Decreased bone density is often a subjective sign in attempting to diagnose osteoporosis. This is strongly dependent on radiographic technique; under- or overexposure can result in erroneously increased or decreased bone density, respectively. A fair number of false positive and false negative diagnoses may result if assessment of bone density is used solely.

Objective radiographic assessment of osteoporosis can be made by evaluating the relative corti-cal thickness of the third metacarpal. The combined cortical thickness measured at the mid-shaft should total at least 50% of the entire thickness of the metacarpal at the same level (Fig. 1).

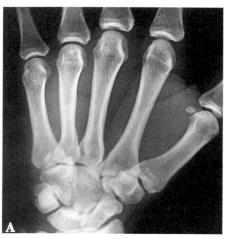 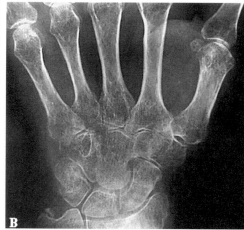

FIGURE 1.   *A,* Note the normal cortical thickness at the third metacarpal shaft in this 30-year-old. The sum of the cortical thickness greatly exceeds 50% of the entire width of the bone, measured at mid-shaft. *B,* The cortices of this elderly osteoporotic woman are markedly thinned, adding up to about 35% of the entire width of the bone. The bones are also more radiolucent; however, this sign is subjective and is dependent on technical factors.

8. What is the Singh trabecular index?

Singh described a method of assessing the trabeculae of the femoral neck to quantify osteoporo-sis. He divided the trabeculae at the neck into compressive and tensile trabeculae and demonstrated the predictable changes in them as osteoporosis progresses. Unfortunately, this technique, while of historical value, is highly subjective and has been replaced by newer, highly sensitive densitometry modalities.

9. Is CT more sensitive than conventional radiographs for evaluating bone mineral density?

Yes. In fact, quantitative CT (QCT) software is available so that bone mineral density can be measured on standard CT scanners. While this technique has been shown to have high sensitivity and precision (particularly in the spine), other methods of assessment based on relative absorption of photons (SPA, DPA) or x-rays (DXA) are usually preferred.

10. What are some indications for measuring bone density?

- Monitoring changes in bone mass in patients being treated for osteoporosis.
- Evaluating postmenopausal or estrogen-deficient women for possible hormone replacement therapy.
- Evaluating bone loss in patients with hyperparathyroidism or hypercortisolism from glucocor-ticoid therapy.
- Determining if osteopenia is present in patients with vertebral deformities or in those in whom osteopenia is suspected on the basis of radiographs.

While many of the conditions and diseases associated with osteoporosis cannot be cured, pre-ventive measures can be taken to avoid such factors as estrogen deficiency, lack of exercise, poor calcium intake, and some endocrine disorders in addition to medication adjustments. The measure-ment of bone mineral density is known as "bone densitometry." Those with significant risk factors should be evaluated before symptoms and signs develop so that early intervention can be made. Bone densitometry not only provides an absolute measurement of bone mineral density, but also de-termines the fracture risk relative to the young normal (age 20–40) and age-matched controls.

11. What is single and dual-photon absorptiometry?

Single photon absorptiometry (SPA) was developed in the 1960s as a means for quantitative assessment of the bone mineral content at various sites of the peripheral skeleton. A highly collimated photon beam from a radionuclide source (I-125) is used to measure photon attenuation, usually at the distal radius. This technique is most accurate when soft-tissue thickness is constant.

The primary disadvantage of SPA is its inability to provide accurate measurements at sites of variable soft tissue thickness and composition (e.g., spine, hip). This limitation was overcome by utilizing dual photon absorptiometry (DPA). DPA utilizes radiation of two distinct energies, one high-energy beam and one of low energy. A high-purity, high-activity Gadolinium-153 source is utilized, providing photons with energies of 44 keV and 100 keV. The low-energy beam is attenuated to a greater degree than the high-energy beam.

In both bone and soft tissue the low-energy beam (44 keV) is attenuated more than the high energy beam (100 keV), but to a much greater extent in bone. Therefore, bone yields a higher contrast at low energies than at high energies. DPA exploits this difference in contrast; entering these attenuation profiles into a mathematical equation allows accurate calculation of the bone mineral density of the spine and hip.

12. What are the units of measurement of bone mineral content and density?

Bone mineral content (BMC) is measured in grams (of bone ash or hydroxyapatite). Bone mineral density is expressed as a function of BMC relative to the area: grams/cm^2.

13. What are the disadvantages of DPA?

The study takes a relatively long time to perform (20–45 minutes for the lumbar spine), anatomic resolution is limited, and radionuclide decay can result in decreased accuracy if proper quality control measures are not taken.

14. What is dual x-ray absorptiometry (DEXA)?

This technique utilizes the same physical principles as DPA, except that the radionuclide source is replaced with an x-ray tube. Two distinct energy x-ray beams are utilized (usually 70 kVp and 140 kVp) and the same types of calculations used in DPA are applied. DEXA is considered the state-of-the-art examination for the diagnosis and follow-up of osteoporosis.

15. What are the advantages of DEXA over DPA?

Shortened examination time due to greater photon flux of the x-ray tube (lumbar spine evaluation takes 5–10 minutes as compared to 20–45 minutes for DPA), better anatomic resolution, greater accuracy and precision, and decreased cost.

16. What sites of the skeleton are routinely assessed on a DEXA scan?

The lumbar spine, from L1 or L2 to L4 and the proximal femur (regions of interest in the femoral neck, trochanteric region, and Ward's triangle (Fig. 2). Ward's triangle is a site at the proximal femur where bone mineral loss is thought to occur first.

17. How can large osteophytes and sclerotic changes in a patient with lumbar degenerative disease affect bone densitometry assessment?

On an anteroposterior (AP) evaluation of the lumbar spine, the osteophytes and sclerotic changes in the vertebrae cause an erroneous elevation of the bone mineral density. This can result in the BMD of an osteoporotic patient appearing falsely normal. This problem is overcome by newer DEXA equipment that allows lateral scanning of the lumbar spine.

18. What other modalities are currently being evaluated for the assessment of osteoporosis?

Ultrasound scanners are available that can measure the patella or calcaneus for bone mineral density. This is accomplished by measuring the velocity of ultrasound through the bone and by measuring the attenuation of the ultrasound wave travelling through the bone (called broad-band

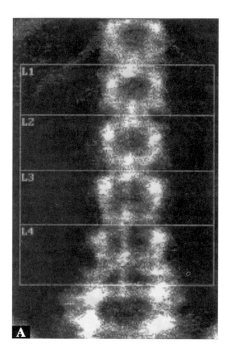

BMD (Ll–L4) = 1.120 g/cm²

REGION	BMD	T (30.0)	Z
L1	1.059	+1.22 114%	+2.15 129%
L2	1.124	+0.88 109%	+1.92 123%
L3	1.184	+0.91 109%	+2.01 123%
L4	1.113	–0.03 100%	+1.10 112%
L1–L4	1.120	+0.67 107%	+1.74 121%

* Age and sex matched
T = peak bone mass
Z = age matched

FIGURE 2. Dual x-ray absorptiometry (courtesy of Dr. Fukat Onseng). *A,* Bone mineral density (BMD) is assessed at each individual vertebral level (L1–L4). *B,* BMD values at each level are compared to normal 30-year-old controls (T) and age-matched individuals (Z). The relative fracture risk is calculated based on these comparisons. The same is done for the proximal femur (hip).

ultrasound attenuation). Ultrasound assessment of the calcaneus can potentially provide quantitative information that may correlate with hip or lumbar spine fracture risk. Ultrasound assessment of bone shows promise as a screening procedure because the equipment is relatively inexpensive and there is no ionizing radiation. Currently, this modality is used as a research technique and is not yet approved for clinical practice.

MRI evaluation of osteoporosis is still in its early stages. BMD assessment is based on the loss of vertebral bone mineral and concomitant increase in fatty marrow occurring in osteoporosis. BMD and the amount of intertrabecular fatty marrow are inversely related; this may potentially allow a future role for MR in assessing bone mineral density.

BIBLIOGRAPHY

1. Grampp S, Jergas M, Gluer CC, et al: Radiologic diagnosis of osteoporosis: Current methods and perspectives. Radiol Clin North Am 31:1133, 1993.
2. Greenspan A: Orthopedic Radiology: A Practical Approach, 2nd ed. Philadelphia, Lippincott-Raven, 1993.
3. Jergas M, Genant HK: Current methods and recent advances in the diagnosis of osteoporosis. Arthritis Rheum 36:1649–1662, 1993.
4. Lang P, Steiger P, Faulkner K, et al: Osteoporosis: Current techniques and recent developments in quantitative bone densitometry. Radiol Clin North Am 29:49–76, 1991.
5. Schneider R, Math KR: Bone density analysis, an update. Curr Opin Orthop 5:66–72, 1994.
6. Wehrli FW, Ford JC, Haddad JG: Osteoporosis: Clinical assessment with quantitative MR imaging in diagnosis. Radiology 196:631, 1995.

47. MRI OF THE MUSCULOSKELETAL SYSTEM

Kevin R. Math, M.D.

1. What advantages does MRI offer over other imaging modalities for evaluation of the musculoskeletal system?

- Assessment of bone marrow abnormalities. MRI can accurately detect subtle derangements in the composition of bone marrow. Any marrow-replacing process (e.g., infection, tumor) is detected as a diffuse (Fig. 1) or focal (Fig. 2) loss of the normally hyperintense fatty marrow signal on T1-weighted images.
- Detection of occult fractures and bone contusions
- Visualization of tendons, ligaments, and cartilage
- Staging of musculoskeletal tumors

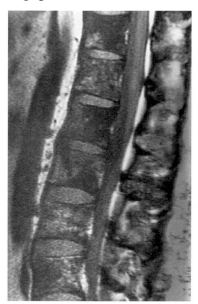 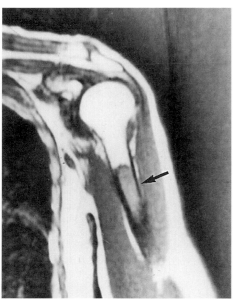

FIGURE 1 *(Left)*. Metastatic prostate cancer—lumbar spine. T1-weighted sagittal MR image demonstrates generalized heterogeneous abnormal marrow signal reflecting marrow replacement by tumor. On T1-weighted images, the vertebrae are normally "brighter" than the intervertebral disc, owing to the hyperintense fatty marrow.

FIGURE 2 *(Right)*. Metastatic lung cancer—humerus. T1-weighted image reveals a focal marrow-replacing lesion at the proximal humeral shaft (arrow). There is intermediate signal intensity replacing the normally hyperintense fatty marrow.

2. For which of the following disease processes has MRI replaced conventional radiographs: neoplasm, fracture, or arthritis?

None of the above. Plain films are definitely the most informative study for each of these diseases. MRI has not replaced conventional radiographs but supplements plain films in further defining the presence and extent of these processes and associated complications.

3. What is the normal appearance of bone marrow on MRI?

Fatty and hematopoietic marrow differ in MR appearance. The adult skeleton, containing mostly fatty (yellow) marrow, appears uniformly hyperintense on T1-weighted images (like fat).

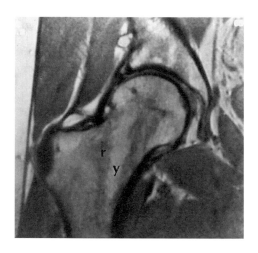

FIGURE 3. Red and yellow marrow, proximal femur. This T1-weighted coronal image demonstrates the normal heterogeneity of marrow signal at the proximal femur. This is not a pathologic condition but rather represents the normal distribution and different signal characteristics of hematopoietic (red—'r') and fatty (yellow—'y') marrow.

Hematopoietic (red) marrow, containing much less fat than fatty marrow, has lower T1 signal (Fig. 3). Hematopoietic marrow predominates in children and in the axial skeleton of adults. The proportion of red marrow in adults becomes relatively increased in chronic anemia (red marrow reconversion). Hematopoietic marrow also may undergo hyperplasia, particularly in smokers, obese women, and high-performance athletes, occasionally resulting in a striking appearance of decreased T1 signal.

4. Before the advent of MRI, which imaging study was routinely performed for evaluation of suspected internal derangement of the knee?

Arthrography, which is done by injecting iodinated contrast and air into the joint, followed by conventional radiographs in different projections. Before MRI, arthrography was done routinely for evaluation of suspected meniscal or cruciate ligament tears and for diagnosis of rotator cuff tears. MRI is noninvasive, offers superior anatomic information, and diagnoses these injuries with greater accuracy than arthrography. Currently, arthrography is rarely performed; it is reserved for patients in whom MRI is contraindicated.

5. Name the structures labeled on the sagittal MR images of the normal knee in Figure 4.

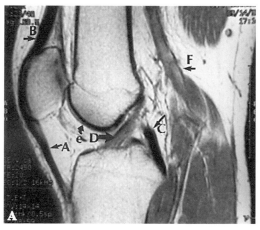
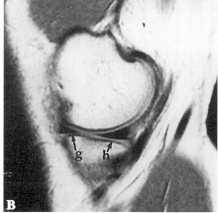

FIGURE 4. *A* and *B,* MRI of the normal knee. A = patellar tendon; B = quadriceps tendon; C = posterior cruciate ligament; D = anterior cruciate ligament; e = articular cartilage, distal femur; F = popliteal vessel; g = medial meniscus, anterior horn; h = medial meniscus, posterior horn.

In the Figure 4B, note that the posterior horn of the medial meniscus is larger than the anterior horn (both horns are equivalent in size at the lateral meniscus). In Figure 4A, note the generalized low signal in the posterior cruciate ligament compared with the normal intermediate signal within the anterior cruciate ligament.

6. Describe the MR features of normal and torn tendons.

Tendons are normally uniformly dark on all MR sequences. They normally appear as tubular or circular low-signal structures on longitudinal and axial images, respectively. Tendon tears result in abnormal size of the tendon (usually increased) and increased internal signal. A complete tear of the tendon results in a focal discontinuity, with the gap often occupied by fluid.

7. What is the "magic angle phenomenon"?

Collagen fibers oriented at 55° to the main magnetic field may result in increased signal within tendons or menisci. Awareness of this artifact avoids confusing it with a pathologic process. The magic angle artifact is most commonly seen in the posterior horn of the lateral meniscus and in the anterior fibers of the supraspinatus tendon and disappears on T2-weighted images.

8. What are the MRI features of a torn meniscus?

Menisci are fibrocartilaginous structures and are normally uniformly dark on MRI, with a triangular configuration. Meniscal tears are manifested by a linear signal that traverses the meniscus and touches the superior or inferior surface or tip of the meniscus (called grade 3 signal) (Fig. 5). Intact menisci may have a globular or linear signal within them that does not touch the surface. This signal is termed grade 1 (globular) or grade 2 (linear) signal and histologically represents myxoid degenerative change within the meniscus, a normal function of aging. Tears also may take the form of blunting of the apex of the meniscus (tip of the triangle).

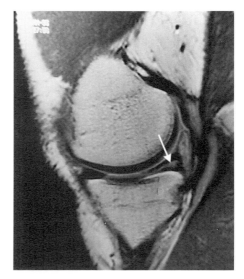

FIGURE 5. Meniscal tear. A linear signal in the posterior horn of the medial meniscus (arrow) touches the inferior surface of the meniscus, consistent with a tear.

9. What is a bucket-handle tear?

A vertical tear of the meniscus in which the inner fragment of meniscus is displaced for a variable distance toward the intercondylar notch (this fragment is the "bucket handle"). The displaced fragment is best visualized on coronal images (Fig. 6).

10. Where do the cruciate ligaments attach?

The anterior cruciate ligament (ACL) extends from the medial (inner) aspect of the lateral femoral condyle to attach about 1 cm posterior to the anterior tibial articular surface, just medial to

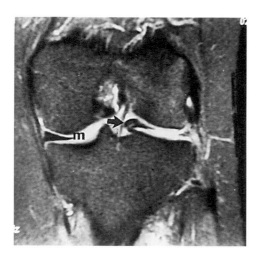

FIGURE 6. Bucket-handle tear, lateral meniscus. A fragment of the posterior horn of the lateral meniscus is displaced into the intercondylar notch (arrow). Note the normal-appearing triangular medial meniscus (m) and the abnormal remaining lateral meniscus.

the midline. The posterior cruciate ligament (PCL) extends from the lateral surface of the medial femoral condyle to the posterior tibia, adjacent to the midline.

11. Which is more commonly torn, the ACL or PCL?
The ACL, by a ratio of at least 9 to 1.

12. Describe the MR appearance of a torn ACL.
Acute ACL tears result in waviness or discontinuity of the ligament, commonly associated with an amorphous heterogeneous signal hematoma at the site of the tear (Fig. 7). The tear most commonly involves the proximal or middle portions of the ACL. Large joint effusions commonly accompany acute ACL tears because of the close proximity to geniculate vessels. Chronic ACL tears may have a variable appearance, ranging from nonvisualization of the ACL to an abnormal horizontal orientation of the ligament.

FIGURE 7. Anterior cruciate ligament (ACL) tear. The ACL is poorly defined, with a heterogeneous signal hematoma near the site of its femoral attachment. The dashed line shows where one would expect to find a normal intact ACL.

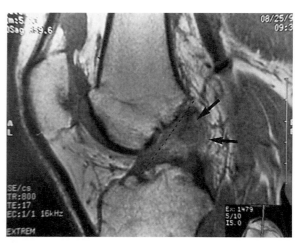

13. Where are the two characteristic sites of bone contusion associated with acute ACL tears?
Contusions typically occur at the anterior aspect of the lateral femoral condyle and at the posterior aspect of the tibial plateau (lateral > medial) (Fig. 8). This is due to excessive anterior translation of the tibia relative to the femur and the resultant impaction injury at these two sites.

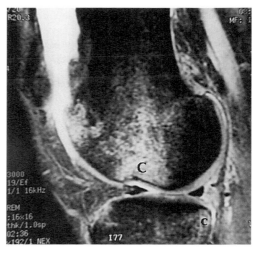

FIGURE 8.   ACL tear—bone contusions. Focal bone contusions are seen in the lateral femoral condyle (C) and posterior tibial plateau (c), manifested by areas of hyperintense T2 marrow signal. Bone contusions at these sites are highly specific for ACL tears.

14. How sensitive and specific is MRI in diagnosing meniscal and ACL tears?
Most reports have found the sensitivity and specificity of MR to be over 90% for the diagnosis of meniscal tears and complete ACL tears.

15. What is O'Donoghue's unhappy triad?
ACL tear, MCL tear, and medial meniscal tear. Up to 70% of ACL tears are associated with other intraarticular injuries.

16. Name the three components of the lateral collateral ligament complex.
From anterior to posterior: iliotibial band, fibular collateral ligament, and tendon of the biceps femoris muscle. Each of these can be identified on MR images.

17. Can MRI estimate the severity of a medial collateral ligament (MCL) tear?
Yes. The MCL is normally visualized as a low-signal structure extending from the medial femoral condyle to the medial tibial plateau. Mild injuries result in edema around the intact ligament, whereas more extensive injuries result in disruption of a variable degree of the visualized ligament fibers (Fig. 9).

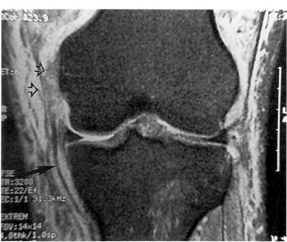

FIGURE 9.   Medial collateral ligament (MCL) tear. Note the hyperintense signal and poor definition of fibers at the femoral attachment of the MCL (open arrows). This represents a large partial tear. Note the intact low signal ligament fibers near its tibial attachment (solid arrow).

18. What is Pelligrini-Stieda disease?

The calcification or ossification sometimes seen in the soft tissues at the medial aspect of the medial femoral condyle after a chronic MCL tear.

19. What is the diagnosis on the sagittal MR image in Figure 10?

Quadriceps tendon tear. Note the discontinuity of the tendon and the increased signal at the site of injury.

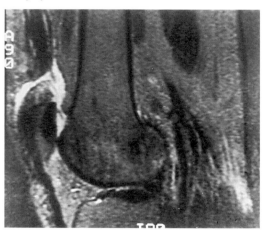

FIGURE 10.   Quadriceps tendon tear. Note the focal discontinuity of the quadriceps tendon near its patellar attachment. The site of the tear is occupied by fluid on this T2-weighted image. Compare with the normal continuous patellar tendon.

20. Name the four muscles of the rotator cuff.

The mnemonic **SITS** may help to remember these muscles: **s**upraspinatus, **i**nfraspinatus, **t**eres minor, and **s**ubscapularis.

21. Where do the rotator cuff tendons insert?

The subscapularis tendon inserts on the lesser tuberosity of the humerus. The remaining three tendons insert on the greater tuberosity.

22. Which tendon of the rotator cuff is most commonly torn?

Supraspinatus.

23. What MR imaging planes are used for evaluating the shoulder?

Because the rotator cuff muscles and tendons course in an oblique fashion, oblique imaging planes must be used to image them tangentially. Therefore, oblique coronal images are performed along the plane of the supraspinatus (posteromedial to anterolateral). Oblique coronal images provide the most information about the integrity of the rotator cuff and are commonly supplemented by oblique sagittal (90° to oblique coronal) and axial images.

24. Describe the typical MR appearance of a rotator cuff tear.

Tears are manifested by increased signal within the tendon or a focal tendinous discontinuity (Fig. 11). Most tears occur in the critical zone of the supraspinatus tendon, a relatively hypovascular area of the tendon approximately 1–2 cm proximal to its greater tuberosity insertion.

25. Are there any other causes of increased signal in the cuff tendons?

Yes. Tendon degeneration is a normal accompaniment of aging and results in increased intratendinous signal. This is termed "tendinosis" or "tendinopathy" and is usually asymptomatic. Cuff tears usually can be differentiated from tendinosis by the T2 signal characteristics; tendon tears show high T2 signal, whereas the T2 signal abnormality in tendinosis is mild to moderate if present at all. The magic angle phenomenon and volume averaging artifact also may result in increased signal.

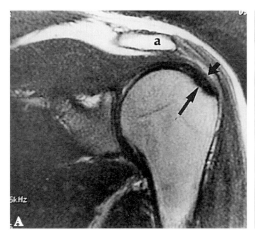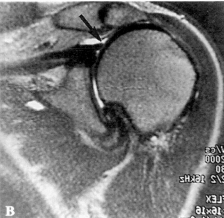

FIGURE 11. *A,* Normal shoulder MRI. The supraspinatus tendon is uniformly low signal and continuous (arrows). The space between the humeral head and the acromion (a) is maintained. *B,* Chronic rotator cuff tear. The supraspinatus tendon is completely torn and retracted to the level of the glenohumeral joint (arrow), where it is surrounded by fluid. Note the high-riding humeral head, in close proximity to the acromion. This is due to the atrophy of the cuff muscles associated with chronic tendon tears.

26. Which MR feature indicates that a rotator cuff tear is chronic?

Muscle atrophy, which results in a high-riding humeral head with the superior humeral head in close proximity to the acromion process. This sign also allows diagnosis of a chronic rotator cuff tear on conventional radiographs.

27. Which disease predisposes patients to chronic rotator cuff tears?

Rheumatoid arthritis.

28. Which other shoulder injuries can be diagnosed on routine shoulder MR?

Glenoid labral tears, biceps tendon injuries, and occult bony injuries.

29. What is a SLAP lesion?

SLAP is an acronym that stands for **s**uperior **l**abrum **a**nterior and **p**osterior. Labral tears are seen in throwing athletes or following shoulder trauma and have an increased incidence of associated rotator cuff and biceps tendon tears. Subtle SLAP lesions may be difficult to diagnose on MRI; MR-arthrography increases the sensitivity for detecting these injuries.

30. How sensitive is MR for diagnosing rotator cuff and labral tears?

Sensitivity and specificity vary with the technical quality of the study and the experience of the radiologist. However, most studies report that the sensitivity and specificity of MR for diagnosis of cuff tears are above 90%. Sensitivity for labral injuries is more variable, ranging from 75% to above 90%.

31. What is the most commonly injured ankle tendon?

Achilles' tendon.

32. Describe the MR appearance of Achilles tendon tears.

The Achilles' tendon is normally uniformly low in signal, with a slightly concave anterior margin, resulting in "kidney bean" appearance on axial images. Tears most commonly occur about 2–6 cm above the calcaneus where the tendon has relatively decreased vascular supply and crossing tendon fibers. Tears result in thickening of the tendon with increased internal signal and a convex anterior margin (Fig. 12). Complete tears can be accurately differentiated from partial tears by a focal tendinous discontinuity, best appreciated on sagittal images.

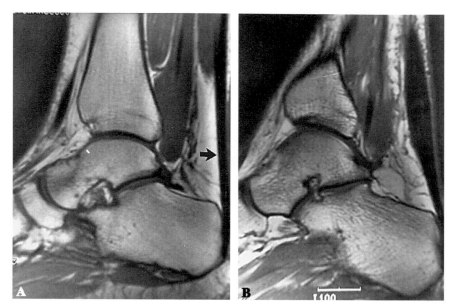

FIGURE 12. *A*, Normal ankle MRI—sagittal plane. The Achilles tendon (arrow) is uniformly low signal with uniform thickness and a straight anterior margin. *B*, Achilles tendon tear. Note the fusiform thickening of this chronically torn Achilles tendon. This is due to an old partial tear of this structure with subsequent healing and fibrosis.

33. Name the three flexor tendons at the medial aspect of the ankle.

The three flexor tendons can be recalled through the mnemonic **T**om, **D**ick, and **H**arry: **t**ibialis posterior, flexor **d**igitorum longus, and flexor **h**allucis longus (Fig. 13).

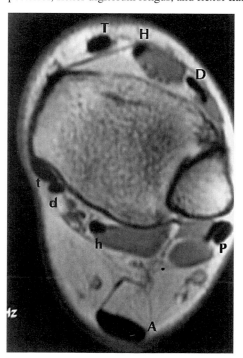

FIGURE 13. Normal ankle MRI–axial plane. Normally 9 tendons at the ankle can be readily visualized on axial images. The flexor tendons are located at the medial aspect of the ankle; tibialis posterior (t), flexor digitorum longus (d), and flexor hallucis longus (h). The neurovascular bundle is located between "d" and "h." The extensor tendons are seen anteriorly: tibialis anterior (T), extensor hallucis longus (H), and extensor digitorum longus (D). Note that the hallucis muscles are associated with their low signal tendons. The peroneal tendons (P) are posterior to the distal fibula at the lateral aspect of the ankle (peroneus longus is lateral or posterior to peroneus brevis). The Achilles' tendon (A) is seen posteriorly at the ankle; note its straight anterior margin.

34. Which of the flexor tendons is most commonly torn?
Tibialis posterior (Tom). It is the second most common tendon tear at the ankle and results in progressive flatfoot deformity. Tears of the tibialis posterior tendon are well seen on MR.

35. Name the three lateral supporting ligaments at the ankle.
Anterior talofibular, posterior talofibular, and calcaneofibular ligaments.

36. Which of these three ligaments tends to tear first?
Anterior talofibular ligament. Tears are best seen on axial images of the ankle.

37. Where is the triangular fibrocartilage (TFC)?
The TFC is a fibrocartilaginous structure at the wrist which extends from the ulnar styloid to the ulnar aspect of the distal radius.

38. How sensitive is MRI for diagnosis of TFC tears?
MR sensitivity is quite variable; sensitivities ranging from 72% to over 90% have been reported.

39. What is the role of MRI in evaluation of the carpal tunnel syndrome?
Carpal tunnel syndrome is readily diagnosed by clinical and electromyographic criteria, and MRI is rarely necessary. MRI demonstrates an enlarged median nerve with increased internal T2 signal and occasional bowing of the adjacent flexor retinaculum. MR is most useful when a mass is suspected clinically or for more difficult clinical diagnoses.

40. What is the most sensitive imaging modality for diagnosing avascular necrosis of the hip?
MRI.

BIBLIOGRAPHY

1. Beltran J (ed): The Ankle and Foot. MRI Clin North Am 2(1):1–153, 1992.
2. Berquist TH: MRI of the Musculoskeletal System, 2nd ed. New York, Raven Press, 1996.
3. Fitzgerald SW (ed): The knee. MRI Clin North Am 2(2):325–499, 1994.
4. Gusmer PB, Potter HG, Schatz JA, et al: Labral injuries: Accuracy of detection with unenhanced MR imaging of the shoulder. Radiology 200:519–524, 1996.
5. Mink JH, Reicher MA, Crues JV III, Deutsch AL: MRI of the Knee, 2nd ed. Philadelphia, Lippincott-Raven, 1993.
6. Pavlov H: Athletic injuries. Radiol Clin North Am 28:435–443, 1993.
7. Rafii M (ed): The Shoulder. MRI Clin North Am 1:1–195, 1993.
8. Sartoris DJ: Principles of Shoulder Imaging. New York, McGraw-Hill, 1995.

48. ARTHRITIS

Kevin R. Math, M.D.

1. What imaging modality is best for diagnosis and follow-up of arthritic disease?
Plain films are usually the only study needed for accurate diagnosis and follow-up. More advanced modalities such as MR and CT are reserved for suspected complications of arthritis (e.g., cord compression, avascular necrosis, fracture).

2. What is an inflammatory arthritis?
Inflammatory arthritides include rheumatoid arthritis and the rheumatoid variants (psoriatic arthritis, Reiter's disease, ankylosing spondylitis). The feature common to all of these disorders is inflammatory pannus that erodes articular cartilage and bone.

3. **What radiographic features must be assessed in attempting to classify an arthropathy?**
   - **Polyarticular vs. monoarticular involvement.** Monoarticular involvement implies a localized process and is commonly posttraumatic, degenerative, or infectious. Polyarticular involvement is seen with systemic diseases such as rheumatoid arthritis (RA), psoriatic arthritis, and gout.
   - **Distribution of joint involvement.** Some arthritides have a predilection for the hands and feet (rheumatoid arthritis, gout), whereas others more severely affect the spine and proximal large joints (ankylosing spondylitis).
   - **Symmetry.** Rheumatoid arthritis is bilaterally symmetrical, whereas degenerative joint disease (DJD) is unilateral or bilaterally asymmetrical.
   - **Erosions.** The presence of erosions implies an inflammatory (RA, infection) rather than a degenerative process.
   - **Joint space narrowing.** The presence and degree of joint space narrowing reflect the loss of articular cartilage. Inflammatory arthritides such as RA result in uniform diffuse joint space narrowing, whereas in degenerative disease the joint space narrowing is localized or uneven.
   - **Osteoporosis.** Osteoporosis is a feature of RA and septic arthritis typically resulting from the hyperemia associated with inflammatory processes. DJD, gout, and psoriatic arthritis usually maintain normal bony mineralization.
   - **Bony alignment.** Ulnar deviation at the metacarpophalangeal (MCP) joints is a feature of RA and lupus arthropathy (reversible in the latter).
   - **Soft tissue abnormalities.** RA—periarticular soft tissue swelling (STS); psoriatic arthritis—fusiform (sausage-like) STS, skin and fingernail changes; scleroderma—calcifications at fingertips (distal tufts).

4. **What is a synovial joint?**

   Synovial joints are characterized by two opposing bones covered with hyaline cartilage at their articular surfaces. The joint is bound by a fibrous joint capsule that is lined by a synovial membrane.

5. **Why do erosions in inflammatory arthropathies such as RA initially occur at the peripheral margins of the joint?**

   Not all surfaces of bone within the synovial joint capsule are covered with articular cartilage. These bare areas, located at the peripheral margins of the articular surfaces, are more susceptible to erosion by proliferating inflammatory tissue (pannus). These marginal erosions occur relatively early, whereas the more central bony erosions occur only after erosion of articular cartilage and joint space narrowing.

6. **Which of the following are synovial joints?**

a. Interphalangeal joint	e. Facet joints	i. Lamboid suture (skull)
b. Acromioclavicular joint	f. Intervertebral disc space	j. Sacroiliac joint
c. Temporomandibular joint	g. Anterior atlantoaxial joint	k. Costovertebral joint
d. Symphysis pubis	h. Hip	

   Answers: a, b, c, e, g, h, j (lower ½ only), k

7. **What is the difference between degenerative joint disease (DJD) and osteoarthritis (OA)?**

   None. These terms are used interchangeably. Some favor osteoarthrosis over osteoarthritis because "-itis" implies an inflammatory process. Inflammation may accompany DJD but is not a primary feature of the disease.

8. **List the radiographic features of DJD.**
   - Nonuniform, asymmetric joint space narrowing
   - Osteophyte formation
   - Reactive subchondral sclerosis (eburnation)
   - Subchondral cysts (degenerative cysts, geodes)
   - No erosions
   - Normal mineralization
   - Intraarticular loose bodies (joint mice)

9. What are the most common sites of involvement of OA?

Knee—medial compartment > patellofemoral > lateral compartment (Fig. 1)
Hip—usually superolateral joint space narrowing
Hands—first carpometacarpal joint, distal interphalangeal (DIP), and proximal interphalangeal (PIP) joints
Feet—metatarsophalangeal (MTP) joint of great toe, midtarsal joints
Shoulder—glenohumeral and acromioclavicular (AC) joints

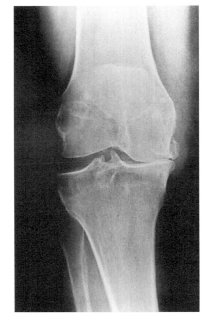

FIGURE 1. Degenerative joint disease—knee. Significant joint space narrowing at the medial compartment of the knee is combined with osteophyte formation at the medial tibial plateau and femoral condyle. The joint space narrowing results in varus alignment at the knee (normally slight valgus).

10. Where are Heberden's and Bouchard's nodes?

Heberden's nodes are at the DIP joints of the hand and Bouchard's nodes are at the PIP joints. These nodes are actually areas of osteophyte formation and soft tissue swelling secondary to DJD.

11. What is the differential diagnosis for premature development of OA?

- Trauma (most common)
- Neuropathic arthropathy
- Osteonecrosis (following collapse of the articular surface)
- Acromegaly (abnormally thickened articular cartilage, normally receiving its blood supply by diffusion, becomes inadequately nourished by the synovial fluid)
- Calcium pyrophosphate deposition disease (CPPD)
- Dwarfism: articular surfaces in diseases such as achondroplasia and epiphyseal dysplasia become incongruent, leading to premature OA
- Developmental dysplasia of the hip (DDH)

12. What is erosive OA?

Erosive OA is a degenerative disease of the interphalangeal joints of the hands with inflammatory and erosive components. This disease primarily affects postmenopausal women and is self-limited. Erosions occur at the center of the articular surface, resulting in a "gullwing" configuration (Fig. 2).

13. What is the typical age and sex predilection for RA?

Age, 25–55 years; female-to-male ratio of 3:1.

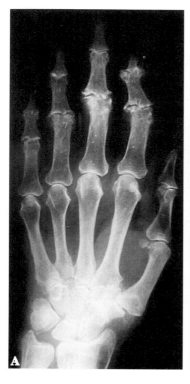
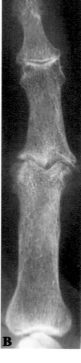

FIGURE 2.   Erosive OA. *A*, Note the joint space narrowing, osteophyte formation, and central erosions at all interphalangeal joints except the thumb. *B*, This magnified view of a finger from the contralateral hand shows the classic central erosion at the distal articular surface of the proximal phalanx and the "gull-wing" configuration at the base of the middle phalanx.

14. Describe the characteristic radiographic features of RA.
- Uniform joint space narrowing
- Bilaterally symmetrical distribution
- Periarticular soft tissue swelling
- Marginal erosions
- Juxtaarticular osteoporosis
- No new bone formation
- Subluxations
- Synovial cysts

15. What joints are most commonly affected by RA?
Hands and feet, with a predilection for proximal joints (carpal/tarsal, MCP, MTP) (Fig. 3).

16. What is a swan-neck deformity? A boutonniere deformity?
Both are finger deformities seen in RA. A swan-neck deformity involves hyperextension at the PIP joints and flexion at the DIP joints. In boutonniere deformity the fingers are flexed at the PIP joints and hyperextended at the DIP joints (as if pushing a button through a buttonhole).

17. What is the direction of deviation of the fingers in RA—ulnar or radial?
Ulnar deviation is seen in 25–50% of patients.

18. Why is ulnar styloid erosion such a common finding in RA?
Two main reasons: (1) pannus proliferation in the prestyloid recess of the radiocarpal joint results in early erosion of the adjacent styloid process, and (2) the extensor carpi ulnaris tendon also runs in close proximity to the ulnar styloid. Tenosynovitis with distention of this tendon sheath, a common finding in RA, may lead to pressure erosion of the adjacent styloid.

19. What level of the spine is most commonly affected by RA?
The cervical spine is by far the most common level. Thoracolumbar involvement is uncommon.

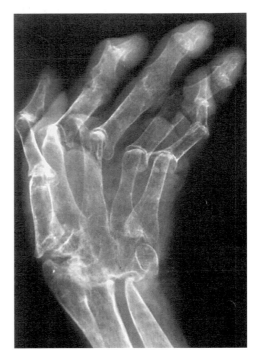

FIGURE 3. Advanced rheumatoid arthritis—hand and wrist. Bony ankylosis at the wrist, penciling of the distal ulna, and marked erosive changes at the metacarpophalangeal (MCP) joints with ulnar deviation of the fingers are classic RA findings. Also note the more severe involvement of the carpus and MCP joints; interphalangeal joints are typically less severely affected.

20. What is the most common cervical spine abnormality in RA?

Atlantoaxial subluxation, which is due to laxity of the transverse ligament of the dens and pannus proliferation at the atlantoaxial joint (Fig. 4), is seen in 25% of patients with RA. Subaxial subluxation (at C2–C3) is the second most common manifestation. Eventually, one may see anterior subluxations at all levels, resulting in a "stepladder" appearance on lateral radiographs.

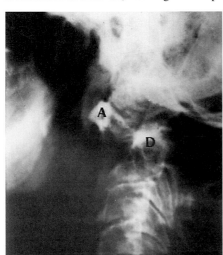

FIGURE 4. Atlantoaxial subluxation—RA. There is marked widening of the space between the anterior arch of the atlas (A) and the margin of the dens (D).

21. How does juvenile RA (JRA) differ from adult RA?

Aside from the younger age, JRA is commonly monoarticular or pauciarticular, whereas adult RA is always polyarticular. JRA may resolve spontaneously (in up to 50% of cases), whereas adult

RA is marked by relentless progression to severe deformity and disability. Adult RA most commonly involves the hands and feet in addition to the larger joints (knees, hips, shoulders, and elbows), whereas JRA is commonly limited to the central larger joints such as hips and knees. Periostitis sometimes occurs in JRA but is rare in adult RA. Because of the immature skeleton in patients with JRA, this disease is commonly associated with growth disturbances (accelerated growth due to hyperemia, epiphyseal overgrowth, premature growth plate fusion).

22. List the radiographic features of rheumatoid involvement of the chest.

- Distal clavicle erosion (bilateral)
- Pleural effusion or thickening (most common finding)
- Interstitial fibrosis (lower lung fields)
- Pulmonary nodules
- Pericardial effusion

23. Is rheumatoid lung more common in men or women?

Although RA affects more women than men, a larger percentage of men suffer from intrathoracic involvement.

24. What is Caplan syndrome?

Caplan syndrome is a pneumoconiosis (inhalational lung disease) that develops in coal workers with RA.

25. What complications should be suspected for each of the following clinical signs in a patient with RA? Which imaging study is most appropriate?

- Palpable popliteal mass—popliteal cyst; diagnosed most cost-effectively with ultrasound.
- Sudden-onset, painful flatfoot deformity—posterior tibial tendon tear; best diagnosed with MRI of the ankle.
- High-riding shoulder deformity—chronic rotator cuff tear; plain film findings of superior migration of the humeral head with resultant decreased space between it and the acromial process are diagnostic (Fig. 5); no further imaging is necessary.

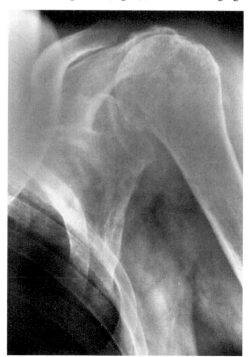

FIGURE 5.   Chronic rotator cuff tear—RA. Chronic tear of the rotator cuff tendons results in retraction of the tendons and atrophy of the cuff muscles; the humeral head ascends to lie in close proximity to the undersurface of the acromial process.

• Severe hip pain after walking up several flights of stairs—stress fracture; the osteopenia commonly present in RA results in an increased incidence of stress fractures with normal activities (insufficiency fractures). MRI or a bone scan is diagnostic.

26. What are the seronegative spondyloarthropathies?
Seronegative spondyloarthropathies and RA share certain features. Both are inflammatory arthritides. This group includes psoriatic arthritis (PA), Reiter's disease (RD), ankylosing spondylitis (AS), and inflammatory bowel disease-associated (IBD) arthropathy (enteropathic arthritis). These entities, formerly called the "rheumatoid variants," are rheumatoid factor-negative; hence the term seronegative.

27. What HLA factor is commonly present in patients with seronegative spondyloarthropathies?
HLA B-27 is present in the majority of patients (96% of AS).

28. What clinical triad is usually present in patients with Reiter's disease (RD)?
Arthritis, uveitis, urethritis. Mnemonic: Can't see, can't pee, can't climb a tree.

29. What diseases usually precede the development of RD?
RD (also termed reactive arthritis) is usually preceded by an infectious illness, most commonly venereal disease or intestinal dysentery (*Shigella* sp.). It is more common in men.

30. What percentage of patients with psoriasis develop arthritis?
About 5%.

31. Can psoriatic arthritis precede the onset of skin lesions?
Yes, in about 20% of patients.

32. In which type of arthritis are "pencil-in-cup" deformities described?
Psoriatic arthritis. Pencil-in-cup deformities refer to advanced bony changes in the hands and feet. The eroded, deformed base of a phalanx is telescoped into the erosive defect at the adjacent distal articular surface, like a pencil in a cup.

33. Are the seronegative arthropathies more common in women or men?
Men.

34. What radiographic features distinguish seronegative arthropathies from RA and from each other?
1. New bone formation is commonly seen in the seronegative arthropathies but absent in RA. It is manifested by bone proliferation at tendon and ligament insertions ("whiskering") and osteophytes. Erosive changes and bony productive changes commonly occur concurrently at affected joints (Fig. 6). Periosteal new bone formation is not uncommon. Bone proliferation is most pronounced and erosive change least evident in AS, whereas in PA and RD these changes are more balanced.
2. Spine and SI joint involvements are common in seronegative arthropathies, and the thoracolumbar spine is affected more commonly than the cervical spine. SI joint involvement is bilaterally symmetric in AS and IBD and bilaterally asymmetric in PA and RD.
3. Osteoporosis is uncommon in the seronegative arthropathies but common in RA and, when present, occurs late.
4. Seronegative diseases are more common in young and adolescent men, whereas RA is much more common in women and increases in frequency with age.
5. Because RA and the seronegative arthropathies belong to the inflammatory arthritis family, findings shared by these diseases include erosions and uniform joint space narrowing. Severe deformity may result in the end stage of any of these diseases (also known as arthritis mutilans).

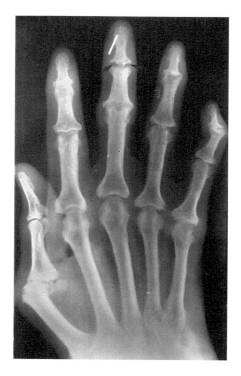

FIGURE 6.   Psoriatic arthritis—hand. Note the marginal erosions and osteophytes at the distal interphalangeal joint of the middle finger (arrows). A metallic foreign body is in the soft tissues of the distal phalanx.

35. What joints are always abnormal in AS?

The sacroiliac joints are always involved; involvement is bilateral and symmetrical. Spine involvement may then progress in an ascending fashion, always affecting the lumbar spine before the thoracic and cervical spine. Proximal large joints (shoulders, hips, knees) may or may not be involved, and involvement of the hands and feet is uncommon.

36. What disease may have SI joint arthritis that is identical to AS?

Inflammatory bowel disease. About 5% of patients with IBD have arthropathy similar to AS. The activity of the arthritis parallels the activity of bowel disease and resolves with remission.

37. Findings diagnostic of a seronegative arthropathy are evident on hand radiographs. Which disease is more likely—PA or RD?

PA. RD involves the feet and not the hands, whereas PA can involve both.

38. What is a syndesmophyte?

Syndesmophytes are vertical ossifications bridging the margins of two adjacent vertebral bodies. This type of ossification involves the outermost fibers of the anulus fibrosus (Sharpey's fibers).

39. What is a bamboo spine?

This descriptive name refers to the appearance of the spine in advanced AS. Squaring of the vertebral bodies is combined with thin, bridging syndesmophytes and occasional bony fusion (ankylosis) of the facet joints. Ossification of the longitudinal and interspinous ligaments also may occur, contributing to the bamboo appearance (Fig. 7).

40. What complications of AS should be suspected for each of the following signs or symptoms? What imaging study is appropriate for further evaluation?

• Acute-onset low back pain—pseudarthrosis (fracture through area of bony ankylosis): plain films (Fig. 8). If negative, MRI.

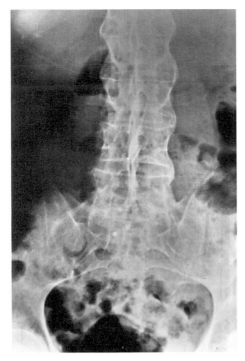 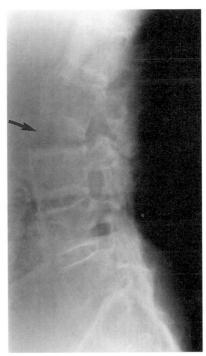

FIGURE 7 *(Left).*   Ankylosing spondylitis—bamboo spine. Note the lateral marginal syndesmophytes and the longitudinal ligament calcification resulting in the bamboo appearance. The SI joints are indistinct.

FIGURE 8 *(Right).*   Ankylosing spondylitis—pseudarthrosis. A fracture through the ankylosis at the L2–L3 level (arrow) causes localized hyperextension of the spine at this level. This is typically associated with severe pain. (Courtesy of Bernard Ghelman, M.D.)

- Lower extremity long tract signs with neck flexion—atlantoaxial subluxation; seen in 2% of patients with AS; C-spine study with flexion and extension lateral views.
- Respiratory difficulty—pulmonary fibrosis; uncommon complication of AS with a predilection for the upper lobes; chest radiographs.
- Urinary incontinence—cauda equina syndrome; MRI.

41. What crystal is responsible for development of gouty arthritis?
Monosodium urate.

42. Differentiate primary gout from secondary causes of gout.
Primary gout is idiopathic and is due to an inborn error of metabolism that results in hyperuricemia. Secondary gout results from diseases that cause increased production or decreased excretion of uric acid, such as myeloproliferative disorders, chemotherapy or radiation therapy, multiple myeloma, and chronic renal failure.

43. Is gout more common in men or women?
Men.

44. What is podagra?
Gouty involvement of the great toe at the metatarsophalangeal joint. The great toe is the most common site of involvement of gout in the skeleton.

45. Do radiographically visible bony changes usually accompany the initial attack of gout?

No. Bony changes of gout usually ensue 5–10 years after the first episode. This explains the drastically decreased prevalence of gouty arthritis over the past 10–20 years; aggressive early treatment of hyperuricemia prevents development of skeletal changes.

46. Describe the radiographic findings of gouty arthritis .

- Tophi (most common at extensor surfaces of joints) (Fig. 9)
- Well-defined erosions, with overhanging edges
- No osteoporosis
- Joint space narrowing (late in disease)
- Most common sites: feet, ankles, knees, hands

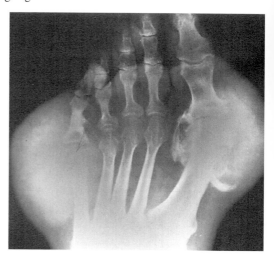

FIGURE 9.   Large calcified gouty tophi centered at the metatarsophalangeal joints of the first and fifth toes obscure the underlying bony abnormalities.

47. What is pseudogout?

Pseudogout is another type of crystal deposition arthropathy. The offending crystal is calcium pyrophosphate dihydrate, a rhomboid crystal with weakly positive birefringence under polarized light. Pseudogout is one of the clinical manifestations of calcium pyrophosphate deposition disease (CPPD). In contrast, monosodium urate crystals in gout are negatively birefringent.

48. What is chondrocalcinosis?

Chondrocalcinosis is the deposition of calcium pyrophosphate in hyaline cartilage and fibrocartilage. This is the hallmark of CPPD. Cartilage is normally radiolucent; abnormal calcium deposition is best seen at the knee (menisci) and wrist (triangular fibrocartilage) (Fig. 10).

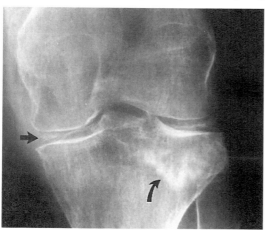

FIGURE 10.   Calcification is seen at the medial (arrow) and lateral joint spaces, representing chondrocalcinosis of the fibrocartilage (menisci). This patient also has a stress fracture at the lateral tibial plateau (curved arrow).

49. What two diseases are associated with CPPD?
Hyperparathyroidism and hemochromatosis.

50. What is the most common location of calcific tendinitis? What crystal is associated with it?
The shoulder is the most common site (Fig. 11), and the offending crystal is calcium hydroxyapatite.

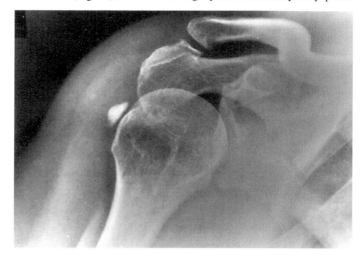

FIGURE 11. Calcific tendinitis—shoulder. There is a focal area of calcification adjacent to the greater tuberosity, at the site of the supraspinatus tendon insertion.

51. What is a Charcot joint?
Charcot joint is an eponym synonymous with a neuropathic joint (originally described in association with syphilis). Both terms refer to the abnormalities of bones and joints related to neurologic deficits.

52. What are the six Ds of a neuropathic joint?

Destruction	Distention
Dislocation	Disorganization
Debris	(Discombobulation)
Density (increased)	

These findings result from repetitive trauma to a joint lacking adequate pain and proprioceptive sensation (Fig. 12).

53. What is the most common cause of neuropathic arthropathy?
Diabetic neuropathy. Charcot joints are seen in 5–10% of diabetics.

54. List six causes of neuropathic arthropathy and the most common sites of involvement.

Diabetes mellitus—foot and ankle	Alcoholism—feet
Tabes dorsalis—lumbar spine, knee	Congenital insensitivity to pain—knee, ankle, foot
Syringomyelia—shoulder	Meningomyelocele—ankle, foot

55. What collagen vascular disease can give rise to a deforming nonerosive arthropathy of the hands?
Systemic lupus erythematosus (SLE). Rheumatoid-like deformities such as ulnar deviation and swan-neck deformity may occur. Unlike RA, there are no associated erosions, and the deformities are reversible; the deformities are due to ligamentous laxity and are voluntarily correctable.

56. What is Jacoud's arthropathy?
Chronic joint deformity following rheumatic fever. Findings are similar to SLE.

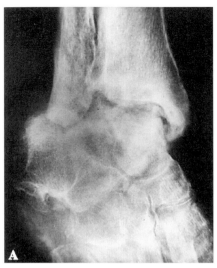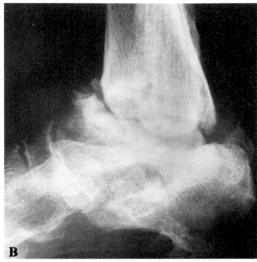

FIGURE 12. Neuropathic arthropathy—ankle. Frontal *(A)* and lateral *(B)* views of the ankle show the advanced destructive articular abnormality in this diabetic foot. Note the collapse of the posterior half of the talus seen on the lateral view and the marked joint space narrowing.

57. Which collagen vascular disease may result in multiple erosions at the interphalangeal joints of the hands, resorption of tufts, and soft tissue calcifications at the fingertips?
  Scleroderma.

58. A patient with lung cancer presents with painful swollen wrists and knees and digital clubbing. Radiographs reveal symmetric periosteal elevation. What is your diagnosis?
  Hypertrophic pulmonary osteoarthropathy (HPOA). This disease is manifested by bilateral periosteal new bone formation along the diaphyses of the long bones. The etiology of this condition is unknown. Pulmonary diseases are most commonly associated with HPOA, including lung cancer, pleural tumors, lung abscesses, and cystic fibrosis. It also may occur in association with inflammatory bowel disease, Whipple's disease, and other liver diseases. Clinical symptoms and radiographic signs of HPOA typically resolve after resection of the thoracic tumor.

59. Construct a table classifying the major arthritides.

Osteoarthritis	**Connective tissue arthropathy**
Primary	Scleroderma
Secondary	Systemic lupus erythematosus
Trauma	**Crystal deposition arthropathy**
Osteonecrosis	Gout
Acromegaly	Calcium pyrophosphate deposition disease
Inflammatory arthritis	**Infectious arthritis**
Neuropathic arthropathy	Pyogenic
Erosive osteoarthritis	Tuberculous
Inflammatory arthritis	Other
Rheumatoid arthritis	
Seronegative spondyloarthropathies	
Psoriatic arthritis	
Reiter's disease	
Ankylosing spondylitis	
Enteropathic arthritis	

BIBLIOGRAPHY

1. Brower A: Arthritis in Black and White. Philadelphia, W.B. Saunders, 1988.
2. Helms CA: Fundamentals of Skeletal Radiology, 2nd ed. Philadelphia, W.B. Saunders, 1995.
3. Kaye JJ: Arthritis: Roles of radiography and other imaging techniques in evaluation. Radiology 177:601–608, 1990.
4. Weissman BN: Spondyloarthropathies. Radiol Clin North Am 25:1235–1262, 1987.
5. West SG: Rheumatology Secrets. Philadelphia, Hanley & Belfus, 1997.

49. BONE TUMORS

Kim Kramer, M.D., and Kevin R. Math, M.D.

1. What radiographic features can be used to differentiate between benign and malignant bone tumors?

• Zone of transition between normal and abnormal bone
• Cortical destruction
• Sclerotic margin
• Periosteal reaction
• Soft tissue mass

Benign or nonaggressive lesions have a sharp zone of transition between the lesion and normal bone (i.e., a sharp border), whereas the zone of transition for malignant lesions is ill-defined.

Benign lesions sometimes cause thinning of the adjacent cortex; however, frank cortical destruction is much more typical of malignant lesions.

A well-defined sclerotic margin is typical of benign lesions and rare in malignant lesions.

The character of the periosteal reaction rather than its mere presence is the feature that is most helpful. Periosteal reaction in slow-growing benign lesions is typically thick, uniform, or wavy because of the layering and bony remodeling that are allowed to occur with nonaggressive processes. Malignant lesions typically have a more amorphous, irregular lamellated (onion-skin) or sunburst type of periosteal reaction. Some benign lesions may have more malignant-appearing periostitis; all features of the lesion must be considered in attempting to judge the aggressiveness of a bone tumor.

2. What is Codman's triangle?

Codman's triangle describes the triangular appearance of the periosteal elevation and new bone at the cortical margins of an aggressive lesion (Fig. 1). It results from the bone's inability to lay down continuous periosteal new bone across a rapidly growing lesion. The sides of the triangle are formed by the periosteum, underlying cortex, and margin of the tumor mass. Although this radiographic finding is consistent with an aggressive process (e.g., osteosarcoma), it is not specific for a malignant lesion and may be seen in benign conditions such as osteomyelitis.

3. Which imaging study is most useful in arriving at an accurate differential diagnosis for a bone tumor?

Plain film evaluation is clearly the most important imaging study and usually all that is necessary to establish an accurate differential diagnosis.

4. What is the role of CT and MRI in the evaluation of bone tumors?

CT and MRI are useful for determining the relationship of the lesion to the surrounding soft tissues (nerves, vessels, muscle). They should be ordered after complete plain film evaluation and are most helpful for staging and preoperative planning of bone tumors. MRI with intravenous contrast is also useful for follow-up evaluation of tumors after chemotherapy or surgery.

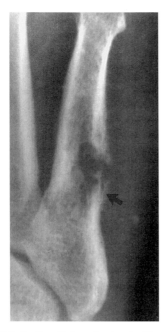 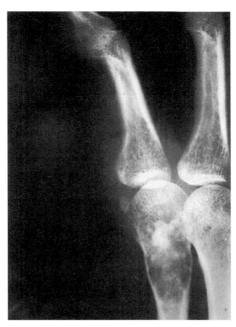

FIGURE 1 *(Left)*.   Codman's triangle. Note the triangular periosteal elevation at the proximal and distal aspects of this lytic 5th metatarsal lesion, indicating that it is aggressive but not necessarily malignant. In fact, this is a case of acute osteomyelitis.

FIGURE 2 *(Right)*.   Enchondroma, second metacarpal. There is coarse, "popcorn-like" calcification in this lesion consistent with chondroid (cartilaginous) matrix.

5. How can calcifications in a bone lesion assist in its diagnosis?

Calcification within a lesion can be cartilaginous (chondroid) or osseous. Chondroid calcification is coarse, having the appearance of "dots and commas" or "rings and broken rings." Identification of this type of calcification leads to a differential diagnosis of cartilaginous lesions, such as enchodroma (benign) or chondrosarcoma (malignant) (Fig. 2). Osteoid calcification is more cloudy, homogeneous, and coalescent; this would favor osseous lesions such as osteosarcoma in the differential diagnosis.

6. Aside from the intrinsic features of a lesion, what other clinical and radiographic features are important?

The age of the patient and the location of the lesion in the skeleton (axial vs. appendicular skeleton) and within the bone (epiphysis, metaphysis, diaphysis).

7. What does FEGNOMASHIC mean?

This commonly used mnemonic helps to remember lytic skeletal lesions:
Fibrous dysplasia
Enchondroma, eosinophilic granuloma
Giant cell tumor
Nonossifying fibroma
Osteoblastoma, osteoid osteoma
Metastasis, multiple myeloma
Aneurysmal bone cyst
Solitary bone cyst
Hyperparathyroidism (brown tumor)
Infection
Chondroblastoma, chondromyxoid fibroma

This long list can be substantially narrowed by considering the patient's age and the location and appearance of the lesion.

8. How are bone tumors classified?

Osseous lesions:	Osteosarcoma	Fibrous lesions:	Fibrous dysplasia
	Osteoid osteoma		Fibrosarcoma
	Osteoblastoma		Nonossifying fibroma
Chondroid lesions:	Chondrosarcoma	Cysts:	Aneurysmal bone cyst
	Enchondroma		Solitary bone cyst
	Osteochondroma	Infection/Other:	Brodie's abscess
	Chondroblastoma		Eosinophilic granula
	Chondromyxoid fibroma		Brown tumor

9. Which two primary bone tumors tend to involve the epiphysis most commonly?

Chondroblastoma and giant cell tumor. Usually they can be differentiated by the age of the patient; chondroblastoma occurs in children prior to skeletal maturity, whereas giant cell tumors almost always occur after growth plate closure.

10. What are the two most common sites of involvement of giant cell tumors?

The knee is the most common site; the wrist is second most common site.

11. What are the classic radiographic features of a giant cell tumor?

Giant cell tumors invariably involve the epiphysis, abut the articular surface, and are eccentrically rather than centrally located (Fig. 3). The lesion has a sharply defined nonsclerotic zone of transition and is seen after growth plate closure in contrast with its childhood epiphyseal counterpart, chondroblastoma.

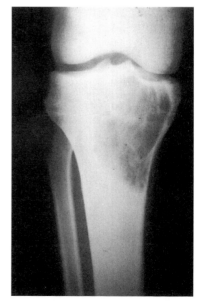

FIGURE 3. Giant cell tumor, proximal tibia. This lytic lesion involves both metaphysis and epiphysis of this young adult, typical of these tumors. Note the extension of the lesion to the articular surface.

12. What is the difference between a nonossifying fibroma (NOF) and a fibrous cortical defect?

Histologically, these relatively common benign lesions are identical. They differ in size; a fibrous cortical defect (FCD) is < 2 cm in length, whereas a nonossifying fibroma is > 2 cm. These asymptomatic lesions are usually encountered incidentally and are readily diagnosed by their characteristic appearance.

13. Describe the radiographic appearance of an NOF.

NOF lesions are lytic, cortical-based lesions located in the metaphysis or diametaphysis of long bones. They typically are well defined, with a scalloped, sclerotic border (Fig. 4). Larger NOFs may be associated with pathologic fractures.

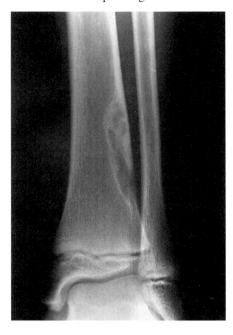

FIGURE 4. Nonossifying fibroma, distal tibia. This lesion is located in the distal tibial diametaphysis, has a sclerotic, well-defined margin, and is cortical based. Its radiographic appearance is diagnostic; biopsy of these common benign lesions is not necessary.

14. Why are NOFs so common in children but never found in people over 30 years of age?

NOF lesions routinely heal with sclerosis and eventually disappear.

15. What are the two most common malignant primary bone tumors in children?

Ewing's sarcoma and osteosarcoma.

16. What is the most common primary malignant bone tumor in adults?

Multiple myeloma.

17. What is the most common malignant skeletal tumor overall?

Metastases. Skeletal metastases account for at least 95% of all bone tumors and should therefore be considered in the differential diagnosis of all lesions.

18. What are the most common primary neoplasms that metastasize to bone?

Lung, breast, kidney, prostate, and thyroid are the most common. Using the first letter of each of these, two helpful mnemonics can be constructed: Lead (**PB**) **Ke**T**t**L**e** and **BLT** and a **K**osher **P**ickle.

19. Which tumors most commonly result in osteoblastic metastases?

Prostate cancer in men and breast cancer in women (Fig. 5). Less common causes of purely osteoblastic metastases include medulloblastoma, transitional cell carcinoma, gastrointestinal malignancies, and lymphoma.

20. What causes the increased bone density in osteoblastic metastases?

The metastatic tumor cells stimulate new bone formation, which is laid down on top of cancellous bone, resulting in an osteoblastic lesion. The density of the metastatic tumor cells themselves do not contribute significantly to the blastic lesion.

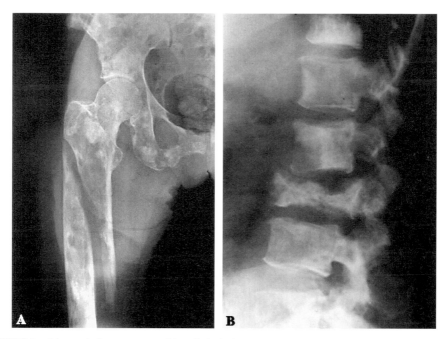

FIGURE 5. Metastatic breast cancer with pathologic fractures. *A*, There are numerous osteoblastic lesions throughout the pelvis and proximal femur with a displaced pathologic proximal femur fracture. *B*, Pathologic fracture of a lumbar vertebral body in a different patient with osteoblastic breast metastases.

21. What are the most common bones to be affected by skeletal metastases?

The axial skeleton (spine, pelvis, skull) and proximal femur and humerus account for 90% of lesions, usually with multifocal involvement. Metastases distal to the knees and elbows are rare.

22. What pediatric bone tumor most commonly metastasizes to other bones?

Ewing's sarcoma. Other causes of pediatric skeletal metastases include neuroblastoma, leukemia, lymphoma, soft tissue sarcomas, retinoblastoma, medulloblastoma, and Wilms' tumor.

23. A 70-year-old woman presents with right hip pain. Her hip radiograph is shown in Figure 6. What is the most likely diagnosis? What test should be ordered next?

Statistically, metastasis is clearly the most likely diagnosis. A radionuclide bone scan should be performed next to assess for multiple lesions, which would further support a metastatic etiology (Fig. 7). If the lesion is not "hot" on the bone scan, myeloma or plasmacytoma would be more strongly considered.

24. What percentage of metastatic lesions detected on bone scans are not seen on radiographs? Why?

About 30%. In order to visualize a lesion on plain films, more than 50% of the bone must be destroyed. The bone scan is much more sensitive; lesions are identified by virtue of increased regional blood flow and increased bone remodeling, which cause "hot spots."

25. What percentage of metastatic lesions detected on radiographs are missed on bone scans?

About 2%. The most common bone tumors associated with false-negative bone scans include anaplastic thyroid carcinoma, neuroblastoma, and eosinophilic granuloma.

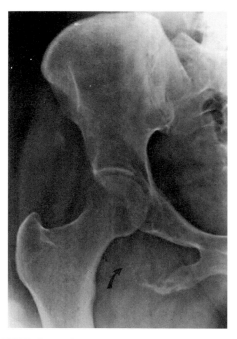 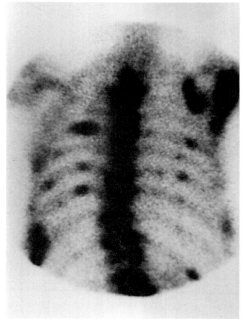

FIGURE 6 *(Left)*.   Metastatic lung cancer, inferior ischium (curved arrow).

FIGURE 7 *(Right)*.   Bone scan—metastatic prostate cancer. There are numerous "hot spots" throughout the thoracic spine, ribs, and left scapula, indicating metastatic disease.

26. Which malignant skeletal lesion is more sensitively detected on radiographs than bone scan?

Multiple myeloma. If this diagnosis is suspected, a metastatic skeletal survey rather than a bone scan should be performed. This survey includes radiographs of the most common sites of involvement (skull, spine, pelvis, femur, humerus). Radiographs typically show multiple well-defined "punched-out" lytic lesions (Fig. 8). Bone scans are often normal because of the inhibition of new bone formation by myeloma cells. About 20% of patients with myeloma have normal plain films and a normal bone scan.

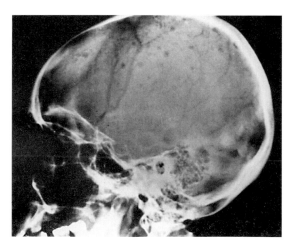

FIGURE 8.   Multiple myeloma—skull. Classical punched-out lytic lesions throughout the skull. These lesions were not demonstrated on a radionuclide bone scan.

27. What do bone metastases from renal cell carcinoma and thyroid carcinoma have in common?
Both may give rise to aggressive, hypervascular lytic expansile lesions. Melanoma also may result in these "blown-out" hypervascular metastases.

28. What is the most common benign primary bone tumor of the hand?
Enchondroma. These tumors are often discovered incidentally or as a result of pathologic fracture. Unlike enchondromas elsewhere in the body, chondroid calcification in hand lesions is much less common.

29. What is the most common primary tumor to metastasize to the hands?
Metastases to the hands are rare. Lung cancer is the most common primary tumor; breast carcinoma is the second most common.

30. What is the differential diagnosis of a sclerotic ("ivory") vertebral body?
Metastasis, Paget's disease, lymphoma, and chronic infection. Paget's disease and metastasis are much more common than lymphoma and chronic infection. Paget's disease sometimes can be differentiated from metastasis by its propensity to enlarge the involved bone and the typical thickened endplates and coarsened trabeculae (Fig. 9). The mnemonic **LIMP** (**l**ymphoma, **i**nfection, **m**etastasis, **P**aget's disease) can help to recall the differential diagnosis.

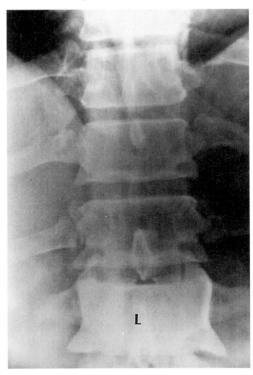

FIGURE 9. Paget's disease—ivory vertebra. There is generalized sclerosis of the L1 vertebral body (L). While this is a nonspecific finding, the enlargement of this vertebra relative to the others and the thickened cortex of the left transverse process are diagnostic of Paget's disease.

31. Which tumor contains physaliphorous cells?
Chordomas. This tumor, arising from notochordal remnants in the midline of the axial skeleton, most commonly occurs at the sacrococcygeal region and base of the skull.

32. Which primary bone tumor may present with symptoms that mimic osteomyelitis?
Ewing's sarcoma. Patients often present with fever, pain, elevated sedimentation rate, and occasional leukocytosis.

33. Which primary bone tumor has a classic "onion skin" type of periosteal reaction?
Ewing's sarcoma (Fig. 10).

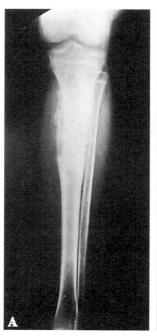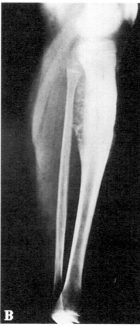

FIGURE 10. Ewing's sarcoma—tibia. There is a permeative lesion involving the proximal tibial shaft with an "onion-skin" periosteal reaction noted at its medial and posterior aspects.

34. How can osteosarcoma and Ewing's sarcoma be differentiated radiographically?
Osteosarcoma (or osteogenic sarcoma) is a bone-forming tumor; exuberant amorphous new bone is laid down at the site of the tumor, often perpendicular to the bone of origin, resulting in a characteristic "sunburst" appearance (Fig. 11). Ewing's sarcoma typically presents with a large soft tissue mass at the site of the tumor and may display the typical "onion skin" type of periostitis. Unfortunately, there is considerable overlap of the two tumors both clinically and radiographically, and radiographic differentiation is often not possible.

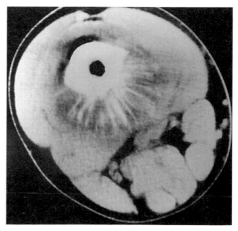

FIGURE 11.   Osteogenic sarcoma-sunburst periosteal reaction.

35. Where do osteosarcoma and Ewing's sarcoma most commonly metastasize?
Both metastasize most commonly to the lungs.

36. What is the most common benign skeletal neoplasm?
Osteochondroma.

37. Which characteristic feature is unique to the growth of an osteochondroma?
Osteochondromas, which may be sessile (broad based) or pedunculated (on a stalk), characteristically arise from the metaphysis and always point away from the end of the bone (Fig. 12).

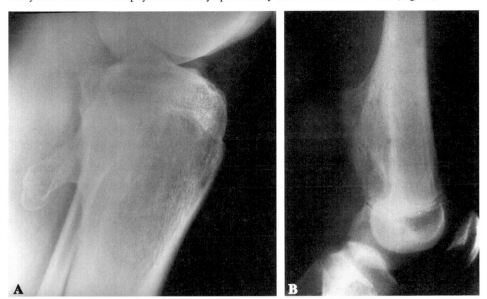

FIGURE 12. *A*, Pedunculated and *B*, sessile osteochondromas. Note the continuous cortex surrounding the pedunculated lesion.

38. Which clinical and radiographic features suggest malignant degeneration of an osteochondroma?
Pain, growth after skeletal maturity, discontinuous cortex around the lesion, and calcification outside the margins of the lesion. The thickness of the cartilage cap of these lesions correlates with an increased risk of malignant degeneration. The cap of an osteochondroma is well visualized on MRI.

39. Which primary bone tumor has the characteristic history of pain at night, relieved by aspirin?
Osteoid osteoma, which occurs most commonly in the long bones. The lesion is a small lucent nidus, usually associated with pronounced surrounding sclerosis (Fig. 13); this sclerosis often masks the nidus, resulting in an appearance similar to a stress fracture.

40. Which imaging study is best for diagnosing an osteoid osteoma?
CT is considered the most accurate study for identifying the lucent nidus and establishing the diagnosis (Fig. 14). This is the only bone tumor for which CT is considered preferable to MRI. These lesions are focally "hot" on bone scans. The lucent nidus must be completely resected to avoid recurrence.

41. What is the fallen fragment sign?
The fallen fragment sign is characteristic of a solitary bone cyst. Pathologic fracture of a simple bone cyst may give rise to a flake of bone (fragment) situated dependently in the fluid-filled cyst cavity (Fig. 15). This sign is present in about 20% of all bone cysts.

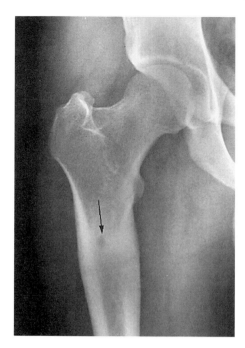

FIGURE 13.   Osteoid osteoma. There is a focal lucent lesion in the medullary cavity of the proximal femoral shaft (arrow) representing the nidus of the lesion. Note the reactive sclerosis surrounding the lesion, sometimes masking its visualization.

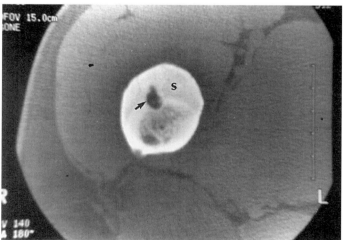

FIGURE 14.   Osteoid osteoma—CT. The nidus of the lesion is clearly visualized (arrow), in addition to the pronounced rind of reactive sclerosis.

42. What is a brown tumor? How did it get its name?

Brown tumors, also known as osteoclastomas, are lytic lesions in patients with hyperparathyroidism. They are most common in the diaphyses of long bones and in the mandible. They are named not as a tribute to Dr. Brown but rather for the brown fluid contained within them, which represents old and recent hemorrhage. Recognition of the numerous additional radiographic features of hyperparathyroidism permits differentiation of these lesions from metastases.

43. Which disease is associated with a pseudotumor as a result of intraosseous hemorrhage?

Hemophilia.

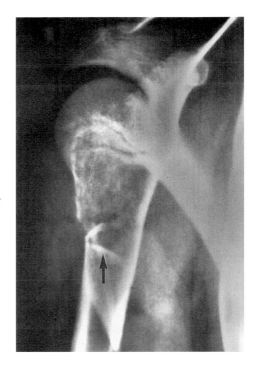

FIGURE 15. Unicameral bone cyst. There is a large lytic lesion in the proximal humeral metaphysis. This is the most common location for a unicameral bone cyst. The "fallen fragment" of cortical bone is seen dependently within the lesion (arrow). (Courtesy of Bernard Ghelman, M.D.)

44. Which lesions can cross the growth plate of a child to involve both the epiphysis and metaphysis?

Osteomyelitis, chondroblastoma, and eosinophilic granuloma.

45. What is a bone island?

Also known as an enostosis, a bone island is an island of cortical bone lying within trabecular bone (Fig. 16). Bone islands may occur in virtually any bone, and usually their long axis is aligned with that of the involved bone. Commonly encountered as incidental findings and measuring < 1 cm, these clinically insignificant lesions must be differentiated from other sclerotic skeletal lesions such as metastases.

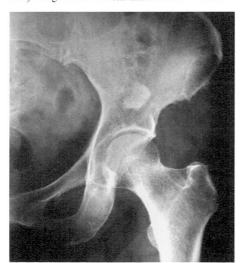

FIGURE 16. Bone island. A rounded sclerotic lesion is seen in the right ilium, having the "brush border" typical of a bone island. An osteoblastic metastasis can present a similar appearance; a bone scan is helpful in these cases (see text).

46. What is fibrous dysplasia?

Fibrous dysplasia is an uncommon bone lesion marked by hamartomatous involvement of the marrow by lesions composed primarily of woven bone and fibrous tissue. This process results in a ground-glass appearance of the involved bone. The lesion is usually solitary (monostotic) and most commonly involves the long bones (long lesion in a long bone), ribs, and craniofacial bones. Involvement of the proximal femur often results in a classic "shepherd's crook" deformity.

47. What is the McCune-Albright syndrome?

McCune-Albright syndrome is the triad of polyostotic fibrous dysplasia, café-au-lait spots, and endocrine disturbances (most commonly precocious puberty).

48. What is Ollier's disease? Mafucci's disease?

Ollier's disease is characterized by multiple enchondromas throughout the skeleton, most numerous in the extremities and ribs. It is not inherited and carries a significant increased risk (~25%) of malignant transformation of enchondromas into sarcomas. Mafucci's disease is also characterized by multiple enchondromas in addition to multiple soft tissue hemangiomas. Malignant transformation in this rare disease exceeds 50%.

49. Which of the following carries an increased incidence of skeletal malignancy: high-dose radiation therapy, bone infarction, Paget's disease, or chronic osteomyelitis?

All of the above. This complication, however, is uncommon.

50. What is the average time interval for development of a radiation-induced sarcoma?

Most tumors develop 10–15 years after radiation exposure (e.g., radiation therapy), usually after exposure exceeding 3000 rads.

51. What are the most common types of radiation-induced sarcomas?

Osteosarcoma and fibrosarcoma.

52. What is the most likely diagnosis for each of the following clinical presentations?

1. 6-month-old infant with chronic otitis media, eczematous rash, multiple lytic bone lesions, and normal bone scan
2. 50-year-old woman with multiple osteoblastic lesions throughout the spine and pelvis
3. 16-year-old girl with retinoblastoma as an infant and a large painful mass involving the knee
4. 4-year-old child with abdominal mass and multiple lytic skeletal lesions
5. 50-year-old man with hematuria and a large expansile lytic lesion of the left iliac wing
6. 16-year-old boy with fever, anemia, anorexia, and leukocytosis; radiographs reveal a large lytic lesion at the distal femur with a large soft tissue mass
7. 61-year-old man with renal failure, recurrent infections and bone pain; radiographs show osteopenia; bone scan is normal
8. 56-year-old smoker with a painful swollen index finger; radiographs reveal a lytic aggressive lesion of the proximal phalanx
9. 22-year-old man with pain in popliteal region; radiographs reveal a stalk-like lesion arising from the proximal tibia, pointing inferiorly
10. 25-year-old woman with dull aching pain in the wrist; radiographs reveal a well-defined expansile eccentric lesion at the distal radius, extending to its distal articular surface
11. 40-year-old woman with renal stones, hypercalcemia, and a focal lytic lesion at the proximal femur

Answers:

1. Eosinophilic granuloma	5. Metastatic renal cell carcinoma	9. Osteochondroma
2. Metastatic breast cancer	6. Ewing's sarcoma	10. Giant cell tumor
3. Osteosarcoma	7. Multiple myeloma	11. Brown tumor
4. Metastatic neuroblastoma	8. Metastatic lung cancer	(hyperparathyroidism)

53. What is the study of choice for evaluation of soft tissue tumors?
MRI.

54. How sensitive is MRI for differentiating between benign and malignant soft tissue lesions?
Not sensitive enough. For the majority of soft tissue tumors, accurate assessment of the metabolic activity of a lesion is not possible. For example, a malignant tumor can be small, well-circumscribed and have homogeneous signal intensity while a benign lesion (classically myositis ossificans) can have heterogeneous signal and be fairly large and enhance with contrast irregularly. Lesions containing homogeneous fat signal can be confidently labeled as lipomas; accurate determination of benignity is also possible with hemangiomas, plantar fibromatosis, and pigmented villonodular synovitis. In view of the nonspecific nature of MR for evaluating soft tissue tumors, one should keep in mind that "benign" features of a soft tissue mass should not obviate pursuing a histologic diagnosis (Fig. 17).

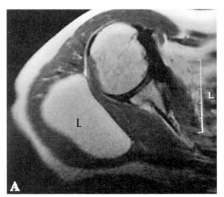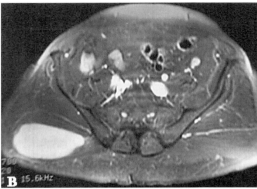

FIGURE 17. Soft tissue tumors—MRI. *A*, On this T1-weighted image a large hyperintense lesion (L) is seen between the deltoid and infraspinatus muscles. The homogeneous fatty signal of this lesion (compare with subcutaneous fat) indicates that this is a lipoma. *B*, On this fat suppressed T2-weighted image, a well-circumscribed, homogeneous, hyperintense lesion is seen in the right gluteal region. The well-marginated homogeneous nature of this lesion may lead the uninitiated to falsely assume that this myxoid liposarcoma is a benign lesion.

BIBLIOGRAPHY

1. Bullough PG (ed): Atlas of Orthopedic Pathology. New York, Gower Medical Publishing, 1992.
2. Greenfield GB, Arrington J: Imaging of Bone Tumors. Philadelphia, Lippincott-Raven, 1995.
3. Helms CA: Fundamentals of Skeletal Radiology, 2nd ed. Philadelphia, W.B. Saunders, 1996.
4. Kransdorf M, Murphey MD: Imaging of Soft Tissue Tumors. Philadelphia, W.B. Saunders, 1996.
5. Kricun ME: Imaging of Bone Tumors. Philadelphia, W.B. Saunders, 1993.
6. Moser RP Jr (ed): Imaging of bone and soft tissue tumors. Radiol Clin North Am 31:237–247, 1993.
7. Resnick D: Diagnosis of Bone and Joint Disorders, 3rd ed. Philadelphia, W.B. Saunders, 1995.

50. MUSCULOSKELETAL INFECTION

Kevin R. Math, M.D., and Bernard Ghelman, M.D.

1. What is the earliest radiographic sign of osteomyelitis?
Soft tissue edema with loss of the normally well-defined fat planes. This sign is nonspecific and also may occur with soft tissue inflammatory processes such as cellulitis.

2. How long does it take before characteristic plain film skeletal findings of osteomyelitis develop?

After about 7–10 days from the onset of infection, ill-defined areas of lucency are seen within the infected bone, often accompanied by a periosteal reaction (Fig. 1).

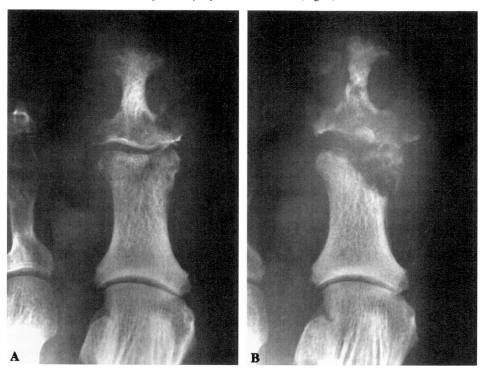

FIGURE 1. *A*, Early osteomyelitis of the great toe. There are vague areas of lucency seen at the medial base of the distal phalanx with slight joint space narrowing. There is also soft tissue swelling. *B*, Four weeks later, there has been progressive bony destruction of the proximal and distal phalanges of the great toe on both sides of the interphalangeal joint.

3. What is meant by the following terms: sequestrum, involucrum, cloaca, and Brodie's abscess (Fig. 2)?

A **sequestrum** is a dead piece of bone within an area of osteomyelitis. As the infection progresses to involve the subperiosteal region and medullary cavity, the periosteum is elevated, resulting in loss of arterial flow to the underlying bone. This devitalized piece of cortical bone persists within the infection as a focal sclerotic density and may harbor living organisms that give rise to recurrent flare-ups of osteomyelitis once the acute infection subsides. The cloak of periosteal new bone that surrounds the dead osteomyelitic bone (sequestrum) is called the **involucrum**. Eventually, the infectious process within the medullary bone can penetrate through an opening within the involucrum called the **cloaca**. The sequestrum and granulation tissue may be discharged through the cloaca and travel through sinus tracts or fistulas to the skin surface. **Brodie's abscess** is a bone abscess of variable size that represents a subacute or chronic focus of active infection.

4. Which nuclear imaging modality can effectively diagnose early osteomyelitis?

A triple-phase radionuclide bone scan. Technetium 99m-labeled diphosphonates are hydroxyapatite analogs; when injected intravenously, they reflect the regional blood flow to the bone and the new bone formation (remodeling).

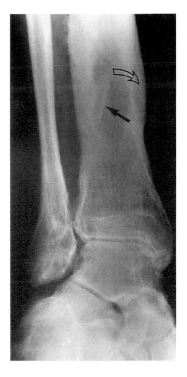

FIGURE 2. Chronic osteomyelitis of the distal tibia. The lytic lesion in the distal tibial shaft represents a *Brodie's abscess*. The linear area of sclerosis within the lesion (solid arrow) is a bony *sequestrum*, and the thick surrounding periosteal new bone (open arrow) is the *involucrum*.

5. When is each set of images obtained for a three-phase bone scan?

For the first phase of the study (radionuclide angiogram), images are obtained every 5 seconds for the first 1 minute after injection. For the second (blood pool) phase, images are obtained approximately 5 minutes after injection. Images for the third (delayed) phase are taken 2–3 hours after the initial injection.

6. Describe the bone scan findings of cellulitis and osteomyelitis.

Cellulitis demonstrates increased uptake on the first two phases of the study because of hyperemia and soft tissue inflammation. The increased uptake in cellulitis dissipates or resolves on the delayed (third) phase.

Osteomyelitis demonstrates virtually identical features as cellulitis on the first two phases of the study. On the delayed phase, however, the abnormal uptake becomes more intense and focal over the infected bone.

7. What is the role of MRI in evaluation of musculoskeletal infection?

MRI is as sensitive as a radionuclide bone scan in the diagnosis of osteomyelitis. In addition to depicting accurately the presence and extent of early osteomyelitis, the regional soft tissues also may be evaluated for soft tissue abscesses, which is not possible on a bone scan. Generally speaking, a bone scan should be done first in evaluating a previously normal bone for osteomyelitis, because it is both accurate and cost-effective. MRI should be reserved for more complicated cases such as suspected osteomyelitis at sites of recent surgery, trauma, chronic infection, or arthritis. For these cases, injection of intravenous contrast and enhancement characteristics may be useful in assessing patients for acute active infection superimposed on chronic infection or postoperative changes. Intravenous contrast also makes soft tissue fluid collections more conspicuous. For suspected spinal infection, MRI is the study of choice in all patients. MR accurately defines the levels of involvement and the presence of an associated paraspinal or epidural abscess and cord compression (Fig. 3).

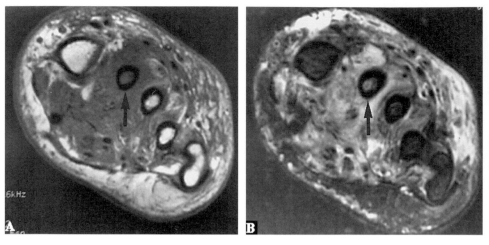

FIGURE 3.　Osteomyelitis of the second metatarsal—MRI: (*A*) T1-weighted and (*B*) T2-weighted axial images through the metatarsals show decreased T1 signal and increased T2 signal within the second metatarsal (arrow), indicative of bone marrow edema. This finding is consistent with osteomyelitis. Note similar signal abnormality infiltrating the surrounding soft tissue consistent with deep soft tissue infection.

8.　Which of the following foreign bodies are radiopaque: wood, plastic, aluminum, sheet metal, glass?

Sheet metal and some types of glass are radiopaque. Wood, plastic, and aluminum are typically radiolucent.

9.　What imaging modality is useful for evaluating suspected soft tissue foreign bodies not visible on conventional radiographs?

Ultrasound is effective in visualizing radiolucent foreign bodies such as wood and glass based on their reflection and attenuation of sound waves.

10.　What are the four main routes through which osteomyelitis is acquired?

- Hematogenous spread
- Contiguous spread from an adjacent infection (sinusitis, cellulitis, dental infection)
- Direct implantation (e.g., puncture wounds)
- Postoperative infection

11.　What are the most common organisms that cause osteomyelitis in pediatric and adult populations?

Neonate/infant: *Staphylococcus aureus*, group B Streptococcus, *Escherichia coli*
Children > 4 years: staphylococci
Adults: staphylococci, gram-negative organisms (particularly in intravenous drug abusers)

12.　What disease has an increased incidence of *Salmonella* osteomyelitis?

Sickle cell disease.

13.　Why is epiphyseal osteomyelitis rare in children after 1 year of age?

The prevalence of epiphyseal osteomyelitis and articular infection in infants and its rarity after 1 year of age is directly related to blood supply (Fig. 4). From birth until about 1 year of age metaphyseal vessels penetrate the cartilaginous growth plate, extending and branching into the epiphysis. These transphyseal vessels permit hematogenous spread of infection to the epiphysis until about 1 year, when they are obliterated.

From 1 year until growth plate closure, the terminal metaphyseal branches of the nutrient arteries turn sharply at the growth plate, and there is slow flowing turbulent blood flow at the junction of these capillaries with the large sinusoidal veins. The growth plate forms a barrier preventing hematogenous spread of infection to the epiphysis. This barrier, combined with the sluggish blood flow in the metaphysis, explains the frequency of metaphyseal osteomyelitis in this age range. In the mature skeleton, after growth plate closure, vascular communication between the epiphysis and metaphysis is reestablished, permitting hematogenous infection at the ends of bones and secondary infectious arthritis. Rarely, an aggressive osteomyelitis crosses the growth plate in a child; this occurs more commonly with tuberculous than pyogenic osteomyelitis (Fig. 5).

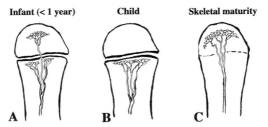

Infant (< 1 year)   **Child**   **Skeletal maturity**

A   **B**   **C**

FIGURE 4.   This diagram illustrates the anatomic basis for preferential involvement of the metaphysis by osteomyelitis between 1 year of age and growth plate closure.

FIGURE 5.   Osteomyelitis of the distal tibia. There is a focal area of lucency in the distal tibial metaphysis representing osteomyelitis. The infection has crossed the growth plate to involve the epiphysis. This is unusual between 1 year of age and growth plate closure.

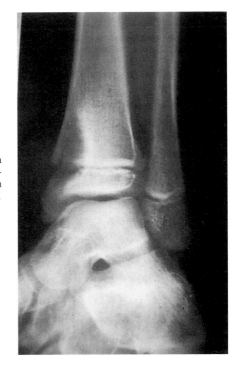

14. Describe the route of transmission and radiographic appearance of infectious arthritis.
   Infection can reach the joints through the following routes:
   • Hematogenous spread: seeding of the synovial membrane.
   • Contiguous spread of infection: from adjacent epiphyseal, metaphyseal, or soft tissue infection.
   • Direct implantation: penetrating trauma, arthrography.
   • Postoperative infection: after arthroplasty or arthroscopy.

The radiographic abnormalities parallel the pathophysiologic processes at the joint. Hyperemia results in osteoporosis at the involved joint. Synovial inflammation and edema result in a joint effusion and soft tissue swelling. Intraarticular inflammatory tissue (pannus) destroys cartilage and erodes bone resulting in joint space narrowing and articular erosions, respectively. As in rheumatoid arthritis, these erosions are initially marginal, at the bare areas of the bone, and later progress to central erosions.

15. What are the two most common sites of involvement of septic arthritis?
Knee and hip.

16. What is the differential diagnosis of an "irritable hip" in a child?
Septic arthritis, transient (toxic) synovitis, fracture, and Perthe's disease.

17. Describe the appropriate imaging work-up of a child with a suspected septic hip.
The imaging work-up should be based on the preference and experience of the clinician and radiologist. Conventional radiographs should be performed first in an attempt to exclude noninfectious causes of hip pain such as fracture and avascular necrosis. Plain film findings of septic arthritis include osteopenia (secondary to hyperemia), widening of the medial joint space (due to joint effusion), and regional soft tissue swelling, often associated with bulging of the fat planes about the hip. Plain films are often normal or equivocal, and aspiration of the joint is usually required for cases in which infection is considered. Some centers proceed to ultrasound of the hip to attempt to identify a joint effusion that can subsequently be aspirated under ultrasound guidance. Alternatively, the joint can be aspirated under fluoroscopic guidance. Iodinated contrast is injected into the hip joint to confirm that the needle is intraarticular. Although MRI and nuclear imaging have a role in evaluating suspected infection, joint aspiration is usually required for definitive diagnosis and identification of the offending microorganism.

18. What is Phemister's triad?
Phemister's triad describes the characteristic radiographic findings of tuberculous arthritis: periarticular osteoporosis, peripheral bony erosions, and gradual narrowing of the joint space. The delayed or gradual loss of the joint space is the hallmark of the more indolent tuberculous arthritis and distinguishes it from pyogenic arthritis, in which the joint space loss is more rapid. Tuberculous arthritis is most commonly secondary to an adjacent tuberculous osteomyelitis and is a monoarticular disease.

19. What is Pott's disease?
Pott's disease is the eponym applied to tuberculous spondylitis. Spinal involvement is present in up to 60% of cases of skeletal tuberculosis. Although the L1 vertebra is most commonly involved, the infection commonly affects other levels of the spine and usually progresses to involve multiple levels. The affected vertebral body may eventually collapse, resulting in an angular kyphosis (gibbus deformity).

20. Describe the radiographic features of infectious spondylitis (Fig. 6)?
Infection typically spreads to the spine hematogenously, seeding the anterior aspect of the vertebral body near the disc. The infection spreads to involve the adjacent disc and eventually the contiguous vertebral body. Involvement of two contiguous vertebral bodies and the intervening disc is seen in the majority of patients; more than one disc level may become involved if the infection is not treated. These events are manifested radiographically as decreased disc height combined with poor definition of the endplate(s) on either side of the disc and occasional osteolytic destruction of the adjacent vertebral body. Long-standing infection may lead to reactive sclerosis of the involved vertebrae, particularly in pyogenic infections. A paraspinal mass is commonly associated with infective spondylitis. These masses can grow quite large in tuberculous infections, in which cord compression and paraplegia may result.

21. What are the MR findings of infectious spondylitis?
Conventional radiographs often underestimate the extent of a spinal infection; MR is the appropriate imaging modality for demonstrating the abnormal marrow signal in the infected vertebral

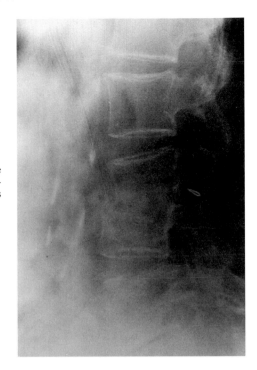

FIGURE 6. Septic spondylitis, lumbar spine. The pyogenic infection in this case results in narrowing/destruction of the involved disc space and osteomyelitis of the adjacent vertebral bodies.

body or bodies. This abnormal signal usually also involves the intervening disc(s). Moreover, MR effectively depicts the presence of associated paraspinal or epidural abscesses commonly associated with spinal infections and effectively excludes spinal cord compression (Fig. 7).

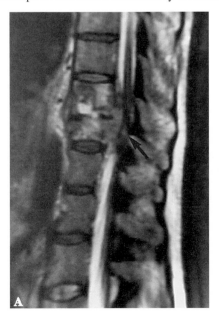

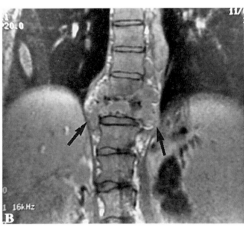

FIGURE 7. Tuberculous spondylitis. *A*, This sagittal T2-weighted image shows an infectious process involving a lower thoracic disc space with the abnormal signal extending into the adjacent vertebral bodies. Note the paraspinal inflammatory mass extending anteriorly and posteriorly at this level, resulting in spinal cord compression (arrow). *B*, Coronal 'balanced MR image clearly shows the lobulated bilateral paraspinal masses (arrows) associated with the spinal infection. Note the narrowed ill-defined disc space compared with normal levels.

22. Can infection involve the intervertebral disc, sparing the adjacent vertebrae?

Yes. Isolated intervertebral disc infection, or discitis, is primarily seen in children; it is rare in adults. Disc infection also may be a complication of invasive procedures such as discography or discectomy.

23. What features distinguish tuberculous spondylitis from pyogenic spondylitis?

Accurate differentiation between these two entities is often not possible, because they share many of the same imaging features. The following findings favor tuberculosis over pyogenic infection:

- Delayed destruction of the disc space
- Large paraspinal mass (commonly calcified, often involves the psoas muscle)
- Absence of sclerosis
- Pulmonary manifestations of tuberculosis

24. Is there any risk of malignancy at sites of chronic musculoskeletal infection?

Yes. Epidermoid carcinoma develops in at least 0.5% of patients with chronic infections and draining sinus tracts. The latent period is usually at least 20 years, and the tumor typically develops deep within the sinus tract, sometimes affecting the adjacent bone. Other types of secondary neoplasm also have been described.

BIBLIOGRAPHY

1. Brower AC: Septic arthritis. Radiol Clin North Am 34:293–309, 1996.
2. Gold RH, Hawkins RA, Katz RD: Bacterial osteomyelitis: Findings on plain radiography, CT, MR and scintigraphy. AJR 157:365, 1991.
3. Jaramillo D, Treves ST, Kasser JR, et al: Osteomyelitis and septic arthritis in children: Appropriate use of imaging to guide treatment. AJR 165:399, 1995.
4. Morrison WB, Schweitzer ME, Bock GW, et al: Diagnosis of osteomyelitis: Utility of fat-suppressed contrast-enhanced MR imaging. Radiology 189:251, 1993.
5. Resnick D: Diagnosis of Bone and Joint Disorders, 3rd ed. Philadelphia, W.B. Saunders, 1995.

51. OSTEONECROSIS

Kevin R. Math, M.D.

1. List the causes of osteonecrosis (also called avascular necrosis [AVN]).

More common causes
    Trauma (fracture)
    Steroid therapy
    Sickle cell disease
    Idiopathic (Legg-Perthe's disease)

Less common causes
    Alcoholism
    Gaucher's disease
    Pancreatitis
    Radiation therapy
    Caisson's disease ("the bends")
    Systemic lupus erythematosus (SLE)

These diseases can be grouped into diseases that result in impaired vascular supply due to vascular disruption (e.g., trauma), intravascular obstruction (e.g., sickle cell disease), vasculitis (e.g., SLE), or increased marrow pressure from infiltrative disease (e.g., Gaucher's disease).

2. What are the radiographic signs of osteonecrosis?

The most common finding is increased density (sclerosis) at the site of AVN (Fig. 1), which is due primarily to the summation effect of new bone (repair) laid down on top of dead bone. This sclerotic new bone is also known as the "zone of creeping substitution." Eventually, this weakened bone may fracture, resulting in collapse of the articular surface. When the fracture occurs in the subchondral bone at an articular surface, it has a crescentic appearance ("crescent sign") (Fig. 2). Eventually,

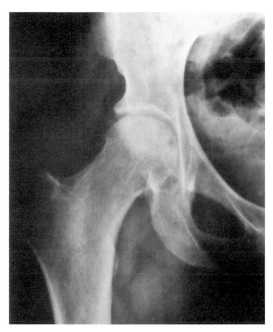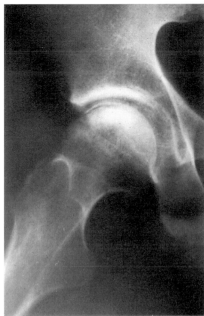

FIGURE 1 *(Left)*.   Osteonecrosis of the femoral head—increased radiographic density. There is generalized sclerosis of the superior half of the femoral head with vague areas of lucency at its medial aspect.

FIGURE 2 *(Right)*.   Osteonecrosis of the femoral head—crescent sign. Note the crescentic lucency at the superolateral articular surface of the femoral head, indicating a subchondral fracture.

this weakened articular surface can collapse (Fig. 3), and ultimately result in secondary degenerative disease. These signs may take months to develop. Earlier, radiographically occult stages of AVN may be detected on a radionuclide bone scan or MRI (Fig. 4).

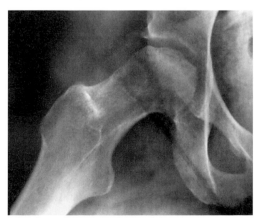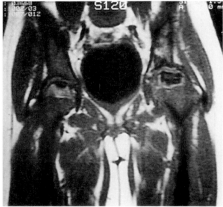

FIGURE 3 *(Left)*.   Osteonecrosis of the femoral head—articular surface collapse. There is flattening and irregularity of the superior articular surface, representing an advanced stage of AVN.

FIGURE 4 *(Right)*.   Bilateral osteonecrosis of the femoral head—MRI. Note the abnormal signal at the superior articular surface of both femoral heads (left greater than right). Radiographs of the right hip were normal. There is generalized decrease in the bone marrow signal (normally hyperintense from fatty marrow elements) secondary to red marrow hyperplasia in this child with sickle cell disease.

3. At what skeletal site is AVN most commonly seen?
The femoral head.

4. Which fracture type is more commonly complicated by AVN of the femoral head, subcapital femur fracture, or intertrochanteric fracture?
As many as 25–50% of subcapital femur fractures are complicated by AVN (Fig. 5). These fractures occur at the junction of the femoral neck and head. AVN is uncommonly associated with intertrochanteric fractures. The relatively high prevalence of AVN with subcapital fractures is due to the fact that the arterial branches of the femoral artery that supply the femoral head (retinacular vessels) course through the joint capsule and subcapital (intracapsular) fractures are commonly associated with injury to these vessels. Greater angulation and displacement of subcapital fractures carry an increased risk for AVN; this explains the therapeutic decision to treat significantly displaced subcapital fractures with joint prostheses rather than internal fixation. Intertrochanteric fractures, which are extracapsular, rarely have a significant effect on arterial blood supply.

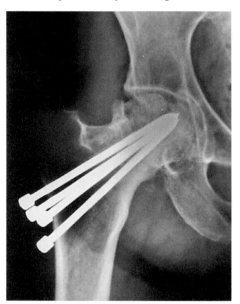

FIGURE 5. Osteonecrosis of the femoral head following subcapital fracture. Despite pin fixation of this nondisplaced subcapital fracture, osteonecrosis eventually developed; note the irregularity of the femoral head articular surface.

5. Name two other fractures in which AVN is a notorious complication.
Talus: displaced talar neck fractures are complicated by AVN in up to 80–90% of cases (Fig. 6).
Scaphoid: scaphoid waist fractures result in AVN of the proximal fragment (Fig. 7).

6. Which imaging modality is more sensitive for diagnosing early AVN—MRI or bone scan?
Although radionuclide bone scan has a high sensitivity for the diagnosis of AVN, it lacks specificity and has poor anatomic resolution. Bone scans usually show abnormal, increased uptake at the femoral head due to the increased flow and remodeling associated with the reparative response to osteonecrosis. Unfortunately, other processes such as trauma, arthritis, and neoplasm also demonstrate increased uptake on a bone scan, making the finding of increased activity difficult to interpret. Furthermore, bilateral AVN may have symmetric increased uptake at the hips, which may be overlooked.

MRI is more sensitive for detection of AVN and provides information about the precise location and extent of the AVN. In addition, MRI can differentiate AVN from other causes of hip pain such as fracture, tumor, and transient osteoporosis.

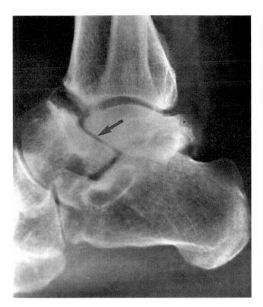 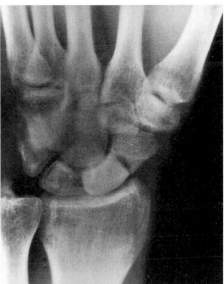

FIGURE 6 (Left). Talar neck fracture with osteonecrosis of the posterior fragment. There is a persistent lucent fracture line at the neck of the talus (arrow), indicating nonunion. Note the generalized sclerosis of the necrotic posterior fracture fragment. (Courtesy of Bernard Ghelman, M.D.)

FIGURE 7 (Right). Scaphoid fracture with avascular necrosis of the proximal fragment. There is generalized sclerosis of the necrotic proximal fracture fragment.

7. What are the stages of AVN of the femoral head?

Several staging systems have been described, and it is more important to remember the progression of radiographic abnormalities than the specific numerical stage.

Stage 0: clinical symptoms (pain), normal radiographs, positive MRI or bone scan.
Stage I: subtle areas of lucency and sclerosis on radiographs.
Stage II: subchondral fracture ("crescent sign").
Stage III: collapse (flattening) of the articular surface.
Stage IV: secondary degenerative joint disease.

Once the disease has progressed to stage II, progression to advanced stages is inevitable. Prompt diagnosis of early AVN is crucial so that the offending agent can be removed. Some surgeons attempt core decompression of the femoral head at early stages to attempt to stimulate revascularization and to relieve elevated marrow pressure; however, the results and indications of this procedure are controversial.

8. What is the "double-line sign"?

The double line is a commonly seen MRI sign of AVN. Most cases of AVN are easily detected on MRI as a focal crescentic, oval, or linear area of abnormal marrow signal in the subchondral bone adjacent to the articular surface. The crescent of abnormal signal often has a characteristic bright inner margin next to a dark outer margin on T2-weighted images (Fig. 8). This sign is seen in up to 80% of cases of AVN of the femoral head. Histologically, the dark line represents sclerosis and fibrosis, whereas the bright line is caused by granulation tissue, edema, and necrosis.

9. A patient on chronic steroid therapy develops radiographically evident AVN of the right hip. Is further evaluation with MRI indicated?

Yes. No further evaluation of the right hip is necessary, because the diagnosis is already evident on plain films. However, MRI of the contralateral hip should be done to attempt to detect less advanced occult AVN of the left hip.

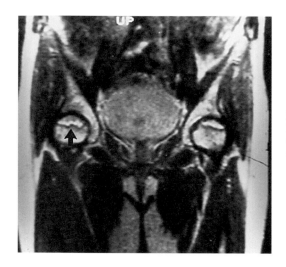

FIGURE 8. Osteonecrosis of the femoral head—"double-line sign." There is bilateral AVN of the femoral heads with the characteristic double line sign (arrow).

10. **List four causes of the increased bony density on radiographs of patients with AVN.**
    • Summation density of new bone plus dead bone.
    • Hyperemia associated with the injury results in osteopenia at adjacent well-vascularized bones. (This results in relative sclerosis of the hypovascular osteonecrotic bone.)
    • Trabecular microfractures of the weakened osteonecrotic bone.
    • Saponification (fat necrosis) of the osteonecrotic marrow fat.

11. **A 50-year-old man presents with severe left hip pain. Radiographs reveal severe osteoporosis of the femoral neck and head. The T2-weighted MRI is shown in Figure 9. What is the likely diagnosis?**

    If you said osteonecrosis, you are wrong. There is diffuse increased signal throughout the proximal femur rather than a well-demarcated subchondral signal abnormality as seen in AVN. This patient has transient osteoporosis, a poorly understood, relatively uncommon cause of hip pain. Originally described in young women in the third trimester of pregnancy, this disease is probably ischemic in etiology, is actually more common in men, and results in diffuse marrow edema in the

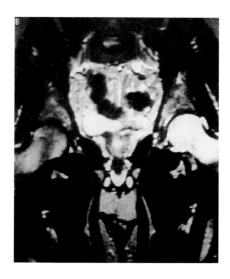

FIGURE 9. Transient osteoporosis of the left femoral head. There is generalized increased signal within the femoral head and neck on this T2-weighted image. This completely resolved within one year.

femoral head and neck. Unlike AVN, this disease is self-limited; clinical and radiographic findings usually resolve in 3–6 months.

12. What do the following diseases have in common: Kienböck's, Kohler's, and Panner's disease?

Each is a specific site of posttraumatic osteonecrosis; they are grouped together as the osteochondroses. Kienböck's (Fig. 10), Kohler's, and Panner's disease occur at the lunate, tarsal navicular, and capitellum (elbow), respectively.

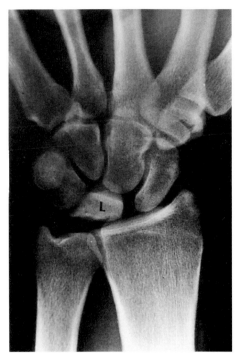

FIGURE 10.   Kienböck's disease. There is generalized sclerosis of the necrotic lunate bone with an irregular contour. This patient also has widening of the space between the scaphoid and lunate from prior ligamentous injury.

13. Describe the radiographic appearance of a medullary bone infarction.

Infarction of the medullary bone at the diametaphyseal region of long bones can occur as an isolated finding or in association with osteonecrosis at the epiphyseal articular region at other sites. Common sites include the knee (distal femur, proximal tibia), distal tibia, and proximal humerus. The classical appearance is that of an irregular serpiginous region of peripheral calcification encircling the infarcted medullary bone (Fig. 11). The calcifications associated with enchondromas, lesions that occur at similar sites as bone infarctions, are distributed diffusely throughout the lesion, allowing differentiation of these lesions from each other (Fig. 12).

BIBLIOGRAPHY

1. Frohberg PK, Braunstein EM, Buckwalter KA: Osteonecrosis. Transient osteoporosis and transient bone marrow edema: Current concepts. Radiol Clin North Am 31:273–291, 1996.
2. Mitchell DG, Rao VM, Dalinka MK, et al: Femoral head avascular necrosis: Correlation of MR imaging, radiographic staging, radionuclide imaging and clinical findings. Radiology 162:709–715, 1987.
3. Potter HG, Moran M, Schneider R, et al; Magnetic resonance imaging in diagnosing transient osteoporosis of the hip. Clin Orthop 280:223–229, 1992.
4. Vande Berg BE, Malghem JJ, Lahaisse MA, et al: MR imaging of avascular necrosis and transient marrow edema of the femoral head. Radiographics 13:501–520, 1993.

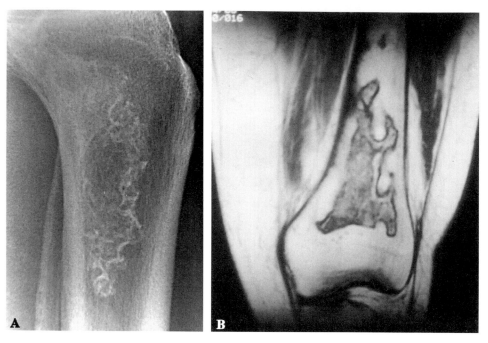

FIGURE 11. *A,* Bone infarction in the proximal tibia. There is peripheral serpiginous calcification in the proximal tibia of this alcoholic individual. *B,* Bone infarction in the distal femur—MRI. This T1-weighted MR image shows the abnormal marrow signal within the infarcted medullary bone, surrounded by the low-signal peripheral serpiginous rim of calcification.

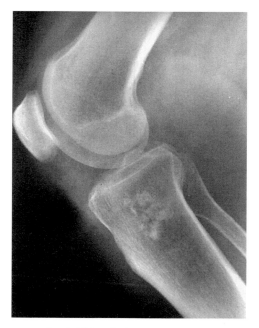

FIGURE 12. The diffuse coarse chondroid (cartilaginous) calcifications within this proximal tibial enchondroma differ from the serpiginous peripheral calcifications of a bone infarction.

52. METABOLIC BONE DISEASE

Kevin R. Math, M.D.

1. What is the difference between osteomalacia and osteoporosis?

Osteoporosis is a decrease in the amount of normally mineralized bone, commonly seen in older women. Osteomalacia is marked by abnormal mineralization of bone; the amount of osteoid is typically normal or may even be increased. Both diseases result in weakening of the bone and associated pathologic fractures.

2. Describe the radiographic findings of osteoporosis.

Conventional radiographs are insensitive for detection of early osteoporosis; this diagnosis is best made with bone densitometry studies. The hallmark of osteoporosis is decreased density of the visualized bones (bones appear darker). This sign is often subjective and may be caused by technical errors such as overexposure; similarly, radiographic underexposure may cause the bones to be abnormally radiodense. One helpful objective sign is measurement of the relative thickness of the cortex of the third metacarpal bone. The total width of both cortices measured at the mid-metacarpal shaft should be at least 50% of the width of the entire bone at the same level. A cortical width of less than 50% is consistent with osteoporosis.

3. What is osteopenia?

Osteopenia is a general term describing a decreased amount (paucity) of bone. It is manifested radiographically as decreased radiodensity. Both osteoporosis and osteomalacia may result in radiographic osteopenia.

4. What is considered the best screening examination for osteoporosis?

Dual x-ray absorptiometry (DEXA) is the most sensitive examination for detection of demineralization (osteoporosis). Nuclear imaging techniques such as dual photon absorptiometry (DPA) are also highly sensitive for objective assessment of bone mineral density and serial changes between two examinations.

5. Why do patients with chronic renal failure get osteomalacia?

There are two main causes. First, renal dysfunction results in defective hydroxylation of vitamin D, leading to abnormal bone mineralization. Secondly, renal failure is commonly accompanied by hyperphosphatemia and hypocalcemia, resulting in secondary hyperparathyroidism (HPT). Elevated parathormone levels result in widespread bony demineralization.

6. Which disease is characterized by osteomalacia in children?

Rickets.

7. List five causes of rickets.

Inadequate dietary intake of vitamin D
Inadequate sun exposure
Abnormal intestinal absorption of vitamin D
Renal or hepatic dysfunction (abnormal hydroxylation)
Phenobarbital—increased breakdown of vitamin D by the liver

8. What are the radiographic signs of rickets?

Fraying, flaring, and cupping of the metaphysis and widening of the growth plate (zone of provisional calcification) (Fig. 1)
Osteopenia
Expansion of rib ends ("rachitic rosary") (Fig. 2)

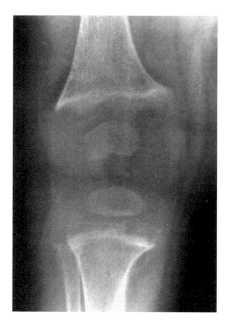

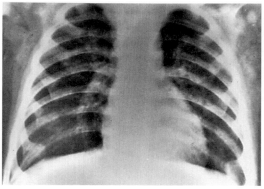

FIGURE 1 *(Left).* Rickets—knee. Note the growth plate widening at the distal femur and proximal tibia, and the fraying and flaring of the metaphyses.

FIGURE 2 *(Right).* Rickets—chest. The rib ends are flared and bulbous, producing clinically palpable nodules (rachitic rosary).

9. Why are the radiographic signs of rickets more evident at the wrists and knees than at the elbows and hips?

Signs of rickets are most evident at sites of active growth. In the upper extremity, growth at the proximal humerus and distal forearm contributes most to limb growth (proportionate growth at the proximal and distal humerus is about 80% and 20%, respectively; growth at the proximal and distal forearm is about 20% and 80%, respectively). Proportionate growth for the entire lower extremity is as follows: distal femur, 40%; proximal tibia, 30%; distal tibia, 20%; proximal femur, 10% (i.e., 70% of lower extremity growth occurs at the knee).

10. What is a "rugger jersey spine"?

This term describes the appearance of the spine in hyperparathyroidism. A thick band of sclerosis at the superior and inferior endplates is separated by a wider intervening area of lucency (Fig. 3). This pattern resembles the appearance of a jersey worn in rugby.

11. What is the difference between primary and secondary hyperparathyroidism?

Primary hyperparathyroidism is usually caused by a parathyroid adenoma, resulting in increased production and circulating levels of parathyroid hormone. Secondary hyperparathyroidism is usually due to renal failure, resulting in increased levels of parathormone as a response to hyperphosphatemia and hypocalcemia. Secondary hyperparathyroidism is also called renal osteodystrophy. Both conditions result in characteristic skeletal findings.

12. Which tumor is associated with hyperparathyroidism as a paraneoplastic syndrome?

Squamous cell carcinoma of the lung.

13. Describe the radiographic findings of hyperparathyroid bone disease.

Osteopenia	Subperiosteal bone resorption
"Salt-and-pepper skull"—due to granular demineralization of skull	Bony resorption at tendon and ligament insertion sites, distal clavicles, sacroiliac joints, and symphysis pubis
Rugger-jersey spine	Erosion of the lamina dura of the teeth (normally seen
Pathologic fractures	as a white line paralleling the margin of the teeth)
Brown tumors	Soft tissue calcifications (2° > 1°)

14. What are brown tumors? Are they more common in primary or secondary hyperparathyroidism?

Brown tumors are lytic skeletal lesions associated with hyperparathyroidism. They contain chronic hemorrhage, which accounts for the brown color of the fluid (hence the name). These lesions are encountered in a higher percentage of primary than secondary HPT; however, more patients with brown tumors have secondary HPT because of the significantly greater number of patients with this disease.

15. Where is the best place to look for subperiosteal bone resorption when hyperparathyroid bone disease is suspected?

Radial aspect of the middle phalanges of the index and middle fingers (Fig. 4).

16. Which radiographs comprise a metabolic skeletal survey?

Radiographs of sites with the highest yield for characteristic pathologic skeletal findings should be performed. These sites include the entire spine (anteroposterior and lateral views), pelvis, chest (including acromioclavicular joints), skull, and hands.

FIGURE 3 *(Right)*. Rugger-jersey spine. The thick bands of sclerosis at the endplates separated by lucency at the mid-vertebral body resemble the stripes of a rugby jersey.

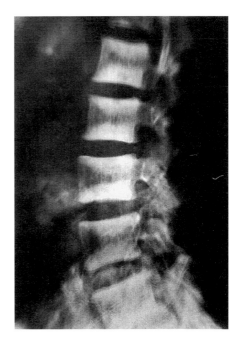

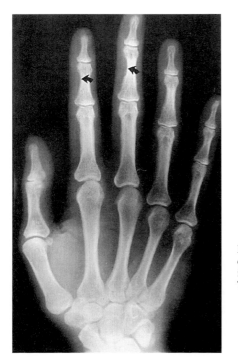

FIGURE 4 *(Left)*. Hyperparathyroidism—hand. Note the concavity at the radial aspect of the middle phalanges of the index and middle fingers, a classical location of this finding. This results from subperiosteal bone resorption.

17. What are "lead lines"? Why do they occur?

"Lead lines" refer to the dense sclerotic line or band at the metaphyses of children with chronic lead intoxication. Contrary to popular belief, they are not due to deposition of lead in the bone at these sites; they are probably due to inhibition of osteoclasts and relative decrease in bone resorption at sites of growth. As in rickets, bony changes are most evident at the wrists and knees (Fig. 5).

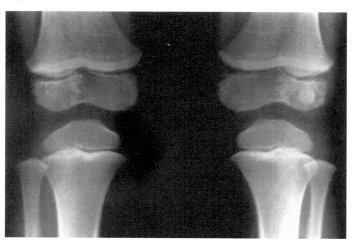

FIGURE 5. Chronic lead intoxication. There are dense metaphyseal lines ("lead lines"), most apparent at the distal femora and proximal tibiae.

18. Aside from wrist radiographs, which x-ray study is helpful for evaluating a child with suspected lead poisoning?

An abdominal radiograph may reveal radiopaque lead in the gastrointestinal tract from an acute ingestion (Fig. 6). Dense metaphyseal bands reflect chronic lead intoxication.

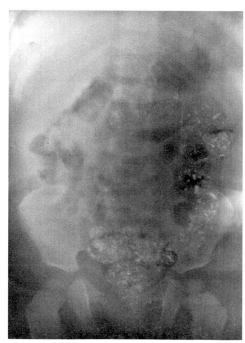

FIGURE 6. Acute lead ingestion. There are innumerable metallic foci seen over the left abdomen and pelvis, representing lead chips in the colon and rectum.

BIBLIOGRAPHY

1. Murphey MD, Sartoris DJ, Quale JL, et al: Musculoskeletal manifestations of chronic renal insufficiency. Radiographics 13:357, 1993.
2. Rosenberg AE: Pathology of metabolic bone disease. Radiol Clin North Am 29:19, 1991.
3. Tigges S, Nance EP, Carpenter WA, Erb R: Renal osteodystrophy: Imaging findings that mimic those of other diseases. AJR 165:143–148, 1995.

53. PAGET'S DISEASE

Kevin R. Math, M.D.

1. Describe the radiographic findings of Paget's disease.

Paget's disease, described by Sir James Paget in 1877, is characterized by thickening of the bony cortex, coarsening of trabeculae, and enlargement of the affected bones (Fig. 1). Radiographic abnormalities reflect the accelerated bone turnover in the lytic, blastic, and mixed phases.

2. What percentage of people over 80 years have Paget's disease?

About 10%.

3. What is the cause of Paget's disease?

Most authorities favor a viral etiology, based on identification of intranuclear inclusion bodies. This theory is unproven.

4. How does Paget's disease present clinically?

The disease is often asymptomatic and discovered incidentally on radiographs obtained for another reason. Pain and bony enlargement are the most common clinical symptoms. An increasing hat size is a classic historical clue to Paget's disease. Patients also may present with neurologic complications of the disease (see below).

5. Is Paget's disease more common in blacks than whites?

The disease is much more common in whites. Paget's disease is quite rare in blacks and Asians and is most common in Northern Europe.

6. What laboratory values may be abnormal in Paget's disease?

The increased osteoblastic activity in Paget's disease is associated with an elevated alkaline phosphatase level. Acid phosphatase tends to be slightly elevated in the lytic phase of Paget's. Urinary and serum hydroxyproline levels are often elevated.

7. Which skeletal sites are most commonly affected by Paget's disease?

Lumbar spine. Increased density of the entire vertebral body or its margins results in the classic "ivory vertebra" or "picture-frame vertebra," respectively.

Skull. Multiple rounded areas of increased density result in the classic "cotton-wool spots" on skull radiographs.

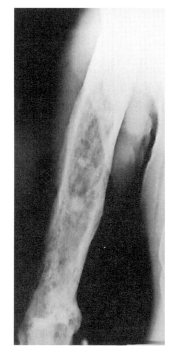

FIGURE 1. Paget's disease—humerus. There are extensive Pagetic changes throughout the entire humerus, marked by cortical thickening, sclerosis, and bony enlargement.

Pelvis. Thickening of the iliopectineal line is considered to be both specific and sensitive for Paget's disease. Involvement of the entire pelvis or an entire hemipelvis is common (Fig. 2).

Femur, tibia. When long bones are affected, involvement typically starts at the end of the bone and eventually progresses to involve the entire bone. The leading edge of the lytic phase of the disease has a characteristic flame shape or "blade-of-grass" configuration. The blastic phase of the disease soon ensues, characterized by cortical thickening, coarsening of trabeculae, and increased bony density. Bowing of long bones is also common (Fig. 3).

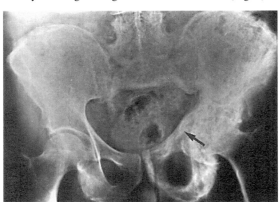 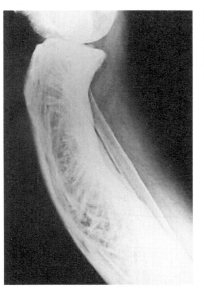

FIGURE 2 *(Left)*.   Paget's disease—pelvis. The entire left hemipelvis is involved, and there are arthritic changes of the left hip. Note the classic thickening of the iliopectineal line (arrow).

FIGURE 3 *(Right)*.   Paget's disease—tibia. There is marked coarsening of trabeculae, and there is anterior bowing of the tibial shaft. Note the marked enlargement of the tibia relative to the fibula.

8. Paget's disease of long bones almost invariably starts at the end of the bone, but in one bone involvement may occur initially at the mid-portion. Which one?

The tibia.

9. What is osteoporosis circumscripta?

Rarely, the early phase of Paget's disease gives rise to a lytic skull lesion that may be quite large. This well-marginated osteolytic area has been termed osteoporosis circumscripta.

10. What is a "banana fracture"?

Pathologic fracture is a known complication of Paget's disease. Such fractures usually are incomplete, involving the convex side of bowed long bones. Also known as fissure fractures, they resemble the incomplete breaks that result from bending a banana (Fig. 4). Pathologic fractures may also be complete and displaced, owing to the relatively weak Pagetic bone (Fig. 5).

11. What are the bone scan findings of Paget's disease?

Since activity on a radionuclide bone scan depends on regional blood flow and bone turnover, both increased in this disease, it is not surprising that the active phase of Paget's disease will typically appear "hot" on a bone scan. Activity may be normal in the quiescent phase of the disease.

12. Describe the appearance of Paget's disease on MRI.

It is variable. Most cases are associated with markedly abnormal, heterogeneous marrow signal which can be mistaken for a malignant neoplasm if not correlated with plain films. Hence, the significance of the MR findings of Paget's disease should be approached with caution, and plain films are mandatory when this diagnosis is being considered. A CT scan is superior to MRI for demonstrating the classic skeletal findings of Paget's disease.

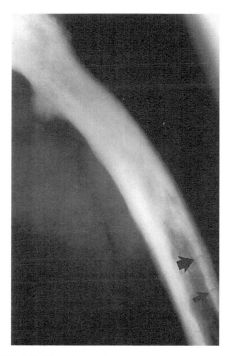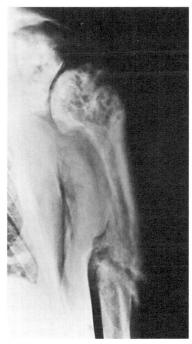

FIGURE 4 *(Left)*.   Fissure fractures. Transversely oriented linear lucencies traverse the cortex at the convex side of the bowed femoral shaft (arrows).

FIGURE 5 *(Right)*.   Paget's disease—humeral fracture. There is an ununited fracture of the mid-humeral shaft with Pagetic changes of the humerus and scapula.

13. How can a sclerotic vertebral body involved by Paget's disease be distinguished from an osteoblastic metastasis?

Enlargement of the involved vertebra and cortical thickening are the most reliable differentiating signs.

14. What neurologic complications may be associated with Paget's disease?

Spinal stenosis, nerve root compression, and cord compression may result from bony expansion of vertebrae. In addition, cranial nerve palsies may result from skull base involvement.

15. What is Paget's arthritis?

There is a high incidence of arthritis in the joints adjacent to pagetic bones. It is most commonly seen at the hip (followed by the knee) and is characterized by concentric joint space narrowing (see Fig. 2). Patients often require joint replacements; surgery may be complicated by the potential of these hypervascular bones to hemorrhage.

16. Which primary bone tumor is associated with Paget's disease?

Giant cell tumor of bone is associated with Paget's disease in rare cases.

17. What is the incidence of malignant (sarcomatous) degeneration in Paget's disease?

Generally, this complication arises in < 1% of patients. However, those with extensive skeletal involvement have a proportionately increased risk, as high as 5–10%.

18. What is the most common malignant cell type when this unfortunate complication occurs?

Osteosarcoma accounts for more than half of these cases, followed by fibrosarcoma and chondrosarcoma.

19. What are the radiographic signs of malignant degeneration of Pagetic bone?

Lytic or destructive areas within regions of prior radiodense bone, new calcifications in the adjacent soft tissues, and increasing pain (Fig. 6).

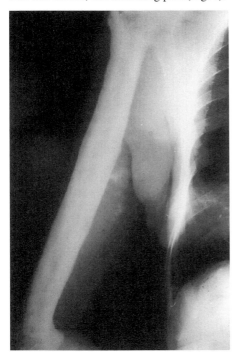

FIGURE 6. Paget's sarcoma—humeral shaft. There are calcifications in the medial soft tissues adjacent to the humerus with a palpable soft tissue mass, representing sarcomatous degeneration.

20. Do Paget's sarcomas tend to be high grade or low grade?

Very aggressive and high grade; they are commonly metastatic at the time of diagnosis and have a very poor prognosis.

BIBLIOGRAPHY

1. Griffiths HJ: Radiology of Paget's disease. Curr Opin Radiol 4:124–128, 1992.
2. Kaufmann GA, Sundaram M, McDonald DJ: Magnetic resonance imaging in symptomatic Paget's disease. Skeletal Radiol 20:413, 1991.
3. Mirra JM, Brian EW, Tehranzadeh J: Paget's disease of bone: Review with emphasis on radiologic features, Parts 1 & 2. Skeletal Radiol 24:163–171, 173–180, 1995.
4. Moore TE, Kathol MH, El-Khoury GY, et al: Unusual radiological features of Paget's disease. Skeletal Radiol 23:257, 1994.
5. Potter HG, Schneider R, Ghelman B, et al: Multiple giant cell tumors and Paget's disease of bone: Radiographic and clinical correlations. Radiology 180:261, 1991.
6. Resnick D: Bone and Joint Imaging. Philadelphia, W.B. Saunders, 1989.

54. JOINT PROSTHESIS IMAGING

Kevin R. Math, M.D., and Giles R. Scuderi, M.D.

1. Name the two most commonly replaced joints.
Hip and knee.

2. Name three common pathologic conditions requiring joint arthroplasty.
Severe arthritis (most commonly degenerative joint disease and rheumatoid arthritis).
Post-traumatic: For severe fractures (comminuted, displaced) that have a poor chance of healing by internal fixation and a high incidence of avascular necrosis (e.g., displaced varus angulated subcapital femur fractures are commonly treated with hemiarthroplasty rather than surgical fixation).
Bone tumors: Extensive resection of osseous neoplasms often require complex endoprostheses; these prostheses are usually custom-made and attempt to replace the resected bone and provide a functional articulation.

3. What are the two most common methods of fixation of joint prostheses?
Most prostheses are embedded in cement, resulting in interfaces between the cement and the prosthetic components and the cement and the adjacent bone. Polymethyl methacrylate (PMMA) is the type of cement most often used. Current cement is radiopaque and is easily visualized on postoperative radiographs. Cementless prosthetic components are currently popular; these prostheses have a textured surface, composed of small metal beads (or mesh) which carpet the surface of the metal. The beads provide a lattice for the ingrowth of bone; bone grows into the interstices between the beads. These prostheses require a tighter fit ("press fit") to allow for bone ingrowth.

4. What are the three most common causes of prosthesis failure?
Infection is a common cause of failure, occurring in less than 1% of primary joint arthroplasties (it is more common in revision arthroplasties). Component loosening and polyethylene wear are the other two most common causes of failure. Loosening can occur secondary to infection; differentiating infectious loosening from mechanical loosening is sometimes challenging.

5. What are the radiographic signs of prosthesis loosening?
The most accurate sign is a shift in position of the prosthesis (Fig. 1). Any change in position of the components from one study to another indicates loosening. Subsidence is the sinking of the prosthesis into the adjacent bone and is indicative of loosening (Fig. 2). Other signs include progressive widening of radiolucent lines at the interface between the cement and bone and lucency between the metal prosthesis and cement (Fig. 3). An interval increase in the width of lucency at these interfaces from one examination to the next is more significant than the absolute measurement of the lucent interface. Fracture of the cement mantle also implies loosening.

6. Following total joint arthroplasty, when would you expect a bone scan to return to a normal level of activity?
For hip arthroplasty activity returns to normal or to a mildly increased baseline level of activity about 6–12 months following surgery. During this time the bone scan lacks specificity, as it is difficult to distinguish normal postoperative activity from pathologic increased uptake. For knee arthroplasty increased activity can persist indefinitely, making interpretation of these studies even more challenging.

7. A patient has a painful total hip replacement with suspected loosening, and normal radiographs. What more sensitive study would you order for further evaluation?

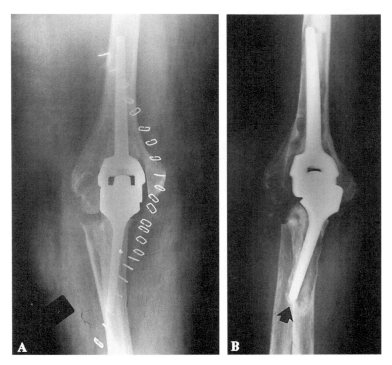

FIGURE 1. Immediate postoperative (*A*) and 3-year postoperative (*B*) radiographs of a total elbow replacement. Note that the metallic stems are well positioned within the central medullary cavity of the distal humerus and proximal ulna in (*A*). The follow-up radiograph (*B*) reveals radiolucency surrounding these metallic stems suggesting loosening. The ulnar stem has penetrated the lateral cortex of the ulna (arrow); this change in position confirms loosening of the prosthesis.

A radionuclide bone scan is highly sensitive for demonstrating increased uptake around a loose prosthesis before radiographic signs develop.

8. List six complications of total hip arthroplasty.

Infection, prosthesis loosening, fracture of prosthesis or bone, heterotopic bone formation, dislocation, and osteolysis.

9. What is the most common cause of a dislocated total hip arthroplasty?

The cause of dislocation varies depending on the time since surgery. Dislocation in the immediate postoperative period is usually due to laxity of the supporting soft tissue structures. Dislocation occurring months after surgery is most often due to prosthesis malposition (Fig. 4). The acetabular cup should be laterally tilted by about 40–50° relative to a line drawn across the ischial tuberosities, and should be tilted anteriorly (anteverted) by about 15–20°. These angles can be assessed on conventional radiographs; retroversion of the acetabular cup is associated with a posterior hip dislocation.

10. A patient with a total hip replacement presents with a radiographically loose and painful femoral component. What complication must be considered prior to contemplating revision surgery?

Infection. It is impossible to differentiate mechanical (aseptic) from infectious prosthesis loosening based on radiographs alone. Furthermore, an infected total joint replacement may present with fairly normal-appearing conventional radiographs with the exception of soft tissue swelling; normal radiographs do not exclude infection. Infection can occur in the immediate postoperative period, but is much more commonly seen 6 months or longer after the surgery due to hematogenous seeding of the prosthesis from a distant source.

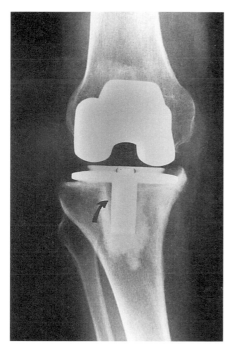

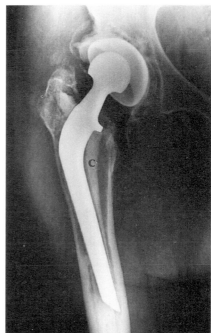

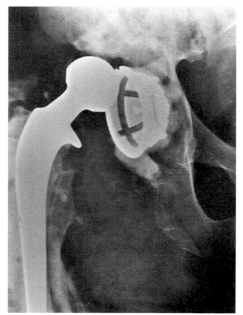

FIGURE 2 *(Above left)*. Total knee replacement—subsidence. The medial aspect of the tibial plateau component has sunk into the tibia, with a rim of bone at its medial aspect. This finding, combined with the radiolucency at the lateral metal–cement interface (curved arrow), indicates loosening of the prosthesis.

FIGURE 3 *(Above right)*. Total hip replacement—loose femoral component. There is a wide area of lucency between the opaque cement (C) and the adjacent bone at the medial aspect of the proximal femur, in addition to the area of lucency at the metal–bone interface. Also noted is lucency at the cement bone interface surrounding the acetabular prosthesis. These were new findings, indicative of loosening of both components.

FIGURE 4 *(Right)*. Total hip replacement—dislocation. The femur has dislocated superiorly and laterally relative to the acetabulum. This dislocation is due to abnormal (vertical) position of the acetabular cup which occurred as a result of loosening (see widened cement–bone interface).

11. How can mechanical loosening be distinguished from infectious loosening clinically and radiographically?

The joint should be aspirated, and fluid sent for gram stain, culture and sensitivity, and cell count. Blood is evaluated for C-reactive protein (CRP) levels and erythroid sedimentation rate (ESR), both commonly elevated with infection. A radionuclide bone scan is sensitive for loosening, but like plain films cannot differentiate between mechanical and infectious loosening. This study should be combined with an inflammation-specific study such as an indium-labeled leukocyte scan or a gallium scan. If the leukocyte scan is normal the findings are compatible with aseptic loosening (i.e., the negative predictive value is high). If the scan is positive, the white cell scan and bone scan are compared for degree of and distribution of activity. Scans are considered "incongruent" if leukocyte activity is greater in degree or at different sites than bone scan uptake; this is specific for infection (Fig. 5). Congruent scans (matching uptake on both scans) are associated with a low incidence of infection.

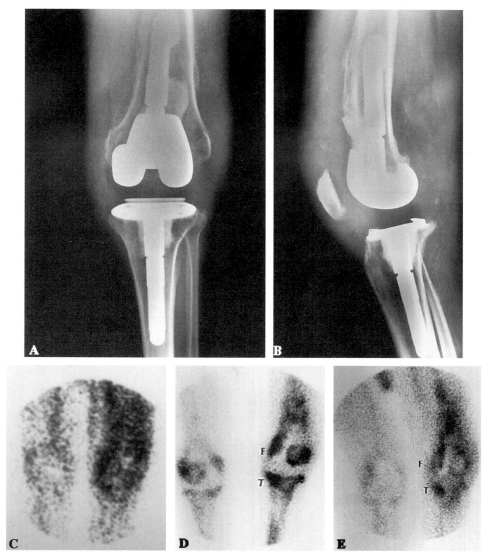

FIGURE 5.   AP (*A*) and lateral (*B*) views of a painful left total knee replacement show soft tissue swelling anterior to the distal femur and associated periosteal elevation, both new findings. Due to the suspicion of infection and the equivocal laboratory studies, a bone scan was done. The first (blood flow) phase (*C*) reveals significant hyperemia to the left knee. The third (delayed) phase of the study (*D*) shows increased uptake at the distal femur (F), proximal tibia (T) and patella. These findings are suspicious for infection but are nonspecific. A radiolabeled leukocyte scan was then performed (*E*); the increased uptake on this scan is greater in degree and different in distribution when compared with (*D*). This "incongruence" is specific for infection, which was in fact present.

12. What is osteolysis?

Also known as aggressive granulomatosis, this is an immune reaction to materials used for joint arthroplasty, resulting in a granulomatous reaction and resultant osteolysis. This can occur in response to cement particles, metal particles, or polyethylene particles (hence the name particle disease). It is manifested on radiographs as focal areas of bone resorption around the prosthesis. This is an indolent process and is normally asymptomatic until complicated by a pathologic fracture or loosening of the prosthesis. This pathologic process is more commonly associated with hip arthroplasty than knee arthroplasty.

BIBLIOGRAPHY

1. Allen AM, Ward WG, Pope TL Jr: Imaging of total knee arthroplasty. Radiol Clin North Am 33:289–304, 1995.
2. Cuckler JM, Star AM, Alavi A, et al: Diagnosis and management of the infected total joint arthroplasty. Orthop Clin North Am 22:523–530, 1991.
3. Griffiths HJ, Priest DR, Kushner D: Total hip replacement and other orthopedic hip procedures. Radiol Clin North Am 33:267–288, 1995.
4. Johnson JA, Christie MJ, Sandler MP, et al: Detection of occult infection following total joint arthroplasty using sequential technetium-99m HDP bone scintigraphy and indium-111 WBC imaging. J Nucl Med 29:1347–1353, 1988.
5. Kantor SG, Schneider R, Insall JN, Becker MW: Radionuclide imaging of asymptomatic versus symptomatic total knee arthroplasties. Clin Orthop 260:118–123, 1990.
6. Merkel KD, Brown ML, Fitzgerald RH Jr: Sequential technetium-99m HDP—gallium-67 citrate for the evaluation of infection in the painful prosthesis. J Nucl Med 27:1413–1417, 1986.
7. Weissman BM: Current topics in the radiology of joint replacement surgery. Radiol Clin North Am 28:1111–1134, 1990.

55. SCOLIOSIS

Kevin R. Math, M.D., and William Kennedy Main, M.D.

1. Define scoliosis.

Scoliosis is a coronal plane deformity of the spine.

2. What is the most common cause of scoliosis?

Scoliosis is idiopathic in about 70% of cases, but idiopathic scoliosis remains a diagnosis of exclusion. While an exhaustive diagnostic work-up is not necessary for all patients, consideration must always be given to the presence of an underlying cause of the spinal curvature.

3. Describe infantile, juvenile, and adolescent idiopathic scoliosis.

Infantile scoliosis occurs before age 4, is more common in boys, and resolves spontaneously in 90% of cases. Juvenile scoliosis is diagnosed between 4 and 10 years of age. Adolescent scoliosis is diagnosed between 10 years of age and skeletal maturity, is the most common type of idiopathic scoliosis, is much more common in females and the spinal curvature is usually convex to the right in the thoracic spine.

4. What is the most common cause of congenital scoliosis?

Vertebral anomalies, which include segmentation anomalies ("block vertebra"), hemivertebrae, and butterfly vertebrae.

5. When a congenital scoliosis is detected, what other organic abnormalities must be sought?

Vertebral anomalies are frequently encountered in association with anomalies of other organ systems in the VACTER (or VATER) syndrome, which includes **V**ertebral anomalies, **A**norectal malformations, **C**ardiac anomalies, **T**racheo**E**sophageal anomalies, and **R**adial and renal anomalies.

6. What disease is associated with a classic short segment, sharply angled severe kyphoscoliosis?

Neurofibromatosis.

7. Name four neuromuscular diseases associated with scoliosis.

Cerebral palsy, muscular dystrophy, myelomeningocele, and polio. Other diseases include a broad category of conditions known as SMA (spinal muscular atrophy), and paralytic scoliosis from spinal cord injury.

8. How can radiographs be used to predict the probability of progression of a scoliotic curve?

Since curve progression generally occurs only during skeletal growth, radiographic assessment of skeletal maturity is an important means of predicting the probability of curve progression. Radiographic estimation of skeletal maturity may involve wrist films for carpal development (skeletal age), pelvic films for apophyseal development, and assessment of vertebral ring apophyseal development.

9. What is the Risser sign and what is its role in the management of scoliosis?

The Risser grading system classifies the extent of ossification of the iliac crest apophyses into quarters. A child with Risser grade 1 (0–25% of apophysis is ossified) can be expected to have substantial potential growth and resultant progression of the curve, while a Risser 4 (75–100% ossified) can be expected to have little if any curve progression. Once the apophysis is completely fused to the iliac crest, skeletal maturity has been attained (Risser 5) and no further progression of scoliosis will occur.

10. What films are taken as part of a standard scoliosis series?

Standing AP and lateral views of the entire spine (long film cassette). AP views with lateral bending to each side can help determine if the curve is flexible. Bending films are generally used only to determine the potential for correction when surgery is being considered.

11. What is the difference between structural and nonstructural curves?

Structural curves are fixed deformities that will not reduce with lateral bending. Nonstructural curves are flexible and can completely reduce with lateral bending. They are usually milder in degree than structural curves.

12. What potential risk should be kept in mind when considering the frequency of obtaining radiographs for follow-up of scoliosis?

The potential risk of development of breast cancer in adolescent girls with scoliosis as a result of repeated x-ray exposure. Breast tissue in this age group is highly radiosensitive—more sensitive than bone marrow. Adequate breast shielding and x-ray beam collimation are warranted in these patients. Furthermore, the frequency of imaging and the number of radiographs should be limited. To minimize the direct radiation exposure of the breast, some advocate performing radiographs in the PA projection rather than AP.

13. What is the Cobb angle?

To monitor the stability or progression of scoliosis, an objective measurement of the curve is necessary. The Cobb angle is the angle between the superior vertebral endplate at the top of the curve (where the angle of inclination toward the concavity of the curve is most acute) and the inferior endplate at the bottom of the curve. Lines are drawn tangent to these endplates, and the angle at their intersection is measured. Unless the angle is very acute, the lines will usually intersect on the viewbox rather than on the film; therefore, it is easier to measure the angle between lines drawn at right angles to the endplate lines (Fig. 1).

14. What are compensatory curves?

Nonstructural scoliotic curves that result from the body's attempt to keep the head centered over the pelvis when scoliosis is present at another level, or when there is leg length discrepancy or pathologic pelvic tilt. They are usually not as severe as the primary curve (Fig. 2). These curves may become structural over time.

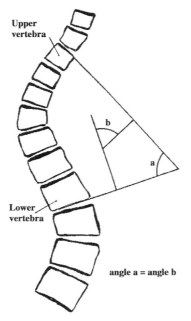

FIGURE 1 *(Right).* Cobb angle measurement.

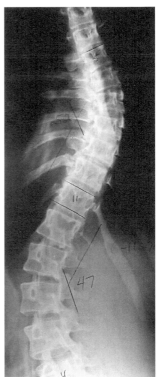

FIGURE 2 *(Far right).*   Idiopathic adolescent scoliosis. There is a primary thoracic dextroscoliosis (convexity to the right side) measuring 52° and a compensatory lumbar levoscoliosis (convexity to the left side) measuring 47°.

15. When a left-sided scoliotic curve is newly appreciated in a 14-year-old boy, what could the diagnosis be?

The possibility of a spinal tumor should always be considered when a new scoliosis is encountered. Idiopathic scoliosis in adolescence is much more common in girls and is much more frequently convex to the right. Therefore, nonidiopathic causes in this adolescent boy must be excluded; MRI is clearly the best imaging modality for excluding secondary causes of scoliosis such as spinal tumor and tethered cord. Syringomyelia is another important cause of a new onset or rapidly progressive scoliosis.

16. When is MRI or other imaging of the spine appropriate in the management of scoliosis?

When there is any reason to suspect that there may be an underlying, treatable cause of the spinal deformity. General indications for MRI include an unusual curve pattern, a clinical history atypical of idiopathic scoliosis, and associated pain or other constitutional symptoms (usually not present in idiopathic scoliosis).

BIBLIOGRAPHY

1. Barnes PD, Brody JD, Jaramillo D, et al: Atypical idiopathic scoliosis: MR imaging evaluation. Radiology 186:247, 1993.
2. Greenspan A: Orthopedic Radiology: A Practical Approach. Philadelphia, Lippincott-Raven, 1993.
3. Schwend RM, Hennrikus W, Hall JE, et al: Childhood scoliosis: Clinical indications for magnetic resonance imaging. Radiology 195:888, 1995.
4. Slone RM, Macmillan M, Montgomery WJ, Heare MM: Spinal fixation part 2: Fixation techniques and hardware for the thoracic and lumbosacral spine. Radiographics 13:521, 1993.
5. Young L: Scoliosis. In Taveras JM (ed): Radiology: Diagnosis, Imaging, Intervention. Philadelphia, J.B. Lippincott, 1989, pp 1–20.

56. LUMBAR SPINE DISEASES

Ralf R. Barckhausen, M.D., and Kevin R. Math, M.D.

1. What are the radiographic signs of degenerative disc disease (DDD)?

DDD is characterized by disc space narrowing, sclerosis of the vertebral body endplates, and osteophyte formation at the vertebral body margins. It may be accompanied by vacuum disc phenomenon (Fig. 1), which is accumulation of nitrogen gas at the affected disc level. On MRI, one can actually see the dehydration of the disc that occurs early in the degenerative process. This dehydration is manifested by low signal in the usually high-signal discs on T2-weighted images (Fig. 2).

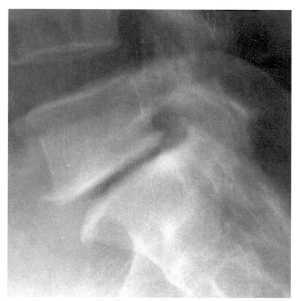

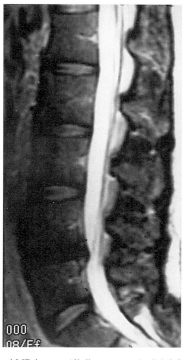

FIGURE 1 *(Above).* Degenerative disc disease (DDD) with vacuum disc phenomenon at the L5–S1 level. Note the anterior and posterior osteophytes at the margins of the vertebral bodies.

FIGURE 2 *(Right).* Disc dehydration and bulge. Sagittal T2-weighted MR image: All discs except the L4–L5 disc are well-hydrated, having the typical "hamburger in a bun" appearance. The L4–L5 disc is dehydrated and bulging, indicating early DDD.

2. What levels of the lumbar spine are most commonly affected by disc pathology?

More than 95% of lumbar disc disease occurs at the L3–L4, L4–L5, and L5–S1 levels.

3. Name the two components of an intervertebral disc.

The nucleus pulposus (centrally) and the anulus fibrosus (peripherally).

4. What is the vacuum disc phenomenon?

Fissures and clefts form within the aging disc; gas released from the surrounding tissues accumulates within these fissures. This gas is composed of 90% nitrogen and results in a linear lucency at the affected level (Fig. 3).

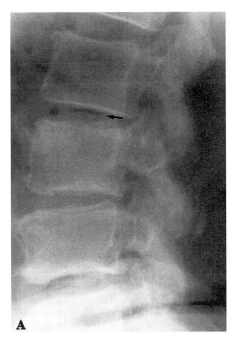

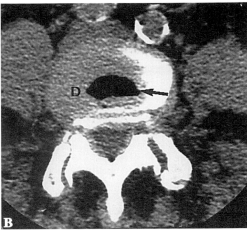

FIGURE 3. Vacuum disc phenomenon. *A*, Lateral view of the lumbar spine showing vacuum disc phenomenon at the L2–L3 level (arrow). *B*, Axial CT image through the disc shows the low (gas) density of the vacuum disc (arrow). The normal disc (D) has soft tissue density.

5. What is a Schmorl's node?

A focal depression in the vertebral endplates caused by intravertebral herniation of the disc. Schmorl's node is a common asymptomatic incidental finding that may affect the superior or inferior endplates, and may be single or multiple (Fig. 4). Conditions that cause weakening of the endplates and subchondral bone have an increased incidence of Schmorl's nodes. Examples include osteoporosis and hyperparathyroidism.

6. What is a limbus vertebra?

A limbus vertebra is a herniation of disc tissue that occurs obliquely at the anterosuperior corner of the vertebral body into the cartilaginous endplate. In the immature skeleton, it results in separation of the corner of the vertebra from the adjacent bone by a linear lucency that persists into adulthood (Fig. 5).

7. Which pediatric spine disease is characterized by multiple limbus vertebrae, Schmorl's nodes, and accentuated kyphosis?

Scheuermann's disease (also called adolescent kyphosis) is marked by weakness in the cartilage growth plate that results in multiple Schmorl's nodes and limbus vertebrae. Anterior wedging of multiple vertebral bodies also occurs, giving rise to the characteristic kyphosis. These findings typically occur in the middle and lower thoracic spine.

8. What is the most common cause of disc calcification?

DDD is the most common cause in adults, whereas the most common cause in children is idiopathic. Other less common causes include ochronosis, hyperparathyroidism, hemochromatosis, acromegaly, juvenile rheumatoid arthritis, ankylosing spondylitis, and spinal fusion.

9. What is a transitional vertebra?

Normally, there are 5 non–rib-bearing lumbar vertebral bodies above the sacrum, easily labeled as L1 through L5. Some individuals have either four or six; those who have four lumbar vertebral bodies are considered to have "sacralization" of the L5 vertebra, whereas those who have six are

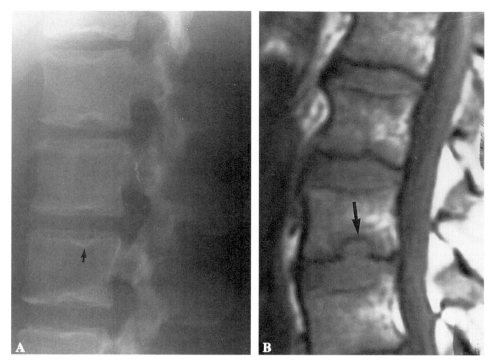

FIGURE 4.   Schmorl's nodes. *A*, Lateral view of the lumbar spine shows Schmorl's nodes at the superior and inferior endplates of all levels (arrow). *B*, Sagittal T1-weighted MR image clearly shows the disc material herniating into the endplate of the vertebra, explaining the appearance on plain films.

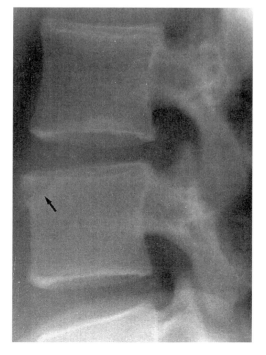

FIGURE 5.   Limbus vertebra. Lateral view of the upper lumbar spine showing the linear lucency at the anterior-superior corner of the vertebral body characteristic of a limbus vertebra.

considered to have "lumbarization" of the S1 vertebra. To avoid the confusing terminology of label-ing the presacral vertebral body L4 or L6, one can simply call this a transitional vertebra and specify the number of non–rib-bearing lumbar vertebral bodies. Recognition of the lowermost lumbar verte-bra as transitional has important implications when lumbar surgery is planned.

10. On a lateral lumbar spine radiograph, the iliac crests overlie what disc level?
L4–L5.

11. Can a transitional vertebra be symptomatic?
Yes. Occasionally, the transitional vertebra has broad transverse processes that may fuse to or articulate with the adjacent sacrum. Rarely, this articulation may result in painful degenerative changes.

12. Can plain films be used to diagnose disc herniation?
No.

13. Then why are plain films routinely ordered for patients with low back pain?
Plain films may reveal the presence of fracture, degenerative disc disease, facet arthrosis, or neoplastic disease, obviating the need for more expensive imaging modalities. In addition, plain film correlaton is often helpful in interpreting MR or CT studies.

14. What is the difference between a disc herniation and disc bulge? Define disc protrusion, extrusion, and sequestration.
A bulging disc is a uniform generalized protrusion of disc material beyond the vertebral body mar-gins and usually occurs concentrically. In a disc herniation, a portion of the gelatinous nucleus pulposus extends through a tear in the anulus fibrosus, resulting in a focal protrusion at the margin of the disc. This focality distinguishes a herniation from a bulge. The herniated disc material usually stays attached to the parent disc (extrusion) or may detach and migrate within the spinal canal (sequestered disc).

15. Why do most discs tend to herniate posteriorly rather than anteriorly?
The nucleus pulposus is eccentrically located closer to the posterior surface of the disc. In addi-tion, the fibers of the anulus fibrosus are thinner and fewer in number posteriorly than anteriorly. Anterior disc herniations are uncommon, and symptomatic anterior herniations are rare.

16. Describe the MR and CT findings of disc herniation.
CT diagnosis of disc herniation is made on thin axial sections through the disc. Normally, the disc should be concave posteriorly with the exception of the L5–S1 disc, which may have a convex posterior margin. A focal protrusion of the soft tissue density disc beyond the margins of the verte-bral endplate is considered a herniation. This usually occurs posteriorly or posterolaterally but some-times occurs laterally. Obliteration of the adjacent epidural fat and compression of the thecal sac are other helpful signs (Fig. 6)
On MR, the protruding disc can be identified both on axial and sagittal images, increasing the sensitivity for detection. The proximity of the herniated disc material to the adjacent nerve roots and thecal sac also can be more accurately determined. Furthermore, disc pathology such as tears of the anulus fibrosus and disc dehydration can be detected on MR but not on CT (Fig. 7).

17. In patients with DDD, what abnormalities of the vertebral endplates are evident on plain films?
Sclerosis of the endplates commonly occurs in DDD. This discogenic sclerosis is sometimes so severe that it is confused with an osteoblastic lesion. On MR, three types of signal alterations in the endplates were described by Modic:
Type 1 (water-like):   decreased T1 signal, increased T2 signal
Type 2 (fat-like):   increased T1 signal, increased T2 signal (Fig. 8)
Type 3 (calcium-like):   decreased T1 signal, decreased T2 signal

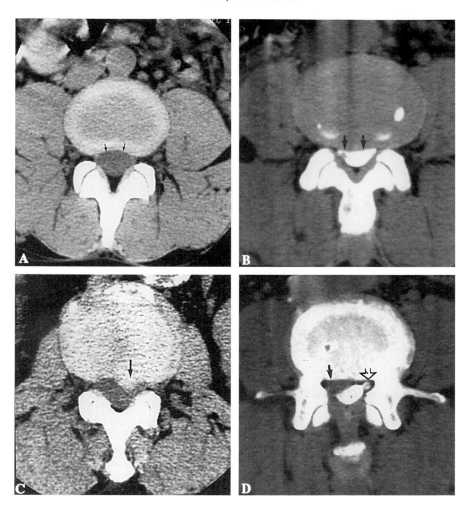

FIGURE 6. *A*, Normal disc. Note the concave posterior margin of the disc (arrows). *B*, Bulging disc. Image from a CT-myelogram showing the broad-based margin of the bulging disc (arrows) pushing on the anterior thecal sac. *C*, Left posterior disc herniation (arrow). *D*, Right posterior disc herniation. The abnormal soft tissue from the herniated disc is seen in the right lateral recess on this CT-myelogram (arrow). Note the normally opacified nerve root sheath on the contralateral side (open arrow).

18. Which nerve roots exit through the L3–L4 neural foramina?

The L3 roots exit under the pedicles of the L3 vertebral body.

19. A right posterior disc herniation at the L4–L5 level may compress which nerve root?

Right L5. The L4 root has already exited through the L4–L5 foramen under the L4 pedicle but above the level of the L4–L5 disc. Thus, the herniation compresses the L5 root, which is still descending in the spinal canal. If the herniation is large enough, the sacral roots may also be compressed. If the herniation at the L4–L5 level is a lateral herniation, the L4 root that has just exited is compressed (Fig. 9).

20. Will the herniated disc material remain indefinitely unless surgically removed?

No. The majority of herniated discs resorb or shrink over time. Most patients with disc herniations can expect gradual improvement in symptoms with conservative treatment. Individuals refractory to conservative treatment may require surgical discectomy.

FIGURE 7. *A (right)*, Herniated discs L4–L5 and L5–S1; the L4–L5 herniation is the larger of the two. There is posterior displacement of the low signal posterior longitudinal ligament (arrow). *B (far right)* and *C (below left)*, Large herniated disc at L4–L5; the gelatinous material from the nucleus pulposus becomes extruded from the disc resulting in root compression and spinal stenosis. On the axial image (c) the disc material can be seen occupying the left lateral recess.

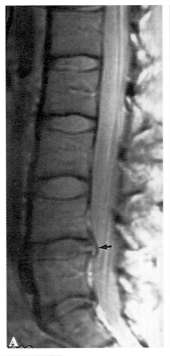
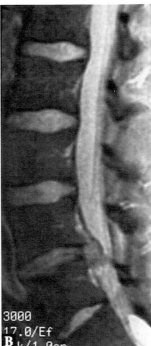

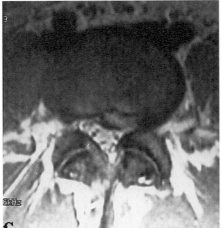

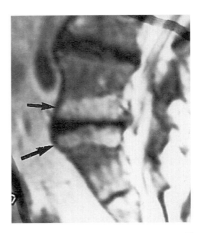

FIGURE 8. Modic type 2 endplate changes. Note the hyperintense (bright) T1 signal at the L5 and S1 endplates, seen in association with degenerative disc disease.

21. What is a myelogram?

Myelography is an invasive method of evaluating the contents of the spinal canal and discs through injection of an opaque contrast medium into the subarachnoid space. This process outlines the spinal cord nerve roots and confines of the spinal canal. Myelography is routinely combined with CT for more thorough evaluation. It is currently reserved as a secondary imaging modality to clarify equivocal findings on MRI and for surgical planning. Headache is the most common complication of myelography (Fig. 10).

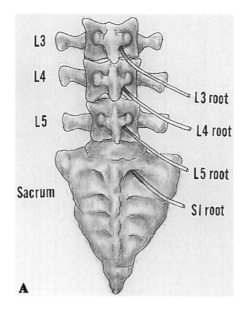

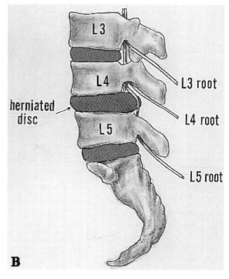

FIGURE 9. These AP (*A*) and lateral (*B*) drawings show the course of the nerve roots as they descend in the spinal canal and exit into the neural foramina under their respective pedicle. The root typically exits above the level of the disc, explaining why a posterior disc herniation affects the root at the level below, while the less common "far lateral" herniation will affect the root at the same level.

22. What is a discogram?

Under fluoroscopic or CT guidance, a contrast agent is injected into a suspected symptomatic disc to attempt to reproduce the patient's symptoms exactly. This provocative test is particularly useful for patients who have several potentially symptomatic abnormal discs or a single abnormal disc of doubtful significance. A discogram is rarely indicated and its use is controversial. Furthermore, the results of the test are somewhat subjective and can be difficult to interpret (i.e., limited specificity).

23. At what level is the conus medullaris (spinal cord termination)?

Usually at L1–L2. The lumbar and sacral roots continue caudally in the spinal canal as the cauda equina.

24. What is the most common cause of lumbar spinal stenosis?

Spinal stenosis is most commonly degenerative, caused by a combination of a posteriorly bulging disc and hypertrophic changes of the facets and ligamentum flavum. The degenerated bulging disc compresses the thecal sac anteriorly, and the hypertrophic bony changes associated with degenerative disease of the facet joints narrows the spinal canal posteriorly and laterally, resulting in a trefoil configuration of the spinal canal (Fig. 11). Vertebral osteophytes and thickening of the ligamentum

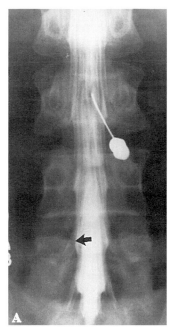 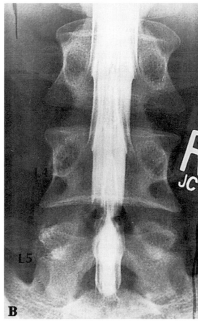

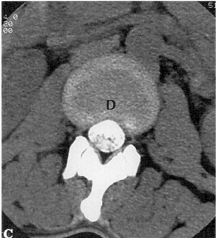

FIGURE 10. *A (Above left)*, Lumbar myelogram. Lumbar puncture was performed at the L2–L3 level (see spinal needle). The nerve roots of the cauda equina appear as longitudinal strand-like filling defects outlined by the contrast material. The right L5 root can be seen exiting (arrow). *B (Above right)*, Spinal stenosis. Note the constriction of the spinal canal at the L4–L5 level. There is lack of visualization of the exiting L5 and S1 roots, indicating nerve root compression. *C (Right)*, Normal CT-myelogram. Note the normal intervertebral disc (D) having a concave posterior margin. The nerve roots in the spinal canal are outlined by contrast, appearing as multiple small dots (filling defects).

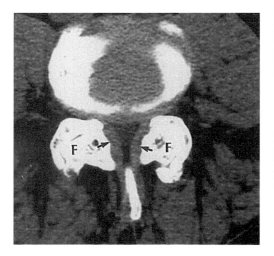

FIGURE 11 *(Left)*. Spinal stenosis. The combination of facet hypertrophy (F), ligamentum flavum buckling and hypertrophy (arrows) and a posteriorly bulging disc result in significant degenerative spinal stenosis.

flavum also contribute to degenerative spinal stenosis. Other acquired causes of spinal stenosis include spondylolisthesis, postoperative epidural fibrosis, trauma, and Paget's disease. Congenital spinal stenosis, which is marked by congenitally short pedicles, occurs in achondroplastic dwarfs but is more often idiopathic. Often, mild degrees of congenital stenosis do not manifest themselves until there is a superimposed disc bulge or facet arthrosis.

25. What are the symptoms of spinal stenosis?

Low back pain commonly accompanied by bilateral lower extremity sciatica or claudication. The pain is typically worse when walking, standing, or hyperextending the lumbar spine and is relieved by lying down, sitting, and flexion of the spine.

26. What type of dwarfism is characterized by lumbar spinal stenosis and a small foramen magnum?

Achondroplasia.

27. What is spondylolisthesis?

Spondylolisthesis is defined as subluxation of one vertebral body on another and most commonly occurs in the lumbar spine region. The degree of spondylolisthesis is based on the percentage of the vertebral body that is displaced: grade 1:0–25%, grade 2, 25–50%, grade 3, 50–75%, and grade 4, 75–100%. Posterior subluxation of a vertebral body on the body beneath is termed retrolisthesis.

28. What are the two main causes of spondylolisthesis?

Degenerative joint disease of the facet joints result in abnormal alignment and motion at these joints and may lead to degenerative spondylolisthesis, the most common cause. The second most common cause of spondylolisthesis is fracture of the posterior elements of the vertebra. In spondylolysis, this occurs through the pars interarticularis (spondylolytic spondylolisthesis) (Fig. 12).

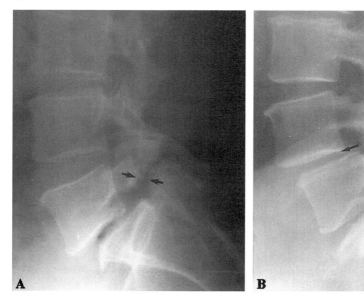

FIGURE 12. *A*, Spondylolisthesis secondary to L5 spondylolysis. The linear lucent pars interarticularis defect is well visualized on this lateral view (arrows). *B*, Spondylolisthesis secondary to degenerative disease of the facet joints. There is sclerosis of the L4–L5 facet joints with degenerative changes, resulting in mild (grade 1) spondylolisthesis (arrows).

29. What is the Scotty dog?

The Scotty dog refers to the resemblance of the vertebra and its processes on an oblique radiograph of the lumbar spine to the shape of a dog. The pars interarticularis is located at the site of the neck of the dog. This is an important reference point in evaluating the spine for spondylolysis, which is a fracture through the pars. Spondylolysis results in a lucent band traversing the neck of the Scotty dog (Fig. 13).

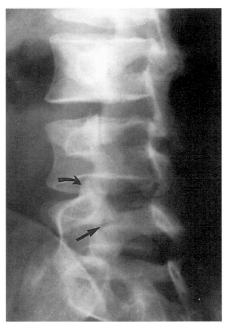

FIGURE 13. Scotty dog spondylolysis. This right posterior oblique radiograph of the lumbar spine demonstrates the linear lucent "collar" at the neck of the scotty dog (straight arrow). The ear of the dog (curved arrow) is the superior articular facet, the foot is the inferior facet, and the head is the right vertebral pedicle.

30. A lateral radiograph of the lumbar spine reveals grade 2 spondylolisthesis at the L4–L5 level. Can this single film determine whether this is due to spondylolysis or degenerative spondylolisthesis?

Close inspection of the alignment of the posterior tips of the spinous processes usually answers this question. In degenerative spondylolisthesis the spinous process of L4 moves anteriorly with the vertebra, whereas in spondylolysis everything posterior to the pars defect (including the spinous process) moves posteriorly. For this reason, patients with degenerative listhesis commonly have spinal stenosis, whereas those with spondylolysis will not (Fig. 14).

31. What is the most common level for spondylolysis in the lumbar spine?

Most common, L5; second most common, L4. Spondylolysis rarely occurs in the cervical spine, where it is most common at the C6 level.

32. Is spondylolysis congenital or acquired?

Most agree that spondylolysis, once thought to be congenital, is a chronic posttraumatic acquired abnormality.

33. What percentage of individuals with spondylolysis have associated spondylolisthesis?

60%.

34. Are the facet joints synovial joints?

Yes. Facet joints are subject to the same degenerative changes present at other synovial joints (sclerosis, subchondral cysts, osteophytes, and joint space narrowing).

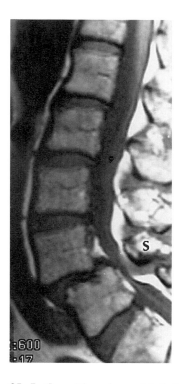

FIGURE 14. Degenerative spondylolisthesis at L4–L5 with spinal stenosis. On this sagittal T1-weighted MR image, L4 has moved anteriorly on L5, and there is associated degenerative disc disease at this level. Note that the L4 spinous process (S) has moved anteriorly as well, and there is secondary spinal stenosis, findings typical of degenerative spondylolisthesis.

35. In the setting of spondylolisthesis, what is the utility of flexion and extension lateral views?

Flexion and extension lateral views assess dynamic instability. In the normal stable spine, the posterior vertebral body margins maintain normal alignment in flexion and extension. Dynamic instability typically shows an increase in the degree of subluxation and widening of the posterior disc space or facet joints with flexion of the spine. Patients with instability are more likely to benefit from surgical posterior fusion of the spine.

36. What is the most common lumbar spine surgery for disc herniation and spinal stenosis?

For disc herniation, a portion of the lamina is removed to gain access to the spinal canal (laminectomy) and the offending disc fragment is removed (discectomy). For spinal stenosis, bilateral laminectomy is performed with or without facetectomies.

37. What is failed back syndrome? What is its incidence?

Failed back syndrome is recurrent or residual low back pain after lumbar disc surgery. The average incidence is approximately 15%.

38. List the most common causes of the failed back syndrome.

Immediate postoperative complications (infection, hematoma, cerebrospinal fluid leak, nerve root trauma)

Arachnoiditis	Residual osteophytes, disc material, or root compression
Epidural fibrosis	Recurrent disc herniation
Mechanical instability	Surgery at the wrong level

39. Which imaging modality is most useful in patients with failed back syndrome?

MRI (with and without intravenous contrast). Intravenous contrast helps to differentiate between scarring and residual or recurrent disc material, the two most common causes of failed back syndrome. These entities look identical on the precontrast study. After intravenous contrast, scar tissue and epidural fibrosis typically enhance, whereas a disc fragment usually does not (although there are exceptions). Differentiation of fibrosis from recurrent disc herniation has important prognostic and treatment implications. Recurrent disc herniations can be successfully treated surgically with good results, whereas postoperative epidural fibrosis has a poor prognosis and may be exacerbated by repeat surgery.

40. What is arachnoiditis? Describe its imaging features.

Arachnoiditis is inflammation of the meningeal layers of the spine. It is an ominous complication of lumbar spine surgery, characterized by persistent low back and leg pain with bilateral motor, sensory, or reflex deficits frequently present at multiple levels. MR and CT-myelogram findings include clumping of the nerve roots of the cauda equina and adherence of the nerve roots to the periphery of the thecal sac (empty sac sign).

41. What is the inverted Napoleon's hat sign?

This sign refers to the appearance of the L5 vertebra on an anteroposterior radiograph in the presence of severe (grade 4) spondylolisthesis. The anterior aspect of the subluxed L5 vertebral body points inferiorly, comprising the dome of the hat, whereas the lateral masses and transverse processes form its brim (Fig. 15).

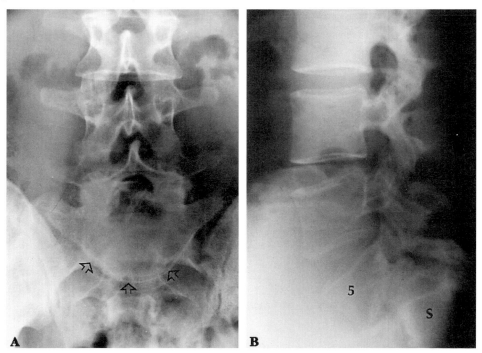

FIGURE 15. Inverted Napoleon's hat sign. *A*, The anterior aspect of the subluxed L5 vertebral body projects inferiorly (open arrows), forming the dome of the hat. *B*, The L5 vertebral body (5) is subluxed significantly anteriorly relative to the sacrum (S), accounting for its hat-like configuration on the AP view.

42. What is DISH?

DISH is an acronym for diffuse idiopathic skeletal hyperostosis (Forrestier's disease). It may be thought of as an ossifying diathesis, with bone forming in the paraspinal regions and at tendon and ligament attachment sites (entheses) of the pelvis and extremities. The classic finding in the spine is flowing ossification along the anterior aspect of at least four contiguous vertebral bodies. Unlike degenerative disc disease, the ossification is separate from the vertebrae (i.e., paravertebral) and the intervening disc spaces are maintained. Other findings include ligament ossification and osteophyte formation throughout the spine, pelvis, and extremities. DISH is more common in men and is typically seen in older patients. The disease is commonly symptomatic, presenting with vague symptoms of low back pain or stiffness and occasional joint pain.

43. What is a conjoined nerve root?

Conjoined nerve roots are congenital anomalies in which two nerve roots emerge from a single dural sheath. The L5 and S1 roots are most commonly affected. Conjoined roots may be mistaken for disc herniations on CT, having the appearance of soft tissue in the anterior spinal canal or neural foramen.

CONTROVERSY

44. A patient with low back pain and right lower extremity sciatica for 2 years visits your office. Which test should you order, CT or MRI?

Although most physicians are likely to choose MRI, some lumbar spine diseases can be diagnosed as effectively (and some more effectively) on CT. Listed below are suspected clinical diagnoses and the best imaging modality for their evaluation.

Disc herniation: Most agree that MRI is better than CT in evaluating suspected disc pathology. Subtle herniations, anular tears, and disc dehydration are seen to better advantage on MR. However, CT is considered highly sensitive for diagnosis of symptomatic disc herniation and may be a reasonable cost-effective alternative or an option in claustrophobic patients.

Spinal stenosis: MR and CT are equivalent in evaluating the size of the spinal canal as well as the anatomic basis for spinal stenosis.

Spondylolysis: CT is more sensitive than MR for diagnosis of spondylolysis (Fig. 16). Most pars defects can be seen on plain films; however, when further imaging is required, this bony abnormality is more effectively diagnosed on CT than MR. Nuclear bone scan with single photon emission CT (SPECT) is an alternative modality in children.

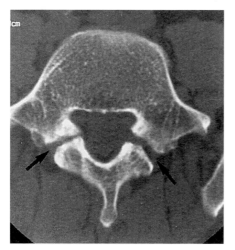

FIGURE 16. Spondylolysis—CT scan. This image, obtained at the level of the mid-vertebral body, shows bilateral lucent defects of the pars interarticularis. Normally at this level a complete bony ring surrounds the spinal canal.

Metastasis: MRI is superior to CT in diagnosing marrow-replacing abnormalities such as neoplasm. Of importance, MR does not replace the radionuclide bone scan in diagnosing the presence and extent of bone metastasis.

BIBLIOGRAPHY

1. Greenspan A: Orthopedic Radiology: A Practical Approach, 2nd ed. Philadelphia, Lippincott-Raven, 1993.
2. Grossman RI, Yousem DM: Neuroradiology: The Requisites. St. Louis, Mosby, 1994.

3. Haughton VM, Eldevik OP, Magnaes B, et al: A prospective comparison of computed tomography and myelography in the diagnosis of herniated lumbar disks. Radiology 137:433–437, 1980.
4. Kricun R, Kricun M: MRI and CT of the Spine. New York, Raven Press, 1994.
5. Modic MT, Masory KT, Boumphrey F, et al: Lumbar herniated disc disease and canal stenosis: Prospective evaluation by MR, CT, and myelography. AJR 147:757–765, 1986.
6. Modic MT, Masaryk TJ, Ross JS: Magnetic Resonance Imaging of the Spine, 2nd ed. Philadelphia, Mosby, 1994.
7. Ross J, Masory KT, Schrader M, et al: Lumbar spine: Postoperative MR imaging with gadopentetate dimeglumine. AJR 155:867–872, 1990.
8. Teplick G: Lumbar spine CT and MRI. Philadelphia, J.B. Lippincott, 1992.
9. Thornbury JR, Fryback DG, Tursk PA, et al: Disc caused nerve compression in patients with acute low back pain: Diagnosis with MR, CT-myelography and plain CT. Radiology 186:731–738, 1993.

57. CERVICAL SPINE IMAGING

Edward Math, M.D., and Kevin R. Math, M.D.

1. Which radiographs are included in a standard cervical spine series?

The standard examination includes anteroposterior (AP), lateral, and open-mouth odontoid views. Bilateral oblique radiographs may be added for visualization of the neural foramina and facet joints.

2. What is a swimmer's view?

A swimmer's view is used when the lower cervical vertebrae, usually C7, cannot be seen on other views, usually because of the patient's inability to cooperate or a large shoulder girdle that obscures visualization of the spine. With the patient in the supine position, the arm is raised over the head, as if taking a freestyle swimming stroke, and the x-ray beam is directed obliquely cephalad through the axilla (Fig. 1).

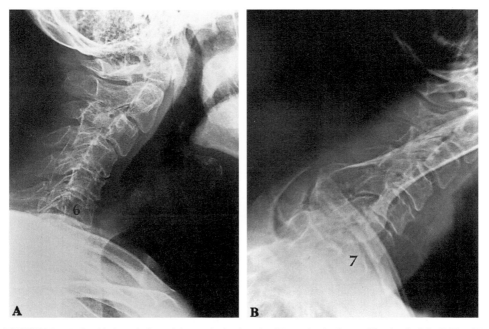

FIGURE 1. *A*, On this lateral view of the cervical spine, the C7 vertebra is obscured by the clavicle. *B*, The C7 vertebra is readily visualized on this swimmer's view.

3. If C7 cannot be visualized on the swimmer's view, can the study be terminated and regarded as a "limited" study?

No. In the setting of trauma, C7 must always be evaluated. If C7 is not seen on the swimmer's or oblique radiographs, a CT scan through this level is necessary.

4. How can the T1 vertebra be readily identified on an AP view of the spine?

Almost always the cervical vertebrae can be counted through C7, and the next vertebra with well-developed ribs is T1. However, the first vertebra with associated ribs is not always T1; in the setting of cervical ribs, it would be C7. Cervical ribs are present in about 0.5% of the population and are often bilateral. The length of cervical ribs is variable; longer cervical ribs may be associated with thoracic outlet syndrome. Knowledge of the fact that the T1 transverse processes point obliquely upward avoids mistaking cervical ribs for T1 ribs.

5. How many cervical nerve roots are there?

There are 8 pairs of cervical roots.

6. Which root exits through the right C5–C6 intervertebral foramen? The left C7–T1 foramen?

The C6 roots exit through the C5–C6 neural foramina. The C8 roots exit through the C7–T1 foramina. In the cervical spine, the exiting nerve root is one more than the superior component of the neural foramen (Fig. 2), whereas in the thoracic and lumbar spine the exiting root is the same number as the superior component of the foramen. For example, the nerve root exiting at the L2–L3 level (under the L2) pedicle is the L2 root, whereas the exiting root at the C2–C3 foramen is the C3 root.

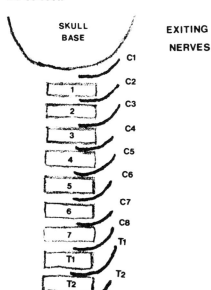

FIGURE 2. This schematic illustration shows which nerve root exits at each specific level. This anatomy is important when attempting to correlate clinical signs and symptoms with imaging findings.

7. Why are the cervical neural foramina best visualized on an oblique radiograph, whereas the lumbar foramina are best seen on a lateral view?

The cervical foramina are angled approximately 45° anteriorly, whereas the lumbar foramina are oriented at 90°. Therefore, when the head is turned to the left for an oblique radiograph, the right-sided foramina are brought into profile and vice versa for the left-sided foramina (Fig. 3).

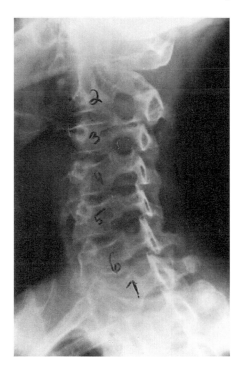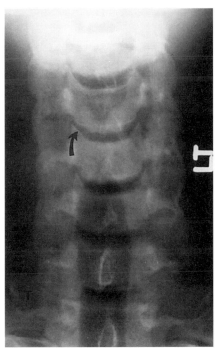

FIGURE 3 (Left). The head is turned to the right (left anterior oblique position), allowing visualization of the left-sided foramina. The foramina to the left side of the vertebral bodies will always be the left neural foramina, and vice versa.

FIGURE 4 (Right). Joints of Luschka. The curved arrow points to the uncinate process of the C5 vertebral body, articulating with the inferior C4 vertebra at the uncovertebral joint (Luschka). Note the upwardly sloping transverse process of the T1 vertebra. This consistent appearance allows one to reliably number the cervical vertebra on an AP radiograph. It is also helpful when assessing for the presence of cervical ribs.

8. Where are the joints of Luschka?

The joints of Luschka, also known as the uncovertebral joints, are the articulations of the uncinate processes (arising from the superolateral aspect of the cervical vertebral bodies) and the inferolateral aspect of the superior vertebral bodies (Fig. 4). These joints are present only at the C3 through C7 levels. Osteophytes arising from the joints of Luschka frequently give rise to neural foraminal narrowing.

9. What is the significance of prevertebral soft tissue swelling on the lateral C-spine radiographs?

Prevertebral soft tissue thickness at the upper cervical spine is usually no more than 7 mm (measured at C2). These tissues are much thicker at the mid and lower cervical spine; at C6 the thickness should be less than 22 mm in adults and less than 14 mm in children. Furthermore, prevertebral soft tissue thickness should not exceed 50% of the anteroposterior diameter of the vertebral body at the same level. Prevertebral soft tissue swelling is a secondary sign of bony or ligamentous injury to the anterior elements of the vertebrae.

10. What is the anterior atlantoaxial interval? What is its normal measurement?

The atlantoaxial interval is the space between the posterior aspect of the anterior arch of C1 and the anterior aspect of the dens. This space should not exceed 3 mm in adults or 5 mm in children and should not vary with flexion and extension. Widening of this space is termed atlantoaxial subluxation and implies laxity or disruption of the transverse ligament of the dens.

11. List the causes of atlantoaxial subluxation.

Trauma (often associated with an odontoid fracture)
Rheumatoid arthritis
Ankylosing spondylitis
Psoriatic arthritis
Retropharyngeal abscess or inflammation
Down's syndrome
Morquio's syndrome

12. Why is atlantoaxial subluxation dangerous? How is it treated?

Atlantoaxial subluxation results in narrowing of the spinal canal and may give rise to cord compression and long tract signs (bowel and bladder incontinence, lower extremity weakness). An anterior atlantoaxial interval of 8 mm or greater is usually regarded as a relative indication for posterior cervical fusion.

13. A patient with rheumatoid arthritis presents with long tract signs and suspected atlantoaxial instability but has a normal lateral radiograph. Which views demonstrate the subluxation with greater sensitivity?

Lateral flexion and extension views. With gentle flexion the widening of the atlantoaxial interval may be elicited (Fig. 5). Long tract signs in a rheumatoid patient also may be caused by subluxation at other levels, which also is detected on the lateral flexion view. Furthermore, a seemingly normally aligned cervical spine may have significant spinal cord compression by pannus at the C1–C2 level; MRI is indicated for evaluation of patients with suspected cord compression, because it readily demonstrates the level, degree, and cause of the compression.

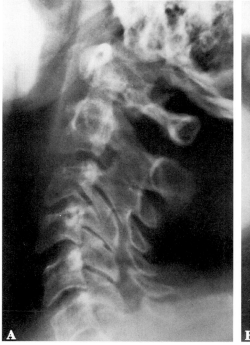 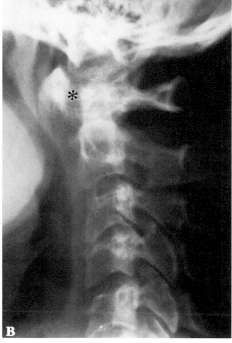

FIGURE 5.   Atlanto-axial subluxation. *A*, Atlanto-axial alignment is normal with the cervical spine extended. *B*, This flexion view of the cervical spine elicits the widening of the atlanto-axial space (*) present in this patient with rheumatoid arthritis.

14. Which lines should be assessed on a lateral cervical spine radiograph to check for normal alignment?

A line drawn longitudinally through the posterior margin of the vertebral body should be gently curved and continuous. The second important line, the spinolaminar line, is drawn longitudinally through the sclerotic line at the junction of spinous process with the lamina (Fig. 6).

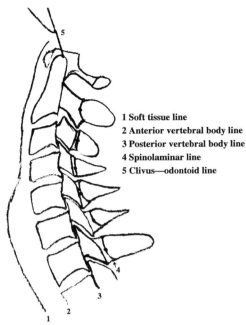

1 Soft tissue line
2 Anterior vertebral body line
3 Posterior vertebral body line
4 Spinolaminar line
5 Clivus—odontoid line

FIGURE 6. Cervical spine alignment. The posterior vertebral line and spino-laminar line are the most important when checking for cervical malalignment. These represent the bony anterior and posterior limits of the spinal canal.

15. On a lateral C-spine radiograph, what are the anterior and posterior limits of the spinal canal?

The anterior and posterior margins of the spinal canal are formed by the posterior vertebral bodies and the spinolaminar line, respectively.

16. What is Chamberlain's line? McGregor's line? McRae's line?

Before the advent of MRI, the position of the dens relative to the foramen magnum was assessed on lateral radiographs by drawing various lines. A high position of the dens may be associated with spinal cord compression (Fig. 7).

Chamberlain's line: line between the posterior aspect of the hard palate and the posterior margin of the foramen magnum. The tip of the dens should be no more than 5 mm above and is usually at or below this line.

McGregor's line: line from the posterior hard palate to the lowest point on the occiput. Tip of the dens should be no greater than 7 mm above this line.

McRae's line: line from the anterior margin of the foramen magnum to its posterior margin. The tip of the dens should never be above this line.

17. What is the os odontoideum?

Separation of the dens from the body of C2. The dens assumes the appearance of a well-circumscribed ossicle with a thin cortical margin and a lucent area that separates it from the adjacent dens. This appearance led to the belief that it is a congenital anomaly. Most authorities now agree that it is more likely an acquired posttraumatic abnormality. It can be differentiated from an acute odontoid fracture by the presence of cortical margins, smaller size of the ossicle than the normal dens, and occasional hypertrophy of the anterior arch of C1. Os odontoideum may be associated with atlantoaxial instability and has an increased frequency in Down's syndrome.

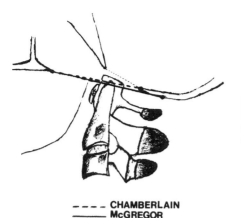

FIGURE 7.   Prior to MRI, the orientation of the atlas to the base of the skull and foramen magnum was routinely assessed by drawing these lines on conventional radiographs.

- - - - **CHAMBERLAIN**
———— **McGREGOR**
············· **McRAE**

18. What is pseudosubluxation? How can it be differentiated from true subluxation?

Anterior pseudosubluxation of C2 on C3 or C3 on C4 is a normal finding on the lateral C-spine of children under 8 years. It is caused by relative laxity of the ligaments combined with shallow facet joints. To distinguish it from true subluxation, one must draw a line from the spinolaminar line of C1 to the spinolaminar line of C3. This is the posterior cervical line (Fig. 8). The spinolaminar line of C2 should not be offset by more than 1 mm.

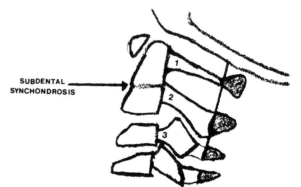

SUBDENTAL
SYNCHONDROSIS

FIGURE 8.   The posterior cervical line permits differentiation of pseudosubluxation from true cervical spine subluxation.

POSTERIOR CERVICAL LINE

19. How can congenital cervical canal stenosis be diagnosed on conventional radiographs?

Canal stenosis is most accurately assessed on CT or MRI. However, on a lateral conventional radiograph, stenosis can be inferred if the anteroposterior dimensions of the canal measure < 16 mm at C1–C2 or < 13 mm at C3 through C7. Furthermore, on a true lateral view, stenosis is usually present if no lamina is visible between the facets and the spinolaminar line.

20. Describe the radiographic findings of degenerative disc disease (DDD). What is meant by cervical spondylosis?

DDD is manifested by disc space narrowing and osteophytes extending from the vertebral body margins, often accompanied by sclerosis of the vertebral body end plates (Fig. 9). Nitrogen gas may eventually accumulate within the degenerated disc (vacuum disc phenomenon). Spondylosis refers to the formation of osteophytes at the site of attachment of the anulus fibrosus. The osteophytes typically form on either side of a bulging disc and are a classic sign of DDD.

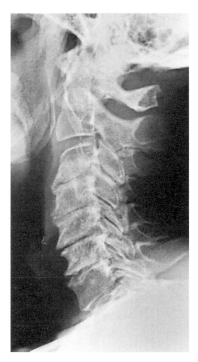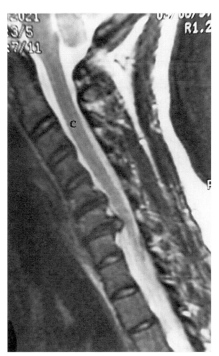

FIGURE 9 *(Left).* Severe degenerative disc disease (DDD). There is marked disc space narrowing with anterior and posterior osteophytes (spondylosis) at the C3–C4 through C7–T1 levels.

FIGURE 10 *(Right).* Cervical disc herniation—MRI. This sagittal T2-weighted image reveals a large disc herniation at the C6–C7 level and a bulging degenerated disc at the C5–C6 level. This patient also had compression of the spinal cord (c). (Courtesy of Dr. Daniel Lefton.)

21. What is the difference between a bulging disc and a herniated disc?

A bulging disc is a **broad-based** extension of anular fibers past the margins of the vertebral body; the nucleus pulposus remains intact. A herniated disc is a **focal** protrusion of the nucleus pulposus through torn fibers of the anulus fibrosus. This gelatinous material may remain attached to the parent disc or may separate from the disc and migrate as a free fragment in the spinal canal. The focality of the protruding disc distinguishes a herniation from a broad-based bulge.

22. What is the most common cervical level affected by DDD? The second most common level?

C5–C6 is the most common level, followed by C6–C7, then by C4–C5. The greatest degree of motion occurs at these levels with flexion and extension.

23. What imaging modality is most effective for evaluation of cervical disc pathology?

MRI is clearly the most useful modality. Discs, canal, foramina, spinal cord, and bone marrow can be accurately assessed (Fig. 10). Occasionally, it may be difficult to differentiate an osteophyte from a protruding disc at the level of the endplate on MRI.

24. If MRI is the imaging study of choice, what role does CT play?

CT is superior to MR in assessing calcifications or bone fragments and is therefore more useful for trauma than for DDD. Vertebral fractures are adequately assessed with CT, and newer technology allows visualization of the fracture in virtually any plane (two- and three-dimensional reconstructions). However, the contents of the spinal canal and the ligamentous structures are much better evaluated on MR. In patients with DDD, CT is primarily useful for differentiating a vertebral osteophyte from a protruding disc; this distinction is occasionally difficult on MR.

25. What is cervical CT-myelography? When is it appropriate?

Since the advent of MRI, CT-myelography has assumed a supplemental role in assessing patients with disc pathology or suspected cord compression. This procedure is reserved for clarification of equivocal findings on MRI or for preoperative patients in whom further information is required by the surgeon. Iodinated contrast is instilled into the subarachnoid space (thecal sac) to provide visualization of the contents and borders of the spinal canal. This can be done either via direct lateral cervical puncture at the C2 level (under fluoroscopic guidance) or by lumbar puncture and tilting the patient into the diving position. The latter technique is much more commonly used to avoid vital structures and potential complications at the upper cervical level. A CT scan is subsequently performed.

26. Which study should be done for suspected cord compression?

MRI evaluates the entire canal and cord in less than 1 hour and is noninvasive. If MRI is contraindicated or unavailable, myelography is necessary. The myelographic sign of cord compression is blockage of cephalad flow of contrast from the lumbar canal to the cervical canal when the prone patient is tilted to the reverse Trendelenburg position. The level of epidural block defines the level of the cord compression.

27. Can patients leave the hospital immediately after the myelogram? Is any preparation necessary?

After myelography, patients must be observed for at least 4–6 hours for complications. The head of the bed is elevated to avoid contrast flow to the cerebral subarachnoid spaces and its associated headache. Complications include headache, dizziness, nausea and vomiting, and seizures. Medications such as tricyclic antidepressants and phenothiazines lower the seizure threshold and should be withheld for 1 or 2 days before and after the procedure.

28. Which operation is most commonly performed for cervical disc disease that is refractory to conservative treatment?

Anterior discectomy with anterior cervical fusion. The offending disc material is resected, along with any associated bony ridges, and a piece of fusion bone (usually from iliac crest or fibula) is placed at the disc space.

29. What is the most common delayed complication of anterior cervical fusion?

Disc disease (herniation, bulge) above or below the level of the fusion may result from increased motion demands and resultant stress at these levels.

30. Which patient population is most prone to ossification of the posterior longitudinal ligament (OPLL)? What are the potential complications of OPLL?

OPLL is much more prevalent in the Japanese. The ossification occurs most commonly in the mid-cervical spine in the sixth or seventh decade of life and may result in spinal canal stenosis with root or cord compression.

BIBLIOGRAPHY

1. Atlas SW: Magnetic Resonance Imaging of the Brain and Spine, 2nd ed. Philadelphia, Lippincott-Raven, 1995.
2. Greenspan A: Imaging of the Spine. St. Louis, Mosby, 1993.
3. Harris JH Jr, Mirvis SE: The Radiology of Acute Cervical Spine Trauma, 3rd ed. Baltimore, Williams & Wilkins, 1996.
4. Kirlew KA, Hathout GM, Reiter SD, et al: Os odontoideum in identical twins: Perspectives on etiology. Skeletal Radiol 22:525, 1993.
5. Runge V, Awh MH, Bittner DF, Kirsch JE: Magnetic Resonance Imaging of the Spine. Philadelphia, Lippincott-Raven, 1995.
6. Smoker WRK: Craniovertebral junction: Normal anatomy, craniotomy, and congenital anomalies. Radiographics 14:255, 1994.
7. Swischuk LE: Emergency Imaging of the Acutely Ill or Injured Child, 3rd ed. Baltimore, Williams & Wilkins, 1994.
8. Wiener JI: MR imaging for the diagnosis of disk-caused nerve compression. Radiology 189:287, 1993.

58. OCCUPATIONAL INJURIES

Kevin R. Math, M.D.

Various occupations and activities are subject to unique injuries. Match the occupation (A–N) with the figure showing the imaging findings that may result.

A. Carpet layer
B. Scuba diver
C. Housemaid
D. Hurdler
E. Baseball player (child)

F. Tailor
G. Skier
H. Golfer
I. Gigolo
J. Ballet dancer

K. Pregnant woman
L. Soldier
M. Radium dial painter
N. Adult baseball player

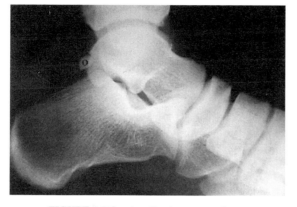

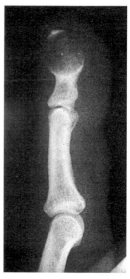

FIGURE 1 *(Above).*   Os trigonum syndome.

FIGURE 2 *(Above right).*
Epidermoid inclusion cyst.

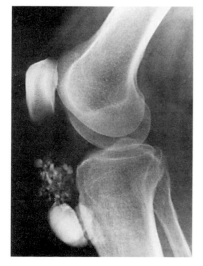

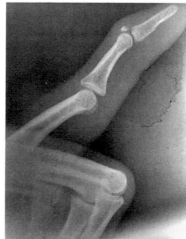

FIGURE 3 *(Above).*   Calcific intrapatellar bursitis.

FIGURE 4 *(Right).*   Mallet finger.

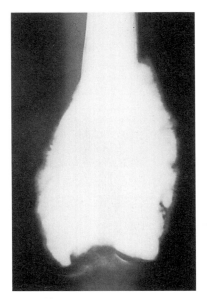

FIGURE 5. Osteosarcoma.

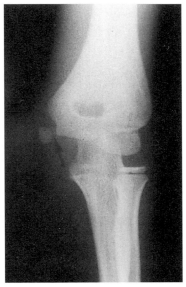

FIGURE 6. Avulsion fracture, medial humeral epicondyle

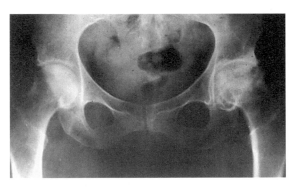

FIGURE 7. Osteonecrosis femoral head.

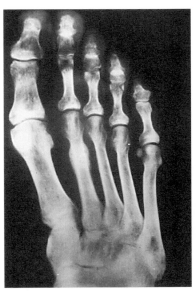

FIGURE 8. Stress fracture.

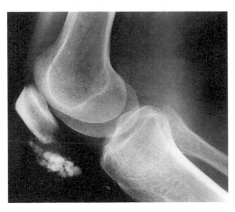

FIGURE 9. Calcific prepatellar bursitis.

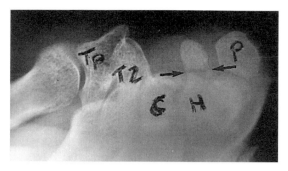

FIGURE 10.   Hamate fracture.

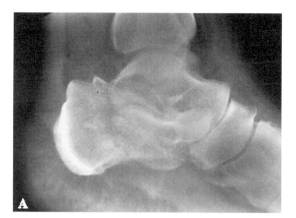

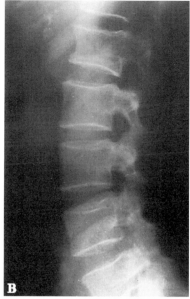

FIGURE 11A and B. Calcaneal fracture and L1 compression fracture.

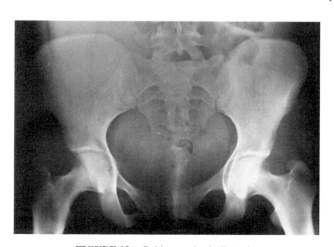

FIGURE 12.   Pubic symphysis diastasis.

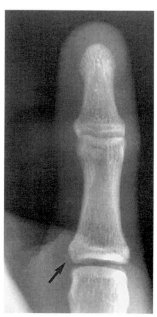

FIGURE 13 *(Right)*.   Avulsion fracture, base of proximal phalanx.

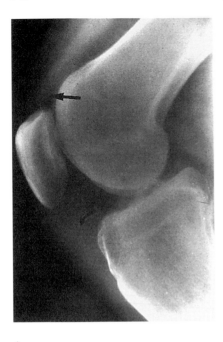

FIGURE 14. Jumper's knee.

Answers

A. Figure 3: Preacher's knee. Frequent kneeling results in inflammation and swelling of the deep infrapatellar bursa (bursitis). This is more commonly seen in tile and carpet layers than preachers. The lateral view of the knee reveals coarse calcifications in the deep infrapatellar bursa, occurring in chronic or recurrent disease.

B. Figure 7: Osteonecrosis of the femoral head. Rapid decompression in scuba divers ("bends") can give rise to nitrogen gas emboli causing avascular necrosis, among other maladies. The typical findings of areas of sclerosis and lucency and articular irregularity seen with osteonecrosis are well delineated.

C. Figure 9: Housemaid's knee. Similar to "A," this term was applied to prepatellar bursitis, encountered as a result of scrubbing floors on one's hands and knees. The coarse calcifications are located in the prepatellar bursa.

D. Figure 14: Jumper's knee—patellar tendon tear or tendinitis. Most commonly seen in younger athletes, this partial tear of the tendon occurs at its junction with the patella. This lateral view of the knee shows the normal soft tissue shadow of the quadriceps tendon (arrow). Note the ill-defined, thickened soft tissue shadow of the torn patellar tendon (curved arrow).

E. Figure 6: Little leaguer's elbow. This is an avulsion fracture of the medial humeral epicondyle, caused by repetitive or excessive valgus stress on the elbow in little-league pitchers. This avulsed epidondyle can become an intra-articular loose body. Note the separation of the medial humeral epicondyle from the adjacent humerus (arrow), combined with regional soft tissue swelling.

F. Figure 2: Epidermoid inclusion cyst. Trauma to the fingertips, as may occur in tailors, can result in implantation of epidermal tissue into the underlying bone, and a characteristic lytic lesion at the tuft.

G. Figure 13: Gamekeeper's thumb. This injury, originally described in gamekeepers when slaughtering wild game, is currently more common in ski-pole injuries. It is an avulsion at the attachment of the ulnar collateral ligament at the base of the proximal phalanx of the thumb. Note the small linear avulsion fragment at the medial base of the proximal phalanx (arrow).

H. Figure 10: Hamate fracture. Fractures of the hook of the hamate are seen in sports such as golf, baseball, and racket sports; they are due to a direct blow to the hypothenar eminence, as may occur with a checked swing in baseball. These fractures are best visualized on a carpal tunnel view or CT scan. The carpal tunnel view reveals a fracture at the base of hook of the hamate (arrows). The other carpal bones seen on this view are trapezium (TR), trapezoid (TZ), capitate (c), and pisiform (P).

I. Figure 11A and B): Lover's fracture. Comminuted compression fractures of the calcaneus result from falling or jumping from a substantial height and landing on the heels. This injury may be sustained by a suitor trying to escape as the husband arrives home (a.k.a. "Don Juan fracture"). This lateral view of the calcaneus reveals generalized compression/flattening of the calcaneus from an axial loading injury. Up to 25% of these calcaneal fractures have associated thoracolumbar compression fractures. Note the compression fracture of the L1 vertebral body.

J. Figure 1: Os trigonum syndrome. An accessory ossicle at the posterior margin of the talus is not uncommon, occurring in up to 8% of individuals. These are usually asymptomatic; in ballet dancers repetitive excessive plantar flexion can cause compression of the os trigonum between the posterior distal tibia and the posterior calcaneus resulting in pain (os trigonum syndrome). The separate bony ossicle is indicated by an "o" within it. On MRI there is often bone marrow edema in this region.

K. Figure 12: Pubic symphisis diastasis. Delivery of a large baby through a relatively small birth canal can result in widening (diastasis) of the symphisis pubis, as seen on this radiograph of the pelvis.

L. Figure 8: March fracture. Metatarsal stress fractures are not uncommon in military recruits subjected to long road marches. The second and third metatarsal shafts are most commonly involved. Radiographically occult stress fractures can be detected with high sensitivity on a radionuclide bone scan. Note the cortical thickening at the painful distal second metatarsal shaft of this long distance runner.

M. Figure 5: Osteosarcoma. Prior to discovering the potentially harmful effects of radiation exposure, watch dials were painted by laborers using paintbrushes and radium so that they would glow in the dark. Painters would place the brushes in their mouths to make them pointed, resulting in chronic radioactive radium ingestion. The incidence of radiation-induced sarcomas in these individuals was substantially increased.

N. Figure 4: Mallet finger. This avulsion fracture at the extensor tendon insertion (dorsally) typically occurs as a result of a baseball striking an extended finger, resulting in forced flexion. The triangular avulsion fragment and associated soft tissue swelling can be seen at the dorsum of the base of the distal phalanx of the index finger.

BIBLIOGRAPHY

1. Bellon EM, Sacco DC, Steiger DA, Coleman PF: Magnetic resonance imaging in "housemaid's knee." Magn Reson Imaging 5:175–177, 1987.
2. Crim MW: Pelvic diastasis in pregnancy. Am Fam Physician 35:185–186, 1987.
3. Gilula LA, Yin Y: Imaging of the Wrist and Hand. Philadelphia, W.B. Saunders, 1995.
4. Gregg PJ, Walder DN: Caisson disease of bone. Clin Orthop 210:43–54, 1986.
5. Norman A, Nelson J, Green S: Fractures of the hook of the hamate: Radiographic signs. Radiology 154:49–53, 1985.
6. Safran MR, Fu FH: Uncommon causes of knee pain in the athlete. Orthop Clin North Am 26:547–549, 1995.

VII. Neuroradiology

59. BRAIN NEOPLASMS: PRIMARY AND METASTATIC

David P. C. Liu, M.D.

1. How are brain tumors classified from a radiologic perspective?

A mass can be classified as intraaxial, meaning that its origin is within the brain parenchyma, or as extraaxial, with its origin outside the brain parenchyma. The differential diagnosis depends on the compartment in which the mass originated.

2. What are the manifestations of metastases to the central nervous system?

Metastasis to the brain parenchyma is the most common manifestation; less common are metastases to the skull, the arachnoid, the subarachnoid space, and the dura. Least common are the paraneoplastic syndromes such as cerebellar atrophy and limbic encephalitis.

3. What is the typical appearance of brain metastases on CT and MR?

More than 80% of parenchymal metastases are multiple, since they are disseminated by hematogenous spread (Fig. 1). They can occur anywhere in the brain, but the gray-white junction is the most common site. Metastases are usually nodular-enhancing or cystic appearing, with a prominent amount of surrounding edema. If a solitary lesion is found, it may be important to identify any

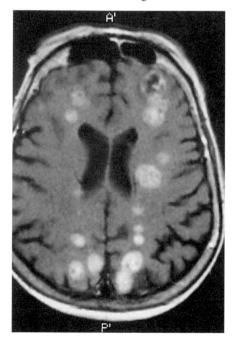

FIGURE 1. Axial T1-weighted MR image of metastases from breast carcinoma following administration of contrast (gadolinium). Multiple nodular enhancing masses of varying sizes are seen. Some have low signal intensity centers signifying necrosis.

additional metastases. The treatment for a solitary metastasis may be surgical resection, while more than one metastasis requires radiation therapy. A double-dose contrast MR or the application of an MR technique called magnetization transfer increases the detection of metastases.

4. Which conditions other than metastases produce multiple small, enhancing parenchymal nodules?

- Disseminated infection (e.g., tuberculosis, cysticercosis, cryptococcus organisms)
- Inflammatory diseases including multiple sclerosis and sarcoidosis
- Primary CNS lymphoma

5. Which primary malignancies produce cystic metastases?

Mucin-producing tumors are usually adenocarcinomas arising from the stomach, the small and large bowel, the pancreas, the ovaries, and the breast.

6. Which primary malignancies produce calcified metastases?

Dystrophic calcifications appear primarily within mucin-producing adenocarcinomas such as those arising from the intestinal tract and from the breasts and the ovaries. Ossified metastases occur with osteogenic sarcoma.

7. Which primary malignancies produce metastases that are hyperdense on enhanced CT?

Hypervascular metastases such as melanoma, renal cell carcinoma, thyroid cancer, choriocarcinoma, bronchogenic carcinoma, and occasionally breast cancer.

8. How does leptomeningeal carcinomatosis present?

Abnormal enhancement in the sulci is the most common finding. Less commonly, small nodules may be identified in the subarachnoid spaces and, occasionally, markedly intense enhancement of the dural margins.

9. How are gliomas classified?

Gliomas constitute a heterogeneous group of tumors, including astrocytomas, oligodendrogliomas, ependymomas, medulloblastomas, and mixed gliomas. Astrocytomas are commonly given grades from I to IV. The low-grade astrocytomas are most common in young adults. The spectrum continues up to high-grade astrocytomas (grade IV), which are called glioblastoma multiforme. Low-grade astrocytomas are classically nonenhancing low attenuation areas and may or may not exert mass effect. As the grade of the tumor increases, there is increased enhancement, and there is usually more mass effect. A glioblastoma multiforme has a central area of low density representing necrosis and is surrounded by a large amount of reactive edema.

10. What does a calcified mass in the brain indicate?

Low-grade astrocytomas should be considered in the differential diagnosis whenever intracerebral calcification is seen. About 10–20% of low-grade astrocytomas contain calcification. Calcification is less common with the higher grade tumors unless the tumor represents malignant transformation from a low-grade lesion. Of the low-grade gliomas, oligodendrogliomas and ependymomas are calcified most frequently.

11. What are the radiographic features of ependymomas?

About 70% of ependymomas arise from the ependymal lining of the fourth ventricle and project into the ventricle (Fig. 2). They are frequently calcified and may have associated cysts or hemorrhage.

12. What are the radiographic features of medulloblastomas?

Medulloblastomas are also most frequently found within the fourth ventricle, since they arise from primitive cells in the roof of the fourth ventricle (the inferior medullary velum) (Fig. 3). Unlike

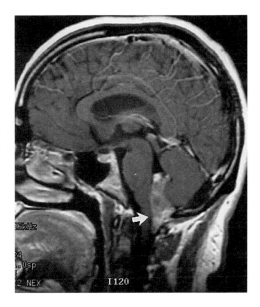

FIGURE 2. Contrast-enhanced sagittal MR image of an ependymoma. This tumor arises from the lining of the fourth ventricle and has grown inferiorly through the foramen magnum (arrow).

ependymomas, medulloblastomas rarely contains cysts or calcifications. Because of their location, both medulloblastomas and ependymomas can cause obstructive hydrocephalus.

13. What other lesions present as intraventricular masses?

In the lateral ventricle, intraventricular masses include meningiomas and ependymomas. In children, choroid plexus papillomas and carcinomas are most commonly found in the lateral ventricle. In adults, however, chorioid plexus papillomas are most commonly found in the fourth ventricle. In the fourth ventricle of adults, other lesions include medulloblastomas, ependymomas, and hemangioblastomas.

14. Which primary CNS tumors commonly metastasize through the cerebrospinal fluid to cause leptomeningeal seeding (i.e., "drop metastases")?

- Medulloblastomas
- Ependymomas
- Other malignant embryonal tumors found in children, such as primitive neuroectodermal tumors (PNET) and pineal tumors
- Malignant gliomas

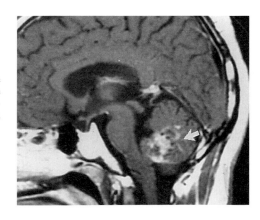

FIGURE 3. Contrast-enhanced sagittal MR image of a medulloblastoma. Because these tumors arise from the roof of the fourth ventricle, they grow posteriorly into the inferior vermis of the cerebellum (arrow).

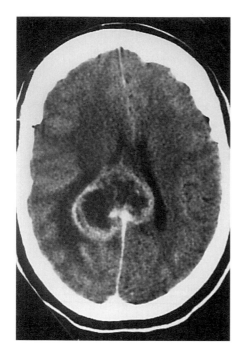

FIGURE 4.   Contrast-enhanced CT image of a butterfly glioma. This tumor has grown from the right side to the left, crossing through the splenium of the corpus callosum.

15. How is the diagnosis of leptomeningeal seeding made?
Cerebrospinal fluid cytology provides definitive evidence. Gadolinium-enhanced MR of the neuraxis is useful and noninvasive but is less sensitive than CSF cytology.

16. Which tumors involve the corpus callosum?
An enhancing necrotic-appearing mass crossing the midline via the corpus callosum has been described as a "butterfly" lesion. The differential diagnosis includes glioma (Fig. 4), lymphoma, and metastases.

17. What are the radiographic and clinical features of CNS lymphoma?
CNS lymphoma is a soft lesion found in a periventricular location (Fig. 5). Most commonly, it is found as multiple, infiltrative, or nodular lesions. CNS lymphoma primarily occurs in immunocompromised individuals, especially those with AIDS. The incidence is also rising in the elderly population.

18. What are common extraaxial tumors?
Extraaxial tumors arise outside the brain parenchyma, from the meninges, the cranial nerves, pituitary, pineal gland, and adjacent bone. Common tumors include meningiomas, neuromas, metastases, lymphoma, pituitary, and pineal tumors.

19. What are the MR and CT features of meningiomas?
They are generally well circumscribed, homogeneously enhancing, and have a broad dural base (Fig. 6). On unenhanced CT, small punctate calcifications can be seen in 20–25% of tumors. The bone windows on CT can also demonstrate thickened adjacent bone (hyperostosis) or bone destruction. On MR, the tumors are typically isointense to gray matter and may demonstrate a "dural tail," which is suggestive of, but not specific for, a meningioma.

20. Where are meningiomas located?
Most commonly, in the parasagittal region. Other locations are high in the convexities, along the sphenoid ridge, the olfactory groove, the parasellar region, and the cerebellar-pontine angle.

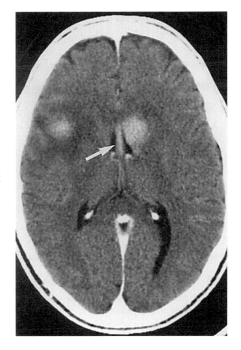

FIGURE 5. Contrast-enhanced CT image of a CNS lymphoma. Often presenting with multiple lesions, the hallmarks are the periventricular location and the poorly defined appearance. Involvement of the septum pellucidum (arrow) is also indicative of the soft, infiltrative nature of the tumor.

21. What are the angiographic features of meningiomas?

Because these tumors are dural-based, they are supplied primarily by meningeal vessels such as the middle meningeal arteries (Fig. 7). A homogeneous, intense vascular blush is identified in the late arterial and capillary phases, which persists into the venous phase (the meningioma is often referred to as the "mother-in-law tumor" because on angiography it "comes early and stays late").

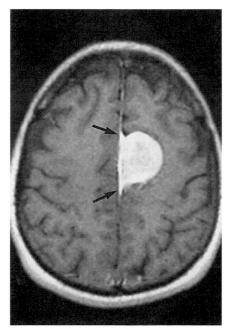

FIGURE 6. Contrast-enhanced axial MR image of a meningioma. This left parasagittal tumor has a broad dural base with the interhemispheric falx. Small anterior and posterior dural tails (black arrows) confirm that the falx is the origin of this lesion.

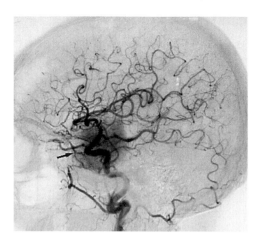

FIGURE 7. Meningioma on angiography. An intense tumor blush in the region of the sphenoid wing is fed by an enlarged middle meningeal artery (arrow).

22. Which primary tumors arise in the pineal region?

Germ cell tumors constitute the most common group of pineal masses. Germinomas are the most common germ cell tumors, and other germ cell tumors include teratomas, embryonal cell carcinoma, choriocarcinoma, and endodermal sinus tumor. Germ cell tumors present as homogeneously enhancing, well-circumscribed masses. Lesions that mimic primary pineal tumors are metastases to the pineal gland, meningiomas that arise from the posterior falx, aneurysms of the vein of Galen, and gliomas arising from the thalamus or the midbrain.

23. Name the most common tumors found in the cerebellopontine angle.

Acoustic neuromas, meningiomas, metastases, and epidermoid tumors.

24. How are acoustic neuromas distinguished from other enhancing tumors such as meningiomas?

The hallmark of an acoustic neuroma is extension of tumor into the adjacent internal auditory canal. This intracanalicular component has been rarely described with other lesions and is most easily recognized on MR rather than CT.

25. What are bilateral acoustic neuromas diagnostic of?

Neurofibromatosis type 2 (Fig. 8).

26. Are there any general distinguishing features of a neuroma?

Like other extraaxial tumors, neuromas present as well-circumscribed homogeneously enhancing masses. They are distinguished based on location rather than any other characteristic in that they arise along the course of a cranial nerve. A trigeminal neuroma, for example, commonly arises from the gasserian ganglion located in Meckel's cave, posterior to the cavernous sinus. As a result, the mass may have a dumbbell appearance, straddling both the middle and posterior fossae.

27. Are there any distinguishing features of an epidermoid?

Yes. Epidermoids are also commonly located in the cerebellopontine angle. These extraaxial tumors are distinguished by their low attenuation and their lack of contrast enhancement (Fig. 9). They must be differentiated from an arachnoid cyst. Epidermoids and arachnoid cysts are easily differentiated from each other on MR; arachnoid cysts are identical to CSF in signal intensity, while epidermoids exhibit signal intensity slightly higher than CSF on all pulse sequences. Epidermoids contain mixed cholesterol and keratin components and are often soft and infiltrating, surrounding vessels and cranial nerves. The other distinguishing feature is the frondlike, irregular surface of epidermoids that renders a cauliflower-like appearance.

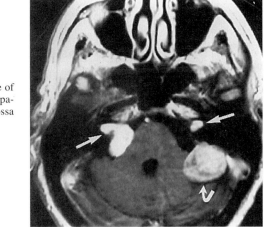

FIGURE 8.   Contrast-enhanced axial MR image of bilateral acoustic neuromas (straight arrows) in a patient with neurofibromatosis type 2. A posterior fossa meningioma (curved arrow) is also present.

28. Which intraaxial tumors are found in the cerebellum?

In adults, the most common cerebellar tumor is a metastasis. The second most common lesion is a hemangioblastoma. In children, gliomas are the most common cerebellar tumors.

29. What are the radiographic features of a hemangioblastoma?

Hemangioblastomas are typically cystic tumors that contain a solid nodule called a mural nodule in its wall (Fig. 10). About 60% of hemangioblastomas have this appearance, while the other 40% exhibit homogeneous solid enhancement. About 80–85% are located in the cerebellum, with the remaining tumors occurring in the medulla or the spinal cord. On angiography, the nodular component stains intensely and persists late into the venous phase. Hemangioblastomas are histologically benign lesions.

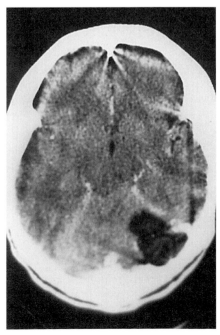

FIGURE 9.   Posterior fossa epidermoid on contrast-enhanced CT. The lesion is lucent and does not enhance with contrast (lesion is dark area adjacent to left cerebellum).

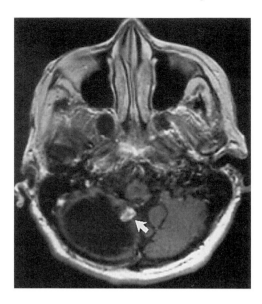

FIGURE 10. Axial enhanced MR image of a cystic hemangioblastoma. An enhancing mural nodule (arrow) is separate from the adjacent unenhancing cyst.

30. What syndrome is associated with cerebellar and spinal hemangioblastomas?
von Hippel Lindau syndrome.

31. What are some causes of intrasellar masses?
Pituitary adenomas are by far the most common intrasellar masses. Other lesions include meningiomas, metastases, cystic lesions, and inflammatory processes such as sarcoid.

32. What are the common clinical presentations of a pituitary adenoma?
Adenomas are clinically classified as hormonally active or inactive. Hormonally inactive lesions are often incidental findings; however, large lesions can extend into the suprasellar cistern and compress the optic chiasm. These patients present with a homonymous hemianopsia. Of the hormonally active tumors, prolactinomas are the most common type of adenoma.

33. What is the radiographic appearance of a pituitary adenoma?
Adenomas smaller than 1 cm are called microadenomas (Fig. 11), and larger adenomas are macroadenomas. Normal pituitary tissue enhances with contrast on both CT and MR. Microadenomas stand out as areas of decreased enhancement; patients must be scanned immediately after contrast injection. Macroadenomas can be solid, cystic, or necrotic, with the solid component enhancing intensely.

34. What are the common suprasellar masses?
• Suprasellar extension of pituitary macroadenomas
• Craniopharyngiomas, which usually have an intrasellar and a suprasellar component
• Aneurysms
• Gliomas—arising from the hypothalamus or optic chiasm
• Meningiomas
• Metastases

35. What are the radiographic features of craniopharyngiomas?
These intrasellar and/or suprasellar masses arise from squamous cells along Rathke's cleft. Most are partially cystic, and they contain calcifications that are better demonstrated on CT. Almost all craniopharyngiomas exhibit nodular or peripheral rim enhancement.

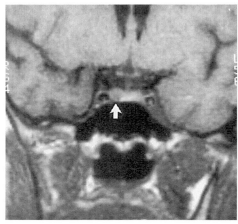

FIGURE 11. Pituitary microadenoma. This unenhanced coronal T1-weighted MR image shows a 6-mm tumor (arrow) creating upward convexity of the gland.

36. What is the differential diagnosis of a mass in the jugular foramen?

The most common mass in this region is a glomus tumor (glomus jugulare tumor). Much less common are metastases and meningiomas.

37. What are glomus tumors?

Also known as chemodectomas or paragangliomas, glomus tumors originate from chemoreceptor cells in the jugular bulb (Fig. 12). Other glomus tumors are found in the middle ear, along the course of the vagus nerve, and in the carotid body. Glomus tumors are markedly hypervascular and enhance intensely on CT, MR, and angiography. On CT, glomus jugulare tumors destroy and erode the bony margins of the jugular fossa. On MR, the bony changes may be subtle, but glomus tumors can be easily identified by their marked intrinsic heterogeneity on all pulse sequences.

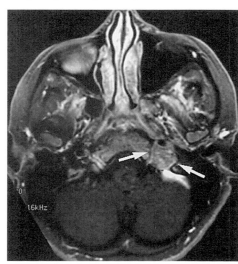

FIGURE 12. Contrast-enhanced axial MR image of a glomus jugulare tumor. Located in the left jugular fossa, this enhancing tumor is heterogeneous and well circumscribed (arrows).

BIBLIOGRAPHY

1. Atlas SW: Adult supratentorial tumors. Semin Roentgenol 25:130, 1990.
2. Bilaniuk LT: Adult infratentorial tumors. Semin Roentgenol 25:155, 1990.
3. Elster AD: Modern imaging of the pituitary. Radiology 187:1, 1993.
4. Harwood-Nash DC: Primary neoplasms of the central nervous system in children. Cancer 67:1223, 1991.

5. Hwang TL, Valdivieso JG, Yang CH, et al: Calcified brain metastases. Neurosurgery 32:451, 1993.
6. Jelinek J, Smirniotopoulos JG, Parisi JE, et al: Lateral ventricular neoplasms of the brain: Differential diagnosis based on clinical, CT, and MR findings. AJNR 11:567, 1990.
7. Olsen WL, Dillon WP, Kelly WM, et al: MR imaging of paragangliomas. AJNR 7:1039, 1986.
8. Siegleman ES, Mishkin MM, Taveras JT: Past, present, and future of radiology of meningioma. Radiographics 11:899, 1991.
9. Tien RD: Intraventricular mass lesions of the brain: CT and MR findings. AJR 157:1283, 1991.
10. Watanabe M, Tanaka R, Takeda N: Magnetic resonance imaging and histopathology of cerebral gliomas. Neuroradiology 35:463, 1992.
11. Zee CS, Chin T, Segall HD, et al: Magnetic resonance imaging of meningiomas. Semin Ultrasound CT MR 13:154, 1992.
12. Zimmerman RA: Imaging of intrasellar, suprasellar, and parasellar tumors. Semin Roentgenol 25:174, 1990.

60. CEREBROVASCULAR DISEASE

David P. C. Liu, M.D.

1. What is the definition of a stroke?

A "wastebasket term," stroke refers to diminished blood supply to brain parenchyma, resulting in a cascade of loss of cell membrane function, which progresses to edema and finally cell death and gliosis.

2. What are different types of strokes?

- Infarct due to arterial or venous occlusion
- Lacunar infarct
- Intracerebral hemorrhage
- Subarachnoid hemorrhage

3. Why is CT the modality of choice for the initial evaluation of stroke?

The role of CT is to exclude the presence of intracerebral hemorrhage. The treatment of an infarct will differ depending on whether hemorrhage is present on CT. CT is also useful in determining if an underlying lesion such as a tumor or a vascular malformation is present. Occasionally, a subdural hematoma may mimic the clinical presentation of a stroke.

4. What are the early changes of an arterial infarct on CT?

Edema, which can be seen as loss of the gray-white matter differentiation and effacement of the adjacent sulci. By 24 hours, the infarcted area appears low in density and is usually wedge-shaped, conforming to the distribution of an artery or arterial branch supplying a portion of the brain (Fig. 1). Hemorrhage may occur any time during this period (Fig. 2).

5. What is the role of MR in the evaluation of stroke?

MR is more sensitive than CT in the evaluation of any kind of edema and for the detection of acute infarction. However, because MR is relatively insensitive to acute hemorrhage, it is not the initial test of choice for acute infarction. More sophisticated MR techniques (e.g., diffusion-weighted imaging) are even more sensitive than conventional MR in detecting stroke.

6. How do early infarcts appear on MR?

Like CT, the earliest changes include loss of the gray-white matter differentiation, edema in the affected gyri (seen as high signal on T2-weighted images), and effacement of the adjacent subarachnoid spaces. The normal signal void in the affected vessels may be lost, indicating thrombus. If intravenous contrast (gadolinium) is given, the meninges adjacent to the infarct may also enhance.

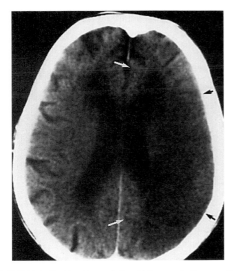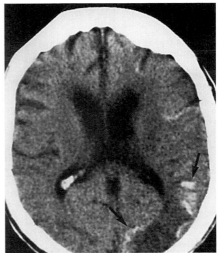

FIGURE 1 *(Left).*   Large left middle cerebral artery infarct, nonhemorrhagic (black arrows) on CT. The sulci have been obliterated by swelling. Note sparing of the brain supplied by the left anterior and posterior cerebral arteries (white arrows).

FIGURE 2 *(Right).*   This small middle cerebral artery branch infarct exhibits hemorrhage along its periphery (black arrows).

7. How do infarcts appear on CT and MR in the subacute phase?

By the third day, the edematous changes and mass effect become increasingly obvious on both CT and MR. If intravenous contrast is given, intense enhancement of the gyri can be seen. This is indicative of breakdown of the blood-brain barrier and may persist up to 8 weeks.

8. How do infarcts appear on CT and MR in the chronic phase?

The hallmark of chronic infarcts is encephalomalacia or volume loss. Focal atrophy and dilatation of the adjacent ventricles and subarachnoid spaces are seen.

9. What are lacunar infarcts?

Small deep infarcts that are the result of compromise of the long, penetrating arterioles, often due to hypertension.

10. Describe the CT and MR appearance of lacunar infarcts.

Because lacunar infarcts are part of a more extensive white matter disease process, they are often multiple and are typically located in the basal ganglia, the thalami, and the periventricular white matter. The infarcted areas contain cerebrospinal fluid and are low in density on CT. On MR, these small infarcts are low in signal intensity on the T1-weighted images and are high in signal intensity on the T2-weighted images.

11. What are "watershed" infarcts?

Infarcts that are the result of generalized hypoxia or anoxia. Because the terminal vessels are most affected, these infarcts occur at the border zones between major arterial territories (the anterior, middle, and posterior cerebral arteries).

12. What are the other radiographic manifestations of generalized hypoxia/anoxia?

If compromise is severe, global cerebral edema is most common, especially in newborns. On CT, the brain is swollen, resulting in obliteration of the cisternal and subarachnoid spaces and loss of the gray-white matter differentiation (Fig. 3). Eventually, the brain undergoes severe atrophy. Less severe hypoxia results in cortical laminar necrosis. Only the superficial cortex is involved.

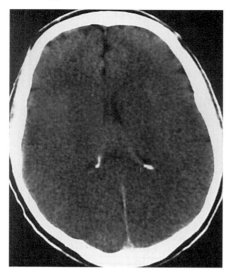

FIGURE 3.   Global ischemia has resulted in diffuse cerebral edema. Note the slit-like ventricles, obliteration of the sulci, and loss of the gray-white matter junction.

13. Why is it important to diagnose carotid stenosis?
In 90% of cases of thromboembolic stroke, atherosclerosis is the underlying cause. A multicenter trial (NASCET, or the North American Symptomatic Carotid Endarterectomy Trial) demonstrated that patients whose internal carotid arteries were narrowed in cross-section by more than 70% benefited from a carotid endarterectomy.

14. What imaging techniques can be used to diagnose carotid stenosis?
The "gold standard" remains selective carotid angiography. However, noninvasive techniques including ultrasound, CT angiography, and MR angiography are playing an increasing role in screening patients and in preoperative planning.

15. What are the technical problems with using ultrasound (or magnetic resonance angiography) as a screening test for carotid stenosis?
Color Doppler, which is used in conjunction with gray-scale imaging and Doppler waveform analysis to image the carotid arteries, tends to overestimate carotid stenosis. For example, a high-grade stenosis may have the appearance of a total occlusion. This is significant, because a patient with a high-grade stenosis is a surgical candidate for endarterectomy and a patient with complete carotid occlusion is not. Likewise, MR angiography tends to overestimate the degree of stenosis. Also, on both ultrasound and MR angiography, it is difficult to visualize tortuous vessels, especially those with sharply angulated turns.

16. What is the major pitfall of CT angiography as a test for carotid artery stenosis?
Calcification, which is commonly associated with atherosclerotic plaque, can obscure the stenosis. Unlike ultrasound and routine MR angiography, CT angiography requires the injection of intravenous contrast.

17. When is carotid angiography necessary?
When precise documentation of a plaque is needed (e.g., for surgical planning, to define the presence or absence of an ulcer, to measure the degree of stenosis), to search for other causes of vascular disease (e.g., vasculitis, aneurysms), and to evaluate existing and potential routes of collateral circulation.

18. What is the "string" sign?

A "string" of contrast may be seen in the internal carotid artery at angiography, which represents a trickle of slow antegrade flow. This signifies a very high-grade stenosis but excludes complete occlusion (Fig. 4).

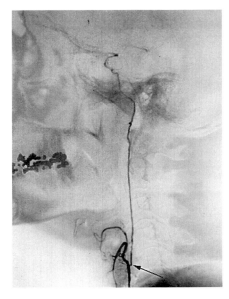

FIGURE 4. A high-grade stenosis is seen at the origin of this internal carotid artery (arrow) on this angiogram. The remainder of the internal carotid artery is stringlike; the vessel is open but is severely narrowed and exhibits slow flow.

19. What is the "subclavian steal" syndrome?

When the proximal subclavian artery is occluded, the blood flow in the ipsilateral vertebral artery reverses (i.e., blood flows antegrade in the contralateral vertebral artery and back down the ipsilateral vertebral artery) to supply the shoulder and arm distal to the obstruction. Patients with this condition can present with brain-stem ischemia and/or diminished or absent pulses in the affected arm.

20. How is the diagnosis of subclavian steal made?

Conventional angiography remains the gold standard; however, magnetic resonance angiography and ultrasound are effective, noninvasive examinations that can suggest or establish this diagnosis.

21. What are some causes of vascular narrowing other than atherosclerosis?

Arterial dissection, vasculitis, vasospasm, secondary narrowing due to adjacent cerebral edema, and encasement by tumor.

22. What causes arterial dissection?

Most commonly, spontaneous disruption of the intima of an artery. Other causes include penetrating or blunt trauma, chiropractic manipulation, and other vigorous activities such as weightlifting. Dysplasias of the arterial wall, including fibromuscular dysplasia and cystic medial necrosis, are also predisposing factors.

23. What portions of the carotid and vertebral arteries are most commonly involved in dissections?

Carotid dissections involve the midcervical segment of the internal carotid artery, narrowing the vessel distal to the carotid bulb, and ending at the base of the skull. Dissections of the vertebral artery are located between the C2 vertebral body and the base of the skull.

24. How is the diagnosis of carotid or vertebral dissection established?
MR is a useful screening study. Conventional MR images obtained in the axial plane may demonstrate subacute blood, which appears as a bright area, in the arterial wall (Fig. 5). MR angiography demonstrates narrowing of the affected segment.

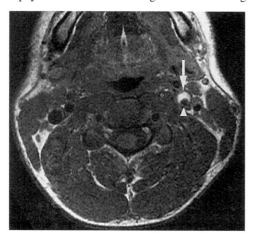

FIGURE 5. On this axial MR image, a high signal crescent-shaped clot is identified within the wall of the left internal carotid artery, representing the false channel of a dissection (white arrow). The true lumen remains dark (white arrowhead), indicative of persistent flow.

25. What are some causes of vasculitis?
Infection, drugs, collagen vascular disease, granulomatous disease, and idiopathic causes.

26. How is vasculitis that affects the CNS classified radiographically?
1. Large-vessel disease, which primarily involves the aortic arch and the great vessels (e.g., in Takayasu's arteritis).
2. Medium-vessel disease, affecting the cervical internal carotid artery (e.g., fibromuscular dysplasia).
3. Small-vessel disease, which affects the intracranial circulation, primarily the distal branches of the anterior, middle, and posterior cerebral arteries.

27. What is the angiographic appearance of vasculitis?
The most extreme example is complete occlusion of a vessel. A nonspecific manifestation is focal segmental stenosis, and a more specific manifestation is luminal irregularity, which has been described as "beading" or a "stack of coins" (Fig. 6).

28. What are some causes of venous thrombosis?
- Dehydration
- Trauma
- Pregnancy
- Oral contraceptives
- Infection, especially associated with sinusitis or mastoiditis
- Tumor with local vascular invasion
- Polycythemia and other hypercoagulable states

29. What is the imaging appearance of venous infarcts?
When the superior sagittal sinus is thrombosed, infarcts are parasagittal, often bilateral, and may become hemorrhagic ("flame-shaped" hemorrhages). Thrombosis of the deep cerebral veins, including the internal cerebral veins and the great vein of Galen, results in infarcted low-density basal ganglia and thalami, with or without petechial hemorrhages. Thrombosis of superficial cortical veins results in nonspecific infarcts since no location is characteristic; the infarcts may occur in the superficial cortex, in the the subcortical white matter, or in areas mimicking watershed infarcts.

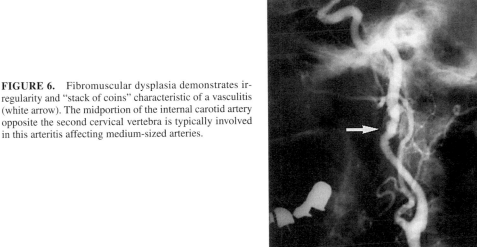

FIGURE 6. Fibromuscular dysplasia demonstrates irregularity and "stack of coins" characteristic of a vasculitis (white arrow). The midportion of the internal carotid artery opposite the second cervical vertebra is typically involved in this arteritis affecting medium-sized arteries.

30. How is thrombosis of a cerebral venous sinus diagnosed on CT?

On unenhanced CT, an intraluminal clot will be hyperdense in the thrombosed venous sinus; this is most obvious in the superior sagittal sinus. Occasionally, thrombosis within superficial cortical veins will be identified as curvilinear areas of high density. Following intravenous contrast administration, the intraluminal thrombus will stand out as a filling defect (Fig. 7) while the adjacent margins enhance intensely. The combination of findings is referred to as the "empty delta sign": the superior sagittal sinus, on cross-section, looks like a triangle, or the Greek letter delta. The peripherally enhancing margins represent engorged and dilated venous collaterals.

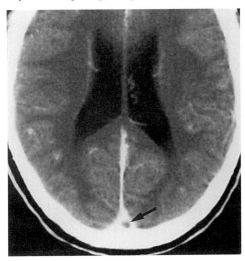

FIGURE 7. Thrombosis of the superior sagittal sinus. A filling defect (arrow) representing clot is seen with an otherwise enhancing sinus on this contrast-enhanced CT image.

31. What are the MR features of venous thrombosis?

Intraluminal clot is easily seen on MR (Fig. 8), making MR the initial study of choice for suspected venous thrombosis. The clot follows the same signal intensity as that of a parenchymal clot. As an acute thrombus evolves into a subacute thrombus, it becomes hyperintense on all pulse sequences. Clot in the chronic stage often undergoes fibrosis and will be surrounded by dilated venous collaterals.

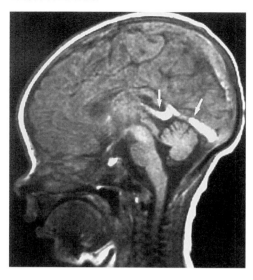

FIGURE 8. Venous thrombosis is seen as a high signal area on MR (sagittal image). The great vein of Galen and straight sinus are involved (white arrows).

32. Aside from hemorrhagic infarcts, what are the common causes of parenchymal hematomas?

1. Hypertension
2. Trauma
3. Coagulopathy
4. Underlying tumor, arteriovenous malformation, or aneurysm
5. Amyloid angiopathy

33. Where are the most common locations for a hypertensive hemorrhage?

The basal ganglia (especially the putamen), the thalamus, the pons, the cerebellum, and the subcortical white matter. In 50% of patients with hypertensive hemorrhage, the force of the bleed results in rupture into the adjacent ventricular system. This latter finding is associated with an especially poor prognosis.

34. What is amyloid angiopathy?

Otherwise known as congophilic angiopathy, it is the most common cause of recurrent intracranial hematomas in the elderly. The walls of the cortical and leptomeningeal arteries are replaced by amyloid beta protein, and hence stain intensely with Congo red. This condition appears to be unrelated to systemic amyloidosis.

35. What is the imaging appearance of amyloid angiopathy?

Hematomas, which are typically multiple and occur at the corticomedullary junction, especially posteriorly.

36. What are the common causes of subarachnoid hemorrhage (SAH)?

• Rupture of a "berry" aneurysm (the most common cause).
• Trauma
• Hypertension
• Coagulopathy
• Dural arteriovenous malformation

37. How is the diagnosis of SAH made?

Radiographically by CT or by lumbar puncture.

38. Where does SAH most often occur when an intracranial aneurysm ruptures?

Because aneurysms frequently occur around the circle of Willis or in the Sylvian fissures, SAH tends to be localized to the basilar cisterns and the Sylvian fissures.

39. What is the role of CT in establishing the diagnosis of SAH?

CT is highly sensitive to acute SAH. Experience from ruptured berry aneurysms indicates that within the first 24 hours, 95% of subarachnoid hemorrhages can be diagnosed. The rate of detection then drops so that only 85% are diagnosed at 48 hours. If clinical suspicion remains high for SAH, a negative CT scan should not preclude a lumbar tap from being performed.

40. What is the role of MR in the diagnosis of SAH?

MR is unreliable in the acute stage. SAH is more easily seen in the subacute stage.

41. How is the diagnosis of a ruptured berry aneurysm made?

Angiography remains the gold standard. The location of the aneurysm, the neck and direction in which it is pointing are essential pieces of information for surgical planning. Angiography can also identify additional aneurysms and the presence of vasospasm; 15–20% of aneurysms are multiple. The right and left carotid arteries and the vertebrobasilar circulation must be injected with contrast for a complete angiographic study.

42. Where are berry aneurysms most commonly located?

At autopsy, aneurysms are most commonly found at the middle cerebral arterial bifurcation (Fig. 9). Although the anterior communicating and posterior communicating aneurysms are less frequent, they are the most likely to bleed.

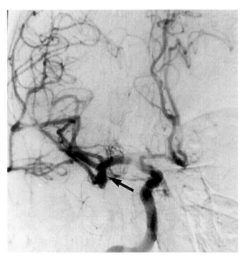

FIGURE 9. AP view of a cerebral angiogram shows a berry aneurysm arising from the right middle cerebral artery trifurcation (arrow).

43. If multiple aneurysms are present, which one has most likely bled?

Extravasation of contrast from the culprit aneurysm is rare but diagnostic. Helpful signs include the size and shape of the aneurysm. Larger aneurysms are more likely to have bled, as are aneurysms that have an irregular, lobulated contour that resembles a nipple. Furthermore, CT is helpful because the region of hemorrhage is a strong indicator of the area in which the aneurysm is located.

44. How do the CT findings help to localize the culprit aneurysm?

Anterior communicating aneurysms typically hemorrhage into the septum pellucidum or the anterior interhemispheric fissure. Middle cerebral artery trifurcation aneurysms typically bleed into the

Sylvian fissure or the adjacent temporal lobe. Posterior communicating aneurysms tend to bleed into the perimesencephalic cistern.

45. Why are follow-up CT scans useful in the evaluation of ruptured berry aneurysms?
The risk of a rebleed is 20–50%, with the highest risk in the first week. Other complications include hydrocephalus and vasospasm, which may or may not result in an infarction.

BIBLIOGRAPHY

1. Bryan RN: Imaging of acute stroke. Radiology 177:615, 1990.
2. Furst H, Harti WH, et al: Color-flow Doppler sonography in the identification of ulcerative plaques in patients with high-grade carotid artery stenosis. AJNR 13:1581, 1992.
3. Goldberg HI: Angiography of extra- and intracranial occlusive cerebrovascular disease. Neuroimag Clin North Am 2:487, 1992.
4. Greenan TJ, Grossman RI, Goldbert HI: Cerebral vasculitis: MR imaging and angiographic correlation. Radiology 182:65, 1992.
5. Litt AW, Eidelman EM, Pinto RS, et al: Diagnosis of carotid artery stenosis: Comparison of 2DFT time-of-flight MR angiography with contrast angiography in 50 patients. AJNR 12:149, 1991.
6. Masaryk TJ, Obuchowski NA: Noninvasive carotid imaging: Caveat emptor. Radiology 186:325, 1993.
7. North American Symptomatic Carotid Endarterectomy Trial Collaborators: Beneficial effect of carotid endarterectomy in symptomatic patients with high grade stenosis. N Engl J Med 325:445, 1991.
8. Osborn AG: Intracranial aneurysms. In Osborn AG: Handbook of Neuroradiology, 2nd ed. St. Louis, Mosby, 1996.
9. Wolpert SM, Caplan LR: Current role of cerebral angiography in the diagnosis of cerebrovascular disease. AJR 159:191, 1992.
10. Yip PK, Liuh M, Hwang BS, et al: Subclavian steal phenomenon: A correlation between sonographic and angiographic findings. Neuroradiology 34:279, 1992.
11. Yuh WTC, Crain MR, Loes DJ, et al: MR imaging of cerebral ischemia: Findings in the first 24 hours. AJNR 12:621, 1991.
12. Zimmerman RD, Ernst RJ: Neuroimaging of cerebrovenous thrombosis. Neuroimag Clin North Am 2:463, 1992.

61. INFECTIOUS, INFLAMMATORY, AND DEMYELINATING DISEASES

David P. C. Liu, M.D.

1. Where can infections occur in the central nervous system?
Everywhere, including the brain parenchyma, the ventricular system, the meninges, and the subdural and epidural spaces. All of these areas can be seeded by the blood; epidural abscesses occur most commonly by extension of infection from adjacent bone or sinus infection. Subdural empyemas are postsurgical complications but may also arise from spread of infection from adjacent osteomyelitis or sinusitis.

2. How are brain parenchymal infections classified?
- Cerebritis, which is generally caused by bacterial infection
- Encephalitis is usually due to viral infection
- Abscess, which usually exhibits a mature capsule

3. What are the imaging hallmarks of a cerebral abscess?
A cerebral abscess forms after a period of cerebritis. Therefore, it has had time to mature and presents on CT (Fig. 1) and MR as a ring-enhancing lesion with a large amount of surrounding white matter edema.

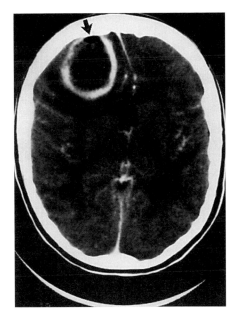

FIGURE 1. Bacterial abscess on contrast-enhanced CT. The smooth, enhancing capsule and surrounding white matter edema are typical, whereas the presence of air (arrow) is much less typical.

4. How can an abscess be distinguished from other ring-enhancing lesions such as tumor?

The enhancing margins of an abscess represent the fibrous capsule that walls off the more central areas of necrosis and pus. The enhancing margin is typically thin and very smooth, versus tumor, which typically appears more irregular and nodular. The capsule of an abscess tends to point toward the ventricles, and this portion of the wall tends to be thinner than the other areas of the capsule. Smaller daughter abscesses may form adjacent to the main abscess.

5. How are cerebritis and encephalitis distinguished from brain abscess?

Cerebritis is indistinguishable from encephalitis radiographically, since they both represent swollen brain. On CT, the involved area is low in density, and on MR, the T2-weighted images demonstrate diffuse areas of nonspecific high signal often involving gray mater and subcortical white matter.

6. What bacterial organisms are responsible for cerebritis and brain abscess?

About 70% of brain abscesses are caused by aerobic and anaerobic streptococci. *Staphylococcus aureus* accounts for 10–15%, and the remaining organisms are usually *Enterobacter* and *Bacteroides* species.

7. What viruses are responsible for encephalitis?

Herpes simplex viruses are the most common cause of nonepidemic acute encephalitis. Herpes simplex type 1 is the most common cause of encephalitis in older children and adults; type 2 is the most common cause of encephalitis in newborns and is acquired during delivery. Less common viruses that may cause encephalitis include cytomegalovirus, Epstein-Barr virus, varicella zoster, and arbovirus. HIV encephalopathy is also becoming increasingly common.

8. How does herpes encephalitis appear on CT and MR?

Encephalitis of all etiologies causes nonspecific edema. MR is much more sensitive than CT in identifying these areas of edema, which are seen as high signal areas on T2-weighted MR images. Herpes, however, has a strong propensity for the medial aspect of the temporal lobes (Fig. 2). In severe cases, small areas of hemorrhage may occur.

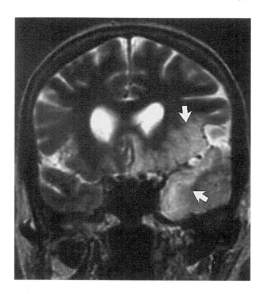

FIGURE 2. Herpes simplex type 1. The high signal edema representing encephalitis is best seen on T2-weighted images and has a propensity to involve the frontal and temporal lobes (white arrows).

9. What are the common intracranial infections in AIDS patients?

HIV encephalopathy is usually a manifestation of endstage AIDS. On MR, the white matter tracts such as the corona radiata, the cerebral peduncles, and the brainstem exhibit poorly defined symmetric areas of abnormal high signal on T2-weighted images (Fig. 3). Generalized cortical atrophy also occurs. Opportunistic infections in AIDS patients include toxoplasmosis, CMV, fungi such as *Aspergillus* and *Cryptococcus* species, and progressive multifocal leukoencephalopathy (PML).

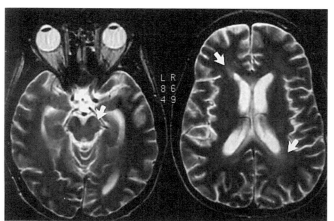

FIGURE 3. HIV encephalopathy. The white matter in the periventricular region (arrows, right image) and cerebral peduncles (arrow, left image) are high in signal on these T2-weighted MR images. The symmetry, diffuse nature, and poorly defined margins are typical.

10. What are the radiographic features of CNS infection by HIV in newborns?

Most CT and MR scans are normal. In a small percentage of newborns with HIV, symmetric, punctate calcifications can be identified in the basal ganglia on CT studies. These calcifications are located in the walls of the lenticulostriate arteries.

11. Are there any features that distinguish toxoplasmosis from other infections in AIDS patients?

Multiple ring-enhancing and nodular lesions are the hallmark of toxoplasmosis (Fig. 4). This appearance is nonspecific and mimics the imaging appearance of multiple brain abscesses, lymphoma, and metastatic disease. Since toxoplasmosis is the most common opportunistic central nervous system infection in HIV-positive persons, patients are treated for presumptive toxoplasmosis if the CT or MR suggests this diagnosis. If the patient does not improve clinically and radiographically, more aggressive diagnostic measures, including biopsy, may be warranted.

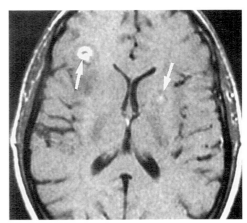

FIGURE 4. Toxoplasmosis in an immunosuppressed patient. Lesions on contrast-enhanced MR may be either ring-enhancing (left arrow) or nodular (right arrow).

12. What is progressive multifocal leukoencephalopathy (PML)?

This indolent infection is caused by the JC virus, which is in the family of papovaviruses. It favors oligodendrocytes, and radiographically the disease involves primarily the white matter tracts. Unlike HIV encephalopathy, this process is typically multifocal. The involved areas usually begin in the subcortical white matter and on the T2-weighted images exhibit nonspecific areas of high signal (Fig. 5). The hallmarks of PML are the lack of mass effect and the lack of contrast enhancement; however, mass effect and contrast enhancement occasionally occur.

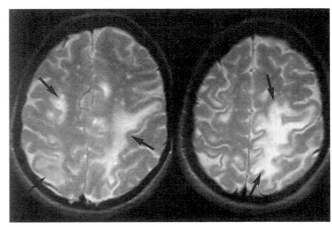

FIGURE 5. Progressive multifocal leukoencephalopathy. The subcortical white matter (arrows) is primarily involved in this patient. The sharply defined margins, multiple areas, and lack of symmetry on this MR examination distinguish PML from HIV encephalopathy.

13. What are the MR features of ventriculitis?

Abnormal enhancement of the ventricular lining (Fig. 6) and high signal around the periphery of the ventricles on proton density and T2-weighted images. In the HIV-positive population, CMV should be ruled out as the primary cause of ventriculitis. Other infectious causes of ventriculitis in the general population include bacterial organisms, especially following rupture of a brain abscess into the ventricular system.

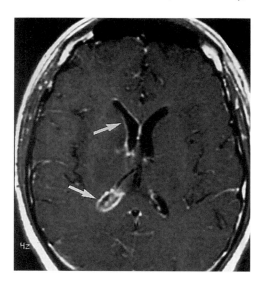

FIGURE 6. Ventriculitis. The abnormally enhancing ventricular margins (arrows) on MR were due to rupture of an intracranial pyogenic abscess.

14. What are some noninfectious causes of ventricular enhancement?
Sarcoidosis, metastatic disease, and lymphoma.

15. What are the radiographic features of a subdural empyema?
Fluid collections in the subdural space are crescent in shape, following the contour of the underlying brain hemispheres. A subdural empyema enhances intensely following the administration of intravenous contrast (Fig. 7). This is in contradistinction to other subdural fluid collections such as hematomas, which enhance but not as intensely as a subdural empyema. The enhancing peripheral rim represents the fibrous capsule that has formed to wall off the infection.

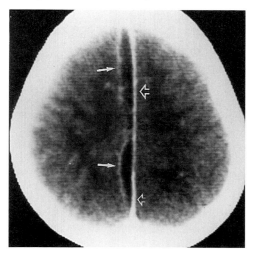

FIGURE 7. Bacterial subdural empyema on contrast-enhanced CT. This collection is a complication of meningitis in a 6-year-old child. One side is outlined by an enhancing interhemispheric falx (open arrows); the other is outlined by abnormally enhancing meninges (straight arrows).

16. What are the features of an epidural abscess?
Unlike subdural empyemas, epidural abscesses are lentiform, or biconvex in shape. The collection exhibits marked rim enhancement. Subdural and epidural empyemas are most commonly caused by sinusitis, and the frontal sinus is the most common source. Both can also cause cortical vein thrombosis with venous infarction.

17. What are the radiographic features of meningitis?

CT and MR are usually normal; the diagnosis of meningitis is a clinical/laboratory one. Advanced cases exhibit intense enhancement of the meningeal surfaces, including the basilar cisterns and the subarachnoid spaces (Fig. 8).

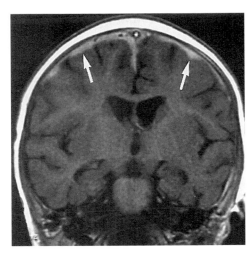

FIGURE 8. Bacterial meningitis. Following contrast, the meninges (arrows) over the high convexities are thickened, enhance abnormally on this MR image, and extend into the interhemispheric fissure.

18. What is cysticercosis?

The most common parasitic infection affecting the central nervous system. It is endemic to Central and South America. In the acute stage, the larvae can incite an intense inflammatory reaction, and cystic or ring-enhanced lesions are seen. In the chronic stage, the lesions appear as punctate calcifications with no enhancement or mass effect (Fig. 9).

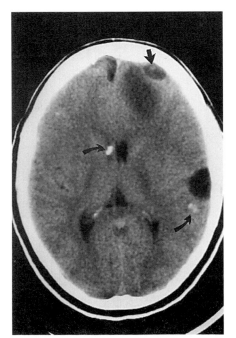

FIGURE 9. An unenhanced CT image demonstrates cysticercosis, a parasitic infection, in various stages. A frontal lesion is active, containing a scolex (straight arrow) and exhibiting surrounding white matter edema. Calcified lesions (curved arrows) are in the chronic stage.

19. What are the radiographic features of tuberculosis in the central nervous system?

The most common manifestation is meningitis, often localized to the basilar cisterns. Since tuberculosis is spread by the blood, multiple parenchymal abscesses representing caseating granulomas can be found anywhere in the brain parenchyma. These abscesses are nodular or ring-enhancing in the acute stage and calcify in the chronic stage.

20. What is the difference between demyelination and dysmyelination?

Demyelinating disorders refer to processes affecting previously normal myelin, of which multiple sclerosis is the prototypical disease. Dysmyelination refers to the formation of abnormal myelin; this group of inherited disorders is also known as leukodystrophies.

21. Why is MR much more sensitive than CT in diagnosing multiple sclerosis?

Demyelination results in swollen, edematous myelin. MR is exquisitely sensitive to changes in brain water content.

22. What are the MR features of multiple sclerosis?

The demyelinating plaques appear as focal discrete areas of abnormal high signal on proton-density and T2-weighted MR images. These plaques are often round or oval and line up along the periventricular region (Fig. 10), especially in the corpus callosum and around the atria of the occipital ventricular horns. The ovoid lesions in the periventricular regions represent plaques along a perivenular distribution and have been termed "Dawson's fingers." About 10% of plaques are located in the posterior fossa, especially in the brainstem and the cerebellar white matter. In optic neuritis, plaques may be identified along the course of the optic nerves or at the level of the optic chiasm.

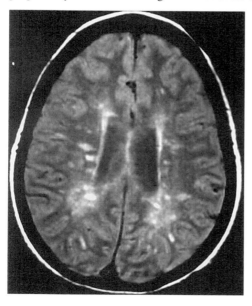

FIGURE 10. Multiple sclerosis on MR. The periventricular distribution and oval shape are typical of demyelination.

23. What is the significance of enhancement of a plaque?

Enhancement represents breakdown of the blood-brain barrier. Although enhancement can be variable and transient, it signifies the presence of active demyelination.

BIBLIOGRAPHY

1. Gean-Marton AD, Vezina LG, Martin KI, et al: Abnormal corpus callosum: A sensitive and specific indicator of multiple sclerosis. Radiology 180:215, 1991.
2. Enzmann DR: Imaging of Infections and Inflammation of the Central Nervous System. Philadelphia, Lippincott-Raven, 1984.

3. Gonzales MR, Davis RL: Neuropathology of acquired immunodeficiency syndrome. Neuropathol Appl Neurobiol 14:345, 1988.
4. Miller DH, MacManus DG, Bartlett PA, et al: Detection of optic nerve lesions in optic neuritis using frequency-selective fat-saturation sequences. Neuroradiology 35:156, 1993.
5. Offenbacher H, Fazekas F, Schmidt R, et al: Assessment of MRI criteria for a diagnosis of MS. Neurology 43:905, 1993.
6. Powell T, Sussman JG, Davies-Jones GAB: MR imaging in acute multiple sclerosis: Ring-like appearance in plaques, suggesting the presence of paramagnetic free radicals. AJNR 13:1544, 1992.
7. Whitley RJ: Viral encephalitis. N Engl J Med 323:242, 1990.

62. NEOPLASTIC DISEASE OF THE SPINE/ CORD COMPRESSION

David P. C. Liu, M.D.

1. How are lesions of the spine classified radiographically?

Lesions intrinsic to the spinal cord are considered intramedullary in location. Lesions within the thecal sac but outside the spinal cord, i.e., in the subarachnoid space, are classified as intradural-extramedullary. Lesions outside the thecal sac are epidural in location.

2. What are the most common epidural lesions?

Vertebral metastases are the most common lesions to result in epidural compression and compromise of the spinal canal. Bony metastases usually originate in the vertebral bodies (Fig. 1) or pedicles and then grow into the spinal canal. Less common epidural tumors include multiple myeloma, lymphoma, and primary tumors of the vertebral column. Non-neoplastic causes of epidural masses include epidural hematoma and epidural abscess, either of which can compress the spinal cord.

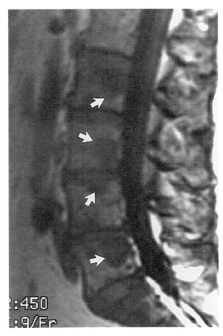

FIGURE 1. Unenhanced T1-weighted MR image of breast carcinoma metastatic to the vertebral bodies. The normal high signal arising from the fatty bone marrow has been replaced by multiple discrete metastatic foci (arrows).

3. Which primary tumors most commonly metastasize to the vertebrae?

Lung, prostate, and breast cancers. Other tumors include gastrointestinal malignancies, renal cell carcinoma, and melanoma.

4. What are chordomas?

Rare, slow growing tumors that arise from notochordal remnants, which explains why most occur near the midline. About half occur in the sacrococcygeal region. Only 10–15% occur elsewhere in the spine (Fig. 2). The remaining 30% occur in the clivus.

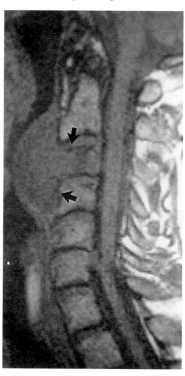

FIGURE 2. Sagittal MR image of chordoma arising from the C2 vertebral body (arrows). The chordoma has projected into the prevertebral soft tissues, compressing the adjacent airway.

5. What are the plain film features of lymphoma in the spine?

The lumbar region is most commonly affected. Lymphoma may appear sclerotic, lytic, or mixed. The classic appearance is a densely sclerotic vertebral body, which is described as "ivory" in appearance. Non-Hodgkin's lymphoma much more commonly affects the spine than does Hodgkin's lymphoma.

6. What is the appearance of an aneurysmal bone cyst in the spine?

The expansile, lytic appearance of an aneurysmal bone cyst (Fig. 3) is similar to giant cell tumors, osteoblastomas, plasmacytomas, and metastases from renal cell cancer, melanoma, and thyroid cancer. These lesions most commonly involve the posterior elements (i.e., the lamina and pedicles) of the vertebrae. The presence of multiseptated cysts with fluid-fluid levels is most characteristic of an aneurysmal bone cyst. The fluid-fluid levels seen on CT or MR represent hemorrhage into the cysts.

7. What are the two most common causes of an aggressive vertebral lesion in an adult older than 40?

Multiple myeloma and metastases.

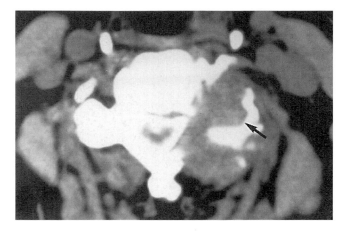

FIGURE 3. This post-myelogram CT of an aneurysmal bone cyst demonstrates an expansile, lytic soft tissue mass arising from the left pedicle and lamina of C5, compressing the thecal sac and displacing it to the right. Hemorrhage may be seen as high-density areas (arrow).

8. A 50-year-old woman with breast cancer presents with normal radiographs and signs and symptoms of spinal cord compression. Has spinal cord compression been excluded?

No. Metastatic lesions can be radiographically occult and can have a significant associated epidural mass and spinal cord compression.

9. What is the best modality for evaluating possible spinal cord compression?

MR, which not only identifies the level of the compression but also the degree of compression (Fig. 4). The same information may be gained from a myelogram followed by a CT myelogram; however, MR has the advantage of being noninvasive. MR also can depict the degree of marrow involvement by tumor, which is often underestimated on CT. Intravenous contrast is helpful in the detection of neoplastic involvement of the spinal cord, nerve roots, and meninges. If metastatic disease to the epidural space is suspected, an unenhanced MR is sufficient.

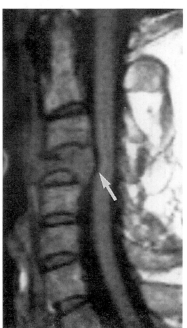

FIGURE 4. Sagittal T1-weighted image of plasmacytoma. Pathologic compression fracture of C3 with mild cord compression (arrow). This is a tumor rather than a benign compression fracture because of the diffuse low signal of the bone marrow, representing tumor infiltration.

10. What is the clinical presentation of spinal cord compression?

Upper motor neuron findings such as extremity weakness may coexist with bladder and bowel dysfunction. Focal back pain suggests focal bony involvement. Hyperreflexia and a sensory level may be noted.

11. Where does the spinal cord end?

Usually at the T12–L1 level. Below L1, any spinal canal compromise affects the cauda equina. As a result, patients with cauda equina compression will present with lower motor neuron symptoms rather than the upper motor neuron symptoms found with spinal cord compression.

12. When is intravenous contrast useful for evaluating spinal lesions or suspected spinal lesions on MR?

For evaluating primary and metastatic epidural tumors, no intravenous contrast is necessary, since there is sufficient contrast between tumor and cerebrospinal fluid. Once a lesion is suspected within the thecal sac (i.e., intradural/extramedullary and intramedullary tumors), gadolinium helps in enhancing the abnormal signal from these lesions, making them more conspicuous.

13. What are common intradural/extramedullary tumors?

Meningiomas, neuromas, and, less commonly, intradural lymphoma and leptomeningeal carcinomatosis.

14. What are the imaging features of spinal meningiomas?

Like intracranial meningiomas, spinal lesions occur primarily in middle-aged and elderly women. These homogeneously enhancing masses occur in the thoracic region or at the level of the foramen magnum (Fig. 5) and have a broad dural base. They commonly calcify and may result in spinal cord compression.

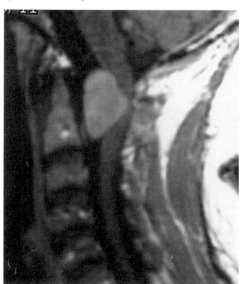

FIGURE 5. This post-contrast MR image of a C1–C2 meningioma demonstrates that this discrete tumor mass (bright ovoid area) arose outside the spinal cord and is compressing and displacing the cord posteriorly.

15. Which spinal tumor can have a dumbbell appearance?

Neuromas. Most neuromas arise from dorsal sensory roots and can occur anywhere along the spinal column. A typical lesion arises in the neural foramen, expanding it, and exhibiting a dumbbell appearance (Fig. 6). This typical appearance is found in only 15% of neuromas; the remaining 85% appear as a nodular, enhancing mass in the thecal sac. A "target" appearance with a hyperintense rim and a hypointense center is often seen.

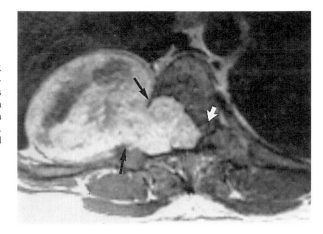

FIGURE 6. T1-weighted axial MR post-contrast image of a right T8 neuroma. Typical dumbbell shape consists of a small intraspinal component and a larger paraspinal mass separated by a widened neural foramen (black arrows). The spinal cord has been compressed and displaced to the left (white arrow).

16. What is the appearance of carcinomatous meningitis?

The intradural nerve roots may be diffusely thickened, clumped, or studded with nodular masses (Fig. 7). The hallmark is the diffuse involvement. The prognosis is poor.

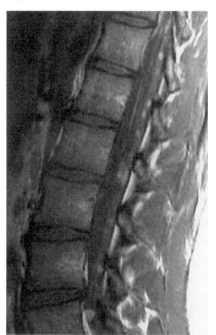

FIGURE 7. Post-contrast sagittal MR image of a leptomeningeal carcinomatosis from small cell carcinoma of the lung. This post-contrast MR image demonstrates multiple small, discrete, enhancing nodular masses scattered throughout the cauda equina.

17. What are the most common intramedullary tumors?

- Ependymoma; more common in the lumbar spine
- Astrocytoma; more common in the cervical spine
- Hemangioblastoma
- Metastases to the spinal cord are very rare; lung and breast are the most common primary sites of metastases.

18. What are the imaging features of an intramedullary mass?

Because these tumors are found in the spinal cord parenchyma, the cord is expanded or distorted in shape. Associated cysts are commonly seen with ependymomas, astrocytomas (Fig. 8), and hemangioblastomas. In hemangioblastomas, the tumor usually consists of a cyst whose wall may contain an intensely enhancing nodule.

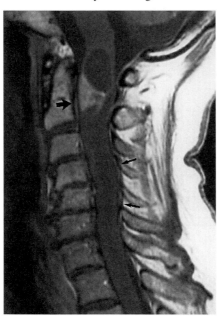

FIGURE 8. Post-contrast sagittal MR image of a cystic astrocytoma at the cervicomedullary junction. An enhancing soft tissue mass (large arrow, bright triangular area) is contiguous with a small cyst (oval dark area). The cord below this mass is abnormally widened by reactive edema (small arrows).

19. A 75-year-old woman with osteoporosis and a history of lung cancer presents with back pain and a fracture of the T10 vertebral body. How can an osteoporotic fracture be differentiated from a pathologic fracture secondary to metastases?

MRI and a radionuclide bone scan can both be helpful. A bone scan showing multiple additional "hot spots" is compatible with metastatic disease, with resultant pathologic fracture. Solitary increased uptake in the fractured vertebra is nonspecific. Increased uptake can persist in elderly patients for up to 2 years, further limiting the usefulness of this finding. MR is ideal for assessing the age of a vertebral fracture; the presence of marrow edema indicates that the fracture is less than 2 months old, while its absence indicates that it is not recent. MR features that favor a malignant etiology of the fracture include abnormal marrow signal in other vertebrae, a convex posterior margin of the vertebral body (i.e., an expanded appearance), and compression of the entire vertebral body, including its posterior third. Features suggesting a benign osteoporotic etiology include normal or mildly abnormal signal in the fractured vertebra, a wedge shape of the vertebral body with sparing of its posterior third, and horizontally oriented low signal paralleling the vertebral body endplate.

BIBLIOGRAPHY

1. Harwood-Nash: Primary neoplasms of the central nervous system in children. Cancer 67:1223, 1991.
2. Lee RR: Spinal tumors. Spine State Art Rev 9:261–283, 1995.
3. Weinstein JN: Differential diagnosis and surgical treatment of primary benign and malignant neoplasms. In Frymoyer JW (ed): The Adult Spine: Principles and Practice, 2nd ed. Philadelphia, Lippincott-Raven, 1997.

VIII. Pediatric Radiology

63. PEDIATRIC CHEST IMAGING

Terry L. Levin, M.D.

1. What is transient tachypnea of the newborn (TTN)?

A cause of respiratory distress in the newborn that occurs in full-term infants within 6 hours of birth and resolves by 3 days of age. The etiology is felt to be retained fetal fluid in the lungs. This theory is supported by its increased incidence in infants delivered by cesarean section, who do not have their lungs "squeezed," as occurs during a normal vaginal delivery. On chest films, there are increased interstitial markings, and the heart size is normal. The lungs are usually slightly hyperinflated (Fig. 1).

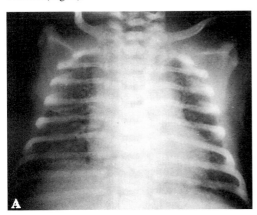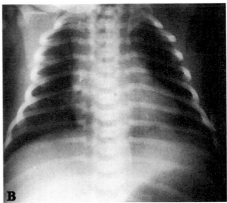

FIGURE 1. Transient tachypnea of the newborn. *A*, Chest radiograph in a full-term infant soon after birth shows increased linear lung markings bilaterally and fluid in the minor fissure. The cardiothymic silhouette is normal in size. *B*, Chest radiograph 6 hours after birth shows marked clearing of the lungs consistent with TTN.

2. What is the cause of respiratory distress syndrome (RDS) in newborns?

Respiratory distress syndrome, or hyaline membrane disease, most commonly affects premature infants. Surfactant, which normally reduces surface tension in the alveoli and prevents end expiratory alveolar collapse, is absent or reduced. Radiographically, the lungs have a granular appearance. Often, the infants require intubation and mechanical ventilation (Fig. 2).

3. What are some complications of respiratory distress syndrome?

"Air-block," or barotrauma, complications result from mechanical ventilation of the stiff lungs of an infant with respiratory distress syndrome. They include
- Pulmonary interstitial emphysema, in which air dissects into the interstitium (Fig. 3)
- Pneumothorax
- Pneumomediastinum
- Pneumopericardium
Bronchopulmonary dysplasia is a long-term complication.

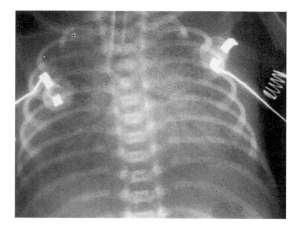

FIGURE 2. RDS. Chest radiograph in a premature infant shows fine uniform granularity distributed symmetrically throughout both lung fields. The baby is intubated.

FIGURE 3. Pulmonary interstitial emphysema. The chest film in this intubated premature infant demonstrates multiple small areas of lucency in the left lung consistent with interstitial air. The heart appears to be in the right chest due to rotation of the infant (note asymmetric appearance of clavicles).

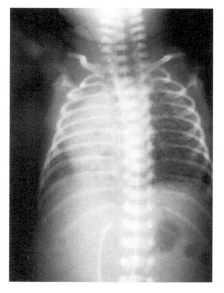

4. What is meant by the "sail sign"?

The sail sign refers to the appearance of the thymus on the frontal film in an infant. Typically, the thymus has a somewhat wavy contour because it is indented by the anterior ribs.

5. What is the typical radiographic appearance of neonatal pneumonia, and what organism causes it?

The radiographic appearance is variable, but patchy or diffuse air-space disease develops. Pleural effusion(s) may occur. The typical responsible organism is group B streptococcus.

6. Which newborns develop meconium aspiration?

Infants who have prolonged or stressful deliveries. Only a relatively small percentage of infants who pass meconium before delivery actually develop clinically significant meconium aspiration. Meconium in the lungs causes a chemical pneumonitis.

7. What is the typical appearance of meconium aspiration?

Hyperinflated lungs with coarse bilateral pulmonary infiltrates (Fig. 4).

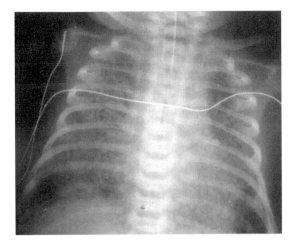

FIGURE 4. Meconium aspiration. Chest radiograph in a full-term infant with a history of a difficult delivery. The coarse bilateral patchy pulmonary infiltrates are typical of meconium aspiration.

8. A frontal chest film of an infant reveals a questionable small pneumothorax. What other views can be obtained to clarify this finding?

A decubitus view, with the side of the patient with the questionable pneumothorax up and the other side down. If this cannot be done, a cross-table lateral can be obtained; the x-ray beam enters the infant on one side—with the infant remaining in the supine position—and the x-ray cassette is placed on the other side.

9. What is the typical clinical and radiographic presentation of Chlamydia pneumonia?

Infants usually present in the first 2 weeks of life. Conjunctivitis is present in 50% of cases. Radiographically there are ill-defined linear markings throughout the lungs, which are hyperinflated.

10. Are congenital diaphragmatic hernias more common on the right or on the left side?

The most common type of congenital diaphragmatic hernia is a left posterolateral hernia, or Bochdalek type hernia. There is resultant herniation of bowel and other abdominal organs into the thorax (Fig. 5).

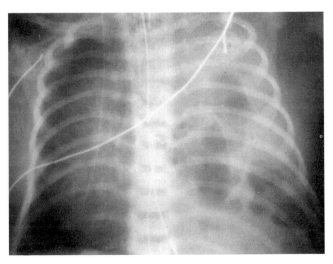

FIGURE 5. Congenital diaphragmatic hernia. Air within bowel loops is present in the left chest in this infant with left-sided CDH. The heart and mediastinum are shifted to the right.

11. What is a congenital cystic adenomatoid malformation (CCAM)?

A hamartomatous lesion of the lung consisting of both solid and cystic elements. The lesion communicates with the tracheobronchial tree. In the newborn period, CCAM may appear as a solid lesion, but as fluid within it is absorbed, it obtains a more air-filled cystic appearance.

12. What are the three types of CCAM?

The three types are classified according to the size of the cysts within it.

Type 1 is the most common type and usually has no associated congenital anomalies. It contains few cysts, which are each larger than 2 cm.

In type 2, which is frequently associated with congenital anomalies, the cysts are more numerous and are smaller than 2 cm.

Type 3 CCAM appears solid but histologically consists of tiny cystic areas.

Most cases of CCAM present in the neonatal period.

13. Which lobe is most commonly affected by congenital lobar emphysema?

The left upper lobe, followed by the right middle lobe and the right upper lobe. Congenital lobar emphysema is the overinflation of a lobe due to a developmental abnormality of the bronchus that supplies that lobe. At birth, the lobe may appear solid on radiographs because it is fluid-filled, but shortly after birth the fluid clears and the lobe appears lucent and expanded (Fig. 6).

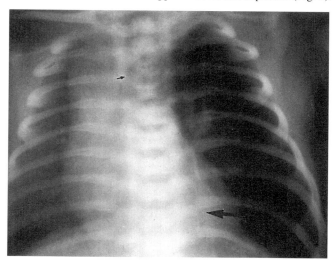

FIGURE 6. Congenital lobar emphysema. The left upper lobe is overexpanded, causing compression of the left lower lobe (large arrow). The hyperexpanded lobe projects over midline (small arrow) and results in shift of the heart and mediastinum to the right.

14. What is the scimitar syndrome?

Also known as hypogenetic lung syndrome, it is a constellation of radiographic findings consisting of a small right lung, a small or absent right pulmonary artery, and a "scimitar" or curvilinear density at the right lung base that represents an anomalous vein that drains all of the right lung or a portion of the right lower lung. The arterial supply to the hypoplastic right lung is systemic (from the aorta).

15. In what location are bronchogenic cysts most common?

In the mediastinum or immediately adjacent to the mediastinum, usually near the carina (Fig. 7). Less commonly, they may occur entirely within the lung. Bronchogenic cysts are often asymptomatic unless they become superinfected.

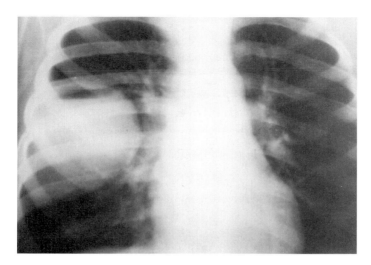

FIGURE 7.   Bronchogenic cyst. The large mass in the right chest represents a bronchogenic cyst. The air-fluid level in the mass indicates communication of the bronchogenic cyst with the tracheobronchial tree.

16. What is the silhouette sign?

On chest films, the margins of the mediastinum, heart, and diaphragm are well demarcated by adjacent air-filled lung. When a portion of the lung becomes nonaerated (due to atelectasis or air-space disease such as pneumonia), the margin of the structure normally demarcated by that area of lung becomes obscured, or silhouetted. For example, the right lower lobe abuts the right hemidiaphragm. If the right lower lobe is opacified, the margin of the right hemidiaphragm will be obscured.

17. Can pneumonia cause abdominal pain?

Yes, occasionally in children a pneumonia that is adjacent to the diaphragm can cause abdominal pain. The lung bases should be carefully examined on abdominal radiographs obtained for abdominal pain.

18. A 3-cm round mass is present in a young child with fever and cough. What is the most likely diagnosis?

Round pneumonia (Fig. 8). The offending organism is usually streptococcus or staphylococcus.

FIGURE 8.   Round pneumonia. Chest radiograph in a child with fever to 101° F: A round mass is present in the left upper lung field, which represents a round pneumonia. The patient received antibiotics and the mass resolved.

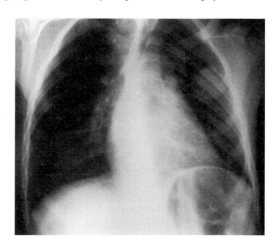

19. What are findings on chest radiographs in children with primary tuberculosis?
- Hilar or mediastinal adenopathy, which is usually unilateral
- Pulmonary parenchymal (air-space) disease
- Pleural disease (effusion)

20. What viral pneumonia can lead to the formation of multiple small calcifications distributed throughout the chest?
Varicella.

21. Who is the typical patient with a spontaneous pneumothorax?
A tall, thin athletic young man in his late teens or 20s. Blebs or bullae may be present at the apices and can "blow out" into the pleural space.

22. What is a pneumatocele?
A thin-walled cyst that may be seen in association with pneumonia (usually staphylococcus), trauma, and hydrocarbon aspiration. They do not represent true cavitary lesions and usually resolve without sequelae.

23. An aspirated foreign body is suspected. Initial chest radiographs are unremarkable. What other imaging studies can be done?
1. An expiratory view. In expiration, the lungs should symmetrically and uniformly decrease in volume, and their density on chest radiographs should therefore be symmetric. In a lobe in which a nonradiopaque foreign body obstructs a bronchus, an expiratory film will demonstrate the presence of air-trapping in the affected lobe.
2. Bilateral decubitus views. Normally, the dependent lung will decrease in volume, but if obstructed, it will air-trap and be larger than the opposite lung on the other decubitus view.
3. Fluoroscopy of the chest. Under real-time observation, air-trapping can be determined.

24. What is acute chest syndrome?
A syndrome that occurs in patients with sickle cell disease. During a crisis, sickling in the pulmonary vasculature causes an outpouring of fluid into the alveoli. Dense areas of lobar consolidation may occur. Superimposed pneumonia cannot be excluded based on the radiographs alone.

25. What is LIP?
Lymphocytic interstitial pneumonia. LIP is characterized by a nodular pattern throughout the lungs. Affected children are usually chronically ill with HIV. The differential diagnosis includes miliary tuberculosis.

26. What are two common types of vascular rings, and how do they present?
Symptomatic vascular rings present with stridor and less commonly with dysphagia. Two common vascular rings are a double aortic arch and a right-sided aortic arch with a left subclavian artery and a persistent ductus.

BIBLIOGRAPHY

1. Blickman JG: Pediatric Radiology—The Requisites. St. Louis, Mosby, 1994.
2. Hilton S, Edwards DK: Practical Pediatric Radiology, 2nd ed. Philadelphia, W.B. Saunders, 1994.
3. Silverman FN, Kuhn J, Girdany B, et al: Essentials of Caffey's Pediatric X-Ray Diagnosis. St. Louis, Mosby, 1990.

64. PEDIATRIC GASTROINTESTINAL RADIOLOGY

M. Patricia Harty, M.D.

1. What is malrotation?

Malrotation is abnormal rotation and fixation of the bowel. During the twelfth week of gestation, the bowel reenters the abdominal cavity and rotates 270 degrees around the axis of the superior mesenteric artery. Normal rotation places the duodenal-jejunal junction (i.e., the ligament of Treitz) in the left upper quadrant and the cecum in the right lower quadrant. The small bowel is anchored on a mesenteric base that extends from the left upper quadrant to the right lower quadrant. If normal rotation does not occur, the duodenal-jejunal junction lies in the midline or right upper quadrant. The cecum lies in the midline or upper abdomen. The base of the small bowel mesentery may extend only several centimeters, allowing the bowel to twist on its mesentery, which can result in midgut volvulus.

2. Why is midgut volvulus a surgical emergency?

As the small bowel twists on a short mesentery, there is obstruction to venous and lymphatic flow, with eventual arterial obstruction. This can occur rapidly, over several hours, and if not surgically repaired all of the bowel supplied by the superior mesenteric artery (from the jejunum to the cecum) will infarct.

3. How does malrotation with volvulus present?

Malrotation may occur at any age, but usually presents in the first few weeks of life. The classic presentation is an infant with bilious vomiting. Bile is found in the vomitus because volvulus usually obstructs the third part of the duodenum, just distal to the ampulla of Vater.

4. Is bilious vomiting always an emergency?

Yes. Duodenal stenosis and distal small bowel obstruction may also present with bilious vomiting. However, volvulus is life-threatening and must be excluded.

5. How is malrotation diagnosed?

An upper gastrointestinal contrast study must be performed if malrotation is suspected, to document the position of the ligament of Treitz. The duodenal-jejunal junction should lie to the left of the spine, at the level of the duodenal bulb (Fig. 1).

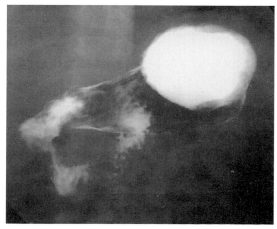

FIGURE 1. Normal upper GI with ligament of Treitz located in the left upper quadrant.

In malrotation, the duodenal-jejunal junction is located in the midline or right upper quadrant. If volvulus is present, there is obstruction of the duodenum, often with a "bird's beak" configuration (Fig. 2).

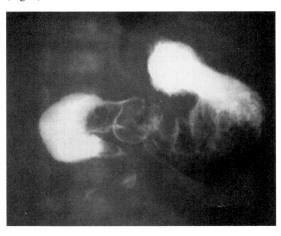

FIGURE 2. Malrotation with volvulus. Transverse duodenum is obstructed, with a "bird's beak" configuration.

6. How is malrotation treated?

Malrotation is treated surgically with a Ladd's procedure.

7. What is intussusception?

Intussusception is one of the most common causes of pediatric bowel obstruction. A proximal section of bowel (the intussusceptum) invaginates into the adjacent distal bowel (the intussuscipiens) and becomes edematous and obstructed (Fig. 3). In a small percentage of cases (about 5%) the intussusceptum contains a lead point such as a Meckel's diverticulum, a polyp, or hypertrophied lymphatic tissue.

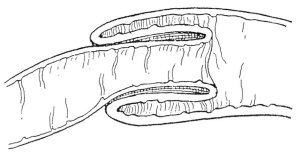

FIGURE 3. Ileocolic intussusception. Diagram shows distal ileum (intussusceptum) invaginating into the colon (intussuscipiens). (From Silverman FN, Kuhn JP: Caffey's Pediatric X-Ray Diagnosis, 9th ed. St. Louis, Mosby, 1993, p 1077, with permission.)

8. Where does intussusception occur?

The most common intussusceptions are ileocolic (the ileum invaginates into the colon) or ileo-ileocolic. Colocolic and ileoileal intussusceptions are infrequent.

9. What are the signs and symptoms of intussusception?

Intussusception is found most commonly in infants and children between three months and four years of age, with the highest incidence between three and nine months. It is more common in boys, and tends to occur most often in the spring and fall. Children present with intermittent, crampy abdominal pain, vomiting, and occasionally fever. The stool may be blood-tinged with mucus, eventually becoming very bloody (which is described as currant jelly stool). Children are often anxious and irritable during the bouts of crampy abdominal pain, and then become apathetic and drowsy.

10. How is intussusception diagnosed?

A plain abdominal radiograph may indicate small bowel obstruction and the intussusception mass may be visible (Fig. 4). However, since the plain film is frequently non-diagnostic, additional imaging is usually required. The intussusception mass is almost always visible on ultrasound.

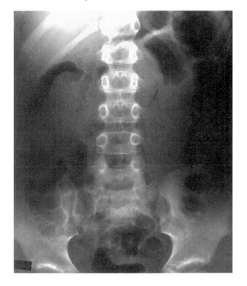

FIGURE 4. Plain abdominal radiograph shows intussusception mass outlined by air in the right upper quadrant.

11. What is the sonographic appearance of an intussusception?

The *donut* and *kidney* signs describe the mass, which is composed of the intussusceptum and the intussuscipiens. The *donut* is the transverse image of the intussusception, and consists of an echogenic center surrounded by a hypoechoic periphery. The *kidney* is the longitudinal view of the intussusception.

12. How is an intussusception treated?

Intussusception is diagnosed or excluded by a contrast enema, and, if present, is also treated at the same time. Before such a study is undertaken, perforation or peritonitis must be excluded. The contrast medium used may be barium, water-soluble contrast, or air. Under fluoroscopic guidance, contrast is introduced slowly into the rectum. If an intussusception is encountered, the pressure generated by the contrast is used in an attempt to "reduce" the intussusception. If air is used the intraluminal pressure used should not exceed 120 mmHg. If a contrast enema is not successful surgery is required.

13. What is the "rule of threes"?

The rule of threes applies to the hydrostatic reduction of an intussusception. The bag containing contrast should be placed no more than three feet above the height of the table, each attempt at reduction should last no more than three minutes. Up to three separate reductions may be attempted.

14. What is the most important indication that a successful hydrostatic reduction of an intussusception has occurred?

Contrast must reflux back into multiple loops of small bowel. Otherwise the intussusception may not have been completely reduced and a distal ileal lead point, such as a Meckel's diverticulum, may have been overlooked.

15. What are the typical presenting features of hypertrophic pyloric stenosis?

Hypertrophic pyloric stenosis is most commonly found in male infants, approximately six weeks of age, who present with progressive projectile vomiting. The vomitus is non-bilious and the infants are often dehydrated on presentation. The hypertrophied pylorus muscle or "olive" may be palpable in the right upper quadrant.

16. How is pyloric stenosis diagnosed?

Pyloric stenosis is frequently diagnosed clinically and is confirmed with ultrasound. Plain abdominal radiographs are of limited value. Therefore ultrasound is the imaging study of choice.

17. What are the sonographic criteria for pyloric stenosis?

The hypertrophied pylorus is identified in the right upper quadrant. The muscle is hypoechoic and the mucosa is echogenic. Various measurements have been reported and the exact numbers are somewhat controversial; however, a pyloric channel length of at least 14 to 17 mm, a mural width of at least 4 mm, and a pyloric diameter of 12 mm are consistent with the diagnosis of pyloric stenosis.

18. What is Hirschsprung's disease?

The absence of ganglion cells in the myenteric and submucosal plexuses in the wall of a portion of the colon. Hirschsprung's disease most commonly involves the rectosigmoid colon (in 70–80% of cases). The entire colon and variable amounts of small bowel may be involved. The agangliotic segment fails to relax, and fecal propulsion is interrupted, leading to a functional obstruction.

19. How does Hirschsprung's disease present?

Most commonly as bowel obstruction in the neonate.

20. How does radiology contribute to establishing the diagnosis?

Plain radiographs show dilated bowel loops, which are frequently filled with stool. A barium enema is the radiologic study of choice. The enema can be used to demonstrate the characteristic finding of a transition zone, which lies between the narrowed aganglionic segment and the distended proximal bowel (Fig. 5). Normally the rectal diameter is similar in size to the cecum; in Hirschsprung's disease, the rectum is narrow. The contrast enema shows the narrow rectal canal, and the larger diameter sigmoid colon. A delayed film at 24 hours is occasionally recommended to show delayed emptying, which may be seen in the disorder.

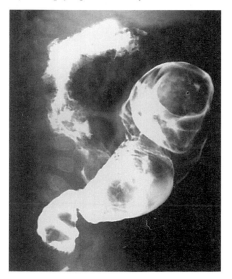

FIGURE 5. Hirschsprung's disease. Lateral radiograph during a barium enema demonstrates the "transition zone" between the narrow rectum and distended sigmoid colon.

21. Does the radiographic transition zone correspond to the histologic transition zone?

The radiologic *transition zone* may lie more distal than the histologic transition zone. Stool may distend the proximal portion of the aganglionic segment. The definitive diagnosis is made by biopsy.

22. What are the types of tracheoesophageal fistulas (TEF), and how common are they?

A. Esophageal atresia (EA) with distal esophageal communication with the tracheobronchial tree accounts for greater than 85% of cases,

  B. Esophageal atresia without a distal communication is the next most common type (5–9%),

  C. "H" type fistulas occur between an otherwise intact trachea and esophagus (2–4%),

  D. Esophageal atresia with both proximal and distal communication with the trachea (1–2%),

  E. Esophageal atresia with proximal communication (1%) is rare (Fig. 6).

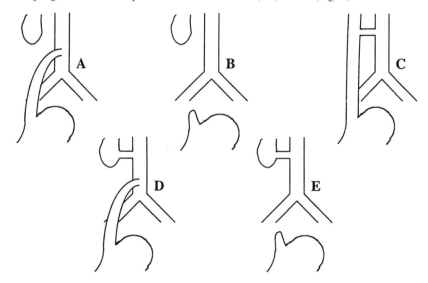

FIGURE 6. Tracheoesophageal anomalies. Esophageal atresia with distal esophageal communication with the tracheobronchial tree (A), esophageal atresia without a distal communication (B), "H" type fistulas between otherwise intact trachea and esophagus (C), esophageal atresia with both proximal and distal communication with the trachea (D), and esophageal atresia with proximal communication (E). (Adapted from Rehbein P: Arch Dis Child 39:131, 1964.)

23. What are the plain film findings in TEF?

Esophageal atresia without a fistula presents with a gasless abdomen. Air or a coiled nasogastric tube may be seen in the proximal esophageal pouch (Fig. 7). Esophageal atresia with proximal TEF also presents with a gasless abdomen. Esophageal atresia with distal TEF and "H" type fistulas may present with a distended abdomen. All patients with esophageal atresia are at risk for aspiration.

24. What is the usual course of the "H" type fistula?

The fistula extends cephalad from the esophagus to the trachea, and occurs most commonly in the lower cervical to upper thoracic trachea.

25. What other anomalies are associated with TEF?

The VACTER spectrum of anomalies: Vertebral anomalies, Anal atresia, Cardiac anomalies, TEF, and Radial and Renal anomalies. Other congenital anomalies are found in approximately 30% of patients with esophageal atresia and TEF, in 17% of infants with esophageal atresia, and in 23% with TEF alone.

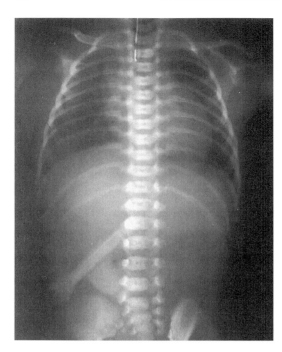

FIGURE 7. Infant with esophageal atresia. No gas is seen in the abdomen and the tip of the NG tube lies in the proximal esophageal pouch.

26. Who is at risk for necrotizing enterocolitis (NEC)?

Premature infants, infants with perinatal stress, and infants with congenital heart disease are at increased risk for NEC. Premature infants account for approximately 80% of patients with NEC.

27. What causes NEC?

Bowel wall ischemia. Factors associated with bowel ischemia include hypoxia, infection, hypoperfusion, stress, umbilical arterial or venous catheterization, and hyperosmolar feedings.

28. What are the plain film findings in NEC?

Since most infants with NEC are too ill to be moved from their beds, plain radiographs are the primary diagnostic imaging tool. The initial radiographic sign is bowel dilatation and straightening of the bowel loops. The characteristic feature of NEC is pneumatosis intestinalis, which is gas within the subserosal or submucosal layers of the bowel wall. Pneumatosis consists of small round or curvilinear lucencies along a segment of bowel. The terminal ileum is the region most frequently involved. Portal venous gas may be seen overlying the liver.

29. What are the complications of NEC?

Bowel perforation and peritonitis. Since patients are usually lying supine, it is important to be aware of the signs of free air on supine radiographs. Free air may be seen under the diaphragm (a *continuous diaphragm* sign may be seen), and in the midline air may be seen outlining the falciform ligament (the *football sign*). Air may be seen on both sides of the bowel wall. On a cross-table lateral, or on a decubitus film, air may be seen between two bowel loops and the peritoneum. Free air requires surgical intervention. Surgery is required to resect necrotic bowel. Strictures commonly develop over time, and the most frequent site for them is the colon.

30. With all the current imaging modalities available, how valuable is the plain abdominal radiograph?

The abdominal film provides a great deal of information. It is important to evaluate the bowel gas pattern, looking for evidence of obstruction, bowel wall edema, and pneumatosis. It is also necessary to look for any evidence of extraluminal gas as in pneumoperitoneum, gas within an abscess cavity, and portal venous or biliary gas. The bones must be examined for the degree of mineralization, and for any evidence of dysplasia, metastases, or fractures. The solid organs and lung bases must also be examined for evidence of organomegaly, pneumonia, and metastases. Radiopaque foreign bodies and abnormal calcifications, such as appendicoliths, calcified tumors, teratomas, and adrenal and pancreatic calcifications must be detected. Plain films are also important for evaluating umbilical, arterial, venous, and inguinal catheter positions.

BIBLIOGRAPHY

1. Kirks DR: Practical Pediatric Imaging: Diagnostic Imaging of Infants and Children, 3rd ed. Philadelphia, Lippincott-Raven, 1997.
2. Fuchs S, Jaffe D: Vomiting. Pediatr Emerg Care 6: 1990.
3. Long FR, Kramer SS, Markowitz RI, et al: Intestinal malrotation in children: Tutorial on radiographic diagnosis in difficult cases. Radiology 198:775–780, 1996.
4. Sheils WE II, Bisset GS III, Kirks DR: Simple device for air reduction of intussusception. Pediatr Radiol 20:472–474, 1990.
5. Silverman FN, et al: Essentials of Caffey's Pediatric X-Ray Diagnosis. St. Louis, Mosby, 1993.
6. Bower AD: The vomiting infant: Recent advances and unsettled issues in imaging. Radiol Clin North Am 26:377–392, 1988.

65. PEDIATRIC URORADIOLOGY

Richard D. Bellah, M.D.

1. What is the role of the radiologist in pediatric urinary tract infection (UTI)?

Urinary tract infections that occur and recur in some children are the result of many interrelated factors, most of which the radiologist cannot assess. Generally speaking, UTI results when bacterial virulence outweighs host resistance. One important factor affecting host resistance that the radiologist can assess is whether there is impairment of unidirectional flow of urine out of the urinary tract, resulting in urinary stasis and predisposing infants and children to UTI.

2. What conditions can be detected radiologically that impair normal urinary flow?

Urinary tract obstruction (congenital), vesicoureteral reflux (VUR), and dysfunctional voiding (e.g., neurogenic bladder) (Fig. 1).

3. Which imaging tests should be used to diagnose these conditions?

Renal and bladder sonography and voiding cystourethrography (VCUG).

4. For what is renal and bladder sonography used?

Renal and bladder sonography should be used to detect hydronephrosis due to obstruction or vesicoureteral reflux, and to assess for any renal parenchymal damage that may have been caused by prior infections.

5. When should renal and bladder sonography be performed?

Sonography should be performed within several weeks after an initial urinary tract infection is diagnosed, but sooner if the child fails to respond to conventional antibiotic therapy. (Also, as a result of the routine use of prenatal sonography, hydronephrosis is often detected in utero, and urinary tract infection can be prevented by prophylactically administering antibiotics to the infant.)

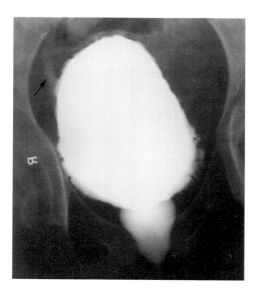

FIGURE 1. Dysfunctional voiding. Fluoroscopic spot view of the bladder and urethra at VCUG show mild bladder wall trabeculation. There is a small amount of vesicoureteral reflux seen on the right (arrow). The urethra has a "spinning top" configuration.

6. How is a voiding cystourethrogram (VCUG) done?

The bladder is catheterized using sterile technique and, under fluoroscopy, the bladder is filled to capacity with iodinated contrast. The catheter is then removed, and the child then voids on the fluoroscopy table. During the procedure, the anatomy of the lower urinary tract and bladder function are examined, a series of radiographic images are obtained, and the presence or absence of reflux of contrast (i.e., vesicoureteral reflux) into the ureters is determined.

7. How is the VCUG modified in infants?

A cyclic study is typically performed. Infants usually void around the small catheter that is placed through the urethra into the bladder; thus multiple cycles of voiding and bladder filling are studied. This also increases the probability that reflux, if present, will be elicited.

8. When should a VCUG be done?

A VCUG should be performed after a first urinary tract infection in both boys and girls, and generally after the bladder infection is treated.

In boys, a routine fluoroscopic VCUG is recommended as the initial examination, particularly to study the urethral anatomy (e.g., to look for valves in the posterior urethra, a common cause of lower urinary tract obstruction in young boys).

In girls, either a routine VCUG can be done or a voiding urethrogram performed by instilling a radionuclide into the bladder. The latter procedure is performed in the nuclear medicine department; images are obtained with a gamma camera, and reflux is detected when the radionuclide (which is diluted in the sterile saline that is placed in the bladder via a catheter) reaches the ureter during the instillation of contrast and/or during voiding.

9. What are the pros and cons of a radionuclide cystogram compared with a fluoroscopic VCUG?

The fluoroscopic VCUG provides anatomic detail but at a much higher radiation dose. The radionuclide cystogram is highly sensitive for detecting reflux because the child is continuously monitored by the gamma camera, but at the expense of good anatomic detail. The radionuclide cystogram is particularly useful for follow-up studies that assess for resolution of previously detected vesicoureteral reflux, and is also useful for screening siblings of patients with known reflux.

10. What is primary vesicoureteral reflux?

Vesicoureteral reflux occurs either primarily or secondarily. Primary reflux is due to "immaturity" or abnormality of the ureterovesical junction that allows urine to ascend into the ureters during bladder filling or voiding. Generally reflux is related to ureteral orifice size as well as the length of the ureter as it tunnels into the bladder.

11. What is secondary vesicoureteral reflux?

Secondary reflux occurs as the result of an abnormality of the ureterovesical junction, such as a distal ureteral diverticulum or a ureterocele (which is an outpouching of the ureter that extends into the bladder). Secondary reflux may also occur as a result of bladder outlet obstruction or due to a neurogenic bladder.

12. How is primary reflux graded?

Primary reflux is graded on a scale from 1 to 5, based on the degree of ureteral and pelvicaliceal (renal collecting system) filling and dilatation (Fig. 2). In addition to providing the referring physi- · cian with a visual description of the degree of reflux, assigning a grade also gives the clinician an idea of the likelihood of spontaneous resolution (e.g., 80% of grade 2 reflux resolves within 3 years).

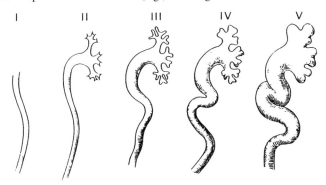

GRADES OF REFLUX

FIGURE 2. Primary vesicoureteral reflux—grading. Reflux is graded according to the degree of ureteral and pelvicaliceal filling. The higher the grade of reflux, the less the likelihood of spontaneous resolution.

13. Is it useful to grade secondary reflux?

Yes, although unlike primary reflux, the grading system does not provide information as to the likelihood of spontaneous resolution of reflux.

14. What is dysfunctional voiding?

Dysfunctional voiding may be due to either a neurogenic bladder or the so-called "pediatric unstable bladder." The bladder may show variable degrees of thickening, trabeculation, and alteration in contour and in storage capacity (see Fig. 1). Bladder-sphincter dyssynergia may be indicated by the presence of a dilated posterior urethra caused by the external sphincter failing to relax as the bladder neck opens. This often leads to high pressure voiding, incomplete emptying, and urine retention.

15. What diagnostic tests are useful in detecting acute and chronic pyelonephritis in children?

Renal cortical scintigraphy (nuclear scan), contrast-enhanced CT, and renal sonography.

Pyelonephritis may be difficult to diagnose accurately, especially in infants and young children who cannot give a history. It may be difficult to distinguish between uncomplicated urinary tract infection and pyelonephritis (with or without subsequent complications such as renal abscess) on the basis of physical examination, history, and laboratory studies. Therefore imaging plays an important role in the workup of children with known or suspected urinary tract infection.

16. What are the findings on a renal nuclear scan in acute and chronic infection?

A renal cortical nuclear scan reveals parenchymal defects in children with acute infection, due to focal areas of edema and inflammation. These revert to normal if the process completely resolves. Residual areas of scar appear as persistent cortical defects on follow-up examinations.

17. What are the CT findings of pyelonephritis?

A contrast-enhanced CT is somewhat less sensitive than a renal cortical nuclear scan for detecting acute infection. Acute infection is seen as wedge-shaped areas of decreased density in the kidney. Areas of scar related to prior infection can also be identified. CT is particularly helpful when abscess formation is suspected.

18. How useful is renal sonography in the workup of suspected pyelonephritis?

Grey-scale sonography is limited in its ability to depict acute pyelonephritis. The sensitivity of ultrasound, however, is increased when power Doppler ultrasound is used (Fig. 3). The latter technique is a relatively new advance in Doppler ultrasound, which depicts normal and abnormal blood flow in a manner that is independent of the direction of the flow; power Doppler is more sensitive than routine color Doppler. Renal sonography may also be used to assess for significant renal scarring due to chronic pyelonephritis.

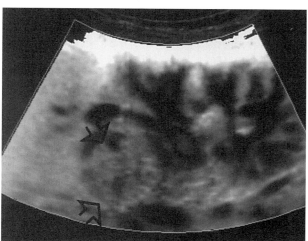

FIGURE 3. Acute pyelonephritis. Power Doppler sonography demonstrates a focal area of decreased perfusion within the upper pole of the kidney (open arrows). This finding corresponds to an area of focal pyelonephritis.

19. Does intravenous urography have a role in the diagnosis of acute pyelonephritis?

No, but it does have a slightly greater sensitivity for detecting renal scars from chronic pyelonephritis than does renal sonography.

20. What are the most common forms of congenital hydronephrosis?

- Ureteropelvic junction (UPJ) obstruction
- Ureterovesical junction (UVJ) obstruction, (commonly referred to as primary obstructive megaureter)
- Vesicoureteral reflux
- Renal and ureteral duplication anomalies
- Posterior urethral valves
- Prune belly syndrome

21. When should a postnatal renal and bladder sonogram be obtained in congenital hydronephrosis?

A postnatal renal and bladder sonogram should be performed on any infant with dilatation of the renal pelvis that is detected prenatally on sonography, if the renal pelvis measures ≥ 4 mm before 33 weeks and ≥ 7 mm after 33 weeks of gestation. A renal pelvic diameter less than 4 mm seen on sonography at birth has been shown to normalize spontaneously within one year. In boys with bilateral hydroureteronephrosis, this sonogram should be done soon after birth, to assess for posterior urethral valves. Otherwise the initial sonogram should be done at 5–7 days after birth (when the glomerular filtration rate is greater than immediately after birth).

22. What are the roles of nuclear medicine, voiding cystourethrography, and intravenous urography in congenital hydronephrosis?

A VCUG should be performed to assess for reflux, and to determine if posterior urethral valves are present (in boys). Utilization of nuclear renal scintigraphy and intravenous urography varies from patient to patient and from institution to institution. Renal scintigraphy provides quantitative information regarding the effect of obstruction on renal function; for example, the function of the obstructed kidney can be compared with the opposite kidney, before and after surgical treatment. The intravenous urogram provides less quantitative information but provides better anatomic detail. It serves best as a "road map" for the surgeon and gives information about anatomy and function following surgery.

23. What are posterior urethral valves?

At the distal end of the verumontanum, several folds, or plicae, arise and pass caudally to encircle a portion of the membranous urethra. These plicae occur normally and vary in the extent to which they encircle the urethra. When they fuse anteriorly they form the most common type of posterior urethral valves (Type 1) (Fig. 4). Type 2 posterior urethral valves are mucosal folds that extend from the proximal end of the verumontanum toward the bladder neck; their very existence is controversial. Type 3 valves refer to a urethral diaphragm that occurs below the caudal end of the verumontanum.

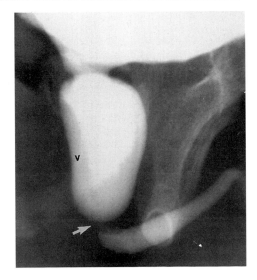

FIGURE 4. Posterior urethral valves. Fluoroscopic spot view shows dilated posterior urethra. Valves (arrows) are identified at the distal end of the verumontanum (v).

24. How are posterior urethral valves detected?

The most common cause of bladder outlet obstruction in infant boys, posterior urethral valves cause changes in the bladder that are detected by sonography and cystography. They include enlargement, thickening, sacculation, and trabeculation of the bladder. Dilatation of the posterior (prostatic) urethra above the valve can be seen on both prenatal and postnatal sonograms, as well as on a VCUG. Hydroureteronephrosis is often present, either due to reflux or due to high pressures in the bladder. If rupture of a caliceal fornix occurs, urinary ascites and/or a urinoma can develop. Posterior urethral valves are confirmed cystoscopically and are treated with fulguration or incision.

25. What is primary obstructive megaureter?

Congenital obstruction at the ureterovesical junction, which occurs more commonly than was previously realized. Primary megaureter results from an abnormal proportion of muscle fibers and fibrous tissue in the distal-most 3–4 cm of the ureter. The degree of obstruction is variable and seems to improve in many cases over time. Most often, this condition is detected incidentally on prenatal sonography. Postnatal sonography and urography reveal a variable degree of dilatation of the ureter and collecting system on the affected side (Fig. 5). Occasionally a short narrow segment of ureter may be seen through sonography at the ureterovesical junction. The VCUG typically shows absence of reflux (although reflux may be present in 10% of cases).

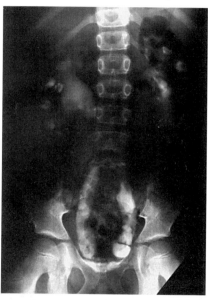

FIGURE 5.   Primary obstructive megaureter. Intravenous urogram shows mild bilateral pelvi-caliectasis. There is moderate ureterectasis most significant in the distal one-half of the ureters.

26. What are common forms of a duplex kidney?

A duplex kidney (duplication of the kidney, collecting system, and ureters) arises from abnormal development of the ureteric bud. Although various degrees of duplication may be present, in the full blown condition the kidney is large and there are separate collecting systems and ureters that drain the upper and lower poles of the kidney.

27. What is the "Weigert-Meyer" rule?

According to this rule, when there is a complete duplication, the lower pole ureter inserts normally into the bladder, and the upper pole ureter inserts ectopically into the bladder medially and to the insertion of the upper pole ureter caudally.

28. Are the collecting systems and ureters dilated in a duplicated system?

The appearance depends on whether there is reflux into the lower pole ureter, and the exact site of the ectopically inserting upper pole ureter. In the typical situation (which is often bilateral), the distal ureters are contained within a common sheath and either come together or insert separately, but are close together in the trigone of the bladder. If the upper pole ureter is associated with a ureterocele (a localized dilatation of the distal ureter), the ureterocele can protrude through the bladder to the urethra and present as a perineal mass. If a ureterocele is present, the upper pole of the kidney may be obstructed (the so-called "drooping lily" effect on the lower pole collecting system), or may be small and dysplastic (causing little or no effect on the lower pole). If a ureterocele is not present, the upper pole moiety may insert in an ectopic location and have a stenotic insertion, causing obstruction (boys and girls) or may present with urinary dribbling (girls only) due to an ectopic insertion into the urethra, vagina, or perineum.

29. What is the most common scrotal mass?

The most common cause of a scrotal mass is probably a hydrocele, which is a collection of fluid outside the testicle, and within the tunica vaginalis, which may be congenital, or may be associated with trauma, torsion, or hemorrhage.

30. What are the main differential considerations of a painful scrotum?

Testicular torsion and epididymitis/orchitis. Testicular torsion is a surgical emergency, and can be confirmed or excluded either with color Doppler ultrasound or with a nuclear scan (using technetium pertechnetate as the radiopharmaceutical). Epididymitis is much more common in the postpubescent male than in younger children, and is identified on sonography by swelling of and increased flow in the epididymis. The cause of epididymitis is often bacterial, and there may be associated infection in the testicle.

31. If epididymitis is present in an infant, what should be suspected as the etiology?

Epididymitis is rare in infants and is usually associated with an anatomic abnormality of the genitourinary system, such as a dysplastic ureter. Renal and bladder sonography as well as a VCUG are therefore indicated.

32. What is the most common testicular tumor in children?

Yolk sac tumors. They occur more frequently than teratomas and are seen primarily during the first two years of life. Most children with yolk sac tumors have elevated AFP levels, whereas those with teratomas do not.

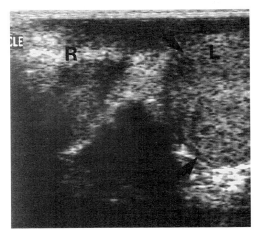

FIGURE 6. Testicular germ cell tumor. Transverse sonogram of the scrotum in an infant shows a normal right (R) testis and massive enlargement of the left (L) testis (arrows).

33. What are the most common testicular tumors in adolescents?

These are also germ cell tumors, but the most common histologic types are seminomas, choriocarcinomas, teratocarcinomas, and tumors with mixed histologies.

34. What urinary problems occur in children with spina bifida?

There is an increased incidence of renal anomalies in children with myelomeningocele, including fusion anomalies (e.g., a horseshoe kidney), renal dysplasia, and agenesis. The most significant problems, however, relate to the abnormal innervation of the bladder.

35. What are the specific problems in spina bifida that are related to the neurogenic bladder?

The neurogenic bladder (Fig. 7) fails to store urine correctly, does not empty properly due to bladder-sphincter dyssynergia, and experiences uninhibited contractions. High-storage pressures result in reflux and hydronephrosis.

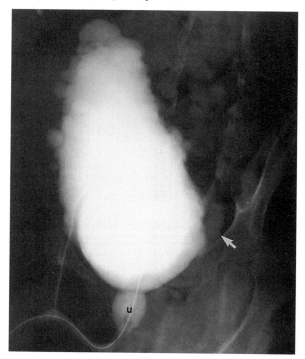

FIGURE 7. Neurogenic bladder. VCUG in patient with meningomyelocele shows a "pine-cone" bladder with marked trabeculation and sacculation. When patient attempts to void, there is dilatation of the posterior urethra (u) with contraction of the external sphincter. A small amount of reflux is seen in the distal left ureter (arrow).

36. What are the goals of therapy for urinary tract dysfunction in spina bifida?

The goals are to decrease storage pressure, either with frequent intermittent catheterization, vesicostomy, and/or bladder augmentation, and to keep the patient "dry" through continent diversion. Cystography is performed to assess bladder size, storage capacity, the volume at which leakage occurs, and to detect any reflux. Renal and bladder sonography are routinely performed every six months to assess for hydronephrosis, stones, and the ability of the patient to empty the bladder with self-catheterization.

37. What is the triad of prune-belly syndrome?

Absent or deficient abdominal musculature, cryptorchidism, and urinary tract abnormalities (Fig. 8).

38. What are the urinary tract abnormalities associated with prune-belly syndrome?

They are diverse, and include marked hydroureteronephrosis as well as marked bladder and urethral dilatation, reflux, renal dysplasia, prostatic hypoplasia, urachal abnormalities, and microphallus. The clinical features often parallel the degree of urinary tract involvement. Newborns with severe renal dysplasia may have Potter's syndrome (oliogohydramnios, pulmonary hypoplasia). Children with urinary tract dilatation and/or reflux need to be closely monitored for infection.

39. What is a basic classification for cystic kidney diseases affecting infants, children, and adolescents?

Cystic renal diseases can be classified as genetic or non-genetic. The most common cause of non-genetic cystic disease is multicystic dysplastic kidney (MCDK).

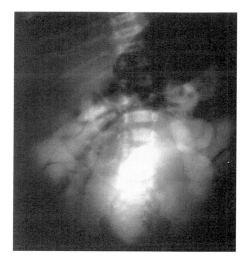

FIGURE 8. Prune-belly syndrome. VCUG demonstrates megacystis as well as bilateral pelvicaliectasis and ureterectasis with significant ureteral tortuousity.

40. What is the most common sonographic appearance of multicystic dysplastic kidney?

Most commonly, MCDK is the result of atresia of the renal pelvis, and the kidney appears on sonography as multiple cysts of varying sizes which do not communicate with each other; there is no definable renal pelvis. The less common form is the hydronephrotic form which has a central renal cyst. MCDK is associated with other abnormalities of the urinary tract, especially a contralateral ureteropelvic junction obstruction, and contralateral vesicourethral reflux.

41. What are the other forms of non-genetic cystic renal disease?

Simple renal cyst (rare in children), medullary cystic disease, caliceal diverticulum, and cystic renal dysplasia (associated with urinary tract obstruction).

42. What are the genetic forms of cystic renal disease?

Autosomal dominant polycystic kidney disease (ADPCKD), autosomal recessive polycystic kidney disease (ARPCKD), glomerulocystic kidney disease, congenital nephrosis, and cystic kidney disease associated with syndromes (e.g., tuberous sclerosis).

43. Does "adult-type" autosomal dominant polycystic kidney disease occur in infants and young children?

ADPCKD has been recognized at sonography both pre- and postnatally. The appearance can closely mimic that of autosomal recessive polycystic kidney disease, in which both kidneys can appear large and echogenic. Small, sonographically resolvable cysts can be seen in either syndrome in the newborn period. More commonly, autosomal dominant polycystic kidney disease is suspected if sonography reveals progressive development of multiple cortical and medullary renal cysts. This may be found incidentally, or in a child referred for hypertension and hematuria. Careful family history as well as sonographic screening of the family is recommended to detect any evidence of cystic kidney disease in parents who may be unaware of their own subclinical disease.

44. What imaging findings may help distinguish autosomal dominant polycystic kidney disease from autosomal recessive polycystic kidney disease, in the infant or young child (Fig. 9)?

The renal sonographic appearances of the two syndromes can be quite similar. The kidneys are often large and echogenic with each type. Careful inspection with sonography can occasionally detect tubular ectasia in echogenic renal pyramids, which is typical of autosomal recessive polycystic kidney disease. Sonographically resolvable cysts are more suggestive of autosomal dominant disease. Additionally, the liver should be examined for abnormal echotexture due to hepatic fibrosis and biliary ectasia, which is often associated with autosomal recessive disease. In adolescents with

ARPCKD, the renal involvement is less marked than the liver disease, which causes portal hypertension and splenomegaly. Excretory urography (or CT) can occasionally be helpful to distinguish the recessive disease from the dominant disease. In the former, there is delay and prolongation of the nephrogram; the contrast is taken up by dilated tubules and has a spoked wheel appearance. These findings are typically absent in the dominant disease in which excretion is prompt.

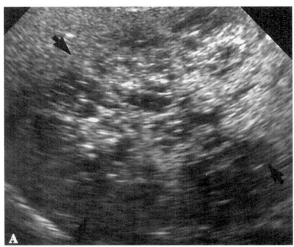

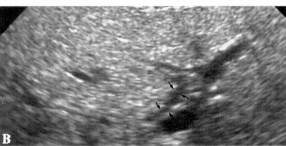

FIGURE 9. Autosomal recessive polycystic kidney disease. *A*, Sagittal sonogram of the right kidney (arrows) shows marked enlargement with heterogeneous echogenicity. Small (1 mm) cystic elements are seen within the renal parenchyma. *B*, Transverse sonogram of liver: parenchyma shows increased liver echotexture due to hepatic fibrosis. Minimal ectasia of the intrahepatic biliary tree (small arrows) can be seen adjacent to left portal vein.

45. What are five hereditary syndromes associated with renal cysts?

Tuberous sclerosis, von Hippel-Lindau, Zellweger's (cerebro-hepato-renal) syndrome, Jeune's syndrome (thoracic asphyxiating dystrophy), and Meckel-Gruber syndrome.

46. What conditions cause echogenic renal pyramids in the infant?

Nephrocalcinosis (due to renal tubular acidosis, hypercalcemia, or furosemide therapy), renal tubular ectasia (ARPCKD), and Tamm-Horsfall protein deposition (transient phenomenon).

47. What is the most common solid renal mass in infants?

The fetal renal hamartoma, also known as the mesoblastic nephroma. Infants usually present with a palpable renal mass. Hematuria, hypertension, and hypercalcemia may also be present. The tumor is composed of monotonous sheets of spindle-shaped cells and usually occupies most of the kidney. The tumor appears large and solid at sonography. The mass is usually resected, and the prognosis is excellent. Less common causes of solitary renal masses in infants include nephroblastomatosis and the malignant rhabdoid tumor.

48. What is the role of imaging infants with ambiguous genitalia?

Evaluation is indicated when the testes cannot be palpated and when there is severe hypospadias, incomplete scrotal fusion, fused labia, a micropenis, or clitoral enlargement. These conditions can be classified as true hermaphroditism, female pseudohermaphroditism, male pseudohermaphroditism, and gonadal dysgenesis, depending on further clinical, laboratory, and surgical investigations. Sonography is the simplest method of identifying the internal anatomy by identifying the presence or absence of a uterus and gonads. This is usually combined with a retrograde genitogram performed under fluoroscopy, that further defines the relationship of the urogenital sinus to the urethra and vagina (Fig. 10).

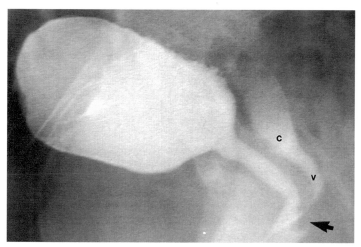

FIGURE 10.   Urogenital sinus in ambiguous genitalia. Retrograde genitogram shows low confluence (arrow) of urethra and the vagina (v) and cervical impression (c).

49. What is nephroblastomatosis?

Multiple or diffuse rests of nephrogenic tissue. They are persistent embryonal remnants in the kidney that are apparent precursors to Wilms' tumor. The involved kidneys are typically enlarged and have a lobulated configuration. Ultrasound, CT, and MR can be used to identify and follow children with nephroblastomatosis (Fig. 11). There are several conditions where children may have

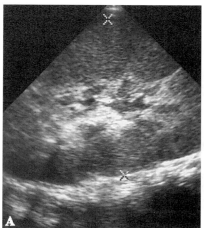
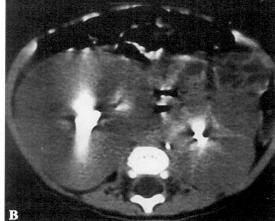

FIGURE 11.   Nephroblastomatosis. *A*, Sonogram of the right kidney shows significant renal enlargement with loss of normal cortical medullary differentiation (the left kidney had a similar appearance). *B*, Computed tomography (enhanced) demonstrates loss of normal intrarenal architecture with diffuse infiltration of both kidneys by intralobar nephroblastomatosis.

nephroblastomatosis and can develop Wilms' tumor: hemihypertrophy, Drash syndrome (pseudoher-maphrotidism), aniridia, and a positive family history of Wilms' tumor/nephroblastomatosis.

50. What are the two major types of nephroblastomatosis?

Perilobar and intralobar. The perilobar form is limited to the periphery of the kidney, while the intralobar form can be found anywhere within a renal lobe as well as within the renal pelvis and collecting system. Nephroblastomatosis may remain dormant, mature, involute, develop hyperplastic overgrowth, or become neoplastic (Wilms' tumor).

51. How can nephroblastomatosis be distinguished from a Wilms' tumor?

With difficulty. Generally, a Wilms' tumor is suggested when a lesion noted by either ultrasound or CT is greater than 3 cm and has a spherical configuration. Many lesions previously thought to be small or medium-sized Wilms' tumors, especially in cases of bilateral or multicentric tumor, may actually represent hyperplastic nephroblastomatosis. Biopsy is of limited value in distinguishing the hyperplastic form from Wilms' tumor, and serial imaging is critical in determining whether surgery should be performed.

52. What is the Mayer-Rokitansky-Kuster-Hauser syndrome?

Vaginal atresia with other variable mullerian duct abnormalities such as a bicornuate or septated uterus. The fallopian tubes, ovaries, and broad ligaments are normal. Unilateral renal or skeletal anomalies are associated in 50% and 12% of cases, respectively.

53. How is pelvic sonography utilized in the evaluation of the child with precocious puberty?

Uterine and ovarian volumes are larger than normal in true isosexual precocious puberty, whereas enlargement of only the ovary has been reported with pseudosexual precocity. True isosexual precocity is due to the premature activation of the hypothalamic pituitary gonadal axis, while pseudosexual precocity refers to pubertal changes occurring independent of these actions, as in the case of a functional ovarian cyst or tumor. Multiple small (less than 1 cm) cysts can be seen in the ovaries of normal children, as well as in children who have precocious puberty. However, the best predictor of true precocious puberty is bilateral ovarian enlargement, while unilateral ovarian enlargement associated with larger cysts is more related to pseudosexual precocity.

BIBLIOGRAPHY

1. Beckwith JB: Precursor lesions of Wilms' tumor: Clinical and biological implications. Med Pediatr Oncol 21:158–168, 1993.
2. Bjorgvinsson E, Majd M, Eggli KD: Diagnosis of acute pyelonephritis in children: Comparison of sonography and Tc99m-DMSA scintigraphy. AJR 157:539–543, 1991.
3. Blickman JG, Lebowitz RL: The coexistence of primary megaureter and reflux. AJR 143:1053–1057, 1984.
4. Corteville JE, Gray DL, Crane JP: Congenital hydronephrosis: Correlations of fetal ultrasonographic findings with infant outcome. Am J Obstet Gynecol 165:384, 1991.
5. Cremin BJ: A review of ultrasonic appearances of posterior urethral valves and ureteroceles. Pediatr Radiol 16:357–364, 1986.
6. Fotter R, Kopp W, Skein E, Hollwarth M, Uray E: Unstable bladder in children: Functional evaluation by modified voiding cystography. Radiology 161:811–813, 1986.
7. Greskovich FJ III, Nyberg LM Jr: The prune belly syndrome: A review of its etiology, defects, treatment and prognosis. J Urol 140:707–712, 1988.
8. Jain M, LeQuesne GW, Bourne AJ, Henning P: High-resolution ultrasonography in the differential diagnosis of cystic diseases of the kidney in infancy and childhood: Preliminary experience. J Ultrasound Med 16:235–240, 1997.
9. Kaplan BS, Kaplan P, Rosenberg HK, et al: Polycystic kidney diseases in childhood. J Pediatr 115:867–879, 1989.
10. King LR, Siegel MJ, Solomon AL: Usefulness of ovarian volume and cysts in female isosexual precocious puberty. J Ultrasound Med 12:577–581, 1993.
11. Lebowitz RL, Mandell J: Urinary tract infection in children: Putting radiology in its place. Radiology 165:1–9, 1987.

12. Nunn IN, Stephens FD: The triad syndrome: A composite anomaly of the abdominal wall, urinary system, and testes. J Urol 86:782–794, 1961.
13. Rosenberg HK, Sherman NH, Tarry WF, et al: Mayer-Rokitansky-Kuster-Hauser syndrome: US aid and diagnosis. Radiology 161:815–819, 1986.
14. Saxton HM, Borzyskowski M, Mundy AR, Vivian GC: Spinning top urethra: Not a normal variant. Radiology 168:147–150, 1988.
15. Sutherland RS, Mevorach RA, Baskin LS, Kogan BA: Spinal dysraphism in children: An overview and an approach to prevent complications. Urology 46:294–304, 1995.

66. PEDIATRIC SKELETAL RADIOLOGY

Terry L. Levin, M.D., and Kevin R. Math, M.D.

1. What is the Salter-Harris classification for fractures?

A classification that refers to fractures that involve the growth plate. It has both descriptive and prognostic utility (Fig. 1).

I	II	III	IV	V

 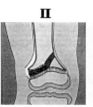 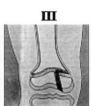 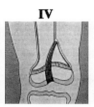 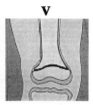

| fracture through growth plate | fracture through growth plate and metaphysis | fracture through growth plate and epiphysis | fracture through growth plate, metaphysis, and epiphysis | compression fracture through growth plate |

FIGURE 1. Salter-Harris Classification of epiphyseal-metaphyseal fractures involving the growth plate.

Salter-Harris	Description
I	Fracture through the growth plate at the zone of hypertrophied cartilage
II	Extends through the growth plate and involves the metaphysis
III	Extends through the growth plate and epiphysis
IV	Extends through the epiphysis, growth plage, and metaphysis
V	Crush injury of the growth plate; carries the worst prognosis

See question 12 in Chapter 70.

2. What is a toddler's fracture?

A spiral fracture of the distal tibia. This injury is common in young children and occurs once the child starts walking.

3. What is the implication of a displaced anterior fat pad at the elbow in the setting of trauma?

Elevation of the anterior fat pad or visualization of the posterior fat pad implies intraarticular fluid. In the setting of trauma, a fracture should be suspected and sought. If no fracture is identified, the child's elbow should be immobilized for 7–10 days, and then radiographs should be repeated to assess for occult fracture. Alternatively, nuclear imaging or MRI can be used immediately following normal radiographs if an immediate diagnosis will alter management.

4. What is the anterior humeral line?

A longitudinal line drawn tangent to the anterior shaft of the humerus should intersect the middle or posterior third of the capitellum of the distal humerus. If this line intersects the anterior third or the junction of the anterior and middle thirds, a supracondylar fracture of the distal humerus should be suspected. A positive "fat pad sign" clinches the diagnosis.

5. Why do most cases of "nursemaid's elbow" present with normal radiographs?

Nursemaid's elbow, or anterior subluxation of the proximal radius, results from excessive traction and torsion force applied to the hand and forearm. Routine radiographs of the elbow require the radiologic technologist to flex and pronate the elbow, the same technique required to manually reduce this injury. Therefore, the technologist often treats the child in addition to providing radiographs.

6. What is pseudosubluxation of the cervical spine?

Pseudosubluxation refers to the normal forward movement of C2 on C3 and less commonly of C3 on C4, which occurs with flexion. This finding is not uncommon in children, is due to relative ligamentous laxity, and is not seen in adults.

7. What is Blount's disease and how is it treated?

Blount's disease, or tibia vara, is a growth disturbance affecting the medial aspect of the proximal tibial metaphysis, resulting in varus deformity at the knee(s). It has two peaks of occurrence: in infancy and adolescence. Infantile tibia vara is usually bilateral and is most commonly diagnosed between age 1 and 3 (Fig. 2). Adolescent tibia vara is usually unilateral, affecting children 8–15 years of age. The adolescent form is less common and usually less severe than the infantile form. The growth disturbance may result in unilateral or bilateral tibial bowing. Although spontaneous resolution may occur, tibial osteotomy may be required for treatment.

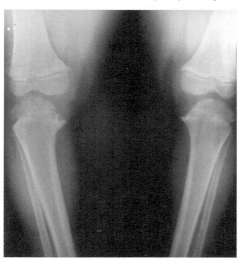

FIGURE 2. Blount's disease. Bilateral tibia vara deformity is present. There is irregularity, inferior displacement, and beaking of the medial aspect of the proximal tibial metaphyses. The medial aspect of the proximal tibial epiphyses are hypoplastic.

8. What is Legg-Calvé-Perthe disease?

Idiopathic avascular necrosis of the femoral head, most commonly affecting children aged 4–8. It is more common in males and rare in blacks. Children may present with a limp or limited range of motion or sometimes knee pain. The condition is bilateral in 10% of cases. Radiographic findings include abnormal mineralization of the capital femoral epiphysis. There also may be a relative decrease in the size of the involved capital femoral epiphysis relative to the normal hip and also a relative widening of the medial joint space. Eventually, characteristic findings of a crescent sign and sclerosis, flattening, and fragmentation of the epiphysis may ensue (Fig. 3). This disease often results in deformity of the femoral head and early-onset osteoarthritis.

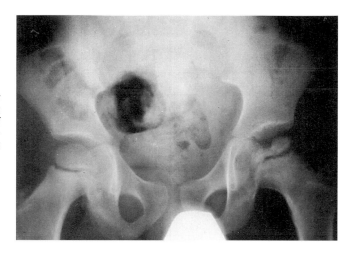

FIGURE 3. Anteroposterior view of the pelvis demonstrates fragmentation and irregularity of the left femoral head in this patient with Legg-Calvé-Perthes disease. The right hip is normal.

9. At what age do the capital femoral epiphyses ossify?
At 3–6 months.

10. What is DDH?
Developmental dysplasia of the hip. Formerly called CDH (congenital dislocation of the hip), DDH is thought to have genetic and developmental etiologies. DDH is more common in girls than boys, has a predilection for involvement of the left hip, and is bilateral in the minority of cases.

11. What complications may develop as a result of failure to promptly diagnose DDH?
Normal development of the hip joint requires the capital femoral epiphysis to be well-seated within the acetabulum. Failure to diagnose DDH will cause dysplasia of the acetabulum with the acetabular line appearing "shallow" (vertically oriented). Furthermore, the femoral head and neck may become malformed. These abnormal articular surfaces will eventually result in secondary deformity and degenerative joint disease, requiring complex osteotomies and sometimes total joint arthroplasty.

12. What are the limitations of conventional radiographs for the diagnosis of DDH?
Since the capital femoral epiphyses do not ossify until 3–6 months, they are radiographically invisible in early infancy, and their location relative to the acetabula must be inferred by assessing the location of the ossified femoral necks. Furthermore, radiographs provide a static assessment of the hip and will not detect dynamic abnormalities.

Plain film findings of DDH in an infant include lateral (and often superior) dislocation/displacement of the proximal femora relative to the acetabula, delay in ossification of the capital femoral epiphysis of the involved femur (Fig. 4), and a shallow acetabulum.

13. What imaging modality is most effective for evaluating suspected DDH?
In experienced hands, ultrasound is highly effective at diagnosing DDH, providing dynamic assessment of the hip through its range of motion. Ortolani and Barlow maneuvers, useful on physical examination, can be combined with ultrasound assessment to provocatively evaluate the dislocatable hip. Absolute measurements of acetabular dysplasia can be provided on ultrasound, and the hip can be serially evaluated during treatment to confirm normal alignment and development.

14. How often is slipped capital femoral epiphysis bilateral?
About 25% of the time. SCFE is more common in boys than girls and predominates in overweight adolescents around the time of the pubertal growth spurt. The epiphysis typically "slips" posteriorly and medially relative to the femoral neck resulting in the appearance of a scoop of ice cream falling off an ice cream cone (Fig. 5).

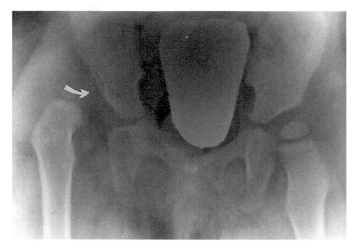

FIGURE 4. Developmental dysplasia of the hip. There is dislocation of the right hip with superior and lateral displacement of the right femoral shaft. The right femoral head is small and the right acetabulum is shallow. A pseudo-acetabulum is present (arrow).

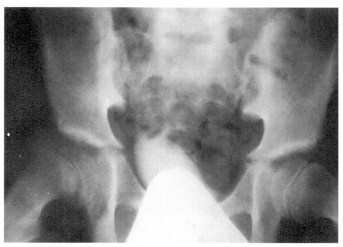

FIGURE 5. Slipped capital femoral epiphysis. The right femoral head is displaced medially and posteriorly relative to the right femoral shaft.

15. What are the complications of SCFE?

Osteonecrosis of the femoral head, the most common complication, increases in incidence with greater degrees of displacement and occurs in up to 25% of cases. Chondrolysis, manifested by narrowing of the joint space within 1 year following the initial injury, is exceedingly rare. Secondary osteoarthritis may occur in early adulthood.

16. What predisposing factors result in an increased incidence of SCFE?

- Rickets/osteomalacia
- Prior radiation therapy, with the hip included in the radiation port
- Hypothyroidism
- Growth hormone therapy

17. What is Caffey's disease?

Caffey's disease, or infantile cortical hyperostosis, is a rare condition of unknown etiology. It is characterized by periosteal new bone formation and cortical thickening in one or more bones, characteristically involving the mandible, clavicles, and upper ribs. The long bones are less commonly involved.

18. What is rickets? Describe its radiographic findings.

Rickets is a failure of mineralization of growing bones. The earliest findings include "fraying and splaying" of the end of the metaphysis and eventual relative widening of the growth plate and metaphyseal cupping. This is due to inadequate mineralization at the zone of provisional calcification and resultant radiolucent unmineralized osteoid. Radiographically, changes are most evident at the ends of rapidly growing bones, such as in the knee and wrist.

19. In hypothyroidism, is bone maturation normal, delayed, or advanced?

Hypothyroidism results in delayed skeletal maturation. Epiphyseal ossification is delayed, irregular, or both.

20. What disease is marked by absence of the clavicles?

Cleidocranial dysostosis. In this condition, the clavicles may be partially or completely absent. Other features include wormian (intrasutural) bones in the skull, a marked delay in ossification of the pubic bones—resulting in the appearance of a widened pubic symphysis—and coxa vara (varus alignment at the hips).

21. What is vertebra plana? What is its differential diagnosis?

Vertebra plana is flattening of one or multiple vertebral bodies. Differential diagnostic considerations include Langerhans histiocytosis (eosinophilic granuloma), leukemia, lymphoma, and storage diseases.

22. What is the most common location of chondroblastoma within a bone?

These benign bone tumors arise in the epiphysis and may extend into the adjacent metaphysis.

23. What is the most common location and radiographic findings of osteosarcoma?

Osteosarcoma occurs most commonly at the knee, including the proximal tibia and distal femur. Osteosarcomas are malignant, bone-producing tumors, resulting in a characteristic mass with cotton-ball appearing homogeneous bony density. Periosteal new bone and a soft tissue mass are also common (Fig. 6).

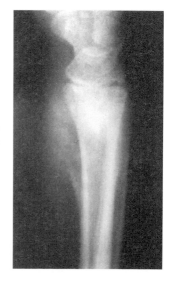

FIGURE 6. There is a dense lesion in the distal metaphysis of the radius with associated bony matrix, periosteal new bone formation, and a soft tissue mass. These findings are typical of osteosarcoma.

24. What are the typical bony findings of sickle cell disease?

These findings reflect the ischemia and infarction that occur as a result of red blood cell sickling. Medullary bone infarctions occur in the shafts of long bones, manifested by a focal oval lesion with serpiginous peripheral calcification. Avascular necrosis of the femoral head or humeral head is also common. The vertebral body endplates have a characteristic concavity or central depression (Fig. 7) secondary to impaired blood supply by the vessels supplying the central portions of the vertebral bodies. This gives rise to "H-shaped" vertebrae. Osteomyelitis, particularly from Salmonella, may complicate the radiographic findings (Fig. 8).

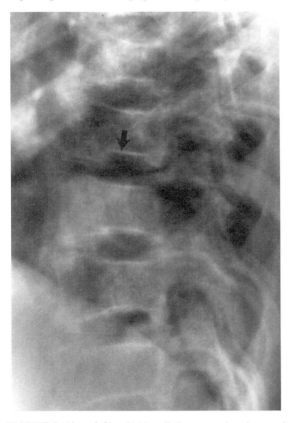 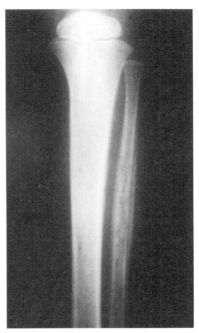

FIGURE 8 (Above right). Anteroposterior view of the tibia and fibula in a patient with sickle cell disease and secondary Salmonella osteomyelitis of the mid-fibula. The findings are indistinguishable from a bone infarction without infection.

FIGURE 7 (Above left). Sickle cell disease—spine changes. Lateral view of the thoracic spine demonstrates a central depression at the end plates of the vertebral bodies (arrow) resulting in "fishmouthing" of the disc spaces.

25. What radiographic skeletal abnormalities are present in lead poisoning?

Chronic heavy metal intoxication produces dense metaphyseal bands. They do not represent deposition of lead in the metaphysis but rather reflect interference of the resorption of the primary spongiosa that normally occurs in growing bones.

26. Which of the following long bone sites are affected most commonly by osteomyelitis: diaphysis, metaphysis, or epiphysis?

Between 1 year of age and skeletal maturity, osteomyelitis primarily involves the metaphysis of long bones. This is due to the terminal capillary loops that are located at this site. Blood flow through these sinusoids is slow, explaining the frequency that organisms lodge at the metaphysis.

27. How is achondroplasia inherited?

Although it is autosomal dominant, 80% occur sporadically without any family history.

28. What is the primary defect present in achondroplasia that results in the extensive skeletal abnormalities?

Defective endochondral ossification. Intramembranous (appositional) growth remains normal. Defective endochondral ossification results in significant shortening of long bones, especially the humerus and femur. Since appositional growth is normal, the metaphyses of bones have a characteristic widened appearance with a V-shaped configuration of the growth plates.

29. What other skeletal abnormalities are seen in achondroplasia?
- Spinal stenosis
- Scalloping of the posterior vertebral bodies
- Short long bones with or without bowing
- Short, stubby digits
- "Trident hand" (middle finger separated from others)
- Large head with frontal bossing
- Rounded iliac bones (lack normal flaring)
- Horizontal acetabular roofs
- "Champagne glass pelvis" due to narrow sciatic notch

30. At what age is osteogenesis imperfecta (OI) usually diagnosed?

It varies with the subtype of the disease. The "congenita" form is diagnosed at birth; the "tarda" form does not occur until early adulthood. OI can be inherited in either autosomal dominant or recessive forms. Infants with the congenital form usually die at birth or in the neonatal period.

31. What is the primary pathologic abnormality in OI?

Abnormal maturation of collagen resulting in defective bone matrix.

32. Name the clinical features of OI.
- Multiple skeletal deformities
- Short stature
- Blue sclerae
- Otosclerosis leading to deafness
- Ligamentous laxity
- Dental abnormalities

33. Name the radiographic abnormalities of OI.
- Severe osteoporosis
- Thin long bones with thin cortices
- Bowing of long bones
- Multiple fractures with or without exuberant callus (Fig. 9)
- Wormian (intrasutural) bones
- Kyphoscoliosis
- Severe skeletal deformities
- Acetabular protrusion (medial bowing of the medial acetabular wall)

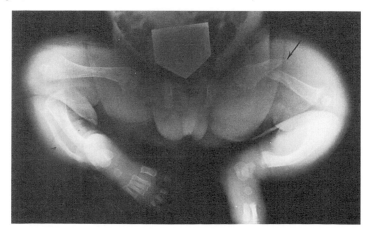

FIGURE 9. Hips and lower extremities in an infant with osteogenesis imperfecta demonstrate fractures (arrow) and bowing of the bones secondary to multiple repetitive subclinical fractures.

34. What is the "shish kabob" technique?

A complex surgical procedure used for correction of severe long bone bowing and deformity in OI. Described by Sofield, the surgery entails performing numerous osteotomies along the shaft of a long bone and threading the multiple short bone segments onto a rod (Fig. 10).

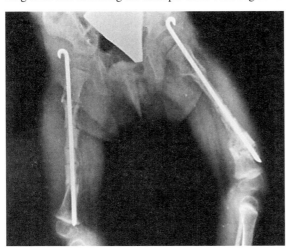

FIGURE 10. The patient has had multiple femoral osteotomies to correct femoral bowing (shish kabob procedure).

35. What is "marble-bone disease"?

Also known as osteopetrosis or Albers-Schönberg's disease, marble-bone disease results from a failure of resorption and remodeling of bone formed by endochondral ossification. Essentially all bones accumulate excessive calcified primary spongiosa in the marrow. This accumulation causes a significant increase in density of all bones on radiographs (Fig. 11) and can result in anemia due to replacement of normal marrow elements with cartilage and immature bone. Severe forms are treated with bone marrow transplantation. Although these dense bones appear strong, they are actually weak and prone to fractures.

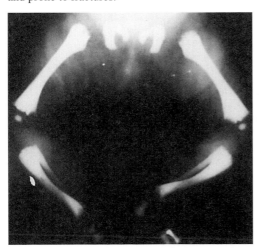

FIGURE 11. Osteopetrosis. The visualized bones in this patient are all extremely dense.

36. What disease did the painter Toulouse-Lautrec have?

Pyknodysostosis. Like osteopetrosis, there is defective resorption of the primary spongiosa causing increased bony density. Individuals with this sclerosing skeletal dysplasia are short in stature, have associated wormian bones, and typically have a characteristic abnormal mandible.

BIBLIOGRAPHY

1. Ozonoff MB: Pediatric Orthopedic Radiology. Philadelphia, W.B. Saunders, 1992.
2. Silverman FN: Caffey's Pediatric X-Ray Diagnosis, 9th ed. St. Louis, Mosby, 1993.
3. Sty JR, Wells RG, Starshak RJ, Gregg DC: Diagnostic Imaging of Infants and Children. Rockville, MD, Aspen Publications, 1992.

67. CHILD ABUSE

Louise B. Godine, M.D.

1. What is child abuse?

Child abuse, the intentional wounding of a child, includes physical, sexual, and emotional abuse as well as neglect. This chapter focuses on some of the common abuse-related skeletal, intracranial, and visceral injuries that can be diagnosed by radiologic imaging.

2. In what age child is skeletal abuse most common?

In infants (less than 1 year old) and toddlers (1 to 3 years old). Half of all fractures occurring in children under 1 year of age are caused by abuse. In fact, most abuse-related fractures occur in infants under 6 months of age.

3. What is the role of radiologic imaging in the diagnosis of child abuse?

Radiologic exams of abused children become legal documents that can provide irrefutable evidence of battering. All imaging modalities are used, including plain film (most common), ultrasound (to document visceral injury), CT (to demonstrate craniocerebral and visceral injury), MRI (to show extent and progression of CNS injury), and nuclear scintigraphy (to identify multiple, old, or unsuspected fractures).

4. Is the "babygram" (a single film of an infant) acceptable as documentation of skeletal abuse?

No! A babygram is unacceptable for many reasons, especially because skeletal injuries from child abuse may be extremely subtle and detection requires high-detail radiographs. Also, a babygram cannot provide the level of detail needed to present a convincing argument in court that child abuse has occurred.

5. If a babygram is inadequate, what is acceptable?

A skeletal survey, which comprises between 10 to 15 separate exposures. This survey should be performed using detail cassettes and should include:

AP (anteroposterior, or frontal view)   AP of the chest
    of each upper extremity   AP and lateral of the entire spine
PA (posteroanterior) of the hands   AP and lateral skull
AP of each lower extremity   AP of the abdomen and pelvis
AP of the feet

6. Should the skeletal survey by supervised and checked by a radiologist immediately after it is obtained?

Yes. The exam should be closely monitored, as any positive findings should be imaged in at least two projections. Furthermore, the study is lengthy and requires careful attention to detail (positioning of the child, labeling of films) and should be performed by a technologist experienced in radiographing children. For these reasons, the study should be performed only during the daytime shift. Finally, the radiologist needs to be present, since the defense lawyer may claim that the films submitted in court do not belong to the child in question.

7. Dr. Paul Kleinman, in his authoritative book on the imaging of child abuse, divides abuse-related skeletal injuries into three categories, depending on the likelihood that a particular injury was caused by abuse. Name the injuries that are highly specific, or pathognomonic, for abuse.

Metaphyseal fractures (bucket handle or corner fractures)
Posterior rib fractures
The "S" fractures: scapular (acromion), spinous process, and sternal

8. What skeletal injuries are moderately specific for abuse?

Multiple fractures, especially when bilateral   Vertebral body fractures and subluxations
Fractures of different ages   Hand and foot fractures (especially of
Epiphyseal separations (Salter-Harris   metacarpals and metatarsals)
   fractures)   Complex skull fractures

9. What common injuries have low specificity for child abuse?

Clavicle fractures, long bone shaft fractures, and linear skull fractures.

10. How does a lesion of low or moderate specificity become one of high specificity?

When there is no explanation for the injury, when the explanation changes, or when the history could not possibly account for the radiographic findings.

11. What are the most common mechanisms of injury for the findings in the high specificity category (in fact, for most skeletal abuse injuries)?

Violent shaking of an infant while holding him or her by the chest, or violent shaking, twisting, pulling, or swinging of an infant while using a limb as a "handle."

12. How old are most victims of high specificity trauma?

Most are under 1 year of age.

13. In an otherwise healthy child, what single skeletal injury is pathognomonic for child abuse?

The metaphyseal bucket handle fracture (Fig. 1) or corner fracture (Fig. 2). These types of fractures do not occur with normal caretaking activities (like feeding, bathing, diapering), roughhousing with older children or adults, or even accidental falls from any height. Nor can the baby cause this type of injury. Remember, one can diagnose abuse by demonstrating a single metaphyseal fracture in a normally mineralized bone.

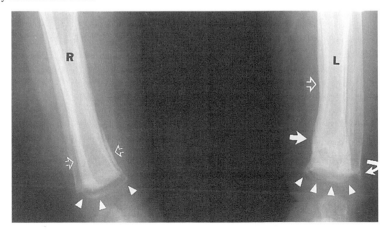

FIGURE 1.   Metaphyseal bucket handle fractures of the distal tibias (arrowheads). Note the periosteal reaction extending proximally along both tibial shafts (open arrows). In addition, there is a corner fracture of the left distal fibula (curved arrow) and a healing transverse fracture of the left distal tibia (heavy arrow).

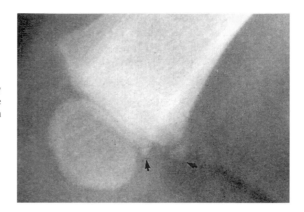

FIGURE 2. Corner fractures: lateral view of the distal femur showing fractures of the metaphysis. The distal femur is a common site of metaphyseal fractures.

14. Where in the metaphysis do these bucket handle and corner fractures occur?

Based on post-mortem histopathologic examination of the metaphyseal lesions, Kleinman et al. determined that these fractures occur in the most immature part of the metaphysis: the zone of provisional calcification of the primary spongiosa. The fracture fragment consists of two invisible layers—the epiphysis and the physis (growth plate)—and this thin, calcified metaphyseal layer of primary spongiosa. As the fracture reaches the periphery of the bone, it goes under the circumferential band of subperiosteal bone that forms the subperiosteal collar.

15. What distinguishes a bucket handle from a corner fracture?

Nothing except the projection of the radiograph and the position of the patient. A corner fracture is just the edge of a bucket handle fracture—it is not a discrete, triangular chip or avulsion fracture.

16. How exactly does this happen?

When the metaphyseal fragment (along with its epiphyseal and physeal components) is viewed perfectly tangentially, it looks like a flat disc of bone separated from the rest of the metaphysis by the lucent fracture line. However, if the joint is slightly flexed or if the projection is not exactly at right angles to the fracture line, the metaphyseal fragment will appear tipped and will then resemble a crescent or bucket handle.

17. What will the x-ray show if the metaphyseal fracture fragment is much thicker at the edges than in the middle?

If viewed tangentially, only the thicker peripheral rim or corner of the fracture fragment will be seen, resembling a triangular bone fragment (hence the name "corner" fracture). Remember, the corner fracture is not a separate triangle of bone, but rather the peripheral, thicker edge (the subperiosteal collar) of the entire metaphyseal fragment (the bucket handle fragment).

18. Are Salter-Harris (epiphyseal separation) injuries common in abuse?

No, except for Salter I fractures (along the relatively weak cartilagenous growth plate, the physis), which usually involve the femur or humerus. These fractures are usually caused by a twisting of the limb.

When a Salter I fracture of the proximal femur occurs in an infant whose epiphysis has not yet ossified, a frontal film of the hips shows what looks like a dislocated hip—that is, lateral displacement of the femoral shaft. This may lead to an erroneous assumption that the unossified femoral head subluxed with it. However, when a Salter I fracture occurs in a baby who has been grabbed by the leg and violently twisted or shaken, the unossified femoral head remains within the acetabulum and only the shaft shifts laterally (Fig. 3).

In a Salter I fracture of the distal humerus, the entire epiphysis is displaced posteromedially while the radius and ulna maintain their normal relationship to the capitellum and trochlea; that is, the long axis of the radius always lines up with the capitellum.

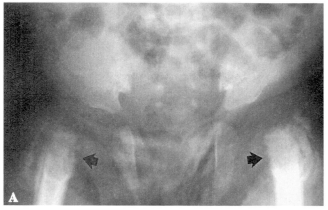

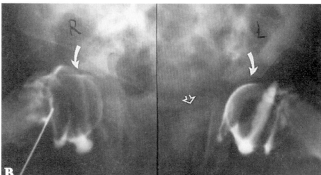

FIGURE 3. Salter I fractures of the hips. *A*, Frontal view of the pelvis and hips in a 2-month-old abused girl demonstrates lateral displacement of the femoral shafts (arrows). Note the abundant calcified subperiosteal hemorrhage and soft tissue calcification surrounding the proximal femoral shafts. *B*, Bilateral hip arthrograms confirm the normal location of the unossified femoral heads within the acetabula and rule out the possibility of bilateral hip dislocations.

19. Why are rib fractures (highly specific injuries for child abuse) most often located posteriorly or laterally?

The distribution of rib fractures in abused infants reflects the position in which the baby was held during the abusive episode(s). Babies are generally picked up under the arms, with the hands of the adult circling the thorax. When the baby is squeezed and shaken violently in this position and the chest forcefully compressed, the palms compress and break the lateral ribs, the fingertips break the posterior ribs at the costotransverse junctions (by levering them over the transverse processes of the spine), and the thumbs break the underlying anterior ribs at the costochondral junctions (Fig. 4).

FIGURE 4. Multiple posterior and lateral rib fractures. Note the vertical arrangement of the posterior rib fractures (arrows) parallel to the spine, corresponding to the placement of the abuser's fingertips while grasping, shaking, and squeezing the baby's chest. Anteroposterior compression also produces the lateral rib fractures (arrowheads). Note the uniform, bulbous appearance of callus at all fracture sites, suggesting that these fractures are at least 3 weeks old.

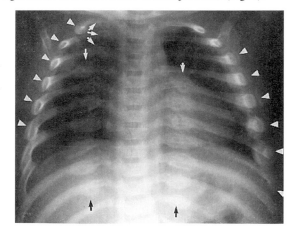

20. Can violent shaking of an infant while holding him or her by the thorax result in injuries at remote sites?

Yes. When an infant is shaken in this manner, the limbs as well as the head flail around uncontrollably. The massive acceleration-deceleration forces generated by the back-and-forth jerking can cause not only extensive intracerebral injury, but also two types of injuries to long bones: metaphyseal fractures and stripping of the loosely attached periosteum from the underlying shaft, leading to subperiosteal hemorrhage. (Periosteal stripping also can occur when a baby is grabbed by a limb and shaken violently.)

21. Which long bone fractures are commonly associated with abuse?
• Humeral fractures—other than the common supracondylar fracture, caused by an accidental fall on an outstretched arm. Remember, however, that a child has to be able to walk or run before he or she can fall on an outstretched arm. Thus **any** humeral fracture in a nonambulatory infant and any humeral fracture other than supracondylar in a slightly older child should be regarded as an abuse fracture until proved otherwise.
• Femoral fractures in pre-ambulatory infants. Children usually start walking alone by 12–15 months. Crawling infants cannot generate the momentum or force needed to break the femur, which is the thickest bone in the body. Once children start to walk and run, accidental femoral fractures become more common.

22. What is the timetable for healing of children's fractures?
0–3 days	Soft tissue swelling
3–7 days	Resolution of soft tissue swelling
10–14 days	Periosteal new bone formation (as early as 4–5 days in young infants)
2–6 weeks	Callus formation and remodeling. It may be difficult to date fractures exactly during this time. Callus forms first as an amorphous blob (around 2–3 weeks after the injury), bridging the fracture site. It then shrinks, becomes denser, and starts to remodel (by 3–6 weeks).
3–12 months	Further remodeling

Prompt bone repair requires immobilization and good nutrition. Metaphyseal fractures take longer to heal than fractures of the shaft.

23. What is the most frequent cause of death from child abuse?

Injury to the central nervous system. It is important to keep this in mind. Skeletal trauma is important for diagnosing child abuse, but it is rarely life threatening.

24. Is there good correlation between the presence of skull fractures and the presence or severity of intracranial injury?

No. Most skull fractures, whether caused intentionally or not, are linear and involve the parietal bone. On the other hand, complex (branching), multiple, bilateral (crossing the midline sagittal suture), depressed, or diastatic (more than 5 mm wide) fractures are more likely to be caused by abuse than by accident and to be associated with intracranial injury.

25. Since head injuries are so common among abused children and can lead to devastating, permanent neurologic damage, how should I work up such a child?

Start with plain films of the skull, which should always be part of the initial skeletal survey. Do head CT next whether or not a fracture is present, since the condition of the brain is what matters most. CT is ideal for documenting intracranial injuries that are less than 48 hours old. MR is best for documenting injuries older than 48 hours, especially hemorrhages (intracerebral or extra-axial) and shearing injuries, both of which are more conspicuous on MR than CT. MR is more sensitive than CT for detecting contusions, traumatic venous thrombosis, and signs of old injury such as encephalomalacia, hemosiderin deposition at sites of old hematomas, and siderosis (meningeal iron deposition).

26. What is the usual cause of skull fractures in child abuse?

A blow to the head with a blunt object or banging the infant's head against a wall or table.

27. Who is at greatest risk for these types of skull fractures?
Children up to the age of 2 years.

28. What are the primary mechanisms of intracranial injury in abused infants?
Blunt trauma and violent shaking. Blunt trauma (with or without fracture) can cause subdural hematomas and cerebral contusion of the coup-contrecoup type. Violent shaking, with its acceleration-deceleration forces, causes the head to whip back and forth, resulting in axonal and vascular shearing injuries.

29. What are the most common intracranial findings on CT/MR in child abuse?
Cerebral contusions and extracerebral fluid collections, especially subdural hemorrhages. Subdural hemorrhages result from tearing of the bridging veins that connect the brain surface to the large superficial venous sinuses.

30. Specifically, where do subdural hematomas localize?
Acute subdural hematomas frequently collect in the interhemispheric fissure and appear on CT as a somewhat thick, high-attenuation stripe with a flat medial border (defined by the falx) and a convex lateral border (Fig. 5). Larger subdural hematomas have the typical crescent or comma-shaped appearance.

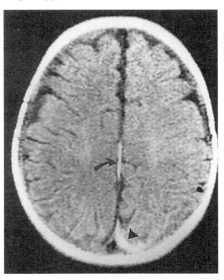

FIGURE 5. Interhemispheric subdural hematoma. A nonenhanced CT scan of the head shows a thick, dense stripe of fresh blood in the interhemispheric fissure (arrow) and in the left parasagittal region (arrowhead). The mother's boyfriend admitted to violently shaking this 4-month-old boy because the baby's cries interfered with his watching TV. Eventually, the mother admitted that both she and her other son had also beeen beaten by this man.

31. What other types of extracerebral hemorrhages occur in child abuse?
Subarachnoid and subdural hemorrhage frequently coexist. Epidural hematomas, on the other hand, are rare and are usually accompanied by skull fractures.

32. Regarding CNS injury: True or false:
- **Cerebral edema is usually caused by direct blows to the head, violent shaking, suffocation, or strangulation.**
- **The CT appearance of diffuse cerebral edema includes (1) loss of normal gray-white matter differentiation and (2) reversal of normal brain density, such that the gray and white matter show decreased density while the cerebellum, thalami, and brain-stem retain their normal, relatively high density.**
- **Long-term sequela of CNS injury include (1) chronic subdural hematomas, (2) progressive ventricular enlargement, (3) cerebral atrophy (focal or diffuse) and (4) cerebral infarcts.**
All true.

33. What is the most common visceral injury in abused children?

Hematomas of the duodenum and jejunum (Fig. 6). The mechanism for this, and virtually all abuse-related abdominal injuries, is blunt trauma from a fist or kick to the abdomen. Such blows compress the anatomically fixed viscera against the spine, resulting in injury to any of the organs lying in the path of force.

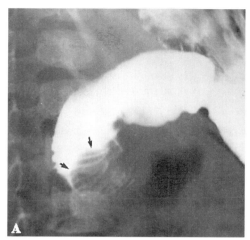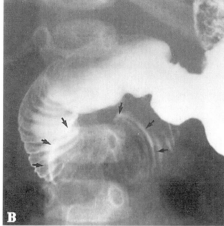

FIGURE 6. *A* and *B*, Duodenal hematoma. Spot films from an upper gastrointestinal series in a boy with intractable vomiting show the typical "coiled spring" appearance of an intramural hematoma (arrows). Note the position of the injury directly over the spine; this results from a blow to the abdomen that compressed the bowel against the spine.

34. What other visceral injuries are associated with abuse?

Pancreatitis (with or without pseudocyst formation) and liver laceration. Trauma is the most common cause of pancreatitis in children—either accidental, as in a handle-bar injury, or non-accidental, as in a blow to the abdomen. Because the liver is also in the direct path of a punch to the abdomen and the liver's edge is unprotected by ribs, a laceration or fracture may occur, often with catastrophic results from silent exsanguination (Fig. 7). Injury to the kidneys and spleen is less common because they are lateral organs and therefore remote from the midline blow.

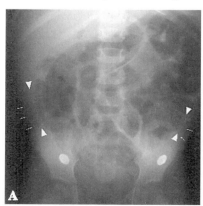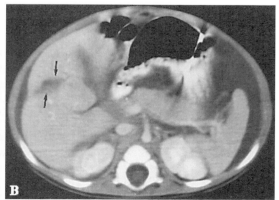

FIGURE 7.   Liver laceration causing hemoperitoneum and fatal exsanguination. This 18-month boy was brought to the hospital dead on arrival with no external signs of abuse. A frontal film of the abdomen (*A*) showed medial displacement of the gas-filled bowel away from the properitoneal fat stripe (arrows), caused by accumulation of intraperitoneal blood (arrowheads) from a large liver laceration. CT from another child (*B*) shows a laceration of the right hepatic lobe (arrows) and ascites.

35. What is the differential diagnosis of child abuse with regard to the skeletal findings?

- Birth trauma
- Osteogenesis imperfecta
- Congenital syphilis
- Physiologic periosteal new bone
- Neonatal osteomyelitis
- Menkes' kinky-hair syndrome
- Drug-related bone changes

36. What are the bones most commonly injured by birth trauma?

The clavicle, humerus, and femur. In fact, the clavicle is the most commonly fractured bone in children. Usually, fractures of the clavicle caused by a difficult delivery are in the midshaft and show definite evidence of callus by the time the baby is two weeks old. Clavicle fractures related to abuse are usually in the distal clavicle and are rarely the only fracture in an abused child.

37. What are the skeletal findings in osteogenesis imperfecta?

Osteogenesis imperfecta (OI) is a group of disorders characterized by frequent fractures as well as by biochemical abnormalities of type I collagen fibers. OI is divided into four types:

Type I. This is the most common type, accounting for 80% of cases. It is transmitted as an autosomal dominant trait. The sclerae are distinctly blue, hearing loss occurs early, and the bones are fragile and prone to recurrent fractures. Abnormal dentition (dentinogenesis imperfecta) occurs in some patients.

Type II. This form is lethal and results in the most severe bone fragility of all four types, with wide, thin bones that look wavy or crumpled like an accordion, caused by multiple fractures sustained in utero. The sclerae are blue. Since these babies die either in utero or in early infancy, this type is rarely confused with child abuse.

Type III. This form is also rare and is similar to type II but less severe. The bones may not be deformed in early life, but the cortex is thin and easily fractured, resulting in bowing. The sclerae may or may not be blue and eventually become normal. Deafness and abnormal teeth are common.

Type IV. This is another rare form characterized by osteopenia and bone fragility of varying degrees. Some of these children do not fracture. Sclerae may be normal or faintly blue. Dental involvement is variable. As in all types of OI, the fractures are in the shafts, not in the metaphyses.

38. How does congenital syphilis mimic child abuse?

Congenital syphilis produces irregularity and fragmentation of the metaphyses of the long bones, producing pathologic fractures that resemble the metaphyseal bucket handle and corner fractures seen in abuse. Whereas syphilitic bone abnormalities will involve every long bone of the body in symmetric fashion, metaphyseal abuse fractures are often asymmetric in distribution and show different degrees of healing. Diaphyseal periosteal reaction (again, involving all of the long bones) is another feature of syphilis. The baby will also have splenomegaly, rhinorrhea (snuffles), a rash, and anemia as well as a positive serologic test.

39. When and where does physiologic new bone occur?

Physiologic periosteal new bone is a thin layer of periosteal reaction that occurs symmetrically along the shafts of long bones and usually disappears by three months of age. It is not associated with fractures.

40. What is Menkes' kinky-hair syndrome?

This is a rare, X-linked disorder of copper metabolism that causes decreased absorption of copper from the gastrointestinal tract. The metaphyses of the long bones develop spurs which may fracture, mimicking corner fractures. However, distinction between abuse and Menkes' is made easier by the following radiographic and clinical features: wormian bones on skull films; corkscrew cerebral and abdominal vessels on angiography; coarse, silvery hair; seizures; mental retardation; and failure to thrive. Low levels of serum copper clinch the diagnosis.

41. What drug used to maintain patency of the ductus arteriosus in infants with ductus-dependent congenital heart disease may cause periosteal reaction in the long bones and ribs?

Prostaglandin E1. The periosteal reaction affects all the long bones symmetrically. The clinical history makes this diagnosis easy.

42. What is the role of a nuclear medicine bone scan in the workup of child abuse?

This is controversial. Most radiologists and clinicians prefer the plain film skeletal survey. Even though the bone scan may be more sensitive for detecting skeletal trauma, the technical demands of producing a high-quality study are often greater than many departments can achieve. For example, documenting a metaphyseal fracture on bone scan may be harder than on plain film, because the fracture may add only a subtle increase in radiointensity to the adjacent tracer-avid growth plate. Bone scans are well suited, however, for detecting rib fractures, for pursuing a strong clinical suspicion of abuse in the face of a negative skeletal survey, and for investigating the older siblings of abused children.

43. What is the responsibility of the radiologist with regard to reporting imaging findings that suggest abuse?

The law is clear: the radiologist is mandated to notify state authorities if there is reasonable suspicion that abuse has occurred. Not reporting such findings puts the physician at risk for criminal sanction. In practical terms, this means that the radiologist must promptly report the findings to the referring physician and notify (or be certain the referring physician notifies) the social service department and child protection workers.

BIBLIOGRAPHY

1. Caffey J: Multiple fractures in the long bones of infants suffering from chronic subdural hematoma. AJR 56:163–173, 1946.
2. Cohen RA, Kaufman RA, Myers PA, et al: Cranial computed tomography in the abuse child with head injury. AJR 146:97–102, 1986.
3. Hilton SV: Differentiating the accidentally injured from the physically abused child. In Hilton SV, Edwards DK: Practical Pediatric Radiology, 2nd ed. Philadelphia, W.B. Saunders, 1994, pp 389–436. This is an outstanding overview of the clinical and radiologic findings in child abuse, with excellent radiographic images and line drawings.
4. Kempe CH, Silverman FN, Steele BF, et al: The battered-child syndrome. JAMA 181:105–112, 1962.
5. Kleinman PK (ed): Diagnostic Imaging of Child Abuse. Baltimore, Williams & Wilkins, 1987. This is the standard reference on the subject.
6. Kleinman PK, Raptopoulos VD, Brill PW: Occult nonskeletal trauma in the battered-child syndrome. Radiology 141:393–396, 1981.
7. Leventhal JM, Thomas SA, Rosenfield NS, Markowitz RI: Fractures in young children: Distinguishing child abuse from unintentional injuries. Am J Dis Child 147:87–92, 1993.
8. Merton DF, Carpenter BLM: Radiologic imaging of inflicted injury in the child abuse syndrome. Pediatr Clin North Am 37:815–838, 1990.
9. Merton DF, Osborne DRS, Radkowski MA, et al: Craniocerebral trauma in the child abuse syndrome: Radiologic observations. Pediatr Radiol 14:272–277, 1984.
10. Radkowski MA, Merton DF, Leonidas JC: The abused child: Criteria for the radiologic diagnosis. RadioGraphics 3:262–297, 1983.
11. Sato Y, Yuh WTC, Smith WL, et al: Head injury in child abuse: Evaluation with MR imaging. Radiology 173:653–660, 1989.

68. PEDIATRIC BRAIN TUMORS

Leo Hochhauser, M.D.

1. What is the difference between an intraaxial and extraaxial brain tumor?

Intracranial tumors are divided into those arising in brain parenchyma (intraaxial, i.e., within the neuraxis) and those arising in a location between the brain and the skull (extraaxial).

2. Where exactly do extraaxial brain tumors originate?

They arise from cells outside the brain, such as the meninges and cranial nerves (Fig. 1).

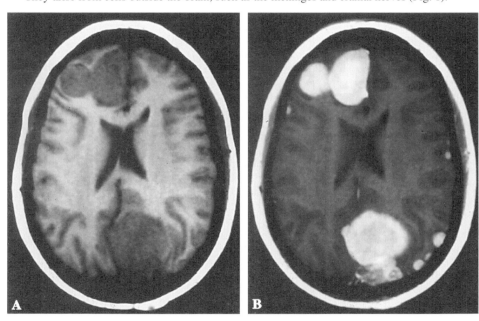

FIGURE 1. Contrast enhancement. T1-weighted image before (*A*) and after (*B*) the intravenous injection of gadolinium shows the advantage of contrast enhancement. The low-signal-intensity tumors (meningiomas, in this patient with neurofibromatosis type 2) become very bright after contrast injection, and additional lesions become visible along the inner table of the skull.

3. Where in the brain do childhood tumors arise?

Almost 50% of all pediatric brain tumors are astrocytomas (which arise from astrocytes), and 60% of these occur in the posterior fossa. Overall, there is no real difference between the numbers of tumors arising above the tentorium (supratentorial) and those arising below the tentorium (infratentorial). However, supratentorial tumors are more common in the first 3 years of life, whereas infratentorial tumors occur more frequently from ages 4 to 11.

4. When does a brain tumor cause clinical symptoms?

A brain tumor declares itself by mechanical effects. Its bulk displaces adjacent tissues and/or obstructs the flow of cerebrospinal fluid. A tumor may cause a neurologic deficit such as a cranial nerve palsy or abnormal excitation leading to pituitary endocrinopathy or seizure.

5. What are other specific signs and symptoms of a brain tumor? How do they differ in infants and older children?

Infants may present with irritability and an enlarged head (macrocephaly), with bulging of the fontanelles and splitting of the skull sutures (visible on radiographs, CT, and MR). There may be failure to thrive. Children may suffer from headache, focal neurologic deficits, blurred vision, weight loss, ataxia, and abnormal gait and balance. Both infants and children may have papilledema, vomiting, and seizures.

6. List the common brain tumors in neonates and children younger than 1 year.

(Suprasellar) malignant astrocytomas	Teratoma
Choroid plexus papilloma	Primitive neuroectodermal tumor (PNET)
Choroid plexus carcinoma	Ependymoma

7. Why is the diagnosis of brain tumors in neonates and young children often delayed?

Because of the immaturity of the brain, focal neurologic deficits are relatively rare. The diagnosis is often delayed because of nonspecific clinical findings.

8. Why is intravenous contrast given with CT or MR for imaging suspected brain tumors?

Intravenous iodine-based dye is injected for CT, and gadolinium is injected for MR. Tumor usually destroys the cell membranes that maintain an equilibrium between extra- and intracellular water (i.e., the blood-brain barrier). The contrast agent leaks from the intravascular space into the intracellular and/or interstitial compartment and enhances the lesion.

9. Why are astrocytomas the most common brain tumor in children?

Astrocytes are the prevalent cells in the central nervous system and therefore contribute to the majority of tumors. The odds of malignant transformation are greater in astrocytomas than in oligodendrogliomas, which arise in cells (oligodendrocytes) that are more sparsely distributed in the brain.

10. What is the WHO classification for astrocytomas?

Astrocytomas are histologically quite heterogeneous. According to the recently revised World Health Organization (WHO) classification of brain tumors, they are divided into four groups that attempt to correlate with survival:

Type 1: Benign and noninvasive pilocytic astrocytoma
Type 2: Fibrillary or low-grade astrocytoma
Type 3: Anaplastic astrocytoma
Type 4: Highly malignant glioblastoma multiforme

11. What was the previous classification system for astrocytomas? What was wrong with it?

The Kernohan classification, which was also four-tiered, described the histologic appearance of astrocytomas, relying on the percentage of atypical nuclei; it assumed that this ratio could predict clinical behavior, which is not always the case.

12. Why do low-grade astrocytomas recur after resection?

Low-grade astrocytomas (type 2) invade the surrounding brain tissue, which precludes complete surgical resection of the tumor. After removal of all visible tumor, a course of radiation therapy is given.

13. What are the four types of intraaxial posterior fossa tumors in children?

Astrocytoma	Ependymoma
Medulloblastoma	Brainstem glioma (a form of astrocytoma)

14. How often do posterior fossa astrocytomas contain cystic components?

Almost 50% of astrocytomas are composed of a cystic structure that contains a nodule in its wall. These tumors are histologically benign and are called pilocytic (Fig. 2). Approximately 40% of astrocytomas are cyst-like tumors in which a rim of enhancing solid tumor surrounds a necrotic center. Solid tumors without cystic components are present in 10%. Most cerebellar astrocytomas arise in the midline; extension to the cerebellar hemispheres is seen in 30%. Fifteen percent arise in the cerebellar hemispheres. Calcification is found in 20%.

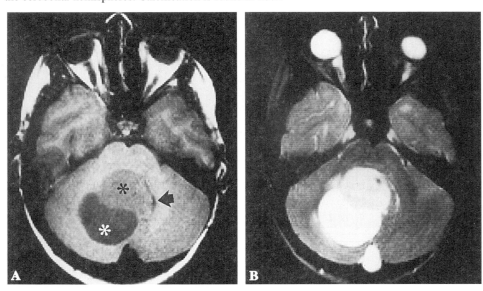

FIGURE 2.   Benign pilocytic astrocytoma of the posterior fossa. *A*, T1-weighted MR image. A tumor (black asterisk) in the vermis obliterates the fourth ventricle (arrow), which is displaced to the left. The mass is associated with a cyst (white asterisk). *B*, T2-weighted image. The tumor and the cyst show different shades of white (high signal intensity), while they are much more easily distinguishable on the T1-weighted image.

15. At what other locations do astrocytomas occur?
Brainstem (Fig. 3), suprasellar region, and optic nerves.

16. Where exactly does a medulloblastoma arise?
The tumor usually arises in the midline from the inferior medullary velum. The tumor bulges into the fourth ventricle and frequently invades the vermis. Occasionally, the tumor is cystic and may be difficult to distinguish from an astrocytoma. About 15% of medulloblastomas contain calcification that is visible on a CT scan.

17. Where exactly do ependymomas arise?
Ependymomas arise from the floor (most commonly) or the roof of the fourth ventricle (Fig. 4). Ependymomas are usually soft and grow through the outlet foramina (Magendie and Luschka) into the cisterna magna and from there through the foramen magnum into the upper cervical spinal canal. Calcification occurs in 30%. The presence of widespread seeding into the subarachnoid space indicates malignancy.

18. Which posterior fossa tumor presents with cranial nerve palsies?
Brainstem glioma. Such tumors impinge on the cranial nerve nuclei. They are frequently inaccessible to surgery or biopsy, and the histological diagnosis is usually made at autopsy.

19. Which posterior fossa tumor presents with vomiting first and headaches later?
Ependymoma. The vomiting center, the area postrema, is located in the floor of the fourth ventricle, where ependymomas arise.

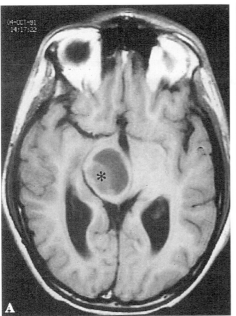 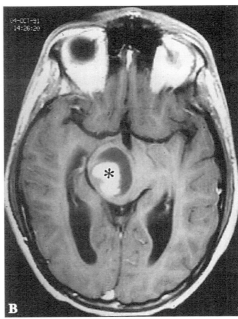

FIGURE 3. Cystic astrocytoma of the brainstem. T1-weighted images without (*A*) and with (*B*) contrast (gadolinium) show the enhancing tumor (asterisk) clearly separate from the unenhancing adjacent cyst, which remains low in signal intensity after contrast administration.

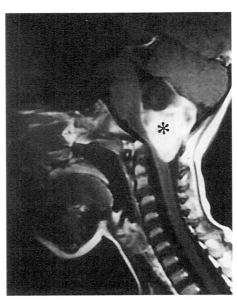

FIGURE 4. Ependymoma. Enhancing tumor (asterisk) extends inferiorly into the cervical canal (on this T1-weighted saggital MR image), a feature found only in ependymomas. A cyst at the rostral end is caused by an associated astrocytic tumor component. Many brain tumors are mixed in histology and derive their name from the most prevalent or the most malignant cell. The cyst partially obliterates the fourth ventricle, which is midline in position.

20. Which posterior fossa tumors present with headaches first and vomiting later?

Astrocytoma of the vermis and medulloblastoma. These tumors may obliterate the cerebral aqueduct, causing ventricular obstruction that results in hydrocephalus and headaches. Astrocytomas originating in the cerebellar hemispheres also cause gait disturbances early in their course.

21. Which extraaxial posterior fossa tumor does not enhance with intravenous contrast on CT and MR?

Epidermoid tumors, which are congenital malformations, present as cystic masses that contain epithelial debris. The lesion is lined by squamous epithelium and insinuates itself into the available space of the brainstem cisterns, therefore causing little mass effect. Epidermoid tumors wrap around the cranial nerves, usually the seventh and eighth. If skin appendages such as hair follicles are present in the tumor, it is classified as a dermoid.

22. Which extraaxial posterior fossa tumor enhances brightly?

Acoustic neuroma (also known as vestibular schwannoma or neurilemmoma) (Fig. 5) and meningioma. These tumors are directly supplied by branches of the internal or external carotid arteries, respectively. Enhancement does not imply breakdown of the blood-brain barrier, because these tumors are extraaxial.

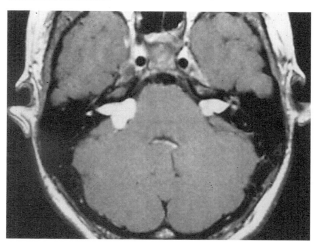

FIGURE 5. Bilateral acoustic neuroma in neurofibromatosis type 2. Axial T1-weighted image after gadolinium administration shows bilateral cone-shaped tumors arising within the internal auditory canals. The right tumor shows exophytic growth into the cerebellopontine angle. The bilaterality of this tumor is due to a chromosomal abnormality (on chromosome 22, which causes neurofibromatosis type 2).

23. What is meant by a primitive neuroectodermal tumor (PNET)?

PNETs (pronounced "peanut" or "pea net") (Fig. 6) may arise anywhere in the brain (i.e., infratentorial, supratentorial, retinal) or the body (e.g., adrenal gland, bone). These tumors arise from small cells that have scant features of differentiation toward mature cells in the brain, such as neurons, glial cells, or ependyma, and mature organ cells, such as adrenal gland or bone in the body. Ewing's sarcoma may be classified as PNET of bone and neuroblastoma as PNET of the adrenal gland (or, if arising in an extraadrenal location, of the sympathetic nervous tissue in that location).

24. So why is the term PNET used?

The clinical behavior of supra- and infratentorial PNETs is similar and requires similar aggressive treatment protocols. Pediatric neuropathologists in association with pediatric neurosurgeons therefore suggested the name primitive neuroectodermal tumor for a group of pediatric tumors with similar outcomes and treatment requirements.

25. How do PNETs spread in the brain?

They have a strong tendency to spread by drop metastases into the spinal subarachnoid space.

26. Medulloblastoma is a PNET of the posterior fossa, yet there are no actual medulloblasts. Why is the term used?

Medulloblastoma (Fig. 7) arises from poorly differentiated cells in the posterior fossa. When Cushing and Bailey, two grandfathers of neurosurgery, described this primitive tumor, they postulated that the cell of origin eventually would be found in the medulla of the central nervous system;

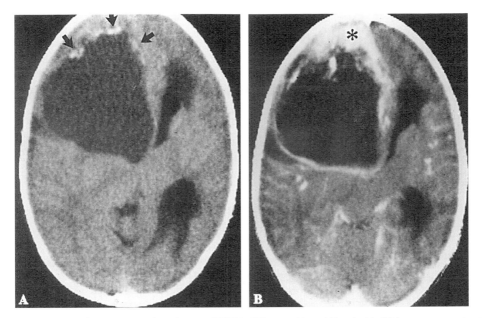

FIGURE 6. Primitive neuroectodermal tumor (PNET). CT scan without (*A*) and with (*B*) intravenous contrast shows a large cystic (low density) mass with a calcified (arrows) anterior rim on the image before contrast injection (*A*). Thick, enhancing tumor becomes visible anteriorly after contrast injection (asterisk), while the remainder of the cyst is enveloped by enhancing tumor tissue. The mass effect of the lesion causes obstruction of the left lateral ventricle at the level of the foramen of Monro. The vessels along the tentorium and in the Sylvian fissures are seen as enhancing lines and dots, which is normal.

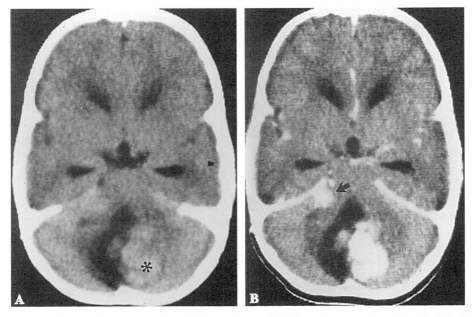

FIGURE 7. Medulloblastoma. Unenhanced CT (*A*) shows a slightly hyperdense mass (asterisk) to the left of the vermis, with an associated cyst on the right. The tumor enhances brightly (*B*). A metastasis is identified along the tentorium on the right (arrow). The tips of the temporal horns are dilated, indicating that there is ventricular obstruction.

hence the name medulloblastoma. Although the medulloblast never materialized, the name remained in honor of the two neurosurgeons. Tumors of primitive cells arising in the supratentorial brain are known by their more traditional names, such as ependymoblastoma and pineoblastoma.

27. Which brain tumors seed into the subarachnoid space and metastasize within the central nervous system?

Pineal germinoma, ependymoma, and medulloblastoma almost always seed early in their course. By the time of diagnosis they have already spread in 25–75% of children. The diagnostic work-up of these lesions therefore requires evaluation of the entire spine, even if no symptoms indicate spinal disease. Treatment involves radiation of the entire brain and spine, with booster doses to levels at which metastases are specifically seen with imaging.

28. What supratentorial tumors occur in the midline?

Pineal region tumors (germinomas, pineoblastomas)
Suprasellar tumors, including craniopharyngioma and astrocytomas

29. Where exactly does a craniopharyngioma develop?

The name denotes its origin from the cranium and the pharynx. The tumor usually arises above the pituitary gland, from congenitally malformed mucosa (Rathke's pouch or cleft), between the posterior and anterior pituitary gland, or along the pituitary stalk. Craniopharyngiomas may affect both children and adults. One-half of all craniopharyngiomas occur in patients younger than 18; they are rare in children younger than 5 years.

30. What is the imaging appearance of craniopharyngioma (Fig. 8).

The mass is commonly cystic and usually fills the entire suprasellar region. The cysts are iso- to hypointense on T1-weighted images and hyperintense on T2-weighted images. The CT and MR appearance reflects the tumor composition of keratinous nodules, fibrous tissue, necrotic debris, and cysts. Calcifications are commonly seen on CT.

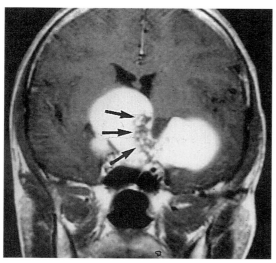

FIGURE 8. Craniopharyngioma. T1-weighted coronal image obtained with contrast enhancement shows a large proteinaceous or oily fluid-containing multilobulated cystic mass in the suprasellar cistern, which elevates the lateral ventricles. The tumor nidus (arrows) is of lower signal intensity than the associated cysts.

31. How do craniopharyngiomas present clinically?

The typical lesion is large, and symptoms are therefore due to mass effect on the optic chiasm, resulting in visual disturbance or compression of the hypothalamus and pituitary gland, with endocrine dysfunction, including diabetes insipidus and amenorrhea. Ventricular obstruction may develop from blockage at the foramina of Monro.

32. What kind of tumors arise from the pineal gland?

The stroma of the pineal gland is composed of germ cells and pineal parenchymal cells. Tumors in the pineal region may arise from the pineal gland or the adjacent tectum. The clinical effects are similar and relate mostly to aqueductal obstruction. Mass effect on the superior colliculi causes inability of upward gaze (Parinaud syndrome). The most common lesions in this location are germinomas, teratomas, and astrocytomas. In addition to germinomas, other germ cell tumors include mature teratoma, embryonal carcinoma, endodermal sinus tumor, and choriocarcinoma.

33. How is ultrasound useful in the diagnosis of central nervous system tumors?

Ultrasound may be used in neonates and infants before closure of the anterior fontanelles, which serve as windows for the ultrasound beam. Lesions may be seen directly, and no radiation is involved.

34. Which is the best imaging test for suspected brain lesions, CT or MR?

CT, although a good initial general screen of the brain, is limited in its evaluation of the posterior fossa because of "hardening" of the x-ray beam when it traverses the temporal bones; this causes streak artifact in the posterior fossa, making complete evaluation difficult. MR is the method of choice because images are easily acquired in multiple planes (which facilitates surgical planning), no radiation is involved, and there are no beam-hardening artifacts in the posterior fossa. A typical MR performed for suspected brain tumor includes images obtained both before and after intravenous contrast (gadolinium).

35. Which brain tumors are hyperdense (bright) on CT before contrast administration?

Tumors with densely packed cells, such as lymphoma and medulloblastoma, and tumors with calcifications, such as ependymoma.

BIBLIOGRAPHY

1. Pizzo PA, Poplack DG: Principles and Practice of Pediatric Oncology, 3rd ed. Philadelphia, Lippincott-Raven, 1997.
2. Pollack IF: Brain tumors in children. N Engl J Med 331:1500–1507, 1994.

---

69. MISCELLANEOUS CONDITIONS OF THE PEDIATRIC CENTRAL NERVOUS SYSTEM

Leo Hochhauser, M.D.

---

1. What is heterotopic gray matter?

The normal migration of neuroblasts from their origin in the germinal matrix in the periependymal region to their final destination in the cortex of the brain may be interrupted for unknown reasons. Clusters of neuroblasts may get literally stuck en route to the cortex in the white matter; mature gray matter then forms in these locations (Fig. 1).

2. What are the symptoms of heterotopic gray matter?

Seizures.

3. How do foci of heterotopic gray matter appear on CT and MR?

On imaging, these nodular lesions are isodense to cortex on CT and isointense to cortex on MR.

4. What is the most common cerebral abnormality in children with a lumbar meningomyelocele?

Hydrocephalus occurs in over 95% of children with a lumbar meningomyelocele because of aqueductal stenosis. These children also almost always have the Chiari 2 malformation.

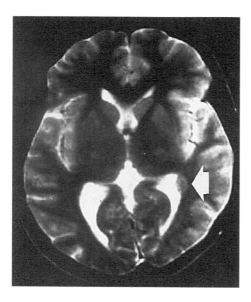

FIGURE 1. Heterotopia. Adolescent girl with long-standing seizure disorder. A group of neuroblasts from the ependymal germ cell layer are situated along the lateral wall of the left atrium (arrow). Normally, neuroblasts are destined to migrate into the cortex, where they become neurocytes. This is an example of arrested migration. A seizure is though to occur during electrical discharge of these cells.

5. What is the Chiari 2 malformation (Fig. 2)?

A complex congenital malformation involving the cranial and caudal ends of the spine. Devastating neurologic deficits result from a lumbar meningomyelocele and a small posterior fossa.

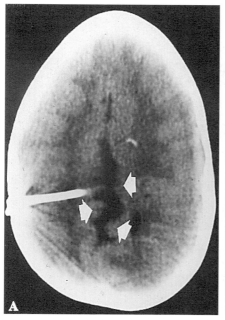

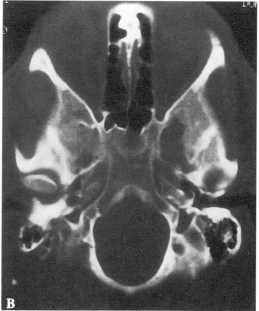

FIGURE 2. Chiari 2 malformation. Complex anomaly of the lower and upper end of the neural tube. The most conspicuous element is the myelomeningocele. Rostral-associated anomalies include ventricular obstruction of the cerebral aqueduct, requiring shunting. Deformities of the tectum and massa intermedia are also present. The falx is either absent or deficient, resulting in the characteristic appearance of interdigitation of the cortical sulci (arrow, *A*). The posterior fossa is small, resulting in both upward and downward displacement of the developing cerebellum, causing the foramen magnum as well as the tentorial notch to be enlarged by the protruding vermis. The axial CT of the skull base shows a large foramen magnum (*B*).

The cerebellum is elongated, with downward herniation of a portion of the cerebellum through the foramen magnum and upward herniation of a portion of the cerebellum through the tentorial notch. The fourth ventricle is elongated and flattened. Although severe neurologic deficits may be present, these children are of normal intelligence.

6. What is meant by a Chiari 1 malformation (Fig. 3)?

Chiari 1 malformation is the caudal descent of the cerebellar tonsils, 5 mm or more below the level of the foramen magnum. Dense arachnoid scarring at the foramen magnum may obstruct the outflow of cerebrospinal fluid from the fourth ventricle and cause hydrocephalus. There is no associated spinal anomaly.

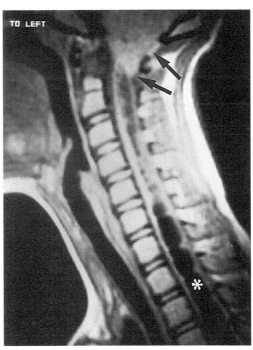

FIGURE 3. Chiari 1 malformation. The more appropriate term is tonsillar ectopia, with or without a syrinx. The disorder may be symptomatic either due to mass effect upon the medulla at the level of the foramen magnum or due to the syrinx, which forms in adulthood. Sagittal T1-weighted image shows the cerebellar tonsils (arrow) and a multiseptated syrinx (asterisk) in a young woman with paresthesias.

7. A child with a ventricular shunt tube presents with headaches. What are two possible reasons?

Ventricular shunts are used to divert cerebrospinal fluid that cannot adequately drain because of obstruction at the level of the ventricle, usually at the aqueduct of Sylvius or outside the ventricular system, most commonly at the level of the arachnoid granulations. Undershunting may result from mechanical obstruction of the proximal shunt tube end in the skull or the distal shunt tube end in the peritoneal cavity (e.g., by an abscess). Rapid enlargement of the ventricles may occur when the sutures are not yet closed. Overshunting may result from the siphon effect in a low-pressure shunt system. The ventricles collapse completely or become slit-like.

8. What is the Dandy-Walker malformation?

Dandy-Walker malformation is a cystic malformation of the posterior fossa. The cyst prevents the normal descent of the transverse sinuses and tentorium. The cerebellum is hypoplastic. Hydrocephalus results from aqueductal obstruction or obliteration of the outlet foramina of the fourth ventricle. The malformation is a spectrum, with the classic Dandy-Walker malformation as the most severe form, and the giant cisterna magna as the mildest form. Between is the Dandy-Walker variant, in which the cerebellum is less hypoplastic than in the full Dandy-Walker malformation.

9. What are the symptoms of Dandy-Walker malformation?

Developmental delay with mental retardation. Seizures result from associated migration anomalies. Agenesis of the corpus callosum is a common associated finding.

10. A child is born with a cleft palate. What may be the associated brain anomaly?

Holoprosencephaly, which is a persistent monoventricle due to absent normal cleavage of the brain. It is a frequent feature of trisomy 13.

11. What is porencephaly?

The result of an intrauterine vascular accident, porencephaly literally means "hole in the brain." The ensuing stroke causes necrosis of the involved segment of the immature brain, which liquefies rather than forming scar tissue.

12. What is the cavum septi pellucidi?

A double-layered membrane between the frontal horns. It frequently fills with cerebrospinal fluid during development but involutes after birth. Up to 80% of neonates have a cavum (cavity) between the layers of the septum pellucidum. A cavum septi pellucidi may extend posteriorly, at which time it becomes a cavum septi pellucidi et Vergae (Verga was an anatomist).

13. What is neurofibromatosis type 1 (NF1)?

A consensus conference of the World Health Organization recognized two forms of neurofibromatosis. NF1 corresponds to the classic von Recklinghausen's disease, which is an autosomally dominant syndrome with an incidence of 1 in 2,500–3,000 births. Over 95% of neurofibromatosis is categorized as type 1.

14. On which chromosome is NF1 found?

Chromosome 17 (there are 17 letters in neurofibromatosis—an easy way to remember this fact).

15. What is the primary brain abnormality in NF1?

Optic pathway glioma, particularly optic nerve gliomas (Fig. 4). This tumor is benign histologically, although the prognosis for preservation of vision is often poor.

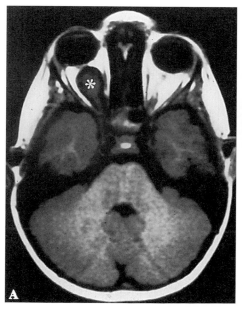

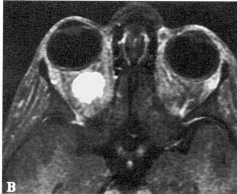

FIGURE 4. Optic nerve gliomas in neurofibromatosis type 1. Axial T1-weighted images without (A) and with (B) gadolinium enhancement. The fusiform enlargement of the right optic nerve is readily identified without contrast enhancement (asterisk). The magnified axial view (B, post-contrast image with fat saturation applied) shows the orbit. The high signal intensity of the orbital fat is suppressed to better distinguish the enhancing tumor.

16. List other central nervous system findings in NF1.

Among the numerous other findings are cerebral astrocytomas; most are juvenile and pilocytic. Spinal findings include scoliosis, intra- and paraspinal neurofibromas, and ectasia of the dura, resulting in lateral meningoceles.

17. What is neurofibromatosis type 2 (NF2)?

NF2 represents less than 5% of all cases of neurofibromatosis, with an incidence rate of 1 in 50,000. It is an autosomal dominant disorder associated with chromosome 22 (also easy to remember). There are numerous central and peripheral findings in both type 1 and type 2 neurofibromatosis.

18. What is the primary brain abnormality in NF2?

Bilateral vestibular schwannomas (also known as acoustic neuromas).

19. List other central nervous system findings in NF2.

Bilateral and multiple meningiomas and multiple spinal schwannomas.

20. What is the tuber in tuberous sclerosis?

Tubers are cortical hamartomas that on pathologic examination feel like potatoes (tuber in Latin).

21. What is the specific tumor that children with tuberous sclerosis get in the brain?

Giant cell astrocytoma. The location of this tumor is almost always at the foramen of Monro, in association with periventricular subependymal hamartomas. These hamartomas appear as calcified small nodules along the ependyma of the lateral ventricles. The giant cell astrocytoma appears on imaging studies as an enhancing mass which obstructs one or both foramina of Monro, resulting in ventricular obstruction.

22. Which imaging modality shows cortical tubers best?

MR, especially T2-weighted images. These show multiple cortical tubers as well-defined areas of high signal intensity. These tubers are low in density on CT and are not as readily seen.

23. Name the intrauterine infections that most commonly cause intracranial calcifications.

Toxoplasmosis, **r**ubella, **c**ytomegallovirus, and **h**erpes (mnemonic: **TORCH**) are the parasitic and viral infections that cause necrotizing vascultitis, resulting in dystrophic calcification of dead brain tissue.

24. Why do infants with TORCH infections present with microcephaly?

The skull is a membranous bone that grows only when the underlying brain grows. Necrotic brain has obviously lost this potential and is no longer available to expand the skull.

25. What is the most common cause for subarachnoid hemorrhage in children and adolescents?

Arteriovenous malformations (Fig. 5) in all age groups may present with subarachnoid hemorrhage. Aneurysms arise at areas of congenital weakness of the walls of intracranial blood vessels and take a long time to develop, so that most patients who present with hemorrhage from an aneurysm are middle aged or older adults. Arteriovenous malformations are present at birth and usually bleed earlier in life than aneurysms.

26. What types of intracranial aneurysms occur during childhood?

Aneurysms in children are usually mycotic aneurysms due to infection. "Mycotic" is a misnomer, as the infection is bacterial and not fungal.

27. What is the best way to image subarachnoid hemorrhage?

An unenhanced CT scan. The high attenuation values of clotted blood stand out well against the background of normal brain density and the low density of the cerebrospinal fluid that is normally present in the subarachnoid space.

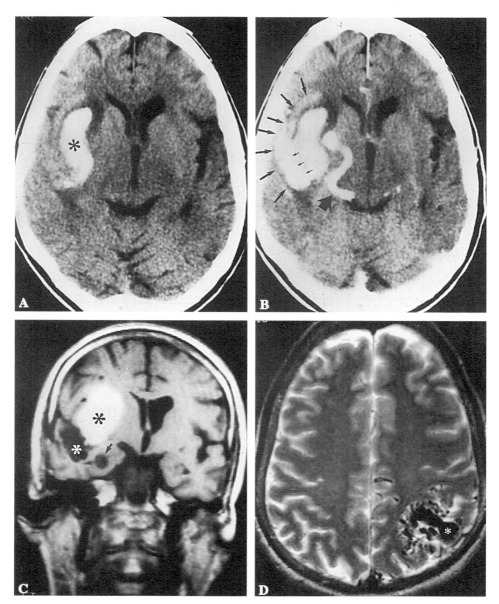

FIGURE 5.   Arteriovenous malformations. CT example (*A*) shows a hemorrhage (asterisk) on the precontrast study. Following intravenous contrast injection, the tangle of abnormal vessels (arrows) becomes apparent, as does the enhancing vein (arrow, *B*). This case underscores the importance of contrast enhancement in cases of unexplained hemorrhage. The coronal T1-weighted MR image (*C*) clearly demonstrates the superiority of MR imaging of these lesions. Although the image was obtained without gadolinium enhancement, it shows all three components of the malformation: high flow in the malformation (white asterisk), hemorrhage (black asterisk), and fast flow in the draining basal vein of Rosenthal (arrow). MR of a second patient with an arteriovenous malformation demonstrates the fast flow (low signal intensity) in a left parietal vascular malformation on T2-weighted axial (asterisk, *D*) and T1-weighted sagittal (asterisk, *E* [following page]) views. A computer reconstructed image of the greatest signal intensities with subtraction of signals from stationary tissues (*F*, following page) shows the arterial supply (small white arrows), the nidus of the malformation (asterisk), and the venous drainage (open arrow).

(Figure continued on following page.)

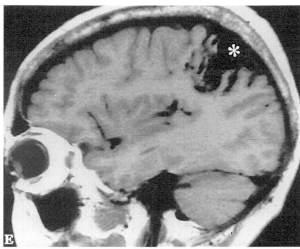

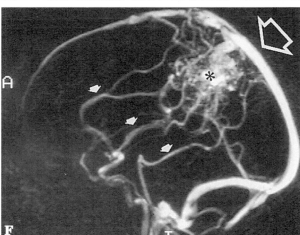

FIGURE 5 *(Cont.).*   See legend on previous page.

28. What are the most common intracranial manifestations of child abuse?

Subdural hematoma (Fig. 6)—from stretching and rupture of bridging veins.

Contusions—from subcortical shearing injury. The densely packed cortex is more rigid than the underlying white matter. The contusions may be hemorrhagic.

Multiple strokes—if the child was strangled, the brain ischemia and edema are preferentially supratentorial in location. The vertebrobasilar circulation is almost always spared.

29. Do strokes occur in children (other than in child abuse)?

Yes, although they are rare. One cause is moya-moya disease, which is occlusion of the supratentorial internal carotid artery. The syndrome was first described in Japan but may occur in any population. The slowly progressive obliteration of the carotid artery results in gradual recruitment of tiny vessels that supply deeply seated areas of the brain, such as the basal ganglia and choroid plexus. On angiography, these vessels appear as a haziness—which is in fact the derivation of the term *moya-moya* (Japanese for "hazy like a puff of smoke").

30. What is the typical appearance of strangulation on a CT scan of the brain?

The supratentorial brain is low in density as a result of bilateral carotid obstruction. The reduced flow to the supratentorial brain causes ischemia, while the vertebral arteries, which are protected by

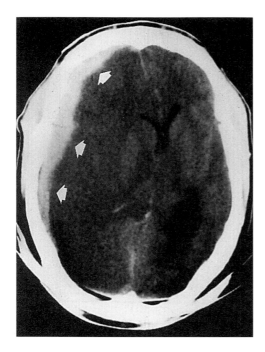

FIGURE 6. Subdural hematoma. Semilunar-shaped hyperdense hematoma (retracted clot) situated along the inner table of the skull on the right. The hematoma is bounded by the falx and the tentorium. There is marked mass effect, with midline shift to the left.

the foramina transversaria in the cervical vertebrae, maintain the flow of oxygenated blood to the infratentorial brain. Obstruction of the venous outflow from compression of the jugular veins results in stasis, which may cause venous infarcts of the supratentorial and the infratentorial brain.

31. What is the cause of moya-moya disease?
The cause is unknown, although it has been postulated that the disease may be immunologically mediated by substances in the cerebrospinal fluid. The carotid arteries become exposed to cerebrospinal fluid when they pierce the dura above the clinoid processes and enter the subarachnoid space. Moya-moya disease is declining in incidence, although the reason is also unknown. The decline may be related to the eradication of smallpox.

BIBLIOGRAPHY

1. Hilton SV, Edwards DK: Practical Pediatric Radiology, 2nd ed. Philadelphia, W.B. Saunders, 1994.
2. Volpe JJ: Neurology of the Newborn, 3rd ed. Philadelphia, W.B. Saunders, 1995.

IX. Trauma

70. EXTREMITY TRAUMA

Kevin R. Math, M.D., and Fred D. Cushner, M.D.

1. Which important radiographic features of fractures should routinely be assessed?

Complete vs. incomplete. Complete fractures traverse the entire width of the bone, penetrating both cortical surfaces. They are described by their orientation as transverse, oblique, or spiral. Incomplete fractures occur primarily in children because of their bony plasticity. These fractures are divided into greenstick (fracture traverses one cortex), torus (one cortex is buckled), and plastic bowing fractures (no fracture line, but long bone is bowed).

Displacement. Displacement describes the location of the distal fragment relative to the proximal one (e.g., dorsal, ventral, medial, lateral). The degree of displacement may be quantified as a measure of the shaft width or as an absolute measurement (e.g., the distal fragment is displaced dorsally by one half shaft width or there is dorsal displacement of the distal fragment by 6 mm).

Angulation. This describes the orientation of the distal fragment relative to the proximal fragment or the angulation at the apex of the fracture. For example, a distal radial shaft fracture with dorsal angulation of the distal fragment = ventral angulation at the fracture site. Either of these is correct, provided that the fracture site or distal fragment is specified.

Comminution. A comminuted fracture has more than two fragments. A "butterfly fragment" is a small separate bony fragment at the site of a comminuted fracture.

2. What is an occult fracture?

A fracture that is present but not radiographically visible. Such fractures are frequently associated with significant symptoms despite normal radiographs. Sites notorious for occult fractures include the scaphoid, sacrum, and femoral neck. Occult femoral neck fractures are an important problem in elderly patients with osteoporosis.

3. What is the rationale for obtaining follow-up radiographs 7–10 days after trauma for a suspected occult fracture?

Hyperemia, inflammation, and resultant bone resorption at the fracture site occur in the earliest stages of fracture healing, allowing demonstration of the lucent fracture line on delayed films (Fig. 1).

4. What other imaging modalities may be used for a more immediate diagnosis of occult bony injury?

MRI or a radionuclide bone scan can promptly diagnose occult fracture and expedite institution of appropriate therapy. MRI offers superior anatomic resolution and greater specificity over bone scanning; however, it is much more expensive.

5. A 75-year-old woman with suspected hip fracture presents with normal radiographs and a normal bone scan. Is hip fracture effectively excluded?

No. The false-negative rate of bone scans for acute femoral neck fractures in elderly patients may be as high as 25% in the first 24 hours after trauma. This is due to the fact that increased radionuclide uptake at traumatic sites depends on increased regional blood flow and bone remodeling, both of which are more sluggish in elderly patients. For this reason, patients are often admitted into the hospital for observation, essentially waiting for the bone scan to become positive in 48–72 hours.

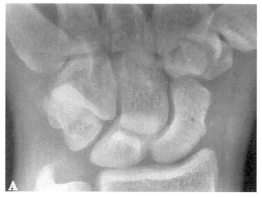
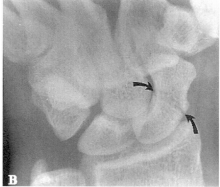

FIGURE 1. Delayed study showing occult scaphoid fracture. *A*, Patient with snuffbox tenderness presents with normal radiographs of the wrist. *B*, A film obtained 10 days later clearly shows the fracture line at the mid-waist of the scaphoid (curved arrows).

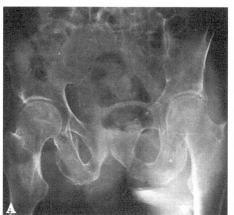
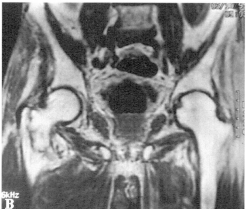

FIGURE 2. Occult hip fracture. *A*, Elderly man with externally rotated right hip and no fracture seen on initial radiographs. *B*, MRI performed on the same day permitted prompt diagnosis of the nondisplaced inter-trochanteric fracture.

MRI is advocated for immediate diagnosis of occult hip fractures in elderly patients (Fig. 2). The examination can be tailored specifically for diagnosis of a hip fracture, and the cost of this "limited" examination can be prorated to become comparable with that of a bone scan. Furthermore, prompt diagnosis results in decreased operative morbidity and decreased length of hospital stay.

6. Differentiate between dislocation and subluxation.

Dislocation involves complete loss of apposition of articular surfaces at a joint, whereas subluxation involves partial contact at the articulation.

7. Why are postreduction radiographs so important after a dislocation?

Postreduction radiographs confirm adequate reduction of the dislocation. In addition, occult fracture and intraarticular fragments are more easily identified after reduction.

8. Is one view of a traumatized bone or joint sufficient in cases with a low index of suspicion for fracture?

Definitely not. It is not uncommon for fractures to be seen on only one view, because the x-ray beam must be perpendicular to a portion of the fracture line to visualize it (Fig. 3). Once the decision

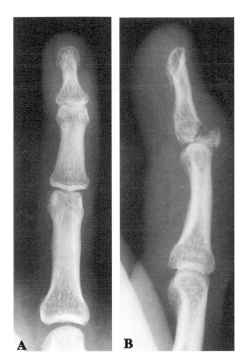

FIGURE 3. *A*, Anteroposterior view of this finger shows no fracture. *B*, The lateral view reveals a significant fracture fragment at the dorsal base of the distal phalanx with intraarticular extension.

to obtain radiographs is made, at least two orthogonal (at right angles to each other) views are essential. Similarly, dislocations may be subtle on one view and obvious on a right-angle view. Most radiology departments have set protocols for each specific examination; thus, it is unnecessary to specify the specific number of views unless a special additional view is needed (e.g., cross-table lateral view of the knee).

9. What is a stress fracture?

Stress fractures are divided into two groups: fatigue fractures and insufficiency fractures. A **fatigue fracture** results from abnormal stress or torque applied to normal bone. A march fracture of the metatarsal shaft in a military recruit is one example. An **insufficiency fracture** occurs when normal or physiologic stresses are applied to abnormal osteoporotic bone. These fractures commonly occur in elderly patients at sites such as the sacrum and pelvis. The anatomic location of stress fractures depends on the nature of the prolonged repetitive activity that caused them. Most stress fractures occur in the weight-bearing lower extremities: metatarsals, calcaneus, and tibial shaft. These fractures can affect medullary (cancellous) bone where they will appear as a band of sclerosis or can involve cortical bone where they result in localized cortical thickening (Figs. 4 and 5).

10. Of the following structures, which is most susceptible to injury in children—(a) metaphyseal bone; (b) epiphyseal bone; (c) growth plate; (d) ligaments; (e) tendons?

The growth plate or physis is the weakest, most susceptible site, accounting for the preponderance of physeal injuries in children.

11. What are the radiographic signs of fracture nonunion?

Sclerosis at the edges of the fracture fragments with a persistent lucent fracture line. There may be sclerotic proliferation of bone at the margins of the fracture; however, this does not bridge the fracture.

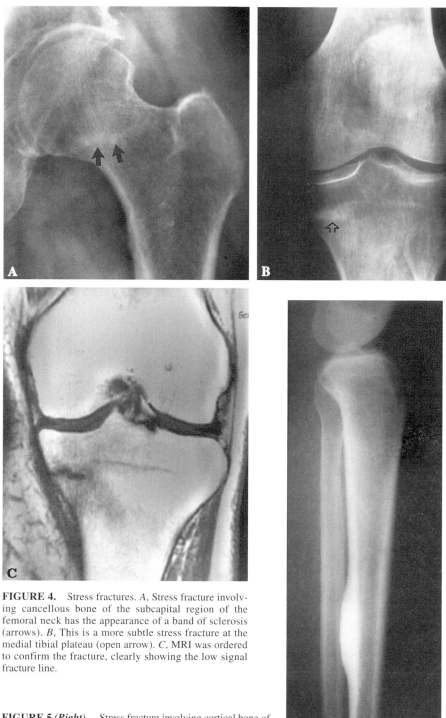

FIGURE 4. Stress fractures. *A*, Stress fracture involving cancellous bone of the subcapital region of the femoral neck has the appearance of a band of sclerosis (arrows). *B*, This is a more subtle stress fracture at the medial tibial plateau (open arrow). *C*, MRI was ordered to confirm the fracture, clearly showing the low signal fracture line.

FIGURE 5 *(Right).* Stress fracture involving cortical bone of the posterior aspect of the mid/distal tibial shaft. Note the segment of posterior cortical thickening.

12. What is the Salter-Harris classification?

A method of classifying types of growth plate injuries that is based on the extent of the injury.

Type I   Only the growth plate is involved; the adjacent epiphysis and metaphysis are intact. This type has the best prognosis.

Type II   Fracture line extends through growth plate and exits through metaphysis, resulting in a metaphyseal corner fragment. This is the most common type, accounting for ~70% of physeal injuries.

Type III   Fracture line involves growth plate and extends into epiphysis; the metaphysis is not involved.

Type IV   Fracture line traverses metaphysis, growth plate, and epiphysis.

Type V   Crush injury at the growth plate without a visible fracture line. This is the least common type (< 1%) and carries the highest association with future growth disturbance.

13. What is osteochondritis dissecans (OCD)?

OCD is a type of osteochondral fracture, resulting in fragmentation of the bone's articular surface. These fragments consist of cartilage alone or cartilage and underlying bone and have varying levels of attachment to the bone. Chondral or osteochondral fragments may remain firmly attached (in situ) and eventually heal or may partially or completely detach, sometimes resulting in intraarticular loose bodies.

14. What is the role of MRI in assessing OCD?

MRI can help to assess the stability of osteochondral fragments; lesions that are large, have fluid extending into the interface with the adjacent bone, or have overlying disrupted articular cartilage and underlying cystic changes are more prone to eventual detachment and are treated more aggressively (Fig. 6).

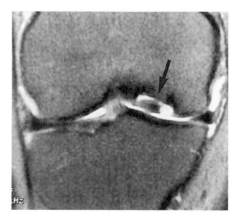

FIGURE 6. Osteochondritis dissecans with loose fragment. Coronal fat-suppressed proton-density MRI shows a loose osteochondral fragment at the medial femoral condyle completely encircled by the hyperintense joint fluid (arrow).

15. Name the most common sites of OCD.

The knee is by far the most common site; 85% of lesions at the knee are at the lateral aspect of the medial femoral condyle (mnemonic **LAME** = lateral aspect medial epicondyle).

The talus is the second most common site, with lesions at the talar dome.

The capitellum of the elbow (humeral articular surface articulating with the radial head) is the third most common site.

16. Which view is best for diagnosing OCD of the knee?

The tunnel view, which visualizes the posterior aspect of the intercondylar notch and depicts this relatively posterior lesion to best advantage (Fig. 7).

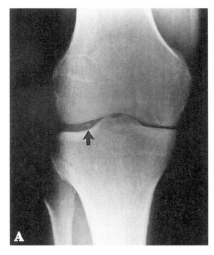
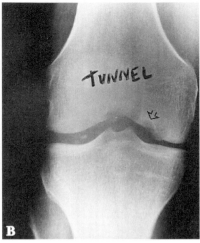

FIGURE 7. Osteochondritis dissecans of the medial femoral condyle with loose body. On the anteroposterior view (*A*) a small calcified loose body overlies the lateral joint compartment (arrow). On the "tunnel view" (*B*) the donor site at the medial femoral condyle is clearly seen (open arrow).

17. Some fractures are so common that they are referred to by commonly used eponyms. Where do the following fractures occur?

A. Boxer's	D. Segond	G. Maissoneuve	J. Bennett	L. Hangman's
B. Colles'	E. Jones	H. Monteggia	K. Jefferson	M. Chance
C. Galeazzi	F. Chauffeur's	I. Lisfranc		

A. 4th or 5th metacarpal neck, from a poorly thrown punch (Fig. 8)

B. Distal radius (wrist), commonly associated with ulnar styloid fracture (Fig. 9)

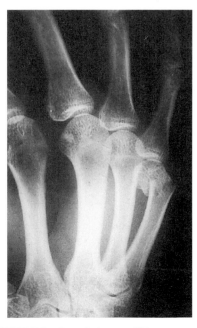
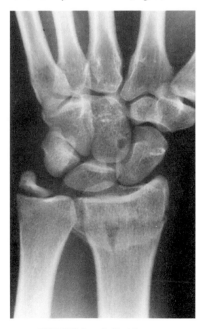

FIGURE 8.   Boxer's fracture, fifth metacarpal.   **FIGURE 9.**   Colles' fracture.

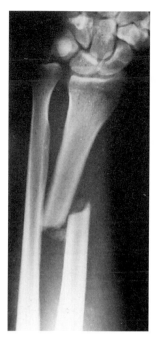

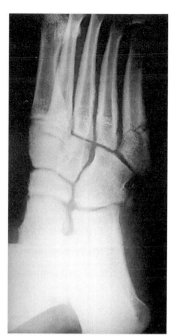

FIGURE 10 *(Right)*. Galeazzi fracture. Note the abnormal alignment at the distal radio-ulnar joint.

FIGURE 11 *(Far Right)*. Jones fracture.

FIGURE 12 *(Bottom Right)*. Chance fracture, L2 vertebral body. The fracture line traverses the spinous process, pedicles, and superior vertebral body.

C. Distal radial shaft, associated with dislocation at the distal radioulnar joint (Fig. 10)

D. Avulsion at the lateral margin of the lateral tibial plateau

E. Proximal 5th metatarsal shaft (Fig. 11)

F. Distal radius (radial styloid); originally described in the 1920s, when it was sustained from backfire of the crank of an automobile engine

G. Medial malleolus and proximal fibular shaft; from eversion injury

H. Proximal ulnar shaft, associated with radial head dislocation

I. Avulsion at medial base of second metatarsal, commonly associated with lateral displacement of the second through fifth metatarsals

J. Base of first metacarpal

K. First cervical vertebra (atlas), secondary to axial loading injury (e.g., diving)

L. Pedicles and posterior elements of the C2 vertebra, secondary to hyperextension

M. Upper lumbar vertebrae, most commonly L2; also known as a "seatbelt injury" secondary to hyper-flexion of the lumbar spine over a fixed fulcrum (seatbelt) (Fig. 12)

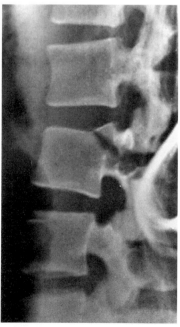

18. What is a fat-fluid level? How is this sign useful in assessing extremity trauma?

A fat-fluid level is the plain film demonstration of the interface between fat floating superiorly and fluid (blood) layering dependently after an intraarticular fracture. This sign is indicative of an intraarticular fracture due to leakage of marrow fat into the joint and interfacing with intraarticular

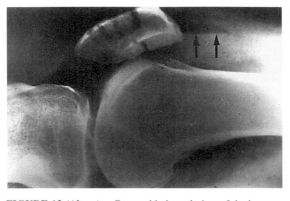
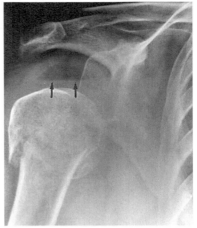

FIGURE 13 *(Above).*   Cross-table lateral view of the knee reveals a fat-fluid level in the suprapatellar region (arrows) secondary to a patellar fracture.

FIGURE 14 *(Above right).*   Erect anteroposterior view of the shoulder shows a fat-fluid level superior to the humeral head (arrows) secondary to a humeral neck fracture.

hemorrhage (hemarthrosis). It is most useful in suspected occult intraarticular fractures at the knee; a cross-table lateral view, obtained with a horizontal x-ray beam and the knee extended parallel to the floor on the x-ray table, readily demonstrates this sign (Fig. 13). A fat-fluid level also may be evident on erect shoulder radiographs in association with intraarticular fractures (Fig. 14). Supine anteroposterior radiographs do not elicit this sign, because the x-ray beam is not parallel to the interface.

19. Which type of fracture is shown in Figure 15? What is its significance?

Figure 15 shows a Segond fracture. This avulsion fracture at the lateral capsular ligament attachment on the lateral tibia has a fairly benign appearance; however, one should be aware of its strong association (> 90%) with tears of the anterior cruciate ligament.

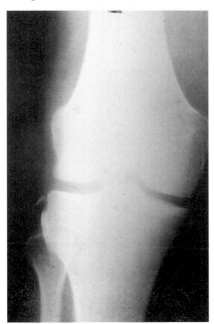

FIGURE 15.   Segond fracture. There is a small linear avulsion fragment at the lateral margin of the lateral tibial plateau.

20. Which study should be ordered after significant extremity trauma and normal radiographs?
MRI is highly effective at detecting occult bony injuries (fracture, contusion); ligament, cartilage, and tendon injuries; and muscle tears not evident on plain films.

21. What is the most commonly dislocated joint?
Shoulder dislocations account for about 50% of all joint dislocations.

22. In which direction does the humeral head most commonly dislocate?
Anteriorly. Anterior shoulder dislocations account for about 95% of all shoulder dislocations, resulting in a subcoracoid location of the humeral head on anteroposterior radiographs (Fig. 16).

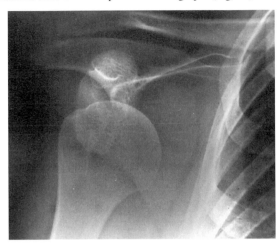

FIGURE 16. Anterior shoulder dislocation. The dislocated humeral head is situated inferior to the coracoid process.

23. What are Hill-Sachs and Bankart lesions?
Hill-Sachs and Bankart lesions are impaction injuries of the posterolateral humeral head and the anteroinferior glenoid, respectively, occurring in association with anterior shoulder dislocations. The dislocated humeral head impacts on the inferior glenoid, resulting in characteristic injuries.

24. Which view best demonstrates the Hill-Sachs defect?
An internally rotated anteroposterior view (Fig. 17).

25. A patient presents to the emergency department with bilateral posterior shoulder dislocations. What is the most likely mechanism of injury?
This type of injury classically occurs in association with seizures. About one-half of posterior shoulder dislocations are due to blunt anterior shoulder trauma, which is typically unilateral. The other half follow motor seizures and are occasionally bilateral.

26. Describe the radiographic findings of a posterior shoulder dislocation.
- Humeral head fixed in persistent internal rotation
- Relative widening of the glenohumeral joint on the anteroposterior view (rim sign: space between the anterior glenoid rim and the medial humeral head ≥ 6 mm)
- Sclerotic line parallel to the medial border of the humeral head secondary to impaction injury (trough line)

Radiographic signs of posterior shoulder dislocations are often subtle and are commonly overlooked (Fig. 18). An axillary view is ideal for optimal assessment of glenohumeral alignment; however, patients often have trouble tolerating this view because of pain. If there is any question of shoulder dislocation on the conventional radiographs, a CT scan is helpful for further evaluation.

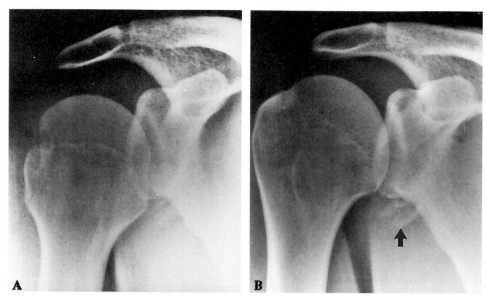

FIGURE 17.   Hill-Sachs defect. *A*, Focal impaction of the superolateral aspect of the humeral head (arrow) is well visualized on the internally rotated view owing to its posterior location on the head. This indicates that there was an anterior dislocation; whether the dislocation was recent or single or multiple cannot be determined. *B*, The Hill-Sachs defect cannot be seen on this externally rotated view. Note the Bankart fracture at the inferior glenoid (arrow).

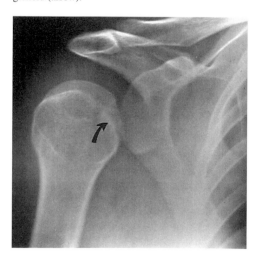

FIGURE 18.   Posterior shoulder dislocation. The shoulder is persistently internally rotated resulting in a "light-bulb" appearance of the humeral head and neck. Note the trough line at the medial humeral head (curved arrow).

27. How are acromioclavicular (AC) joint injuries radiographically diagnosed and graded?
    Anteroposterior views of both AC joints are taken simultaneously and then repeated with weight-bearing stress on the joints. Normal AC joint width is about 3–5 mm, with no more than 3 mm difference between the two sides. The following is the grading system for AC joint injuries:

Type I	Diagnosed clinically; mild ligamentous injury at the joint, usually with normal radiographs
Type II	Rupture of the AC ligaments and joint capsule with AC joint widening
Type III	Same as type II plus disruption of coracoclavicular ligaments with widening of the space between the coracoid and clavicle (Fig. 19)

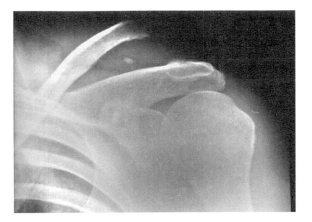

FIGURE 19. Grade 3 acromioclavicular joint dislocation. There is marked superior displacement of the distal clavicle relative to the acromion and coracoid processes.

28. What is the imaging modality of choice for evaluation of suspected sternoclavicular joint injury?

Computed tomography. These injuries are much less common than AC joint injuries and are easily overlooked on routine radiographs. Although the clavicle usually dislocates anteriorly, posterior dislocations are more dangerous, because they can be complicated by injury to the great vessels, esophagus, and trachea.

29. What is inferior pseudosubluxation of the humeral head?

Acute fractures of the humeral head and neck may be complicated by varying degrees of inferior displacement of the humeral head relative to the glenoid (see Fig. 14). This results from a combination of massive hemarthrosis, lax muscle tone, and stretching of the joint capsule; it is not a true inferior dislocation. Humeral head position usually returns to normal after a few months.

30. What is a bipartite patella?

A bipartite patella is either a variant of ossification of the patella or a result of clinically insignificant trauma to the immature skeleton, resulting in a linear fracture-like lucency traversing the patella. It is commonly seen as an incidental finding and should not be mistaken for a fracture.

31. How can a bipartite patella be distinguished from a patellar fracture?

- The lucent line of bipartite patella is almost always at the superolateral aspect of the patella (Fig. 20).
- The two fragments of a bipartite patella have irregular edges, unlike the sharp edges of a fracture, which fit evenly together like a jigsaw puzzle (Fig. 21).
- The coronal width of a bipartite patella is greater than the width of the contralateral normal patella.
- 50% of bipartite patellas are bilateral; when in doubt, image the contralateral knee.

32. Name the five most common sites for avulsion injury at the ankle.

- Lateral malleolus
- Medial malleolus
- Base of the fifth metatarsal (Fig. 22)
- Anterior process of the calcaneus
- Dorsal talonavicular region (capsular attachment)

33. What tendon inserts on the base of the fifth metatarsal?

Peroneus brevis.

34. How does the radiographic appearance of an eversion injury differ from that of an inversion injury?

Eversion injuries result in oblique distal fibular fractures and transverse medial malleolar fractures (either at tip of malleolus or at its base) and may be associated with widening of the medial

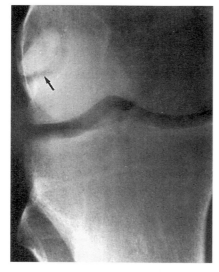

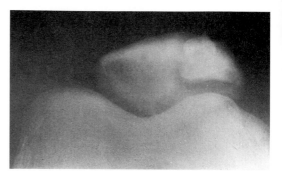

FIGURE 20 (Left). Bipartite patella. Note the curvilinear lucent line at the superolateral patella (arrow).

FIGURE 21 (Above right). Bipartite patella. The two "fragments" do not appear to fit evenly together, as would be expected if this were a true fracture.

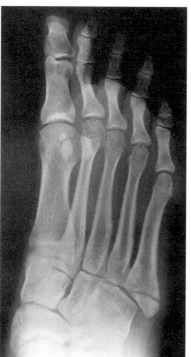

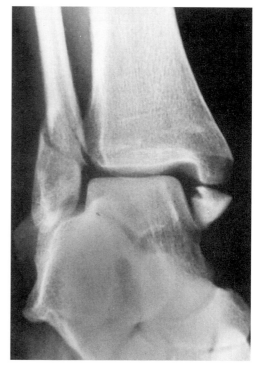

FIGURE 22 (Above left). Avulsion fracture at the base of the fifth metatarsal.

FIGURE 23 (Above right). Eversion injury of the ankle. There is a transversely oriented fracture line at the base of the medial malleolus, and an oblique fracture at the lateral malleolus, characteristic of eversion injury.

ankle mortise if ligaments are disrupted (Fig. 23). **Inversion** injuries result in an oblique fracture of the medial malleolus combined with small transverse lateral malleolar avulsion fragments. Widening of the lateral ankle mortise also may be present.

35. What is Bohler's angle?

Bohler's angle is the angle between lines drawn from the superior apex of the mid-calcaneus (posterior facet) to the anterior process of the calcaneus and from the same site at the mid calcaneus to the posterior calcaneal tuberosity. This angle is normally 20–40°. A decreased Bohler's angle indicates relative flattening of the calcaneus and is a useful sign of calcaneal fracture (Fig. 24).

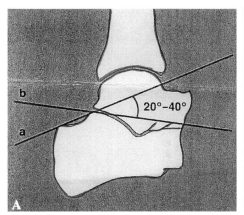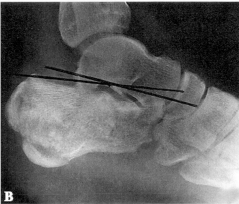

FIGURE 24. Bohler's angle. *A*, Diagram illustrating the points of measurement of this angle. *B*, Bohler's angle in this calcaneal fracture is clearly decreased.

36. What bones compose the hindfoot, midfoot, and forefoot?

The calcaneus and talus compose the hindfoot. The remaining tarsal bones (cuboid, navicular, cuneiforms) compose the midfoot, and the metatarsals and phalanges compose the forefoot. The joint between the tarsal and metatarsal bones is called Lisfranc's joint, and the joint between the hindfoot and midfoot is called Chopart's joint.

37. What is an os trigonum?

An os trigonum is an accessory bony ossicle at the posterior margin of the talus, best seen on the lateral view. It is present in about 8% of individuals and rarely causes symptoms. Ballet dancers may develop symptoms (os trigonum syndrome) from repetitive plantar flexion and resultant compression of this ossicle between the posterior tibia and calcaneus.

38. Who was Lisfranc? What type of injury bears his name?

Lisfranc reportedly was a surgeon in Napoleon's army who gained notoriety for rapid forefoot amputations as treatment for fracture-dislocations sustained after falling off a horse. Forced plantarflexion of the foot (while still in the stirrup) results in this fairly common injury at the tarsal-metatarsal joints (also called Lisfranc's joint). The classic Lisfranc fracture-dislocation is marked by lateral displacement of the second through fifth metatarsals; the medial margin of the second metatarsal, which usually lines up with the medial margin of the middle cuneiform, becomes laterally displaced. There is commonly an associated avulsion fracture at the medial base of the second metatarsal (Fig. 25).

39. What is the sail sign?

This important sign refers to the sail-like appearance of the displaced anterior fat pad on a lateral radiograph of the elbow. This fat pad, normally seen as a thin lucent band anterior to the distal humerus, becomes anteriorly displaced by intraarticular blood or fluid, giving rise to the sail sign (Fig. 26). In the setting of trauma, the sail sign indicates hemarthrosis secondary to intraarticular fracture. The posterior fat pad is not visualized on a normal lateral elbow film, because it lies within the olecranon fossa; its visualization carries the same significance as the sail sign. Visualization of these fat pads implies an intraarticular fracture, even if no fracture line is seen; delayed radiographs

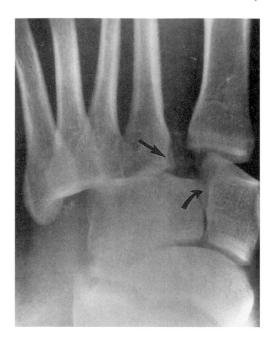

FIGURE 25 (Left). Lisfranc fracture-dislocation. The medial margin of the base of the second metatarsal (solid arrow) is laterally displaced relative to the medial margin of the middle cuneiform (curved arrow), and all other metatarsals are similarly displaced. There are small fracture fragments between the first and second metatarsal bases.

FIGURE 26 (Right). Sail sign. The displaced anterior fat pad has a sail-shaped appearance (straight arrow). The posterior fat pad is visualized (curved arrow). It is always abnormal on technically adequate lateral elbow radiographs.

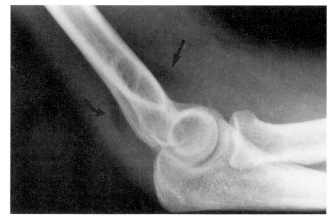

performed in 7–10 days usually delineate occult fractures. Inflammatory arthritides and infection also displace the fat pads with joint fluid or pus.

40. What is the most common direction of radial head dislocation?

The radial head is usually dislocated anteriorly. It is normally aligned with the capitellum of the humerus on all views of the elbow.

41. How is carpal alignment assessed on a posteroanterior radiograph?

All joint spaces at the wrist are normally of uniform width, each about 1–2 mm. Three parallel curvilinear arcs can be drawn to assess carpal alignment (Fig. 27). The first arc is drawn over the proximal articular surfaces of the scaphoid, lunate, and triquetrum; the second is drawn over the distal articular surfaces of these bones; and the third is drawn along the proximal articular surfaces of the hamate and capitate. These arcs are normally smoothly curved; disruption of the arc's continuity implies ligamentous injury and malalignment.

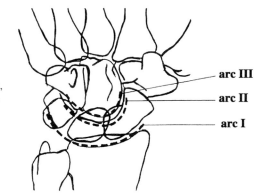

FIGURE 27. These three arcs, described by Gilula, are helpful for detecting occult carpal malalignment.

42. Name the most commonly fractured carpal bone.

The scaphoid. Fractures of the scaphoid account for up to 70% of carpal injuries and usually result from a fall on an outstretched hand. Patients usually have focal tenderness over the snuffbox region. If this fracture is suspected, a special navicular view should be performed. If radiographs are normal but clinical suspicion is high, an immediate diagnosis can be made with a bone scan or MRI. Alternatively, the patient can be treated conservatively and return for follow-up radiographs in about 10 days. Occult fractures are usually visible on a follow-up study.

43. What are the two most common complications associated with scaphoid fractures?

Delayed union or nonunion and avascular necrosis.

44. Which type of fracture has a higher risk of avascular necrosis—proximal scaphoid or distal scaphoid? Why?

Fractures through the proximal third of the scaphoid carry the worst prognosis and highest risk of avascular necrosis. This is directly related to the blood supply of the scaphoid; the middle and distal portions of the scaphoid receive their own direct blood supply, whereas the proximal scaphoid relies on intraosseous perfusion from the middle portion of the scaphoid. Proximal scaphoid fractures commonly result in disruption of this tenuous blood supply and resultant risk of avascular necrosis. Fractures distal to the vessels that penetrate the mid-scaphoid do not significantly affect arterial flow to the proximal scaphoid. Generally speaking, the more proximal the fracture line, the greater the risk for fracture nonunion and avascular necrosis. MRI is ideal for evaluation of clinically suspected avascular necrosis or fracture nonunion, neither of which is clearly demonstrated on conventional radiographs.

45. Which view is best for distinguishing between lunate and perilunate dislocation?

The lateral view. Normally, the distal radius, lunate, and capitate are well-aligned on the lateral view. In perilunate dislocations, the capitate dislocates dorsally from the lunate fossa. In lunate dislocations, the lunate dislocates and tilts ventrally from its normal location at the distal radius (Fig. 28).

46. What is the Terry Thomas sign?

This sign, named after the British comedian with a gap between his two front teeth, refers to the widened space between the lunate and scaphoid bones on a frontal view of the wrist secondary to scapholunate dissociation (Fig. 29). Injury to the scapholunate ligament and other supporting ligaments causes this space to widen to > 2 mm or more than the adjacent intercarpal spaces. Also known as the David Letterman sign, this widening is usually accompanied by abnormal rotation ("rotatory subluxation") of the scaphoid, resulting in a signet ring-like configuration of the bone.

47. Which carpal bone is fractured in Figure 30?

The dorsal fragment in Figure 30 indicates a triquetral avulsion fracture, the second most commonly injured carpal bone.

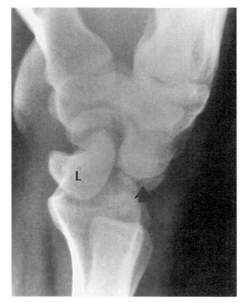

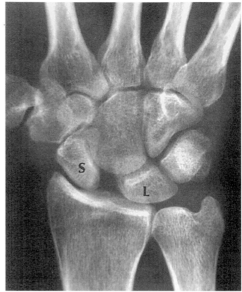

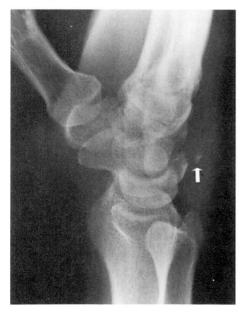

FIGURE 28 *(Above left)*. Perilunate dislocation. The capitate (arrow) and remainder of the carpus are dorsally dislocated relative to the lunate (L), which is normally located.

FIGURE 29 *(Above right)*. Scapholunate dissociation. The space between the scaphoid (S) and lunate (L) is markedly widened, reflecting severe ligamentous injury.

FIGURE 30 *(Left)*. Triquetral fracture. This dorsal fragment (arrow) indicates a triquetral fracture. Note the associated soft tissue swelling.

48. Which view is best for demonstrating a suspected fracture of the hook of the hamate?

A carpal tunnel view, essentially an axial view of the carpus, is best for evaluation of this ventrally projecting process. Cross-sectional imaging with CT is also ideal for evaluating these injuries and can provide information about other bones and soft tissues.

49. What is the most common direction of hip dislocation?

About 85% of all hip dislocations are posterior. Posterior dislocations usually result from dashboard injuries in motor vehicle accidents. The flexed knee strikes the dashboard, driving the femur posteriorly. An associated fracture of the posterior acetabulum is common.

50. Which imaging modality is best for evaluation of complex acetabular or pelvic fractures?

CT. Current technology allows thin sections to be obtained through the fracture sites with computer-generated two- or three-dimensional reconstructed images. The precise extent of the fracture as well as associated soft tissue injuries and intraarticular fragments is well demonstrated on CT and commonly underestimated on plain films.

51. Name the common sites for avulsion fracture at the hip and pelvis and the muscles or tendons that attach at these sites.

Anterior superior iliac spine—sartorius muscle   Lesser trochanter—iliopsoas tendon
Anterior inferior iliac spine—biceps femoris tendon   Greater trochanter—gluteal tendon
Ischial tuberosity—hamstring tendons

52. Define slipped capital femoral epiphysis (SCFE).

SCFE is a growth plate injury at the proximal femoral physis (Salter I), typically seen between 11 and 15 years of age, the period of most rapid growth. The demographic groups most commonly affected are boys > girls, and blacks > whites. Anteroposterior and lateral views of both hips are necessary to demonstrate accurately the posteromedial slippage of the femoral head epiphysis relative to the femoral neck. About 20% of cases are bilateral.

53. What is posttraumatic myositis ossificans?

Myositis ossificans is characterized by an ossifying or calcifying mass within the soft tissues, usually after trauma. Up to one-third of patients recall no significant traumatic event. By the fourth week after trauma, calcifications develop within the mass, progressing to the classic peripheral calcification or ossification by 6–8 weeks. The hallmark of this lesion is its zonal phenomenon of ossification; the lesion progressively ossifies in a centripetal fashion, eventually resulting in a coalescent ossified mass. During this evolution one can see mature trabecular bone at the periphery of the lesion with a lucent center. The zonal maturation pattern, combined with separation of the lesion from the adjacent bone, allows differentiation from parosteal osteosarcoma; sarcomas ossify centrally and diffusely rather than peripherally. Accurate radiographic differentiation is crucial, because *biopsy of these lesions is ill-advised.* Whereas biopsy of the periphery of the lesion yields mature bone, sampling of the more central lesion demonstrates hemorrhage, necrosis, and mitotic figures, potentially resulting in a misdiagnosis of an osteosarcoma (Fig. 31).

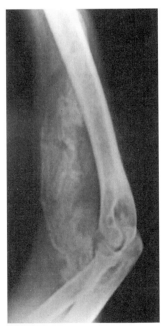

FIGURE 31 *(Right).* Myositis ossificans of the elbow. There is a large ossified mass, bridging the elbow joint in this quadriplegic patient. Identification of trabeculae and cortex is diagnostic of ossification.

BIBLIOGRAPHY

1. Berquist TH: Imaging of Orthopedic Trauma, 2nd ed. New York, Raven Press, 1992.
2. Daffner RH, Pavlov H: Stress fractures: Current concepts. AJR 159:245, 1992.
3. Deutsch AI, Mink JH, Waxman AD: Occult fractures of the proximal femur: MR imaging. Radiology 170:113–116, 1989.
4. Gilula Y, Yin Y: Imaging of the Wrist and Hand. Philadelphia, W.B. Saunders, 1996.
5. Goldman AB, Pavlov H, Rubenstein D: The Segond fracture of the proximal tibia: A small avulsion that reflects major ligamentous damage. AJR 151:1163–1167, 1988.
6. Harris JH Jr, Harris WH: The Radiology of Emergency Medicine, 3rd ed. Baltimore, Williams & Wilkins, 1993.
7. Riddervold HO: Easily missed fractures. Radiol Clin North Am 30:475, 1992.

8. Rizzo PF, Gould ES, Lyden JF, et al: Diagnosis of occult fracture about the hip. J Bone Joint Surg 75A:395–401, 1993.
9. Rubin DA, Dalinka MK, Kneeland JB: Magnetic resonance imaging of lower extremity injuries. Semin Roentgenol 32:194–222, 1994.

71. SPINAL TRAUMA

John J. Wasenko, M.D.

1. What does a complete cervical spinal series consist of?
Lateral, anteroposterior, open-mouth, oblique, and flexion and extension radiographs.

2. Why is the lateral view the most important of the cervical spine series?
Because most significant injuries can be detected on the lateral view, including vertebral body fractures, dislocations, and soft tissue injuries. Often, the lateral view is checked by the radiologist before the other views are obtained.

3. Describe four lines that can be drawn on a lateral radiograph to assess the alignment of the cervical spine.
   1. The anterior spinal line, which is formed by the anterior margins of the vertebral bodies
   2. The posterior spinal line, which is formed by the posterior margins of the vertebral bodies
   3. The spinolaminar line, which is formed by the anterior cortical margin of the spinous processes
   4. A fourth line connecting the tips of the spinous processes

4. What are normal prevertebral soft tissue measurements in adults and children?
In adults, the prevertebral soft tissue in the retropharyngeal area measures a maximal anteroposterior dimension of 3.4 mm on the lateral radiograph, and in the retrotracheal area it measures 14 mm. In children, the prevertebral soft tissues measure 3.5 mm and 7.9 mm in the retropharyngeal and retrotracheal areas, respectively.

5. What is the significance of widening of the prevertebral soft tissues?
In the setting of trauma, this finding indicates that a cervical spine fracture may be present even if one is not clearly seen on the lateral film.

6. What is the normal width of the anterior atlantodental interval in adults and children?
   • 2.5–3 mm in adults
   • 5 mm in children
The anterior atlantodental interval is the distance between the anterior aspect of the dens (the superior portion of the C2 vertebra) and the posterior cortex of the anterior arch of C1.

7. Describe the normal appearance of the articulating facets of the cervical spine.
The inferior articulating facets of the vertebral body above are posterior to the superior articulating facets of the vertebral body below. The appearance is similar to shingles on a roof.

8. What are the normal anatomic relationships at the craniovertebral junction?
The tip of the clivus should intersect the odontoid process at the junction of the anterior and middle thirds. The posterior lamina of C1 should be in alignment with the posterior margin of the foramen magnum.

9. How is pseudosubluxation differentiated from true subluxation due to ligamentous injury?
There is no discontinuity in the spinolaminar line with pseudosubluxation, whereas it is discontinuous with true subluxation.

10. Where does pseudosubluxation occur?

Pseudosubluxation occurs in children as a result of ligamentous laxity and is commonly seen at the C2–3 and C3–4 levels.

11. Describe the appearance of a Jefferson fracture.

On the open-mouth radiograph (a view of the C1–2 region obtained with the mouth open, in the anteroposterior projection), the lateral masses of C1 are displaced laterally and overhang the lateral masses of the C2 vertebral body. There may be widening (> 2.5–3 mm) of the anterior atlantodental interval with soft tissue swelling on the lateral radiograph (Fig. 1).

12. When is a Jefferson fracture considered to be unstable?

When the anterior atlantodental interval is greater than 6.9 mm on the lateral radiograph. This indicates that there has been disruption of the transverse ligament.

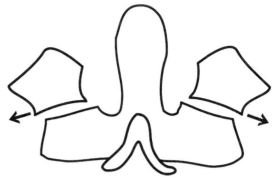

FIGURE 1.   Jefferson fracture. The lateral masses of C1 are displaced laterally with respect to the lateral masses of C2 (arrows).

13. What are the three types of fractures of the odontoid process?

Type I involves the tip of the dens, type II the base of the dens, and type III the superior aspect of the C2 vertebral body.

14. Explain the origin of an os odontoideum.

An os odontoideum is a round, well-corticated bony structure located just superior to the C2 vertebral body. It is through to represent congenital nonunion, incomplete ossification of the dens, or possibly an ununited fracture as the result of previous trauma.

15. Describe the three types of hangman's fracture.

A hangman's fracture is a bilateral fracture of the pars interarticularis of C2; this portion of the vertebra connects the superior and inferior facets. There is minimal displacement of the fracture fragments in type I, anterior displacement of the C2 vertebral body in type II, and anterior displacement of the vertebral body and bilateral facet dislocations in type III (Fig. 2).

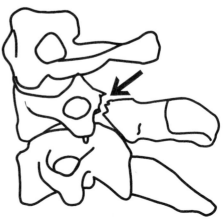

FIGURE 2.   Hangman's fracture. There is a fracture through the pars interarticularis of C2 (arrow).

16. Are unilateral and bilateral facet dislocations stable or unstable injuries?

A unilateral facet dislocation is a stable injury because there is disruption of the ligamentous complex only on the side of the dislocation. A bilateral facet dislocation is unstable due to bilateral disruption of the posterior ligamentous complexes.

17. What injury is present when the lateral masses have a bowtie appearance on the lateral radiograph?

The bowtie appearance results from anterior subluxation of one lateral mass with respect to another. This is a unilateral facet dislocation—the inferior articulating facet of the vertebral body above is dislocated anteroinferior to the superior articulating facet of the vertebral body below (Fig. 3).

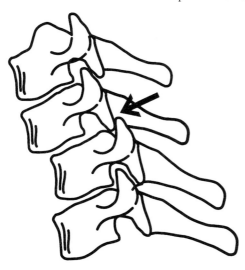

FIGURE 3. Unilateral locked facet. The inferior articulating facet of the vertebral body above is located anterior to the superior articulating facet of the vertebral body below (arrow).

18. What measurement is useful in the diagnosis of dissociation of the occiput from the atlas?

The powers ratio, which is a ratio of the line from the basion to the posterior laminar line of C1 and a line from the opisthion to the posterior surface of the anterior arch of C1. A value greater than 1 is abnormal.

19. How is the laminar space useful in the evaluation of cervical spinal trauma?

Narrowing of the laminar space, the distance between the articular pillars and the spinolaminar line, is a highly accurate sign for unilateral facet dislocation.

20. Describe a burst fracture.

A comminuted fracture of a vertebral body. There is variable displacement of fracture fragments with varying spinal canal compromise.

21. What percentage of fractures detected with CT are not seen with plain radiographs?

About 25%.

22. Is computed tomography of use in the evaluation of spinal trauma?

Yes. It is extremely valuable in the evaluation of known or suspected spinal fractures. CT can detect displaced fracture fragments and neural arch fractures that are not evident on plain radiographs. It also demonstrates the degree of spinal canal compromise by displaced fracture fragments.

23. What is an advantage of MR in the evaluation of spinal trauma?

The ability to visualize the spinal cord, thecal sac, spinal canal, intervertebral discs, and paravertebral soft tissues.

24. Is CT, CT myelography, or MRI the modality of choice for the detection of spinal cord contusion or hematoma?

MR. With its superior spatial and contrast resolution, MR readily demonstrates the spinal cord and depicts nonhemorrhagic and hemorrhagic contusions. MR also demonstrates hemorrhage adjacent to the spinal cord and other ligamentous and soft tissue injuries.

25. What are limitations of MR in the evaluation of spinal trauma?

Limitations include the need for MR-compatible life support equipment, the potential need for sedation to minimize patient motion, and the length of time necessary to perform a complete examination. In addition, fractures are poorly visualized with MR.

26. Is MR useful in the follow-up evaluation of spinal trauma?

MR is useful to follow injuries to the spinal cord such as contusions, which may resolve or result in myelomalacia, and in the detection of a posttraumatic syrinx.

27. What is the probability that a cervical spine fracture is present in an alert patient who has no complaints of pain or neurologic signs or symptoms?

Essentially zero.

28. A patient has normal plain films of the cervical spine but has neurologic symptoms suggesting spinal cord injury. What radiologic study should be performed?

MR.

BIBLIOGRAPHY

1. Anderson LD, D'Alonzo RT: Fracture of the odontoid process of the axis. J Bone Joint Surg 56A:1633–1674, 1974.
2. Berquist TH: Imaging of adult cervical spine trauma. Radiographics 8:667–694, 1988.
3. Effendi B, Roy D, Cornish B, et al: Fracture of the ring of the axis: A classification based on analysis of 131 cases. J Bone Joint Surg 63A:319–327, 1981.
4. Gehweiler JA Jr, Osborn RL, Becker RF: The Radiology of Vertebral Trauma. Philadelphia, W.B. Saunders, 1980.
5. Harris JH Jr, Edeiken-Moore B: The Radiology of Cervical Spine Trauma, 2nd ed. Baltimore, Williams & Wilkins, 1987.
6. McArdle CB, Crofford MJ, Mirfakhraee M, et al: Surface coil MR of spinal trauma: Preliminary experience. AJNR 7:885–893, 1986.
7. Quencer RM, Sheldon JJ, Donovan-Post JM, et al: Magnetic resonance imaging of the chronically injured cervical spinal cord. AJNR 7:457–464, 1986.
8. Tarr RW, Drolshagen LF, Kerner TC, et al: MR imaging of recent spinal trauma. J Comput Assist Tomogr 11:412–417, 1987.
9. Wasenko JJ, Lanzieri CF: Plain radiographic examination in cervical spine trauma. In Camins MB, O'Leary PF (eds): Disorders of the Cervical Spine. Baltimore, Williams & Wilkins, 1992.
10. Young JWR, Resnik CS, De Candido P, et al: The laminar space in the diagnosis of rotation flexion injuries of the cervical spine. AJR 152:103–107, 1989.

72. CHEST TRAUMA

Stuart A. Groskin, M.D.

1. How important is chest trauma from a public health perspective?

Overall, trauma is the third leading cause of death in this country; it is the leading cause of death in individuals younger than 35. Chest trauma is second only to head injuries as a cause of trauma-related death. It is directly responsible for 25,000 deaths each year in the United States and annually contributes to the deaths of another 25,000 trauma victims. Emergency department physicians and surgeons must be familiar with the clinical and radiographic manifestations of chest trauma since they are usually the primary care providers for these patients. However, as the survival and long-term hospitalization of trauma victims becomes more common, it is equally important for pediatricians, intensivists, and internists to be familiar with the acute and chronic problems associated with chest injuries.

2. How are chest injuries categorized?

Usually into two categories: blunt and penetrating. Blunt chest injuries, in which the mechanical integrity of the chest wall is maintained, are more common in civilians and are usually the result of motor vehicle accidents or falls. Penetrating chest injuries include injuries in which a communication exists, even if only momentarily, between the atmosphere and the internal contents of the chest. Penetrating chest wounds are more common in military personnel since they are usually the result of gunshots or stabbings. However, penetrating injuries are being seen with increasing frequency in hospitals in urban centers.

3. What are the most important considerations when evaluating a patient who has chest injuries?

The ABCs—airway, breathing, circulation—are the first priority in all trauma patients. After the patient has been stabilized and immediately life-threatening injuries have been treated, an inventory of other injuries should be taken. Patients with chest trauma should always initially be treated as though they have associated injuries. Head, abdominal, and musculoskeletal injuries are common and contribute significantly to overall mortality. Because these injuries may mask or be masked by associated chest injuries, they must be carefully sought out. Treatment of closed head injuries and significant intraabdominal bleeding may assume precedence in patients with chest trauma.

4. What is the ABCDE approach to guide the radiographic search for thoracic injuries?

Air—extrapulmonary (pneumothorax, pneumomediastinum, pneumopericardium, pneumoperitoneum, subcutaneous emphysema)

Aorta—traumatic aortic rupture

Bones—thoracic spine fractures, and less important fractures of the ribs, scapula, and sternum

Contusions and lung lacerations

Catheter (vascular) and tube placement

Diaphragm—rupture

Effusions—hemothorax

The radiographic search for these injuries should be undertaken only after the patient has been clinically assessed and stabilized. Since most trauma victims are radiographed while supine or semi-recumbent, abnormalities such as pneumothorax and hemothorax may look different than they would on an erect chest radiograph.

5. What is the best way to diagnose a pneumothorax in a trauma victim?

With a CT scan of the thorax (upper abdomen). In at least 20% of victims of blunt thoracoabdominal trauma who undergo abdominal CT scans to evaluate intraabdominal injuries, pneumothoraces are seen on the CT scans that were not seen on the plain chest films. This high incidence of occult pneumothorax in trauma patients is an excellent reason to always view the uppermost images of abdominal CT scans (which should always start at the lung bases) on lung settings (level—400 HU/Window 1500 HU) and on soft tissue settings.

6. Why is it so difficult to diagnose a pneumothorax on a supine or semierect chest radiograph?

Because the interface between the pneumothorax and the adjacent lung is not parallel to the incident x-ray beam. Free air in the pleural space rises to the most nondependent portion of the pleural space. In a supine patient, the most nondependent portion of the pleural space is anterior, medial, and caudal. Air that collects in this part of the pleural space projects over the underlying lung and often cannot be easily seen.

7. If the classic findings of pneumothorax are not present on a supine chest radiograph, what are some clues that may indicate the presence of a pneumothorax?
- The deep sulcus sign: abnormal deepening of the costophrenic angle on the affected side
- The double diaphragm sign: the anterior and posterior interfaces of the diaphragm with air (anteriorly with the pneumothorax, posteriorly with the lung) can be seen, creating the impression of two diaphragms on the affected side
- Visualization of pericardial fat
- Basilar hyperlucency

8. Why are radiographically and clinically occult pneumothoraces in trauma patients important to detect?
Because ultimately 70% require chest tube drainage, often during surgery or when the patient is placed on a positive pressure mechanical ventilator.

9. What is a pneumomediastinum?
Pneumomediastinum (Fig. 1) refers to the presence of free air in the mediastinum. Pneumomediastinum does not usually produce significant physiologic alterations in adults and does not usually require any special treatment because in adults free mediastinal gas usually spontaneously decompresses into the soft tissues of the chest wall, neck, and retroperitoneum.

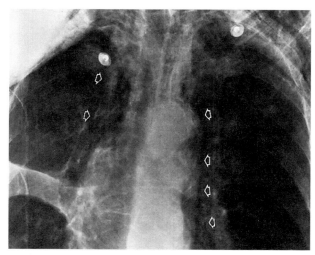

FIGURE 1. Detailed view of pneumomediastinum on a supine frontal chest radiograph. Open arrows point to the mediastinal pleura, which has been elevated away from the mediastinum by mediastinal air.

10. What is the significance of pneumomediastinum in children?
Gas may accumulate in the mediastinum, producing a tension pneumomediastinum associated with life-threatening hemodynamic instability. In this circumstance, a mediastinal drainage catheter may need to be inserted to decompress the mediastinal gas collection. Why adults and children may be affected so differently by a pneumomediastinum has not been completely determined but may involve the incomplete development in children of the connective tissue sheaths that demarcate the interconnected soft tissue compartments of the mediastinum and cervical region.

11. What is the major significance of pneumomediastinum in adults?
It may be a sign of underlying tracheal or esophageal injury, and it can obscure a pneumothorax. Usually, however, pneumomediastinum is a relatively benign finding that is produced by the rupture of the airspaces that release gas into the pulmonary interstitium. If this gas dissects centrifugally, a pneumothorax may result. If it dissects in a centripetal direction, it may gain access to the mediastinum, producing a pneumomediastinum.

12. Traumatic aortic rupture is important to diagnose as soon as possible because high mortality (90%) is associated with delayed treatment. What is the most efficient way to establish or exclude this diagnosis?

This is probably one of the most difficult questions faced by trauma physicians and radiologists. There is no one best way to diagnose or exclude traumatic aortic rupture (Fig. 2). Although the mechanism of injury may suggest the possibility of an aortic tear, the presence of traumatic aortic rupture is usually first suggested by the perception of a widened mediastinum (the mediastinum simply looks too big—there is no reliable specific measurement) or a poorly marginated aorta on the initial frontal chest radiograph. However, most initial trauma chest radiographs are made with the patient supine, and the normal engorgement of the mediastinal veins produced by this position can cause widening of the mediastinal silhouette. In most series, only about 10% of patients whose only radiographic evidence of potential aortic rupture is widening of the mediastinum seen on a supine radiograph are ultimately found to have an aortic injury.

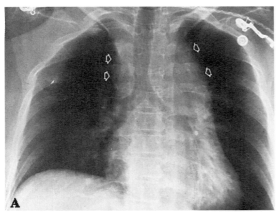
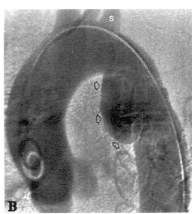
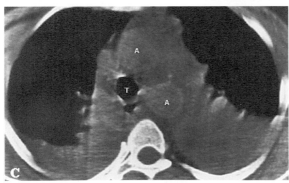

FIGURE 2. Traumatic aortic rupture. *A,* Semierect frontal chest radiograph taken after the patient was involved in a motor vehicle accident. Open arrows demarcate the borders of the enlarged mediastinum, raising the possibility of mediastinal hemorrhage. *B,* Aortography shows a large traumatic pseudoaneurysm (open arrows) arising just distal to the origin of the left subclavian artery (S). *C,* An unenhanced CT scan shows the aorta (A) and trachea (T) surrounded by mediastinal hemorrhage; bilateral pleural effusions (hemothorax) also are present.

13. Is diagnosis easier to make if the radiograph can be repeated with the patient upright?

An upright radiograph cannot be obtained until major spinal injuries are excluded clinically and radiographically. With an upright radiograph, the specificity of the findings of mediastinal widening and aortic contour abnormality increases but remains low. On the other hand, if the mediastinal width and the aortic contours appear completely normal on a frontal chest radiograph, the likelihood of an aortic injury is low and no further tests are usually done.

14. What should be done if the chest radiograph suggests the possibility of aortic injury and the patient is hemodynamically unstable?

If there is no other obvious source of blood loss, direct inspection of the aorta in the operating room is indicated. If there is an apparent extrathoracic source of bleeding, particularly in the abdomen, the patient can undergo a laparotomy, and a transesophageal ultrasound examination of the aorta (TransEsophageal Echocardiography, or TEE) can be performed simultaneously. This test is very sensitive and specific for diagnosing traumatic aortic rupture and can be done portably in the operating room to save time.

15. What should be done if the chest radiograph suggests aortic injury, but the patient is hemodynamically stable?

Evaluation can be performed using one (or more) of three tests: CT scan, TEE, and aortography. The aortogram is considered the gold standard test for diagnosing aortic rupture. Patients who have grossly abnormal mediastinal or aortic silhouettes often go directly to aortography because of the perceived high probability of aortic rupture.

16. What are the disadvantages of aortography?

It is invasive, expensive, and time-consuming. Its use should be limited to situations in which the probability of a positive study is higher than 10%.

17. How should patients with only moderately abnormal chest radiographs be screened before deciding whether to perform aortography?

TEE is highly sensitive and specific when performed by an experienced operator. It can be done in about 15 minutes and can be performed at the bedside, in the emergency room, or in the operating room. However, some patients cannot tolerate the intraesophageal ultrasound probe, and concerns about retching and aspiration have been raised. The ascending aorta cannot be seen well with this technique.

18. What is the role for helical CT of excluding aortic injury?

An increasing number of studies suggest that dynamic contrast-enhanced helical CT of the chest can reliably detect or exclude aortic injury and should be done routinely in all patients with an appropriate mechanism of injury and a suggestive chest radiograph. Helical CT scans can be completed in less than 10 minutes, image the entire thoracic (and, if needed, the abdominal) aorta, and can demonstrate other injuries in the chest and abdomen. Intravenous contrast is required, however, which may lead to (although in very few patients) renal damage, vomiting and aspiration, and a contrast reaction.

19. Can an unenhanced helical scan, without intravenous contrast, be used to to exclude aortic injury?

Although direct evidence of aortic injury may be seen on helical CT scans of the thorax (aortic tears and pseudoaneurysms can be seen when contrast is given), many physicians believe that the presence of blood in the mediastinum, even in absence of other abnormalities, is suggestive enough of aortic injury that an aortogram should be performed. Alternatively, if the scan appears completely normal, showing no evidence of mediastinal hemorrhage, there is some evidence that aortic injury is effectively excluded. If the scan reveals evidence of mediastinal hemorrhage, aortography can be performed for more definitive evaluation (although only about 20% of these cases are positive for aortic injury), or the helical CT scan can be repeated with intravenous contrast. Some data suggest that a normal-appearing aorta on an enhanced helical CT effectively excludes an aortic tear.

20. To sum up, what should be done after determining that a chest radiograph is abnormal?

It depends on the patient's overall physical status and on the resources available at your institution. Generally, unstable patients go to the operating room for TEE or direct inspection during surgery, and stable patients undergo TEE or helical CT prior to or instead of aortography.

21. We spend a lot of time looking for rib fractures on chest radiographs. Is this worthwhile?

Not really. Rib fractures rarely if ever require specific treatment. Also, the presence of rib fractures does not reliably predict the presence of other significant associated injuries. Similarly, the absence of rib fractures does not significantly diminish the likelihood that more ominous injuries are present. Finally, up to 50% of acute rib fractures cannot be seen on chest radiographs. It is far more important to look specifically for findings such as pneumothorax, hemothorax, abdominal visceral injuries, and aortic rupture than to spend a lot of time looking for rib fractures.

22. How common are thoracic spine fractures?

The cervical spine is routinely imaged with plain films in trauma patients; the thoracic spine is not, despite the fact that thoracic spine fractures account for about one-third of all spine fractures and are more frequently associated with complete sensorimotor deficits than are cervical or lumbar spine fractures. They can be difficult to detect clinically and therefore should be carefully looked for with imaging studies. Frontal chest radiographs do not adequately evaluate the thoracic spine (frontal and lateral collimated views of the thoracic spine are minimal requirements for this), but they can provide some helpful information about the spine's mechanical integrity.

23. What are some plain film findings in thoracic spinal fracture?

Apart from obvious vertebral body fracture—anterior vertebral body wedging, cortical discontinuity, free bony fragments—focal bulges should be searched for in the paraspinal lines. In trauma victims, such bumps can indicate the presence of traumatic paraspinal hematomas and should stimulate a more intensive search for underlying fractures.

24. What does a ruptured diaphragm look like?

Rupture of the diaphragm (Fig. 3) is a relatively uncommon injury that can result from blunt or penetrating thoracoabdominal trauma. Although chest radiographs are usually abnormal, the radiographic findings are often nonspecific, indicating pleural effusion and basilar atelectasis. The best plain film sign of diaphragm rupture is intraabdominal contents such as stomach, bowl, and nasogastric tube in the thorax. A portion of the stomach, usually the fundus, can herniate into the chest, through a hole in the diaphragm, while the remainder of the stomach remains in the abdomen. When this happens, patients may be able to eat normally and their radiographic gastric air bubbles may appear to be in normal position. When evaluating these patients, make sure before concluding that all is well that you see all parts of the stomach if you do an upper GI series.

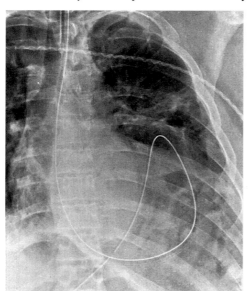

FIGURE 3. Rupture of the left hemidiaphragm. Frontal chest radiograph obtained after the patient was involved in a motor vehicle accident shows loss of definition of the left hemidiaphragm and cranial intrathoracic displacement of the nasogastric tube, consistent with a diaphragm laceration with intrathoracic herniation of the stomach. This diagnosis was confirmed at the time of a subsequent laparatomy.

25. What are the CT and MR findings of a ruptured diaphragm?

CT scans of the thorax and abdomen may show abdominal structures lateral to the border of the diaphragm and may on occasion actually demonstrate the laceration itself. Sagittal and coronal reformatted CT images may be particularly helpful in this regard. MR also has been used to diagnose diaphragm rupture and, although quite effective, is not generally employed in critically ill trauma victims.

26. What happens if a ruptured hemidiaphragm is not diagnosed and treated immediately after the injury occurs?

Most patients with a ruptured hemidiaphragm can fare well for several months to a few years. Unfortunately, the lack of acute problems does not mean that the injury is resolving. Diaphragm ruptures do not usually heal by themselves; positive intraperitoneal pressure favors the continued herniation of abdominal contents into the negative pressure environment of the thorax. After a relatively asymptomatic period, which lasts about 3 years, most patients develop chest or abdominal pain, dysphagia, fever, and cough when the abdominal viscera that herniated into the chest become incarcerated and infarct or become obstructed. This situation is a surgical emergency, but the true source of the patient's acute distress is often initially unrecognized, and valuable time can be lost while trying to establish a diagnosis.

27. What is a pulmonary contusion? How does it differ from a pulmonary laceration?

Pulmonary contusions and pulmonary lacerations occur in the context of blunt or penetrating thoracoabdominal trauma. Traditionally, a pulmonary contusion was defined as a focal area of hemorrhagic pulmonary edema in which the structural integrity of the underlying lung was maintained. Radiographically, pulmonary contusions look like areas of pneumonia or aspiration. Typically, they show significant resolution in 48–72 hours without specific treatment.

A pulmonary laceration is an area in which the substance of the lung is ripped apart. Lacerations typically present as elliptical areas of uniformly increased density that represent focal intraparenchymal hematomas. Occasionally, they present or evolve into gas-filled cystic structures (traumatic pneumatoceles). Lacerations resolve slowly and may leave a permanent scar.

CT evidence suggests that structural lung damage occurs in pulmonary contusions and in pulmonary lacerations, and suggests that these two entities may be part of a continuum of lung damage rather than separate forms of injury.

BIBLIOGRAPHY

1. Daffner R: Imaging of Vertebral Trauma. Rockville, MD, Aspen, 1988.
2. Gavant ML, Flick P, Menke P, Gold RE: CT aortography of thoracic aortic rupture. AJR 166:955–961, 1996.
3. Gavant ML, Menke PG, Fabian T, et al: Blunt traumatic aortic rupture: Detection with helical CT of the chest. Radiology 197:125–133, 1995.
4. Groskin SA: Selected topics in chest trauma. Semin Ultrasound CT MR 17:119–141, 1996.
5. Kang EY, Muller NL: CT in blunt trauma: Pulmonary, tracheobronchial, and diaphragmatic injuries. Semin Ultrasound CT MR 17:114–118, 1996.
6. Meyer S: Thoracic spine trauma. Semin Roentgenol 27:254–261, 1992.
7. Mirvis SE, Young JWR (eds): Imaging in Trauma and Critical Care. Baltimore, Williams & Wilkins, 1992.
8. Smith MD, Cassidy JM, Souther S, et al: Transesophageal echocardiography in the diagnosis of traumatic rupture of the aorta. N Engl J Med 332:356–362, 1995.

73. ABDOMINAL AND PELVIC TRAUMA

Douglas S. Katz, M.D.

1. What is the test of choice for imaging a patient with blunt abdominal and/or pelvic trauma?

If the patient is stable enough to undergo imaging, the test of choice is a CT scan, performed with both oral and intravenous contrast. Oral contrast should be given if at all possible (through a nasogastric tube, if necessary), but imaging should not be significantly delayed, especially if significant trauma is suspected. Plain films of the cervical spine, chest, abdomen, and pelvis (and extremities, if appropriate) are usually obtained before the patient undergoes a CT scan.

2. What if the patient is unstable?

Unstable patients should be managed on clinical grounds and taken to the operating room, if appropriate, for emergency surgery rather than undergoing imaging.

3. How is penetrating trauma to the abdomen and pelvis managed?

Most patients with penetrating trauma to the abdomen and pelvis undergo surgical exploration—especially if the peritoneum has been violated. Management of patients with retroperitoneal trauma (e.g., a stab wound to the flank) should be individualized. Many patients benefit from CT as opposed to immediate surgery (which may not be necessary).

4. What is the disadvantage of performing peritoneal lavage in a trauma patient before obtaining a CT scan?

The role of peritoneal lavage is diminishing, in part because of the accuracy of CT. Free intraperitoneal air and fluid on CT are significant signs of injury in a trauma patient, but because both are introduced into the peritoneal cavity during peritoneal lavage, the detection of free air and fluid on CT is rendered meaningless after lavage.

5. Why should bone and lung (base) windows be examined on the CT scans of every trauma patient?

Bone windows should be viewed to search for bony fractures (e.g., an occult vertebral body fracture or pelvic fracture) that were not seen on plain films. Lung windows should be viewed to search for free intraperitoneal air and occult pneumothorax at the lung bases. Occult pneumothorax is common, because air rises to the lung bases in a supine patient. Thus a pneumothorax missed on a supine chest radiograph may be detected on an abdominal CT.

6. Is a small, occult pneumothorax clinically significant?

In a trauma patient, it may be—especially if the patient is on a ventilator or will be intubated for emergency surgery. A chest tube may need to be placed. Even if a trauma patient is not intubated, the small pneumothorax may enlarge with time and become clinically significant.

7. What are common visceral organ injuries in trauma patients?

The spleen and liver are often injured (Fig. 1). A spectrum of injuries is seen, from contusions (low-density areas on CT, signifying parenchymal injury) to lacerations and shattered organs.

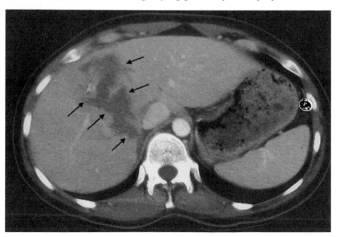

FIGURE 1. Young woman who was involved in a motor vehicle accident. Image from a contrast-enhanced CT shows a large hepatic laceration (arrows).

8. Do all patients with splenic and hepatic injuries need to go to surgery?

Definitely not. Only a minority of patients require surgery. Experience with imaging trauma patients using CT has shown that even injuries that appear to be severe on CT may be managed nonoperatively if the patient remains hemodynamically stable. CT serves to identify and classify injuries and provides a "road map" if surgery is required; coexistent injuries are also found.

9. How do renal injuries appear on CT?

As with splenic and hepatic injuries, a spectrum is seen, from contusions to subcapsular hematomas and severe lacerations involving the main renal vessels and collecting system (Fig. 2). Most severe injuries require surgery.

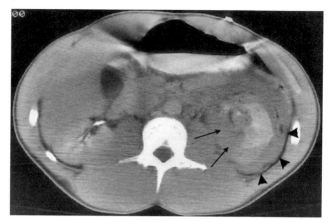

FIGURE 2. Image from a CT demonstrates a left perinephric hematoma in a patient who was involved in a motor vehicle accident. Some functioning left renal parenchyma is present, but there are significant areas of decreased function (hematoma and/or contusion, arrows), and there is left perinephric hematoma (arrowheads). The right kidney is normal.

10. Do any signs on a CT scan indicate that a patient needs to go to surgery immediately?

Occasionally, active extravasation of intravascular contrast is seen. Such patients must usually undergo surgery (or emergency embolization by an interventional radiologist) to prevent exsanguination (Fig. 3).

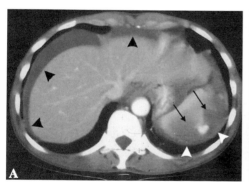
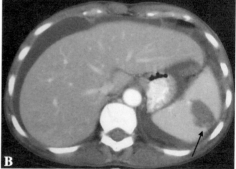

FIGURE 3. Images from a CT show a splenic laceration (arrows) in this patient who is status post a motor vehicle accident (*A*). There is hemorrhage around the spleen and liver (arrowheads). A slightly higher image (*B*) shows active extravasation (arrow) of intravascular contrast from the spleen. This patient was taken to emergency surgery on the basis of the CT findings.

11. On CT, if one of the kidneys does not opacify with intravenous contrast, what should be done?

The vascular pedicle is injured, and emergency surgery is usually indicated to attempt revascularization. This should be done if a relatively short time (< 6 hr) has passed since the trauma (Fig. 4).

12. Is the pancreas commonly injured in trauma?

No. Pancreatic injury (e.g., pancreatic fracture) is unusual and indicates that highly significant trauma has occurred. Associated injuries are common, and surgery is usually required. Much more common is trauma-related pancreatitis without gross pancreatic disruption.

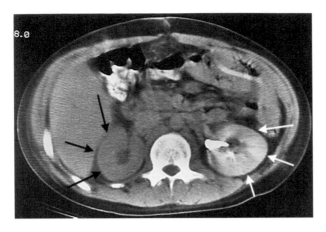

FIGURE 4. CT image reveals no contrast excretion by the right kidney (arrows) due to a traumatic injury to the right main renal artery. Note that the right kidney is smaller than the normally functioning left kidney (white arrows).

13. Can trauma to the adrenal gland occur?

Yes. Adrenal trauma, although relatively uncommon, is manifested by adrenal hemorrhage. On CT, the gland is enlarged and heterogeneous.

14. A patient presents with dilated bowel loops in the left chest and severe pain several months after a significant motor vehicle accident. What has happened?

The patient has a delayed presentation of rupture of the left hemidiaphragm. The diaphragmatic injury occurred at the time of the trauma, but the bowel has acutely herniated through the diaphragmatic defect and is now obstructed and probably strangulated. It may be very difficult to detect a diaphragmatic tear on CT, at the time of the initial injury. Thus this type of delayed presentation is not unusual (Fig. 5).

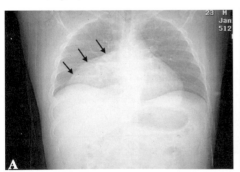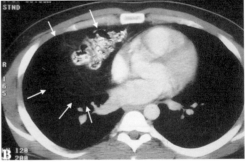

FIGURE 5. A 20-year-old with acute right chest pain and a history of a motor vehicle accident several months prior. Scout digital image (*A*) from a CT shows a large, lucent density along the right heart border (arrows). CT image at the level of the pulmonary veins (*B*) shows a right medial diaphragmatic hernia (arrows), which contains fat and a portion of the colon. Surgical correction was subsequently performed.

15. What are the major radiographic signs of diaphragmatic rupture?

Signs associated with rupture of the diaphragm include pleural effusion, elevation of the diaphragm, rib fractures, and adjacent parenchymal injury (e.g., splenic fracture). Tear of the diaphragm signifies significant trauma, and associated injuries are common. On CT, continuity of the diaphragm should be looked for, although congenital defects in the diaphragm can mimic an acute rupture. The bowel should be examined carefully to ensure that it is located within the abdomen and has not herniated into the chest. It is helpful to perform multiplanar reconstructions on CT to examine the diaphragm in equivocal cases.

16. On which side of the body is diaphragmatic rupture more common? Why?

Diaphragmatic rupture and subsequent herniation of abdominal contents into the chest are believed to be more common on the left side of the body, presumably because the liver protects the right diaphragm and prevents the bowel from herniating through a small defect (although the liver itself may herniate into the chest through a large right diaphragmatic defect). Some authorities believe that in reality the incidence of right- and left-sided rupture is equal, but more right-sided diaphragmatic tears are clinically silent for the reasons described above.

17. Can the small bowel be injured in trauma?

Yes. Small bowel injury, although significant, may be difficult to detect (both clinically and on CT). The duodenum and jejunum are the most commonly injured portions of small bowel, because they are tethered, whereas the more distal bowel is freer to move around the abdomen. Free intraperitoneal air and/or contrast outside the bowel lumen may occasionally be seen in small bowel perforation. Other signs reported to be indicative of small bowel injury on CT include focal thickening of bowel and focal collections of fluid ("interloop fluid"), particularly blood, in the mesentery.

18. What are the two types of bladder rupture?

Intraperitoneal and extraperitoneal.

19. What is the significance of an intraperitoneal bladder rupture?

Intraperitoneal rupture usually occurs when a full bladder is injured. The bladder dome ruptures into the peritoneal cavity. Intraperitoneal bladder rupture is usually an indication for surgical repair (Fig. 6).

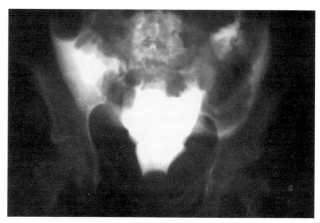

FIGURE 6. Intraperitoneal bladder rupture is demonstrated on this cystogram of an 18-year-old woman. Notice that bowel loops are outlined by contrast. Fractures of the pubis are evident. (Case courtesy of Steven Perlmutter, M.D.)

20. What is the significance of an extraperitoneal bladder rupture?

Extraperitoneal rupture is often associated with pelvic fractures, although the injury may be opposite (or contrecoup) to the site of the pelvic fracture(s). The injury occasionally may be due to direct penetration of the bladder by a bony fracture fragment. Extraperitoneal bladder rupture can often be managed conservatively without the need for operative repair (Fig. 7).

21. How can a bladder rupture be excluded?

Either by cystogram or CT-cystogram. To perform a conventional cystogram, a Foley catheter is inserted into the bladder, and several hundred cc of iodinated contrast are injected under fluoroscopic control into the bladder immediately after a retrograde urethrogram is performed (and is unremarkable). Alternatively, contrast is injected into the bladder through the catheter and a CT is performed. Leakage of contrast outside of the bladder diagnoses a bladder rupture. It is important to distend the bladder optimally under the pressure of direct contrast injection. For this reason, simply scanning the bladder during a routine CT is not an acceptable way of excluding bladder rupture.

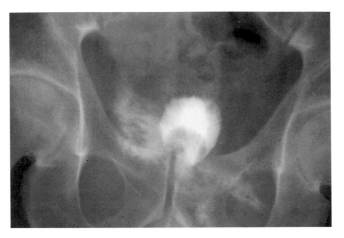

FIGURE 7. A 59-year-old man status post a fall. Post-drainage image from a cystogram, which was performed through a Foley catheter (lucent defect in bladder is from the balloon) shows extravasation of contrast into the extraperitoneal tissues. (Case courtesy of Steven Perlmutter, M.D.)

22. Why is it important to obtain a postvoid (i.e., postdrainage) radiograph when performing a conventional cystogram?

Occasionally a subtle injury may be obscured by the images of the filled bladder, and/or a tear may become manifest only after the bladder is drained.

23. What is meant by the "one-shot IVP"?

The "one-shot" intravenous pyelogram is a study performed on an emergency basis in the emergency department. Intravenous contrast is injected into an unstable patient, and soon after a frontal radiograph of the abdomen and pelvis is obtained. This study provides only a limited overview of the urinary tract and should be discouraged if at all possible. One potential use of the one-shot IVP is in a hemodynamically unstable patient who is headed to the operating room for exploration of the peritoneal cavity. The surgeons ordering the test want to know whether the patient also has a gross renal injury that will require them to explore the retroperitoneum as well.

24. A urethral injury is suspected in a male. What should be done?

A retrograde urethrogram (RUG) should be performed by a radiologist under direct fluoroscopic visualization (if at all possible) (Fig. 8). A Foley catheter is inserted into the urethral meatus, and iodinated contrast is gently injected. If there is no evidence of an injury, the catheter is gently inserted into the bladder, and a cystogram is performed.

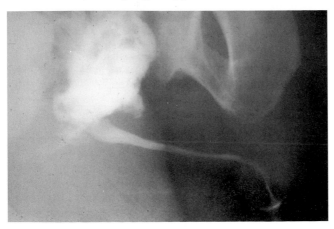

FIGURE 8. Image from a retrograde urethrogram performed on a young man after trauma. There is disruption of the posterior urethra, with significant contrast extravasation.

25. What is the usual cause of an injury to the anterior (distal) urethra?

The typical cause is a straddle injury, such as a fall over a bicycle or fence.

26. CT shows a large retroperitoneal hematoma, and ongoing hemorrhage into this region is suspected. What should be done?

Angiography is the test of choice, both for diagnostic and therapeutic purposes. Surgical exploration in this setting is difficult, and bleeding into the retroperitoneum may be due to multiple and/or bilateral vessels that are difficult to identify. Bleeding vessels identified at angiography are embolized, using various materials such as Gelfoam and metallic coils.

27. Injury to the testicle(s) is suspected as a result of blunt trauma. What is the test of choice in this setting?

Ultrasound. Unfortunately, the ultrasonographic signs of testicular injury may be subtle, and it is often difficult to distinguish a testicular hematoma from a rupture extending to the testicular capsule (the latter is usually an indication for surgery).

28. Free fluid is identified on CT in the peritoneal cavity. What may be the sources of the fluid?

- Fluid from a prior peritoneal lavage
- Hemorrhage from injury to a solid organ, vessel, or bowel
- Urine extravasating from the kidney, ureter, or bladder
- Bile extravasating from the liver or biliary tract
- Lymph extravasating from the thoracic duct or other lymphatic structures

Density measurements of the fluid are very helpful. Hemorrhage usually measures over 20 Hounsfield units, while bile and urine are usually closer to water density (0 Hounsfield units). Lymph may measure less than 0.

CONTROVERSY

29. Does ultrasound have a role in imaging trauma patients?

Most radiologists believe strongly that ultrasound has no proven role in the routine imaging of trauma patients. In addition to the need for extensive training and experience to use the modality appropriately, ultrasound is less sensitive than CT for detecting visceral organ injuries (particularly in adults), and it cannot image the retroperitoneum adequately. There are also numerous reasons why CT is preferable to ultrasound. Bony injuries cannot be evaluated on ultrasound, and density measurements cannot be performed (e.g., on fluid collections).

BIBLIOGRAPHY

1. Becker CD, Spring P, Glattli A, et al: Blunt splenic trauma in adults: Can CT findings be used to determine the need for surgery? AJR 162:343–347, 1994.
2. Gay SB, Sistrom CL: Computerized tomographic evaluation of blunt abdominal trauma. Radiol Clin North Am 30:367–388, 1992.
3. Jeffrey RB Jr, Cardoza JD, Olcott EW: Detection of active intraabdominal arterial hemorrhage: Value of dynamic contrast-enhanced CT. AJR 156:725–729, 1990.
4. Lang EK: Intra-abdominal and retroperitoneal organ injuries: Diagnosis on dynamic computerized tomograms obtained for assessment of renal trauma. J Trauma 30:1161–1168, 1990.
5. McConnell DB, Trunkey DD: Nonoperative management of abdominal trauma. Surgical Clin North Am 70:677–688, 1990.
6. Meredith JW, Young JS, Bowling J, et al: Nonoperative management of blunt hepatic trauma: The exception or the rule? J Trauma 36:529–535, 1994.
7. Pollack HM, Wein AJ: Imaging of renal trauma. Radiology 172:297–308, 1989.
8. Sandler CM, Hall TJ, Rodriguez MB, et al: Bladder injury in blunt pelvic trauma. Radiology 158:633–638, 1986.

74. INTRACRANIAL TRAUMA

John J. Wasenko, M.D.

1. Why is computed tomography the modality of choice for evaluating patients with acute head trauma?

CT rapidly and accurately demonstrates skull fractures, subarachnoid hemorrhage, and lesions requiring immediate surgical attention, such as intraparenchymal hemorrhage and extracerebral hematomas.

2. How should CT scans of patients with head trauma be filmed?

Images routinely should be filmed using three different window settings:
1. Soft-tissue windows to evaluate the brain for hemorrhage and edema
2. At a window setting to detect epidural and subdural hematomas
3. Bone windows to detect fractures

3. Should intravenous contrast be used in the evaluation of head trauma?

No, it should not be used routinely. However, it may be of use if the unenhanced CT is normal and the patient has an unexplained neurologic deficit. Intravenous contrast also may be of use in patients with unexplainable mass effect.

4. Can MR be used routinely instead of CT for evaluating patients with head trauma?

No. There are several disadvantages of MR in this setting. MR is slower than CT and less sensitive for the detection of subarachnoid hemorrhage. Skull fractures also are more difficult to detect than on CT. Trauma patients often have internal or external devices (e.g., ventilators) that may not be MR-compatible. Moreover, MR may be less readily available than CT on an emergency basis.

5. Describe the CT appearance of an intraparenchymal hematoma.

An intraparenchymal hematoma is a sharply marginated, hyperdense mass with a surrounding rim of hypodensity that represents edema. There is variable mass effect, depending on the size of the hematoma. The frontal and temporal lobes are most commonly involved. Intraparenchymal hematomas may be multiple.

6. What is the pattern of evolution of an intraparenchymal hematoma?

An acute intraparenchymal hematoma is initially hyperdense because of clotted blood, with mass effect and surrounding edema. Over several weeks, the hematoma becomes isodense with normal brain. Mass effect persists at this point. The hematoma then becomes hypodense over one to several months. The overlying cortical sulci and the adjacent ventricle become dilated to compensate for the loss of parenchymal volume.

7. What is the characteristic shape of an epidural hematoma?

An epidural hematoma is typically biconvex (or lentiform) in configuration because of the dura, which is firmly adherent to the inner table of the calvarium. The most common location is over the temporal lobe (Fig. 1).

8. Why does an epidural hematoma require immediate surgical intervention?

Most epidural hematomas result from injury to the middle meningeal artery. Because the artery is under pressure, the hematoma may enlarge rapidly to compress vital brainstem structures. Permanent neurologic deficits or death may result.

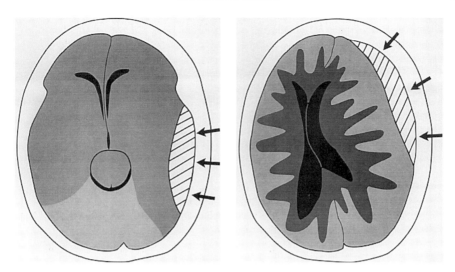

FIGURE 1 *(Left).* Biconvex epidural hematoma overlies the left temporal lobe (arrows).
FIGURE 2 *(Right).* Crescent-shaped subdural hematoma overlies the left frontoparietal region (arrows).

9. Describe the typical appearance of a subdural hematoma on CT.

An acute subdural hematoma is characteristically a hyperdense, crescent-shaped collection with concave medial and convex lateral borders (Fig. 2).

10. Why is a subdural hematoma typically diffuse, overlying a large segment of a cerebral hemisphere?

A subdural hematoma results from tearing of bridging veins within the subdural space. This space offers little resistance to the hematoma, which may expand diffusely, sometimes over an entire hemisphere.

11. Are all acute subdural hematomas homogeneous and hyperdense on CT?

No. The hematoma may be mixed in density as a result of either unclotted blood or cerebrospinal fluid from tears in the arachnoid.

12. Describe the appearance of subarachnoid hemorrhage on CT.

Subarachnoid hemorrhage typically appears as an area of hyperdensity in the basal cisterns, the sulci overlying the cerebral convexities, the sylvian fissure, and the interhemispheric fissure.

13. What are *coup* and *contrecoup* injuries?

A coup injury occurs at the site of impact. Momentary inbending of the skull compresses the adjacent brain, with resultant injury (typically, contusion). A contrecoup injury occurs at a site remote from the site of impact. It is produced by deceleration of the skull as the brain continues in motion and strikes the inner table of the skull.

14. Name the most common sites of cerebral contusions.

Frontal lobes, lateral aspect of the temporal lobes, and inferior surface of the frontal and temporal lobes.

15. Which common vascular injuries may be associated with intracranial trauma?

Dissection (i.e., of the carotid or vertebral arteries)
Lacerations of a vessel

Development of a pseudoaneurysm
Development of an arteriovenous fistula
Thrombosis of a vessel

16. What is the importance of detecting a fracture of the posterior wall of the frontal sinus?

Such fractures may result in a cerebrospinal fluid leak or infections such as epidural or subdural empyema and meningitis.

17. List other potential complications of intracranial trauma.

Hydrocephalus

Cerebral atrophy

Cerebral infarction

Tension pneumocephalus (i.e., extracerebral but intracranial air under tension, typically from a
   skull fracture through which air enters but cannot escape [a ball-valve effect])

18. How is a diffuse axonal injury produced?

Diffuse axonal injury is caused by a rotational force that produces a shear strain, which is maximal at the junction of tissues with different densities, such as the junction of the grey and white matter.

19. Describe the CT and MR appearance as well as the location of diffuse axonal injury.

Diffuse axonal injuries are elliptical or oval lesions that are poorly seen with CT but readily demonstrated with MR. The lesions are hyperintense on T2-weighted images. Most commonly, they are located in the subcortical white matter of the frontal and parietal lobes, the splenium of the corpus callosum, the corona radiata, the internal capsule, and the dorsolateral aspect of the brainstem.

20. What can be seen on a CT scan of a patient who has been shot in the head?

CT shows the bullet, bullet fragments, path of the bullet, and associated skull fractures. It also demonstrates lesions requiring immediate surgical intervention, including intraparenchymal and subdural hematomas.

21. Can MR be used to evaluate patients with gunshot wounds?

No. A gunshot wound is a contraindication to MR because bullets undergo deflection when placed in a magnetic field. The deflection may result in further damage to the brain. In addition, the bullet and its fragments distort the image and degrade its quality.

22. When is MR used in the evaluation of intracranial trauma?

MR is useful to evaluate the subacute and chronic stages of head injury because it is more sensitive than CT for the depiction of hemorrhagic contusions and nonhemorrhagic (diffuse axonal injury) lesions.

23. What is a growing skull fracture?

A growing fracture, formerly called a leptomeningeal cyst, occurs when a fracture is associated with a dural tear and extension of the arachnoid into the fracture. Cerebrospinal fluid pulsations remodel the adjacent bone, resulting in enlargement of the fracture.

24. What is a subdural hygroma?

A subdural hygroma is a hypodense extracerebral fluid collection that is isodense with cerebrospinal fluid. It is caused by a tear in the arachnoid, with resultant leakage of cerebrospinal fluid into the subdural space.

25. Is it possible to distinguish a subdural hygroma from a chronic subdural hematoma?

No. Both fluid collections are similar in appearance; both are isodense with cerebrospinal fluid.

26. Is a chronic subdural hematoma always crescent-shaped?

Characteristically they are crescent-shaped, although occasionally they may be biconvex because of absorption of fluid into the hematoma or formation of adhesions.

27. Which features of skull fractures point to child abuse?

Multiple, bilateral fractures that cross suture lines and fractures in various stages of healing, indicating that they occurred at different times.

28. Is MR of use in the evaluation of intracranial trauma resulting from child abuse?

Yes, because it can help determine the age of blood. Like the detection of fractures in different stages of healing, the detection of blood collections (especially subdural hematomas, most characteristically found in the interhemispheric fissure) of different ages indicates multiple episodes of injury, which is virtually diagnostic of child abuse.

29. Why is MR insensitive for detecting subarachnoid hemorrhage?

The high concentration of oxygen in cerebrospinal fluid impedes the conversion of oxyhemoglobin to deoxyhemoglobin. Deoxyhemoglobin is necessary to produce the signal intensity change that can be visualized with MR. In addition, cerebrospinal fluid pulsations tend to break up clot, which further impedes the degradation of oxyhemoglobin to deoxyhemoglobin.

BIBLIOGRAPHY

1. Bakay L: The value of CT scan in gunshot injuries of the brain. Acta Neurochir (Wien) 71:189–204, 1984.
2. Bradley WG Jr, Schmidt PG: Effect of methemoglobin formation on the MR appearance of subarachnoid hemorrhage. Radiology 159:99–103, 1985.
3. Gentry LR, Godersky JC, Thompson BH: MR imaging of head trauma: Review of the distribution and radiopathic features of traumatic lesions. AJNR 9:101–110, 1988.
4. Gentry LR, Godersky JC, Thompson BH: Traumatic brain stem injury: MR imaging. Radiology 171:177–187, 1989.
5. Hesselink JR, Dowd CF, Healy ME, et al: MR imaging of brain contusions: A comparative study with CT. AJNR 9:269–278, 1988.
6. Meservy CJ, Towbin CJ, McLauren RL, et al: Radiographic characteristics of skull fractures resulting from child abuse. AJR 149:173–175, 1987.
7. Reed D, Robertson WD, Graeb DA, et al: Acute subdural hematomas: Atypical CT findings. AJNR 7:417–421, 1986.
8. Sato Y, Yuh WTC, Smith WL, et al: Head injury in child abuse: Evaluation with MR imaging. Radiology 173:653–657, 1989.
9. Smith AS, Hurst GC, Duerk JL, et al: MR of ballistic materials: Imaging artifacts and potential hazards. AJNR 12:567–572, 1991.
10. Wasenko JJ, Hochhauser L: Central nervous system trauma. In Haaga JR, Lanzieri CF, Sartorius DJ, Zerhouni EA (eds): CT and MRI of the Whole Body. Part I: Imaging of the Brain. St. Louis, Mosby, 1994.

X. Breast Imaging

75. BREAST IMAGING

Julie Barudin, M.D., and Susan Orel, M.D.

SCREENING MAMMOGRAPHY

1. What is a screening mammogram?

Screening mammography is the imaging of asymptomatic women to detect early, clinically occult breast cancer. Because of the screening function that mammography performs, it has a unique role in radiology (Fig. 1).

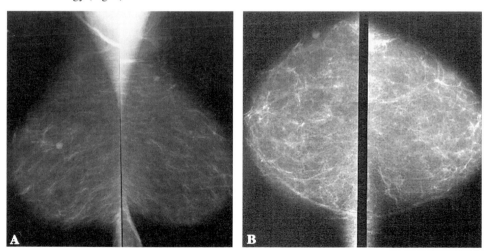

FIGURE 1. A typical routine screening mammogram. Four views are obtained, two of each breast: *A*, oblique views and *B*, craniocaudad views. Note that this particular patient has relatively fatty breasts; that is, the breasts are fairly gray. In this type of background parenchyma, internal visibility is excellent. The smooth nodules on either side represent intramammary lymph nodes.

2. How is a mammogram performed?

The breast is compressed between a compression paddle and a platform (which holds the film) for each view that is taken. Compression must be firm to ensure the best possible visibility. Some women find the necessary compression painful, but for most it is only uncomfortable.

3. What views are taken for a routine mammogram?

The routine views are the craniocaudal (CC) view and the mediolateral oblique (MLO) view, done on each breast (for a total of four films). In the CC view, the breasts are compressed in a plane parallel to the floor, and in the MLO view the breasts are compressed parallel to the woman's pectoralis muscle. Both views are necessary for proper evaluation of the entire breast (see Fig. 1).

4. How common is breast cancer?

Breast cancer is the most common cancer of American women; 183,000 new cases were reported in 1994. It is the leading cause of cancer death in women under age 54, and the second most common in women aged 55–74.

5. What are the risk factors for breast cancer?

The risk factors include advancing age, early menarche, late menopause, nulliparity, family or personal history of breast cancer, and previous biopsy-proven atypical hyperplasia or lobular neoplasia. However, 75% of breast cancers occur in women without known risk factors; thus, *screening is recommended for all women according to age guidelines.*

6. When should a woman have a screening mammogram?

The age guidelines (periodically debated and revised) recommended by the American College of Radiology and the American Cancer Society are yearly mammography for women 50 years and above.

However, for the patient with a first-degree relative who developed premenopausal breast cancer, some suggest that screening should begin when the patient is 10 years younger than the age at which her relative was diagnosed.

7. Are all women in the United States screened according to the guidelines? If not, why not?

Only about one-third of the women in the U.S. are screened according to the above guidelines. The many reasons include fear, availability of mammography, economics, and lack of physician recommendation.

8. How can primary care physicians increase the likelihood that their patients will be screened?

The most important step is to recommend a mammogram. In addition, other important points should be stressed to address the obstacles mentioned above. First, remind the patient that screening is for asymptomatic women and that even if she has no symptoms, she needs a mammogram. Reassure her that mammography should not be painful, although a certain degree of temporary compression is necessary to obtain adequate images. Also reassure the patient that mammography is safe and that the degree of radiation exposure is very low.

9. What other information should the primary care physician give to the patient prior to mammography?

Remind the patient to bring all of her previous mammograms to the imaging center at the time of her next mammogram, if possible. Also, remind her that she may be called back for additional views, depending on how the imaging center is run, and that a call-back does not always mean that something is wrong. (See diagnostic mammography below.)

10. What is the false-negative rate of mammography?

The false-negative rate is approximately 10–15%. Most false-negative results occur in patients who have very dense breasts (Fig. 2). Each mammography report should indicate the density of the patient's breast tissue; if the tissue is dense, the likelihood of a false negative increases. A negative mammographic report should not preclude further evaluation (including biopsy) of a palpable, suspicious mass.

11. Is breast ultrasound (US) useful for screening?

No. Ultrasound is not clinically useful for breast cancer screening. Breast ultrasound should be used only as a directed exam to determine whether a given abnormality (either palpable or detected on mammography) is cystic or solid.

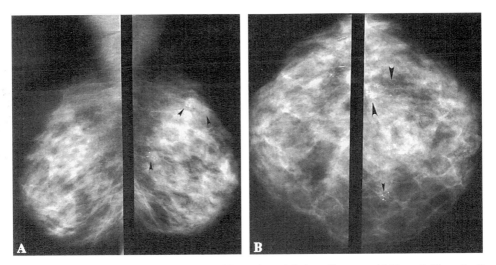

FIGURE 2. Dense breasts: *A*, oblique views and *B*, craniocaudad views. Compare with Figure 1. The patient's mammogram shows breast parenchyma that is fairly white because of increased fibrous or glandular tissue. The density may camouflage noncalcified masses. Some calcifications, however, may still be seen even with dense breasts (arrowheads). Needle localization and excisional biopsy demonstrated hyalinized fibroadenomas.

DIAGNOSTIC MAMMOGRAPHY

12. What is a diagnostic mammogram? How does it differ from a screening mammogram?

Diagnostic mammography is better called a diagnostic imaging examination, for it may include other modalities, such as ultrasound, MRI, or galactography. A diagnostic examination is a directed imaging work-up that seeks to answer a particular question. The question may be related to a particular symptom (see below), or it may seek to answer a question raised by a finding on a previous screening examination. In ordering mammograms, a diagnostic examination should be ordered when the patient has a breast-related symptom.

13. What is meant by call-back?

Screening examinations are checked for technical quality by well-trained, dedicated mammography technologists. In many screening centers, screening is done without the physical presence of a radiologist. Therefore, if the technique is satisfactory, the patient is released before the radiologist has looked at the films. This method allows the greatest patient throughput and helps to decrease the cost of screening. However, it creates the need for a small percentage of women to return for additional imaging, that is, a call-back. Sometimes a highly suspicious finding on the screening views needs additional work-up. However, many women are asked to return to prove that a screening abnormality is *not* worrisome. Patients should be aware that a call-back does not necessarily mean that anything is wrong.

14. Why are additional views sometimes necessary, such as a spot compression view or a magnification view?

Additional views are sometimes necessary for better evaluation of a particular area of the breast. Spot compression refers to compression by a small paddle, which allows greater compression (and therefore greater visibility) of a particular area than the routine compression paddle. A magnification view involves magnifying an area, most often to assess calcifications.

15. Who orders the call-back, and what about the results?

In most centers, it is the radiologist's responsibility to contact the patient directly and to schedule the call-back. Usually a report is issued at the initial reading before the call-back study is performed. A final impression and recommendation are issued after the call-back analysis. The results of a call-back consist of one of three recommendations:

1. Return to routine screening
2. Six-month follow-up for a probably benign finding
3. Biopsy for a suspicious finding

16. What about a patient with a lump?

The work-up of a palpable abnormality depends on the patient's age. Despite some controversy, many radiologists recommend the following guidelines:

1. Under 30 years   Ultrasound (US) first to decide whether the lump is caused by a simple cyst.
2. 30–35 years   Variable; may follow guidelines (1) or (3); often follow (3) in patients with a positive family history
3. 35 years and over   Mammography first, possibly followed by US

Some physicians prefer to attempt aspiration of a palpable abnormality as the first step to determine whether it is caused by a cyst. For a palpable abnormality, in skilled hands, this method is often more efficient and may diagnose as well as treat the palpable abnormality while saving both time and imaging costs. Occasionally, even a simple cyst may not yield fluid upon clinically guided aspiration because of its mobility or because of a particularly fibrous wall. Therefore, imaging is still useful after a negative aspiration attempt of a palpable mass. If a palpable abnormality is proved to be a simple cyst, by either aspiration or imaging, the patient may return to routine screening. The presence of a simple cyst on imaging does not necessitate drainage.

17. What if the patient has a lump, but the mammogram and ultrasound are negative?

Be aware of the false-negative rate of mammography! Do not stop the work-up because a mammogram is negative. If the lump is suspicious clinically, it should be biopsied despite a negative mammogram.

18. What is the differential diagnosis of a spiculated mass?

Unless the patient has had previous surgery in the exact location of a spiculated mass, any spiculated mass must be considered suspicious for malignancy and must be biopsied. In rare cases, a spiculated mass that is not associated with postsurgical change may represent a benign process, such as a radial scar, but most often spiculated masses are malignant.

19. What is the differential diagnosis of a well-defined mass?

Well-defined borders usually suggest a benign process, although some cancers (< 5%) present in this manner. Other possibilities include cysts and fibroadenomas.

20. How do I handle a patient with nipple discharge?

Most of the time, nipple discharge represents benign disease. However, if the discharge is unilateral, especially if it arises from one duct opening only and is bloody or watery, it may indicate malignancy. A unilateral diagnostic imaging work-up may be performed, which includes mammography as well as possible galactography. Galactography consists of injection of a small amount of contrast material into a duct to visualize the draining system.

21. What about the patient with breast pain?

Bilateral, diffuse breast pain is a common symptom, almost always attributable to fibrocystic changes and hormonal influences. Localized breast pain is an extremely unlikely presentation for cancer. However, if the pain is localized, consider a directed ultrasound or unilateral mammogram, which may define the cause of the pain, such as a distended cyst. Ultrasound is not useful for diffuse breast pain.

22. What about the patient with mastitis?

Usually, mastitis is a clinical diagnosis. However, treatment is altered if an abscess is present. This is the one situation in which a total breast ultrasound may be performed in an attempt to locate a breast abscess if it exists and possibly to help guide drainage. If a patient with mastitis does not respond to treatment, mammography should be performed, because mastitis and inflammatory cancer have a similar clinical presentation.

23. What if the patient has had augmentation implants?

Patients who have implants are, of course, still at risk of breast cancer. In addition, often an evaluation is needed to assess the integrity of the implants. Screening mammography should be ordered according to the same guidelines outlined above. However, because the implants obscure portions of breast tissue, extra views are routinely performed (Fig. 3). Even with additional views, however, the sensitivity of mammography is decreased for patients with augmentation implants. The patient should be aware that her examination will take longer than the examination of women without implants. In addition, the examination should be carried out in a facility with a radiologist present. If there is a question about implant rupture and mammography is normal, MRI or ultrasound may be useful imaging adjuncts.

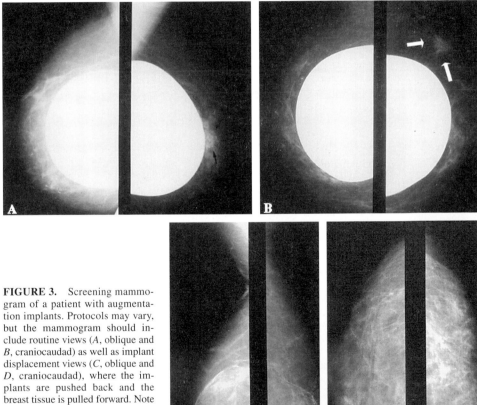

FIGURE 3. Screening mammogram of a patient with augmentation implants. Protocols may vary, but the mammogram should include routine views (*A*, oblique and *B*, craniocaudad) as well as implant displacement views (*C*, oblique and *D*, craniocaudad), where the implants are pushed back and the breast tissue is pulled forward. Note how much breast tissue is still not imaged despite the multiple views. In this case, the patient had a spiculated lesion with malignant calcification (arrows) that could be seen only on the routine views. Biopsy revealed infiltrating and intraductal breast carcinoma (see Fig. 6B).

24. What is the best course of action for a patient who is breastfeeding an infant and has a lump?

Often a palpable abnormality during late pregnancy or lactation is caused by a galactocele. Ultrasound is the most appropriate first step; mammography should be avoided because of the mammographic density in breastfeeding patients. If ultrasound demonstrates a cyst, the work-up is complete. A solid lesion should be biopsied.

25. What if a male patient has a breast lump? Can it be cancer?

Yes. Approximately 1% of breast cancers occur in men. Mammography may be performed in an attempt to differentiate between gynecomastia (which may be unilateral) and carcinoma. However, this differentiation is often difficult (Fig. 4). The decision to biopsy most often must be based on clinical grounds.

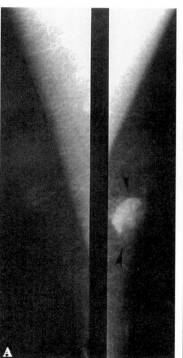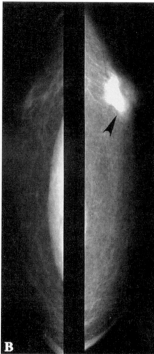

FIGURE 4. A mammogram in a male patient with a right-sided breast lump. *A*, Oblique and *B*, craniocaudad views are shown. The arrows demonstrate an ill-defined mass in the retroareolar position. Biopsy yielded infiltrating breast carcinoma.

BREAST INTERVENTIONAL TECHNIQUES

26. How many surgical biopsies performed in the United States yield benign results?

Approximately 75% of surgical excisional biopsies performed in the U.S., both for mammographically detected and palpable lesions, yield benign histology. One way to decrease the false-positive rate and the associated costs is to use newer procedures that can perform tissue sampling without the need for an expensive operating room visit (see below).

27. How is a biopsy of a mammographically detected, nonpalpable lesion performed?

Options include needle localization and surgical excision as well as needle core biopsy and fine-needle aspiration.

28. How is excisional surgical biopsy of a nonpalpable lesion performed?

Excisional surgical biopsy of a nonpalpable lesion is done by preoperative needle localization. On the day of surgery, the patient first comes to the radiology suite, where a needle is used to place a

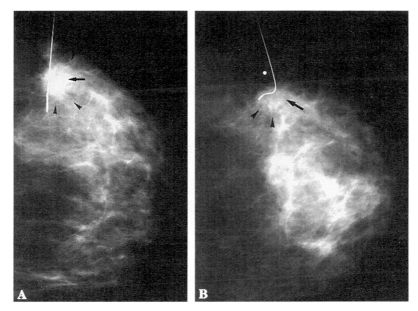

FIGURE 5. Final films from a needle localization (*A*, 90° lateral and *B*, craniocaudad). The films were sent along with the patient to the operating room. An ill-defined mass (arrowheads) and indeterminate calcifications (arrow) were localized. Note that at the end of the wire the hook is not optimally opened, or "sprung." This situation occurs infrequently and is most likely a function of the texture of the surrounding breast tissue. Usually, there is no problem, and the wire remains well-anchored, as in this case (see Fig. 6).

thin wire with mammographic or ultrasonographic guidance. The surgeon then uses this wire, along with films taken after wire placement, as a road map to direct the surgery (Fig. 5).

29. How can the surgeon know that the mammographic lesion has been removed, if it is not palpable?

All needle localizations must be followed by a specimen radiograph. The actual specimen is taken to the radiology suite, where it is imaged to determine whether the mammographic abnormality is indeed present (Fig. 6). This information is immediately relayed to the operating room, where the surgeon and patient have been waiting. Often the specimen is imaged on some type of localizing grid, so that the exact location of the abnormality within the specimen can be relayed to the pathologists. The specimen radiograph is sent to pathology along with the specimen.

30. What is a needle biopsy?

The terminology is slightly confusing. **Needle localizations**, described above, refer to preoperative placement of a guiding wire for an excisional biopsy. During a needle localization, no tissue is actually removed through the needle.

A **needle biopsy** also may be performed. Tissue samples are removed through the needle, and a trip to the operating room can often be avoided. The needle is placed in the proper position using imaging guidance, either with mammography or ultrasound.

Cells can be removed with **fine-needle aspiration** (FNA), using a 25-gauge needle. Problems include frequent lack of adequate sample as well as a limited number of well-trained cytopathologists in the U.S. This technique is often performed in Europe, however.

Another option that is gaining popularity is **core biopsy**. A large gauge (usually 14-G) needle is placed, guided by either ultrasound or stereotactic mammography. A spring-loaded biopsy gun is then used to remove a histologic sample of tissue. Tissue cores are treated by the pathologist in a similar fashion to specimens received from excisional biopsies. Studies have shown greater accuracy

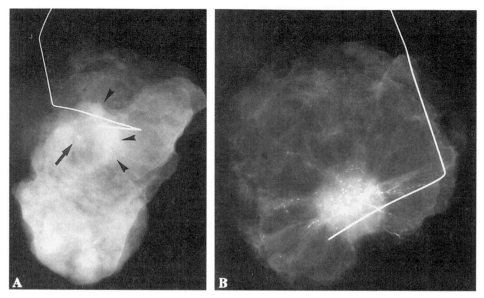

FIGURE 6A and B. *A*, Magnified specimen radiograph. This is the specimen radiograph obtained from the localization above (Fig. 5). The wire is still in place, which is common. Note that the mass (arrowheads) and calcifications (arrow) have been removed successfully. Histology revealed infiltrating lobular carcinoma. *B*, Magnified specimen radiograph from the localization and biopsy of the patient in Figure 3. The spicules and malignant-appearing calcifications are much better seen than on the screening views. Histology revealed infiltrating and intraductal breast carcinoma.

FIGURE 6C. Magnified radiograph of a specimen that has been placed on a grid. This grid is printed onto a stiff card, onto which the specimen is placed in the operating room. Adhesive ensures that the specimen does not move in relation to the grid once it is placed on the cardboard. The radiologist then tells the surgeon that the abnormality (in this case, calcifications) are located at coordinates C2, D2, C3, C4, D4, C5 and D5. This is just one method of localizing the finding within the specimen for the pathologists. Histology yielded intraductal carcinoma (or ductal carcinoma in situ) of the comedo type.

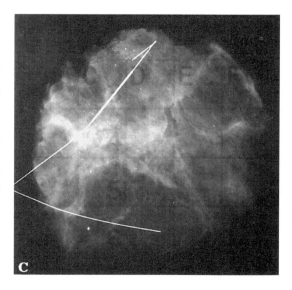

with core biopsies than with FNA. The accuracy of core biopsy and needle localization with excisional biopsy is similar.

31. Define stereotaxis.

Stereotaxis refers to a computerized method of triangulation. A mammographic image of the lesion is obtained using two precise angles of the x-ray tube. A computer then uses geometry to calculate the exact three-dimensional location of the lesion. Stereotaxis can be used to guide needle localizations, needle biopsies, or cyst aspirations. A major advantage of stereotaxis over conventional methods of needle localization is that it can be used for lesions seen in only one mammographic view.

BIBLIOGRAPHY

1. Bassett LW, Kimme-Smith C: Breast sonography. AJR 156:449–455, 1991.
2. Berg WA, Caskey CI, Hamper UM, et al: Diagnosing breast implant rupture with MR imaging, US, and mammography. RadioGraphics 1323–1336, 1993.
3. Breast cancer screening for women ages 40–49. NIH Consensus Statement 1997 15(1):1–35, 1997.
4. Destouet JM, Monsees BS, Oser RF, et al: Screening mammography in 350 women with breast implants: Prevalence and findings of implant complications. AJR 159:973–978, 1992, 1992; discussion 979–981.
5. Homer MJ, Smith TJ, Safaii H: Prebiopsy needle localization. Methods, problems, and expected results. Radiol Clin North Am 30:139–153, 1992.
6. Jackson VP: The role of US in breast imaging. Radiology 177:305–311, 1990.
7. Jokich PM, Monticciolo DL, Adler YT: Breast ultrasonography. Radiol Clin North Am 30:993–1009, 1992.
8. Kopans DB, Swann CA: Preoperative imaging-guided needle placement and localization of clinically occult breast lesions. AJR 152:1–9, 1989.
9. Liebman AJ, Kruse B: Breast cancer: Mammographic and sonographic findings after augmentation mammoplasty. Radiology 174:195–198, 1990.
10. Parker SH, Jobe WE, Dennis MA, et al: US-guided automated large-core breast biopsy. Radiology 187:507–511, 1993.
11. Parker SH, Lovin JD, Jobe WE, et al: Stereotactic breast biopsy with a biopsy gun. Radiology 176:741–747, 1990.
12. Parker SH, Lovin JD, Jobe WE, et al: Nonpalpable breast lesions; stereotactic automated large core-biopsies. Radiology 180:403–407, 1991.

XI. *Vascular and Interventional Radiology*

76. FUNDAMENTALS OF ANGIOGRAPHY

Kenneth D. Murphy, M.D.

1. What is the preprocedural preparation for an angiogram?

Obtain informed consent, review the pertinent laboratory data, limit oral intake to clear liquids only (for a maximum of 8 hours before the procedure), and intravenous hydration (if necessary).

2. What are the laboratory values required for a safe arterial or venous puncture?

Prothrombin time (PT) less than 16 seconds, partial thromboplastin time (PTT) less than 40 seconds, and platelet count in excess of 75,000/mL.

3. What are the contraindications to elective angiography?

The relative contraindications include: recent myocardial infarction, history of severe contrast reaction, renal failure, coagulopathy, pregnancy, and impaired ability of the patient to cooperate or lie flat. An absolute contraindication to elective angiography is a hemodynamically unstable patient.

4. What is the Seldinger technique?

It is a nonsurgical method for percutaneous catheterization of a vessel, which was originally described by Sven Seldinger in 1953. Prior to that time, all arteriograms were performed using surgically placed catheters. The first step in the technique is to localize the vessel by manual palpation and then to clean the overlying skin with povidone-iodine. Local anesthesia is achieved by administering 2% lidocaine. A small superficial incision is made directly over the artery with a #11 scalpel blade. An 18-gauge hollow needle with a sharp stylet is carefully inserted into the vessel. The stylet is removed and the needle withdrawn until pulsatile blood return is obtained. A guidewire is then advanced through the needle into the vessel. The needle is removed and exchanged for the desired catheter (Fig. 1).

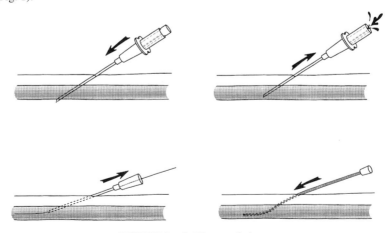

FIGURE 1. Seldinger technique.

5. Where should the femoral artery be punctured?

Over the middle of the medial third of the femoral head. Access at this level is preferred because entry is usually below the inguinal ligament. An infrainguinal puncture is desired because the risk of retroperitoneal hemorrhage is minimized. The femoral vein is also completely medial to the artery at this level (with no overlap). Proximal and distal to this level the vein can lie ventral to the artery. Finally, the femoral head provides a rigid structure to compress the artery against, which facilitates hemostasis at the conclusion of the procedure.

6. What is the risk of a groin puncture that is above or below the femoral head?

A "high arterial" femoral puncture or one that is proximal to the femoral head is associated with an increased incidence of retroperitoneal hemorrhage and formation of a pseudoaneurysm. A "low arterial" femoral puncture or one that is distal to the femoral head may result in a pseudoaneurysm or an arteriovenous fistula.

7. What is the difference in single-wall and double-wall puncture technique?

To perform a single-wall puncture only the ventral wall of the vessel is punctured to gain entry to the vessel. A double-wall puncture is performed by puncturing both the dorsal and ventral walls of the vessel, and subsequently withdrawing the needle until an intraluminal position is encountered.

8. What are the advantages and disadvantages of the single-wall technique?

Single-wall puncture technique is preferred for bypass grafts and for patients at risk for puncture site hemorrhage. The risk of bleeding is minimized as only a single hole is made in the vessel. The disadvantage of the single-wall puncture technique is the increased risk of access site dissection.

9. What sites can be used for arterial access?

The principal sites used to obtain arterial access include the femoral and brachial arteries. Other sites for arterial access include the axillary artery, the popliteal artery, and the abdominal aorta.

10. Why is the left brachial or axillary artery puncture site preferred over a similar puncture site on the right?

Because the catheter does not cross a common carotid artery origin and advancement of the catheter into the descending aorta is easier.

11. What is translumbar aortography?

The technique of directly accessing the abdominal aorta with a catheter or needle from the flank. The procedure is reserved for patients without femoral, axillary, or brachial access. The technique was

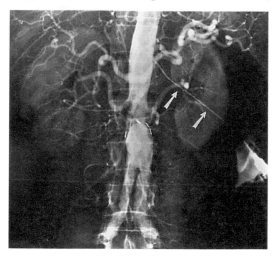

described by dos Santos in 1929. The procedure is performed with the patient in the prone position. A special 18-gauge needle with a 6 French sheath is placed directly into the abdominal aorta percutaneously from the left flank (Fig. 2). The needle can be placed in a "high" position at T12 to L1 for abdominal aortography, or a "low" position at L2 to L3 for pelvic and lower-extremity arteriography.

FIGURE 2. Translumbar aortogram (TLA) in patient with prior aorto-iliac graft. The TLA needle (arrows) enters the aorta at T12.

12. What are the contraindications to translumbar aortography?
Coagulopathy, abdominal aortic aneurysm, abdominal aortic graft, and severe hypertension.

13. What is the gauge system?
A classification system for grading the caliber of a needle. The gauge system defines the outer needle's diameter as how many of the same sized needles lined up side-to-side would measure one inch. Puncture site needles are usually 18 to 19 gauge.

14. What is the design of the basic guidewire?
Guidewires are designed to facilitate safe placement of the desired catheter in a specific vessel. The features of an ideal guidewire include low profile, low thrombogenicity, low friction coefficient, maximum torquability, maximum radiopacity, and an atraumatic tip. The standard guidewire is composed of an outer stainless steel coil wire supported by an inner mandril wire that extends the length of the coil. Tandem to the inner mandril wire is a fine stainless steel safety wire that is soldered to the coil tip (Fig. 3). The safety wire functions to prevent complete guidewire transection should the coil break. The guidewire stiffness is determined by the thickness of the inner core wire. The degree of wire tapering predicts the flexibility and floppiness of the tip.

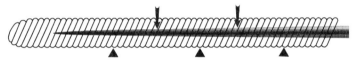

FIGURE 3.   Schematic of standard guidewires composed of an outer stainless steel coil wire (arrowheads) wrapped around an inner mandrel wire (arrows).

15. What is a hydrophilic guidewire?
The hydrophilic wire is a torque wire coated with a hydrophilic polymer that has a markedly reduced friction coefficient when wet. It is composed of a nickel-titanium alloy covered by a polymer. The hydrophilic wire should not be inserted through or withdrawn from a needle, because of the risk of shearing off the outer polymer layer.

16. What are the characteristics of different catheter materials?
Catheters are classified by shape, length, inner diameter, outer diameter, coating, and material. The materials used for catheter construction are polyurethane, nylon, polyethylene, polypropylene, and teflon. Polyethylene (PE) catheters are the most common. These are soft, pliable, and torquable, and maintain their preimprinted shape. PE has a low coefficient of friction and is less stiff than nylon and teflon.

17. What are the advantages of nylon and polyurethane catheters?
Nylon catheters are relatively stiff and can tolerate higher flow rates than polyethylene. Polyurethane catheters are more pliable than polyethylene catheters; this facilitates improved catheter tracking over a guidewire. This pliability is also a drawback, as the catheter is prone to recoil during a contrast injection. The most significant limitation of polyurethane is its high coefficient of friction. In order for polyurethane catheters to be functional they are coated with a low friction material to promote passage over a guidewire.

18. What are the characteristics of teflon catheters?
Teflon catheters are stiffer than catheters made of other materials. They tolerate high injection pressures and have a low coefficient of friction. Teflon is the material commonly used for dilators and sheaths.

19. What does French represent when describing catheter size?
French (F) is a measure of circumference of round tubes. The outer catheter diameter is measured in French units, where 1 French is equal to one third of a millimeter.

20. What is a braided catheter?

A catheter that contains a fine wire mesh within its wall. The reinforcing wire renders the catheter more torquable and radiopaque. Catheter materials compatible with placement of a braid include polyethylene and polyurethane.

21. What makes a catheter radiopaque?

The radiopacity of the standard catheter materials is limited. Radiopacity is enhanced by imbedding the catheter wall with bismuth, barium, or lead. In addition, the wire of a braided catheter renders it more radiopaque.

22. How is the catheter bursting pressure determined?

The bursting pressure of the catheter is equal to the catheter thickness divided by the internal radius multiplied by the tensile strength of the catheter material.

23. What is Poiseuille's law?

It states that the injection volume a catheter can accept is directly proportional to the injection pressure and catheter radius, and inversely proportional to the contrast viscosity and the catheter length. A longer or smaller radius catheter has a reduced maximum injection flow rate. Similarly, contrast agents with higher viscosity (nonionics) result in reduced catheter flow rates when compared to low viscosity (ionic) contrast. The contrast agent's viscosity can be reduced by warming the dye prior to injection.

24. What are the complications of routine angiography?

The incidence of complications varies with the access site, patient's age, and duration of the procedure. Angiograms performed from an axillary approach have a higher incidence of complications than those performed via a femoral access route. Older patients and longer procedure times are additional factors that predispose to an increased incidence of complications. Complications include arterial thrombosis, arterial dissection, arterial rupture, embolization, vasospasm, cardiovascular collapse, stroke, renal failure, infection, contrast reaction, and death. Development of lower profile catheters has reduced the incidence of complications from angiography.

25. What is digital subtraction angiography (DSA)?

A computer-based digital imaging technique. The computer acquires images before and during contrast injection. The image acquired before contrast opacification is referred to as the mask. The noncontrast mask is electronically subtracted from contrast images to erase everything except the contrast-filled vessels. The images from the injection can be immediately viewed on a monitor. As a result, the procedure time is reduced, as delays for film developing are omitted. The contrast resolution of DSA is superior to conventional film-screen angiography. As a result, the contrast can be diluted for DSA studies. The spatial resolution with DSA is less than conventional film-screen angiography.

26. What are the advantages of DSA over conventional film-screen angiography?

DSA reduces contrast volume, procedure time, and film expense, while enhancing contrast resolution. In addition, DSA images can be manipulated after acquisition.

BIBLIOGRAPHY

1. dos Santos R, Lamas A, Pereira-Caldas J: Arteriograia da aorta e dos vasos abdominias. Med Contemp 47:93, 1929.
2. Seldinger SI: Catheter replacement of the needle in percutaneous arteriography. Acta Radiol 39:368–376, 1953.

77. CAROTID IMAGING

Elmer Nahum, M.D., and Kenneth D. Murphy, M.D.

1. What are the four segments of the internal carotid artery?

The four segments of the internal carotid artery (ICA) are the cervical, petrous, cavernous, and supraclinoid (cerebral) (Fig. 1). The cervical ICA arises posterolaterally at the common carotid bifurcation and is devoid of any angiographically identifiable branches. The petrous segment is the portion of the ICA within the carotid canal of the petrous bone. The cavernous segment (carotid siphon) is the S-shaped portion within the carotid sinus that terminates at the level of the anterior clinoid process. (Some authors have divided the cavernous segment into precavernous and cavernous segments.) The supraclinoid portion is the intracranial ICA distal to the anterior clinoid process, after it passes through the dura.

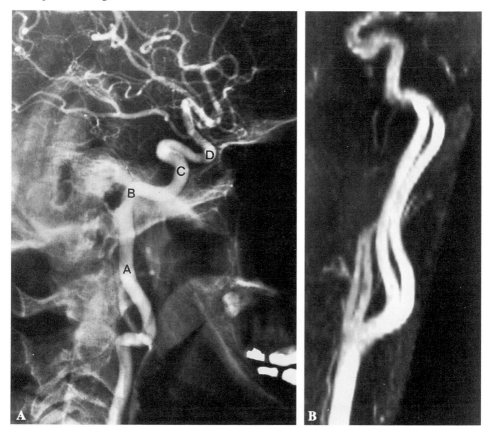

FIGURE 1. *A,* Lateral views of the internal carotid artery on conventional angiogram. Cervical (A), petrous (B), cavernous (C), and supraclinoid (D) segments. *B,* Lateral view of both carotid arteries on MR angiography.

2. What is the most common disease that results in narrowing or occlusion of the cervical carotid artery?

Atherosclerosis.

3. Which portion of the cervical carotid is most affected by atherosclerosis?

The carotid bulb (Fig. 2). The bulb is the fusiform portion of the distal common carotid and the proximal internal carotid. Atherosclerosis typically involves the posterolateral aspect of the bulb initially, and later progresses circumferentially.

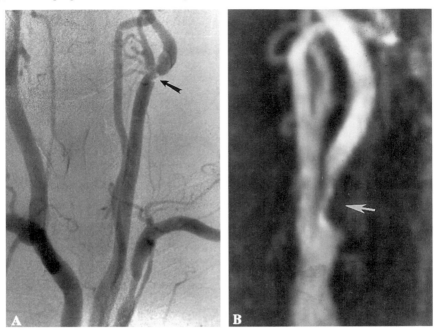

FIGURE 2.   Atherosclerotic plaque involving the posterolateral wall of the left carotid bulb (arrow) on conventional angiogram (*A*) and MRA (*B*).

4. Why is the carotid bulb preferentially affected by atherosclerosis?

The carotid bulb is an elastic artery while the ICA is primarily a muscular artery; the histologic difference in wall composition and flow disturbances at the bulb may explain the propensity for atherosclerosis to develop at that location.

5. Why is accurate imaging of the carotid important if atherosclerotic disease is suspected?

Because carotid endarterectomy can potentially prevent a future stroke, accurate imaging of the carotid artery is essential.

6. How does atherosclerosis of the cervical carotid artery lead to stroke?

Although a carotid stenosis may lead to diminished blood flow with resultant ischemia, most strokes or transient ischemic attacks from cervical carotid disease are believed to be due to emboli. The irregular atherosclerotic surface of the carotid artery serves as a nidus for platelet aggregation, which has the potential for embolization. Plaque rupture can result in release of atheromatous debris that can embolize. Embolization of platelet aggregates, atheromatous debris, or thrombi can lead to a variety of neurological events ranging from ipsilateral cerebral ischemia to transient monocular blindness.

7. What patients may benefit from carotid endarterectomy?

The large multi-center North American Symptomatic Carotid Endarterectomy Trial (NASCET) demonstrated a clear benefit from carotid endarterectomy in symptomatic patients with high-grade (70–99%) stenoses. In patients with a moderate stenosis (30–69%), the NASCET data is still pending.

Patients with mild disease can be managed with a medical regimen including aspirin and dietary modification. Another trial, the Asymptomatic Carotid Atherosclerosis Study (ACAS), has shown that even asymptomatic patients with stenoses greater than 60% benefit from carotid surgery. Despite a lesser degree of luminal narrowing, symptomatic patients with carotid artery ulceration or recurrent symptoms are also candidates for surgical treatment.

8. Can an endarterectomy be performed if complete carotid occlusion is present?

No. Patients with complete carotid occlusion cannot undergo endarterectomy since the ICA above the stenosis will be thrombosed.

9. In addition to atherosclerosis what are the causes of carotid stenosis?

Other causes of stenosis include fibromuscular dysplasia, dissection, inflammatory arteriopathies, and aneurysm.

10. What imaging modalities are available for evaluation of cervical carotid disease?

Ultrasound, MR angiography (MRA), conventional angiography, and CT angiography.

11. What is a cost-effective work-up of symptomatic carotid artery disease?

Carotid duplex ultrasound is generally the first study performed, since it is noninvasive and readily available. If there is only mild disease, then conservative management is warranted. If a moderate to severe stenosis is detected, then MRA can be performed. The findings of MRA and ultrasonography are concordant in up to 84% of cases. With concordant MRA and ultrasound data, some vascular surgeons will operate on a 70–99% stenosis that is symptomatic. If the MRA and ultrasound findings are discordant, conventional angiography is necessary for further evaluation.

12. What is the significance of an ulcerated atherosclerotic plaque of the cervical carotid?

A plaque that ruptures atheromatous material will form an irregular crater that serves as a nidus for platelet aggregation. Patients with ulcerated plaque are at higher risk for stroke or transient ischemic attacks. Unfortunately, it is difficult to accurately diagnose an ulceration in a plaque. The most sensitive and specific examination in this situation is conventional angiography, yet the sensitivity and specificity of angiography for diagnosing an ulceration are only 46% and 74%, respectively (Fig. 3).

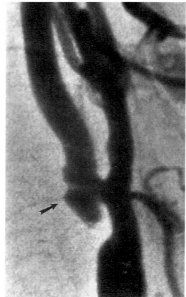

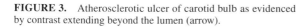

FIGURE 3.   Atherosclerotic ulcer of carotid bulb as evidenced by contrast extending beyond the lumen (arrow).

13. What are the potential risks of carotid angiography?

Puncture site hematoma, contrast reaction, introduction of infection, vascular injury, and stroke. The incidence of stroke during cerebral angiography is < 2%. The causes of stroke during angiography include inadvertent injection of air bubbles or blood clots, or catheter-related problems such as thrombosis, vascular spasm, dissection, or disruption of loose plaque.

14. What are the three components of a diagnostic carotid ultrasound exam?

B-mode imaging, spectral analysis, and color Doppler.

15. What is B-mode carotid imaging?

B-mode refers to the conventional two dimensional gray-scale ultrasound images. A high-frequency 7–10 MHz transducer is typically used to obtain high resolution images.

16. What is the normal appearance of the carotid artery on B-mode imaging?

The normal carotid artery has a thin, echogenic intima, a hypoechoic media, and a hyperechoic adventitia. The intima-media complex should be no greater than 0.8 mm in thickness (Fig. 4). Thickening of the wall corresponds to an atherosclerotic plaque. The plaque is described as fibrofatty or "soft" if it is hypoechoic, or as calcific or "hard" if it is hyperechoic and accompanied by posterior acoustic shadowing.

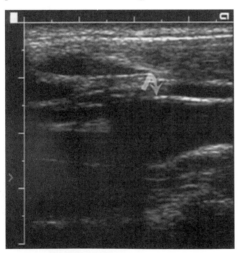

FIGURE 4. Cervical carotid B-mode ultrasound. Note the normal intima-media complex (curved arrow).

17. How is spectral analysis performed?

A pulsed-wave Doppler window is placed over a specific segment of the vessel. The morphology of the resultant waveform is analyzed with the velocity on the y-axis and time on the x-axis (Fig. 5). The external carotid has a high resistance waveform which appears as very low velocity during diastole. The normal internal carotid has a low resistance waveform, since there is limited impedance to intracranial flow. The common carotid has a waveform somewhere in between these two patterns.

18. What are spectral analysis findings when a stenosis is present?

With stenosis of the internal carotid artery or bulb, sampling below the stenosis will demonstrate a waveform that mimics the external carotid artery, due to the increased resistance to flow. At the level of the stenosis and beyond the velocity increases and there is broadening of the wave due to turbulence. Generally the velocity increases as the severity of the stenosis increases. Numerical measurements of the Doppler-based velocities correlates well with the degree of stenosis. For example, a peak systolic velocity of 1.3 meters/second (m/s) and an end diastolic velocity of 1.0 m/s represent a 70% stenosis.

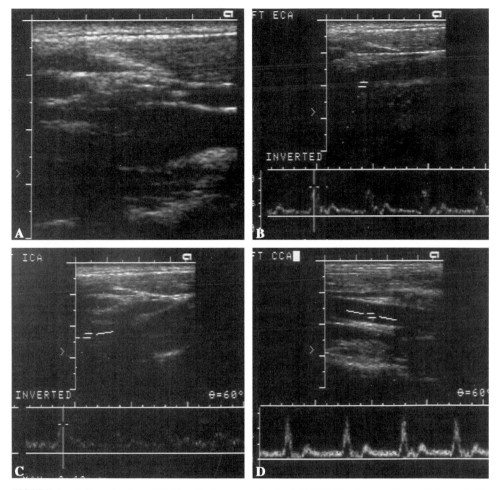

FIGURE 5. *A*, B-mode of carotid bifurcation in a normal patient. *B*, ECA Doppler waveform with low velocity in diastole. *C*, ICA waveform with higher velocity in diastole. *D*, CCA waveform appears as a combination of the ICA and CCA.

19. How are the color Doppler images used when imaging the carotid artery?

The color Doppler images demonstrate flow direction and corroborate any discrepancies on the B-mode and spectral analysis.

20. What are the potential pitfalls of omitting conventional angiography prior to carotid surgery?

One potential pitfall is that additional distal stenoses (or "tandem" lesions) may not be identified. Tandem stenoses occur in approximately 20% of patients who undergo an endarterectomy. The distal stenosis occurs most often in the cavernous segment (the siphon) of the intracranial ICA. MR angiography has limited sensitivity for detecting such lesions. Tandem stenoses may limit the clinical benefit of carotid endarterectomy.

Another potential pitfall occurs when the carotid is imaged with sonography. Flow through a stenosis may be so limiting that the velocity decreases in the area of the stenosis, which then may be underestimated on sonography. While ultrasound may underestimate such a stenosis, MR angiography may give the impression that there is a total occlusion instead of a high grade stenosis. Some institutions now perform CT angiography in such situations, in addition to or instead of MR angiography, since these stenoses are more accurately characterized with CT angiography.

21. What influences the surgeon's decision to operate based only on non-invasive imaging (as opposed to based on conventional angiography)?

This decision is based on many factors including the availability of MR angiography, the experience of the interpreting radiologist, the quality of the sonographic and MR exams, and financial considerations.

22. What patients are affected by fibromuscular dysplasia of the carotid artery?

Fibromuscular dysplasia (FMD) is more common in women than men by a 9 to 1 ratio. Women with this disorder are usually between 50 and 70 years of age when they present with this disorder. FMD is identified on 0.6% of all carotid angiograms.

23. What is the natural course of carotid FMD?

The vast majority of patients found to have FMD on angiography do not develop any sequelae and have a good prognosis.

24. What are the potential complications of FMD of the carotid artery?

Dissection, aneurysm, and emboli.

25. What features distinguish carotid FMD?

FMD of the carotid artery typically involves the ICA above the carotid bulb. The most common type of FMD is medial dysplasia. This form has webs alternating with segments of mural thickening, resulting in the "string-of-beads" appearance (Fig. 6). Less common types of FMD may be indistinguishable from atherosclerosis. Atherosclerosis and FMD can coexist, which may create diagnostic confusion.

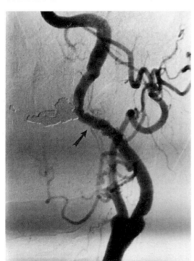

FIGURE 6.   Classic beaded appearance of FMD involving the mid-cervical ICA (arrow).

26. What other vessels can be involved by FMD?

In general, medium-sized muscular arteries that have a long course before branching can be affected by FMD. Renal FMD is the most commonly affected artery. About one-third of patients with renovascular hypertension have FMD. The ICA is the second most commonly affected artery. Iliac and visceral arteries (e.g., the splenic artery) may also be involved. FMD is commonly a bilateral condition. There is an association of carotid FMD with cerebral aneurysms. Evaluation of such aneurysms with MR angiography or conventional angiography should be considered in patients with carotid FMD.

27. What is a standing wave and how can it be distinguished from FMD on angiography?

The standing wave is an artifact in a vessel that creates a beaded or corrugated appearance that may mimic FMD. The exact cause of the phenomenon is unknown, but is thought to be related to the speed of the injection. In a standing wave no portion of the vessel is larger than the normal vessel diameter. In the classic type of FMD, the beaded segments are larger than the normal vessel.

28. In 20–40 year olds, what are the two most common diseases of the cervical carotid that lead to cerebral ischemia?

Premature atherosclerosis and carotid dissection.

29. When does carotid dissection occur?

The true incidence of carotid dissection is unknown but is thought to be the cause of stroke in up to 20% of patients under age 40. While dissection usually occurs following significant trauma, it may occur following a seemingly trivial injury, or even spontaneously. When related to trauma, the injury beings in the superior aspect of the ICA at the level of the C2 vertebra. Dissection can also occur in the vertebral artery with patients presenting with posterior fossa symptoms. Some cases of dissection occur in already weakened vessel walls of patients with FMD or vasculitis.

30. What are the angiographic findings of carotid dissection?

As with any arterial dissection, an intimal flap at the entrance site of the dissection may be seen. As the intimal tear extends into the subintima or media, a double lumen of contrast may be visualized. If the true lumen is obliterated enough to allow only a small amount of contrast to enter, a "string sign" may be seen. Eventually, total occlusion may ensue (Fig. 7A).

MR combined with MR angiography appears to be more accurate than angiography for the diagnosis of dissection and can be performed quickly. Visualization of the double lumen on an axial MR image is the characteristic finding (Fig. 7B).

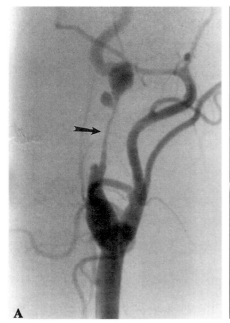 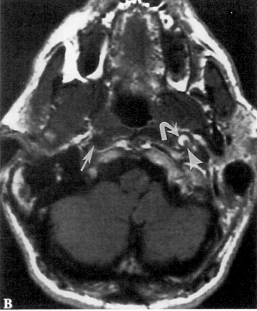

FIGURE 7. *A,* Carotid dissection: string of contrast in true lumen (arrow) of cervical carotid caused by compression by the nonvisualized false-lumen. *B,* Axial T1-weighted spin-echo image at level of dissection showing normal flow void in right ICA (arrow). The left ICA has markedly increased signal in the false lumen (curved arrow) and mildly increased signal in the compressed true lumen (arrowhead).

31. What are the presenting symptoms of carotid dissection?

Besides stroke of TIA, patients may have headache, neck pain, a bruit, cranial nerve palsy, or an incomplete Horner's syndrome. Cranial nerve palsies are thought to be due to direct stretching of the intimately associated nerves around the ICA or to loss of blood supply to these nerves by the small nutrient vessels. The ninth through twelfth cranial nerves and the superior cervical ganglion and its fibers are adjacent to the cervical ICA. The incomplete Horner's syndrome, miosis and ptosis without anhydrosis, may occur; this is known as oculosympathetic paresis. This occurs in dissection because the specific sympathetic fibers that produce miosis and ptosis travel along the ICA, while the fibers producing facial sweating travel adjacent to the external carotid artery.

BIBLIOGRAPHY

1. Corrin LS, Sandok BA, Houser OW: Cerebral ischemic events in patients with carotid artery fibromuscular dysplasia. Arch Neurol 38:616–618, 1981.
2. DeMarco JK, Schonfeld S, Wesbey G: Can non-invasive studies replace conventional angiography in the preoperative evaluation of carotid stenosis? Neuroimaging Clin North Am 6:911–929, 1996.
3. Executive Committee for the Asymptomatic Carotid Atherosclerosis Study: Endarterectomy for asymptomatic carotid artery stenosis. JAMA 273:1421–1428, 1994.
4. Faught WE, Mattos MA, et al: Color flow duplex scanning of carotid arteries: New velocity criteria based on receiver operator characteristic analysis for threshold stenoses used in the symptomatic and asymptomatic carotid trials. J Vasc Surg 19:818–827, 1994.
5. Heiserman JE, Dean BL, Hodak JA, et al: Neurologic complications of cerebral angiography. AJNR 15:1401, 1994.
6. Mattos MA, van Bemmelen PS, Hodgson KJ, et al: The influence of carotid siphon stenosis on short- and long-term outcome after carotid endarterectomy. J Vasc Surg 17:902–910, 1993.
7. North American Symptomatic Carotid Endarterectomy Collaborators: Beneficial effect of carotid endarterectomy in symptomatic patients with high grade carotid stenosis. N Engl J Med 325:445–453, 1991.
8. Patel MR, Kuntz KM, Klufas RA, et al: Preoperative assessment of the carotid bifurcation. Can magnetic resonance angiography and duplex ultrasonography replace contrast angiography? Stroke 26:1753, 1995.
9. Polak JF, O'Leary DH, et al: Sonographic evaluation of carotid or carotid artery atherosclerosis in the elderly: Relationship of disease severity to stroke and transient ischemic attack. Radiology 188:363–370, 1993.
10. Provenzale JM: Dissection of the internal carotid and vertebral arteries: Imaging features. AJR 165:1099–1104, 1995.
11. Stempel M, Groth H, Greminger P, et al: The spectrum of renovascular hypertension. Cardiology 72(suppl 1):1–9, 1985.
12. Stingaris K, et al: Three-dimensional time-of-flight MR angiography and MR imaging versus conventional angiography in carotid artery dissections. Int Angio 15:20–25, 1996.
13. Streifler JY, Eliasziw M, Fox AJ, et al: Angiographic detection of carotid ulceration. Stroke 25:1130–1132, 1994.

78. ANGIOPLASTY

Kenneth D. Murphy, M.D.

1. What is percutaneous transluminal angioplasty (PTA)?

The procedure of dilating diseased vessels that are narrowed or occluded with a balloon catheter. The first such procedure was reported in 1964 by Dotter and Judkins; in their patient, a superficial femoral artery stenosis was dilated percutaneously by passing coaxial catheters of increasing diameter. In 1978 Gruentzig developed a 7 French balloon catheter from polyvinyl chloride, which could be inflated to predetermined diameters. Since these pioneering efforts, technological advances and clinical experience have enabled PTA to become a mainstay in the management of vascular occlusive disease.

2. Is angioplasty limited to arterial lesions?

No. Angioplasty can be performed safely and efficaciously in arteries and veins. Angioplasty is also successful in dilating other vascular conduits, such as bypass grafts, portosystemic shunts, vascular stents, and stent-grafts. The greatest angioplasty experience has been acquired in the arterial system. Knowledge of the normal and abnormal histology of blood vessels is critical to understanding the mechanisms of angioplasty.

3. What are the three types of arteries and what are their functions?

Arterioles, muscular arteries, and elastic arteries. The arterioles are the smallest arteries, whose primary role is to regulate the overall vascular tone. The muscular arteries are intermediate in size and are composed primarily of smooth muscle cells. Their principal function is to regulate the distribution of blood flow. Examples of muscular arteries include the coronary, visceral, and peripheral arteries. The elastic arteries are the largest in diameter. Elastic arteries, such as the aorta and the proximal iliac arteries, contain extensive elastic fibers in their wall, which facilitate diastolic recoil and maintenance of a uniform hydrostatic pressure.

4. What are the basic layers of a vessel?

The walls of arteries and veins are composed of three basic layers. The innermost layer, the intima, is a single layer of endothelium, which rests on a bed of connective tissue that is bound by the lumen and the internal elastic lamina. The second layer, the media, is composed of connective tissue, collagen, and smooth muscle. The media is located between the internal elastic lamina and the external elastic lamina. The adventitia, the outermost layer, is external to the external elastic lamina. It is composed of loose connective tissue, with interspersed elastic fibers, nerves, lymphatics, and nutrient blood vessels.

5. What are the theorized mechanisms of PTA?

Angioplasty restores vessel patency by means of a controlled injury to the vessel wall. Several mechanisms of PTA have been proposed, including pulverization of plaque, compression of plaque, stretching of the vessel wall, and fracture of the plaque with induction of a focal dissection.

6. What is plaque fracture and focal dissection?

The most universally accepted mechanism of PTA. The radial force of the inflated balloon fractures the noncompliant plaque at its thinnest point. As a result, a cleavage plane is formed that can extend through the wall in a circumferential or longitudinal direction. This cleavage plane represents a focal dissection. The plaque disruption and focal dissection can result in dissociation of the plaque with the intima and media, a factor believed to retard the progression of the plaque. Vascular remodeling of the local dissection occurs with time and typically results in a relatively smooth luminal surface. When the iatrogenic dissection of PTA is too extensive, a flow-limiting dissection flap may result. In such cases, an additional intervention such as stent placement or surgery is indicated.

7. What is the role of vessel wall stretching in PTA?

Stretching of the vessel wall from PTA contributes to luminal enlargement. The outward or radial force of the inflated balloon stretches the media and induces smooth muscle necrosis. The damaged media results in a more compliant vessel with improved luminal diameter. The balloon-induced stretching is thought to be an important component of venous angioplasty because venous strictures are associated with a large component of scar tissue.

8. Does plaque compression from angioplasty contribute to restoration of the luminal diameter?

Initially, the mechanism of PTA was thought primarily to be compression of the atheromatous plaque by the balloon with secondary extrusion of the plaque's liquid content. As PTA evolved, more clinical experience and research demonstrated the role of plaque compression to be limited.

9. What are the histologic factors favoring a successful angioplasty?

A small luminal diameter prior to angioplasty, a deep dissection after angioplasty, and vessel wall lesions (plaque) with reduced lipid content.

10. What are the indications for lower extremity balloon angioplasty?

Lifestyle-limiting claudication, extremity pain at rest, tissue loss, and the need for improved inflow or outflow prior to surgical bypass. Patients also may be candidates for PTA if surgery is too risky, their life expectancy is short, or they lack a satisfactory vein for a vascular bypass. In patients in whom an amputation is inevitable, angioplasty may be indicated in an attempt to limit the level of amputation (e.g., an above-the-knee amputation may be converted to a below-the-knee amputation).

11. What are contraindications to angioplasty?
- A hemodynamically unstable patient
- A stenosis immediately adjacent to an aneurysm
- An ulcerated plaque associated with distal embolization
- A stenosis that is not hemodynamically significant

12. What is a hemodynamically significant stenosis?

A stenosis is generally considered significant if the luminal diameter is reduced by 50% and the systolic pressure gradient is in excess of 10 mm Hg across the lesion (Fig. 1). The pressure gradient across a lesion is equally as important as the degree of luminal compromise. A lumen that is diminished by 50% will have a corresponding 75% reduction in cross-sectional area, which reduces the flow rate through this area to a clinically significant level. An exercise state can be mimicked by intraarterial administration of vasodilating agents such as nitroglycerin, tolazoline, or papaverine. A gradient greater than 20 mm Hg is considered significant after such a vasodilatory challenge.

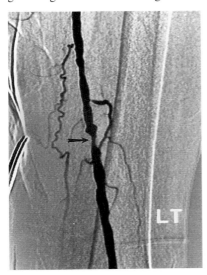

FIGURE 1. Left superficial femoral artery with significant stenosis (arrow).

13. What characteristics of a stenosis are more likely to result in a successful angioplasty?

Successful angioplasty is associated with stenoses that are short, noncalcified, and concentric (Fig. 2). Eccentric stenoses have a reduced PTA response and increased complication rate because the rigid plaque is more resistant to balloon dilatation than the adjacent normal vessel wall (Fig. 3). As a result, the force of the inflated balloon dilatation will be transmitted primarily to the normal vessel wall, placing it at risk for disruption and rupture. Stenotic lesions respond more favorably to angioplasty than complete occlusions. For iliac and femoropopliteal stenoses, an intact distal runoff (calf vessels) is also predictive of PTA success.

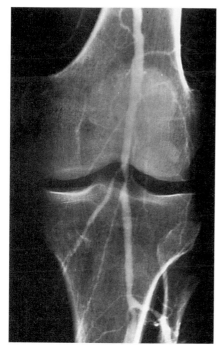
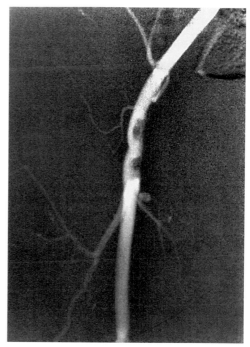

FIGURE 2 *(Left)*. Short, concentric popliteal artery stenosis: a favorable lesion for angioplasty.

FIGURE 3 *(Right)*. Common femoral arteriogram demonstrates an eccentric plaque: an unfavorable lesion for angioplasty.

14. What is the Law of Laplace?

The Law of Laplace describes the outward force a balloon generates on a vessel wall. The law states that the outward force (F) on the vessel wall at the site of the stenosis is proportional to the balloon pressure (P) and radius (R) of the inflated balloon: $F = P \times R$. Thus, the outward force or tension a balloon creates is linearly related to the inflation pressure if the diameter remains fixed. Similarly, if the inflation pressure is fixed, a balloon with a diameter half that of a larger balloon will generate half the dilating force. A greater dilating force is generated by a balloon inflated against a high-grade stenosis than against a lower-grade lesion. The inflated balloon has a typical "dog bone" configuration with the central "waist" representing the stenosis. As the waist on the balloon is effaced with inflation, the radial force on the stenosis diminishes.

15. What is the basic design of the modern angioplasty balloon?

Several models are available, but their fundamental design is similar. The basic design consists of a double-lumen catheter with an oblong balloon at its tip (Fig. 4). The larger central lumen is for the guidewire, and a smaller second lumen is present for inflation of the balloon chamber. The chamber is usually inflated with dilute contrast. The composition of the balloon material is variable and determines its properties and performance. Most modern balloons are constructed from polymers such as polyvinyl chloride, polyethylene teraphtahlate, and nylon-reinforced polyurethane.

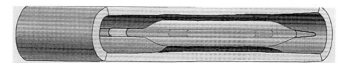

FIGURE 4. Schematic of prototype balloon catheter.

16. How is an angioplasty performed?

The technique is relatively well established; the initial step is percutaneous access via the Seldinger technique. Typically, a transfemoral approach is used for arterial dilatation. Venous stenoses can be accessed from a variety of locations. An introducer sheath is placed at the access site; the sheath site varies with the balloon diameter required for the lesion. The lesion is crossed using a guidewire with a floppy or tapered tip. Heparin is administered to prevent thrombosis at the angioplasty site. A catheter is advanced across the lesion to facilitate exchange for a stiffer wire. The balloon is passed over the wire and centered on the lesion. The balloon is inflated (up to several times), typically for about 45 seconds for each inflation for arterial stenoses and longer for venous stenoses. The patient should experience a mild degree of discomfort with inflation that subsides with deflation.

17. What are the final steps of angioplasty?

An angiogram is performed to evaluate the technical success of the procedure. Postangioplasty pressure measurements are made across the lesion.

18. How is balloon size determined?

The controlled dissection of angioplasty requires the balloon diameter to be 10–15% greater than the true luminal diameter. The luminal diameter can be estimated by measuring the adjacent nondiseased vessel or the same vessel on the contralateral side. These measurements can be made accurately with modern digital subtraction angiography units. If traditional film-screen angiography (i.e., "cut" film) is used, direct measurements can be made on the initial films with the realization that, due to geometric magnification, the true vessel lumen is magnified by 15% on the radiographs. The balloon length should match the lesion length. The balloon should not extend more than 1 cm beyond the stenosis because dilatation of the adjacent normal vessel can lead to complications such as dissection, thrombosis, or accelerated atherosclerosis.

19. What constitutes a technically successful angioplasty?

- Restoration of luminal diameter with less than a 30% residual stenosis
- A transstenotic pressure gradient of less than 5 mm Hg
- Absence of dissection or vessel rupture (Fig. 5)
- Relative reduction in number and caliber of collaterals if a venous stenosis was angioplastied

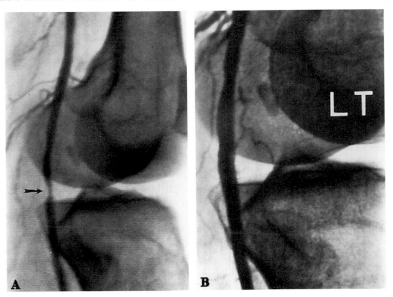

FIGURE 5. Popliteal artery stenosis (*A*) before (arrow) and (*B*) after successful angioplasty.

20. What are the complications of angioplasty?

The type and incidence of complications vary with the lesion's location and morphology. Complications include spasm, dissection (Fig. 6), embolization, thrombosis, vessel rupture, access site trauma, renal dysfunction, contrast allergy, and death.

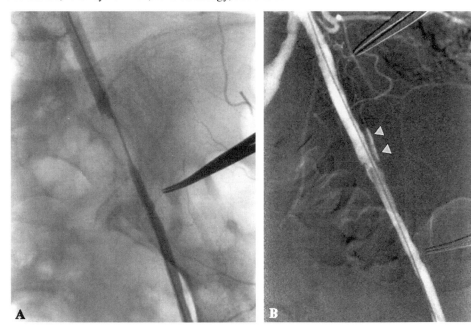

FIGURE 6.   Pelvic arteriogram demonstrates (*A*) high-grade left common iliac artery stenosis pre-angioplasty and (*B*) dissection (arrowheads) after angioplasty.

21. What is the most frequent complication?

Access site complications, especially the development of a hematoma at the puncture site. The hematoma is typically self-limited and is treated with additional compression. If the axilla was used for vascular access and a hematoma develops, the brachial plexus may be compressed and secondary palsy may develop. Prompt surgical evaluation is necessary to avoid permanent nerve injury. Other puncture site complications include balloon catheter impaction, nerve injury, arteriovenous fistula, and pseudoaneurysm.

22. How are the other complications treated?

The remaining complications are more significant but less common. They can be minimized with attention to procedural detail and technique. Spasm is treated pharmacologically with intraarterial vasodilators such as nitroglycerin. Angioplasty-induced dissections that limit flow are initially treated by repeat balloon dilatation. If that fails, stent placement or surgery is indicated. Distal embolization is rare and typically necessitates aggressive thrombolytic therapy or surgical embolectomy. Angioplasty site thrombosis is treated by thrombolytic therapy or surgical thrombectomy. Vessel rupture is a severe, life-threatening complication that requires prompt intervention. In such cases, the balloon should be reinflated at the site of rupture to temporarily tamponade the bleeding. The vessel can then be repaired surgically or by endovascular placement of a covered stent. Postangioplasty renal dysfunction can be minimized by aggressive hydration and by minimizing the contrast load.

23. How common are complications from angioplasty?

In a review of 6,620 aortoiliac angioplasties, the overall complication rate was 8.1% and the major complication rate was 2.7%. Complications require treatment in only 2.0–2.5% of extremity arterial balloon angioplasties.

24. Describe a technically unsuccessful angioplasty and its management.

An unsuccessful angioplasty is defined as a residual stenosis greater than 30%, a residual trans-stenotic pressure gradient greater than 5 mm Hg, or the presence of a significant flow-limiting dissection. In some instances the dissection flap can be "tacked-up" with repeat balloon inflation. If that fails, surgery or percutaneous intravascular stent placement should be considered. Likewise, if there is a significant residual stenosis or gradient, stent placement or surgery should be performed (Fig. 7).

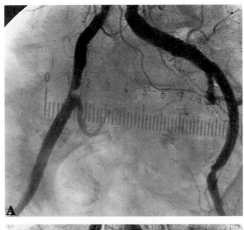

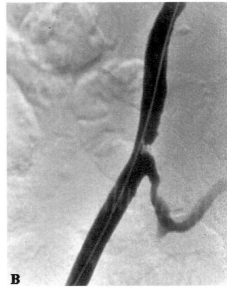

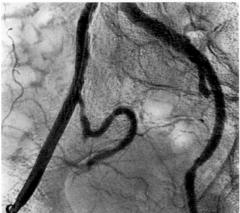

FIGURE 7. Right external iliac artery stenosis (*A*) pre-angioplaty, (*B*) post-angioplasty with marked recoil, and (*C*) post-stent.

25. How successful is arterial angioplasty?

The patency rate following arterial angioplasty varies with the length of follow-up and location of the lesion. The primary patency rate for abdominal aortic angioplasty has been reported to be 93% at 4 years of follow-up. The primary patency for femoropopliteal artery angioplasty has been reported to be 47% at 1 year and 42% at 3 years.

26. What is the function of a sheath?

An introducer sheath facilitates multiple guidewire, catheter, and balloon catheter exchanges without trauma to the entry site. The sheath also can be used to measure pressures, inject pharmaceuticals, and obtain blood samples.

27. How is vasospasm managed?

If untreated, vasospasm can lead to acute thrombosis at the angioplasty site. A prophylactic measure to minimize the risk and severity of vasospasm is the administration of sublingual nifedipine 15–30 minutes preprocedure. Also, intraarterial nitroglycerin can be administered in doses of

50–100 µg during the procedure. The administration of all vasodilators is carefully titrated to the patient's blood pressure.

28. What patients should be heparinized after angioplasty?

Anticoagulation with heparin after angioplasty is recommended for hypercoagulable patients, patients with low-flow states, femoropopliteal or tibial artery PTA, angioplasty following thrombolysis, angioplasty complicated by significant dissection, and lower extremity angioplasty with impaired distal runoff. Heparinization can be restarted 6–12 hours after sheath removal, at 1000 units per hour. Typically, the loading bolus of heparin is omitted.

29. What is the "kissing balloon" technique?

This technique, which is advocated for dilatation of a complex bifurcation stenosis, involves the simultaneous inflation of separate balloon catheters positioned at the bifurcation stenosis. If narrowings are present in both bifurcation branches, simultaneous balloon inflation will serve to expand both stenoses. If the narrowing is limited to a single vessel at a bifurcation, the technique is still advocated to "protect" the nonstenotic branch from inadvertent balloon compression and secondary luminal compromise.

30. For what is the kissing balloon technique most commonly used?

For treatment of bilateral common iliac arterial artery stenoses. Similarly, bilateral common iliac stents can be deployed using the kissing technique (Fig. 8).

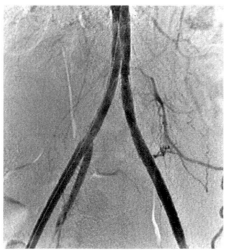

FIGURE 8. Pelvic angiogram after deployment of right and left common iliac artery stents using "kissing" technique.

31. What is an intravascular stent?

A metallic conduit designed to be placed percutaneously in blood vessels to maintain or restore their patency. The most common application is in the treatment of atherosclerotic occlusive disease. Two major stent designs have been developed for clinical use. The Palmaz balloon-expandable stent (Cordis-Johnson and Johnson Interventional Systems, Miami, FL) is a stainless-steel device that is expanded by balloon inflation. The Palmaz stent was the first stent approved for arterial use. The second design is the Wallstent (Schneider, Minneapolis, MN), a self-expanding device that is less rigid but more flexible than the Palmaz stent. The Wallstent has received approval by the FDA for arterial placement. Several other stent designs are under investigation.

32. Where can intravascular stents be placed?

Intravascular stents have been deployed in several locations, including the aorta, iliac, femoral, popliteal, subclavian, brachial, coronary, and carotid arteries. Stents also have played a significant role in the treatment of central venous occlusive disease. Currently, FDA approval is restricted to iliac and coronary artery stent placement. The other sites of placement remain investigational. The greatest experience has been accumulated with stent placement in the iliac arteries. The clinical patency rate of balloon-expandable stents in the iliac arteries has been reported to be 86% at 4 years.

33. What is the primary indication for intravascular stent placement?
A failed angioplasty.

BIBLIOGRAPHY

1. Becker GJ, Katzen BT, Dake MD: Noncoronary angioplasty. Radiology 170:921–940, 1989.
2. Dotter CT, Judkins MP: Transluminal treatment of arteriosclerotic obstructions: Descriptions of a new technique and a preliminary report of its application. Circulation 30:654–670, 1964.
3. Gruentzig A, Hopff H: Die perkutane rekanalisation chronischer arterieller verschlusse mit einer neuen dialtationskather: modifikation der Dotter-technik. Dtsch Med Wochenschr 99:2502, 1974.
4. Hallisey MJ, Meranze SG, Parker BC, et al: Percutaneous transluminal angioplasty of the abdominal aorta. J Vasc Interv Radiol 5:679–687, 1994.
5. Losordo DW, Rosenfield K, Pieczek A, et al: How does angioplasty work? Serial analysis of human iliac arteries using intravascular ultrasound. Circulation 86:1845–1858, 1992.
6. Matsi PJ, Manninen HI, Vanninen RL, et al: Femoropopliteal angioplasty in patients with claudication: Primary and secondary patency in 140 limbs with 1–3 year follow-up. Radiology 191:727–733, 1994.
7. Murphy KD, Encarnacion CE, Le VA, Palmaz JC: Iliac artery stent placement with the Palmaz stent: Follow-up study. J Vasc Interv Radiol 6:321–329, 1995.
8. Rholl KS, VanBreda A: Percutaneous intervention for aortoiliac disease. In Standness DE, Van Breda A (eds): Vascular Diseases: Surgical and Interventional Therapy. New York, Churchill Livingstone, 1994, pp 433–466.
9. Schwarten DE, Tadavarthy SM, Castaneda-Zuniga WR: Aortic, iliac, and peripheral arterial angioplasty. In Castaneda-Zuniga WR, Tadavarthy SM (eds): Interventional Radiology. 2nd ed. Baltimore, Williams & Wilkins, 1992, pp 378–421.

79. EMBOLOTHERAPY

Kenneth D. Murphy, M.D.

1. What is embolotherapy?
A therapeutic procedure in which blood vessels and vascular spaces are deliberately occluded by injecting material into them using imaging guidance.

2. What are the indications for embolotherapy?
Embolotherapy is an evolving technique that can be performed for a wide variety of clinical conditions. Indications include uncontrolled hemorrhage, aneurysms, preoperative devascularization of lesions to reduce operative blood loss, and therapeutic or palliative treatment of benign and malignant tumors including vascular neoplasms.

3. What lesions are amenable to preoperative devascularization using embolization techniques?
Preoperative embolization of selective hypervascular lesions has been performed in an attempt to minimize operative blood loss. Conditions that can be embolized preoperatively include hypersplenism and renal cell carcinoma. Embolization of primary and secondary osseous masses have proven successful in reducing blood loss during surgery. A common bone lesion responsive to this technique is metastatic renal cell carcinoma (Fig. 1).

4. What bleeding conditions are amenable to embolization?
Embolization to treat bleeding is indicated when medical therapy is unsuccessful and the risks of surgery are prohibitive. Such conditions include bronchial artery hemorrhage, gastrointestinal bleeding, obstetric hemorrhage, and traumatic bleeding from the liver, spleen, kidneys, or pelvis.

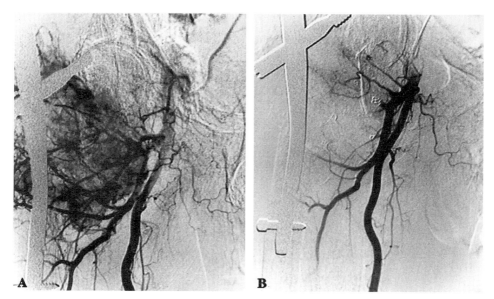

FIGURE 1. Metastatic renal cell carcinoma to femur. *A,* Diagnostic angiogram demonstrates a large hypervascular metastasis in the proximal right femur. *B,* Post-embolization angiogram demonstrates near complete ablation of the tumor vascularity. The patient subsequently underwent revision of the prior internal fixation with minimal blood loss.

5. What neoplastic conditions are amenable to embolotherapy?

The role of embolotherapy for neoplasms ranges from primary treatment of the tumor to palliation. Selected hepatic neoplasms, such as unresectable hepatocellular carcinoma, can be treated primarily with embolization in combination with chemotherapy. Other tumors and tumor-like conditions amenable to embolization include soft-tissue arteriovenous malformations, pulmonary arteriovenous malformations (Fig. 2), and primary bone tumors (Fig. 3).

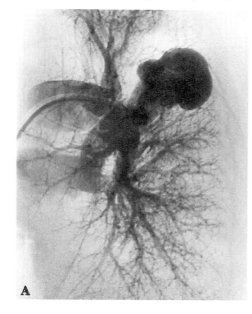

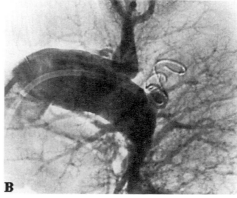

FIGURE 2. Pulmonary arteriovenous malformation (PAVM). *A,* Left pulmonary arteriogram demonstrates a large PAVM in the left upper lobe. *B,* Post-embolization angiogram demonstrates occlusion of the PAVM by metallic coils.

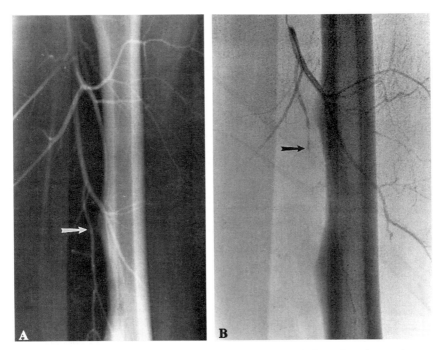

FIGURE 3. Left femoral aneurysmal bone cyst. *A*, Selective left profunda femoral arteriogram demonstrates a terminal branch (arrow) supplying the mildly hypervascular lesion. *B*, Post-embolization arteriogram demonstrates complete occlusion of the primary feeding vessel (arrow).

6. What aneurysms are amenable to embolization?

In select cases, arterial and venous aneurysms can be embolized in an effort to prevent rupture or limit the effects of rupture. The aneurysms suitable for embolization include visceral, cerebral, and neoplastic aneurysms, and post-traumatic pseudoaneurysms. The primary embolic agent for aneurysm occlusion is the metallic coil.

7. What is the most common visceral arterial aneurysm?

The splenic artery aneurysm (Fig. 4*A*). Visceral aneurysms occur less frequently in the hepatic, superior mesenteric, and celiac arteries.

The splenic artery aneurysm is usually solitary and is more common in women. They are located in the distal third of the splenic artery in over 75% of cases, and they occur at bifurcation points, suggesting an underlying abnormality of the vessel wall.

8. What are predisposing factors for the development of a splenic artery aneurysm?

Portal hypertension, pancreatitis, trauma, atherosclerosis, pregnancy, and fibromuscular dysplasia.

9. How do splenic artery aneurysms present? How can they be treated?

Most splenic artery aneurysms are clinically silent. The most significant complication is rupture and intraabdominal hemorrhage. The risk of splenic artery aneurysm rupture is increased during pregnancy. Treatment of splenic artery aneurysms is indicated for lesions greater than 1.5 to 2.0 cm in diameter. Therapeutic options include spleen-preserving transcatheter embolization (Fig. 4*B*) or surgical splenectomy and aneurysmectomy.

10. What are the principal embolic agents?

Gelatin sponge, polyvinyl alcohol foam, metallic coils, absolute alcohol, microfibrillar collagen, sodium tetradecyl sulfate, tissue adhesives, and glue.

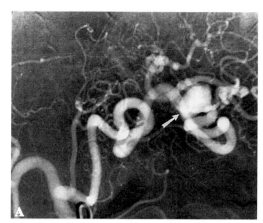

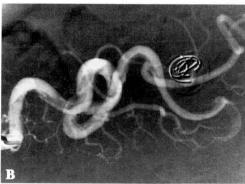

FIGURE 4. Splenic artery aneurysm. *A*, Celiac arteriogram demonstrates a 2 cm aneurysm in the distal splenic artery (arrow). *B*, Selective splenic arteriogram demonstrates thrombosis of the aneurysm after embolization with coils.

11. What are the features of an ideal embolic agent?

The ideal embolic agent should be sterile, nontoxic, widely available, biocompatible, radiopaque, inexpensive, and easily prepared and delivered.

12. What is a metallic coil?

A permanent embolic agent composed of stainless steel or platinum. Some coils have Dacron fibers attached to promote thrombogenicity. The coils are available in a variety of lengths, diameters, and configurations. The coils are deployed via the catheter by pushing a guidewire or coil pusher. The catheter material of choice for coil deployment is polyethylene. Polyethylene catheters have the least friction at the interface between the catheter and the coil. Correct sizing of the coil with respect to the target vessel is important to prevent coil migration into a nontarget vessel.

13. Which coils are MR compatible?

In general, platinum coils are MR compatible as they are not subject to magnetic torque and do not generate significant MR artifacts.

14. What is polyvinyl alcohol foam?

An inert particle that incites an inflammatory response in the target vessel with resultant thrombosis. Although considered a permanent embolic agent, recanalization of thrombus can occur over time. PVA particles are available in sizes ranging from 100 to 1,500 microns. The particles are suspended in minimally dilute contrast, and deployed via a catheter by syringe injection. PVA has been used successfully for bronchial artery embolization, as well as for embolization of tumors. PVA is generally not used for gastrointestinal hemorrhage as the agent's small size predisposes to end arteriole thrombosis with resultant bowel necrosis.

15. What is the role of ethanol as an embolic agent?

Dehydrated ethanol is a liquid embolic agent that is readily available. The alcohol denatures plasma proteins, dehydrates endothelial cells, and incites an intense thrombosis. The agent is radiolucent and its deployment must be carefully controlled as nontarget embolization can lead to pain, nerve injury, and necrosis of normal tissues. Occlusion balloon catheters are used to deliver alcohol in order to minimize reflux into adjacent nontarget areas. Transcatheter ethanol embolization can be effective in treatment of slow flowing arterial-venous malformations, as well as in treatment of renal cell carcinoma.

16. What is sodium tetradecyl sulfate?

A liquid embolic agent used primarily for venous malformations and extremity varicosities. The agent acts as a powerful sclerosant.

17. What is microfibrillar collagen?

A particulate embolic agent that causes immediate vascular occlusion. The principal limitation of this agent is its rapid degradation with resultant vessel recanalization and target reperfusion.

18. What are the complications of embolotherapy?

The complications vary with the agent, the technique of administration, and the site of embolization. Complications include postembolization syndrome, nontarget embolization, abscess, vasospasm, renal failure, coil migration, and death.

19. What is nontarget embolization?

Inadvertent embolization of site remote from the desired target. Secure catheter position proximal to the target is paramount to avoid catheter dislodgment during the procedure, and resultant nontarget organ embolization. An unstable catheter position is a contraindication to transcatheter embolization.

20. What is the postembolization syndrome?

A syndrome characterized by fever, pain, nausea, vomiting, and leukocytosis. The symptoms appear shortly after the procedure, and usually resolve in three to five days. The volume of tissue embolized correlates with the severity and the duration of symptoms. The clinical syndrome is a response to tissue necrosis.

21. What is the appropriate treatment for the postembolization syndrome?

Conservative management with analgesics for pain, and antiemetics for nausea and vomiting.

22. What is the significance of gas in the target organ postembolization?

The detection of gas in the target organ after embolization is not infrequent. The gas is usually a subclinical finding (Fig. 5). The source of the gas is thought to be tissue necrosis. The presence of

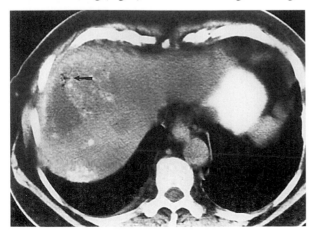

FIGURE 5. Post-embolization gas (arrow) within a hepatic mass after chemoembolization.

gas does not usually imply an abscess. Unless there are other signs of infection, this finding can be followed conservatively. The resorption of gas may take several weeks, due to the devascularization of the target organ.

23. What findings suggest that postembolization gas is due to infection?

Persistent fever and a fluid level in the embolized area. The C-reactive protein value may also serve as an index for infection. Typically, the C-reactive protein rises after the embolization, and begins to normalize after five days. A continual rise in the C-reactive protein level after five days suggests the presence of infection.

24. What is an arteriovenous malformation?

An arteriovenous malformation (AVM) is an abnormal communication between the arterial and venous circulations. While the pathogenesis is incompletely understood, the AVM appears to be the result of focal failure of normal vascular development in utero, with persistence of primitive vascular communications. The AVM is an isolated anomaly which is present at birth but is usually not clinically apparent until adolescence or adulthood.

25. What are the signs and symptoms of an AVM? What are the complications of an AVM?

The AVM is typically a warm, nontender mass that pulsates. AVMs may occur anywhere, but characteristically occur in the extremities. Clinical symptoms of an AVM include disfigurement, pain, swelling, distal ischemia, and venous insufficiency. Complications of AVMs include bleeding, skin ulceration, limb overgrowth, pain, and high-output congestive heart failure. In general, AVMs are not treated until they are symptomatic or a complication occurs.

26. What are the diagnostic imaging findings of an arteriovenous malformation?

Plain radiographs of an AVM will occasionally reveal phleboliths or bone demineralization adjacent to the AVM. Doppler ultrasonography can demonstrate high-velocity arterial signal within the mass. MR imaging is an ideal imaging modality because it is noninvasive, can detect arteriovenous shunting, and can demonstrate the depth and relationship of the AVM to adjacent muscle and bone.

27. What are the angiographic findings of an arteriovenous malformation?

Angiography is reserved for cases where intervention is indicated. Angiographic evaluation requires selective catheterization and rapid contrast injection with rapid filming. The standard angiographic appearance of an AVM is a hypervascular mass with feeding arteries and draining veins (Fig. 6). It is important to demonstrate the size and caliber of all the feeding and draining vessels. It is equally crucial to define the calibers of the actual arteriovenous communication, as this will determine the size and type of embolic agent that is used to treat the AVM.

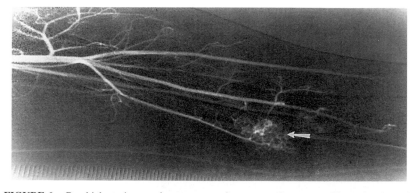

FIGURE 6.   Brachial arteriogram demonstrates a forearm arteriovenous malformation (arrow).

28. What are the therapeutic options for an arteriovenous malformation?
Despite surgical and interventional radiologic advances, the treatment of AVMs remains a challenge. Therapeutic options include conservative medical management, surgery, and embolization. The choice and timing of optimal therapy remains to be defined. An asymptomatic AVM is best managed with conservative care. Surgical treatment or embolization is reserved for symptomatic patients. Surgical resection is ideal for focal, superficial lesions. Surgery for large or deep-seated AVMs can be complicated by significant intraoperative bleeding and postoperative AVM recurrence. For these lesions, embolotherapy has been advocated.

29. What are the agents used for embolization of AVMs?
The principal agents are polyvinyl alcohol particles, absolute alcohol, sodium tetradecyl sulfate, and various glues and tissue adhesives. The advantage of PVA is its wide availability. Unfortunately, vessels occluded with PVA can recanalize, leading to recurrence of the AVM. Variable success has been reported with absolute alcohol and tissue adhesives.

30. What is the technique for transcatheter embolization of arteriovenous malformations?
The vessels feeding the AVM are selectively catheterized, and the embolic agent is delivered. The embolic material should eradicate the nidus of the AVM without passage through the venous system.

31. What may happen if only the proximal feeders of an AVM are embolized, and not the nidus?
Analogous to surgical ligation of proximal feeding vessels, collateral vessels will develop to supply the AVM, with recurrence of symptoms.

32. What is hypersplenism?
A disorder in which pancytopenia is associated with splenomegaly. There is leukopenia, thrombocytopenia, and anemia, with hyperplasia of the marrow precursors. After splenectomy, the cell counts return to normal. In hypersplenism, the spleen is massively enlarged and often painful. The etiologies of hypersplenism include lymphoproliferative disorders, myeloproliferative disorders, inflammatory diseases, and passive splenic congestion.

33. What is the role of embolotherapy in hypersplenism?
Embolization of a portion of the spleen corrects hypersplenism while preserving immune function. The procedure is performed by selective catheterization of the splenic artery. The catheter tip must be positioned distal to the principal pancreatic branches, to avoid nontarget embolization and resultant pancreatitis. The preferred embolic agents are gelfoam and polyvinyl alcohol. Approximately 40% of the splenic volume is embolized. The most significant complication of splenic embolization is sepsis and formation of an abscess. The risk of postembolization infection is minimized by meticulous aseptic technique, periprocedure antibiotics, and administration of the pneumococcal polysaccharide vaccine before the procedure.

34. What is hepatic chemoembolization?
An evolving technique of treating hepatic neoplasms. The tumors amenable to chemoembolization include unresectable hepatocellular carcinoma, colorectal metastases refractory to chemotherapy, and a variety of other secondary liver tumors, including carcinoid, pancreatic carcinoma, and cholangiocarcinoma.

35. What is the theorized mechanism of transcatheter embolization for uncontrolled hemorrhage?
Temporary or permanent occlusion of the vessel supplying the bleeding lesion. Vessel occlusion decreases the pulsatile pressure head, allowing the patient's own coagulation factors to facilitate hemostasis. The technique involves transcatheter deployment of the embolic agent proximal to the bleeding point.

36. What are the indications for angiography and embolization in patients with pelvic trauma?

Open pelvic fracture, expanding pelvic hematoma, and transfusion requirement greater than 4 units over 24 hours.

37. What is the angiographic technique for evaluating patients with pelvic trauma?

Evaluation of suspected arterial injuries in pelvic trauma requires a diagnostic abdominal aortogram and a pelvic angiogram. Selective hypogastric artery injections are necessary to detect small but significant bleeding sites originating off terminal branches. The superior gluteal artery is a common site for arterial injury and hemorrhage.

38. What is the technique of pelvic arterial embolization for bleeding?

The angiographic findings of vessel injury include contrast extravasation (Fig. 7A) and vessel transection, represented by an abrupt vessel cutoff. Both findings warrant immediate transcatheter embolization (Fig. 7B). The preferred embolic agent is gelfoam, although metallic coils are effective. The embolization agent is typically administered as a pledget just proximal to the bleeding site. In cases of multiple bleeding sites with hemodynamic instability, a scatter embolization or proximal hypogastric artery coil blockade should be considered. A scatter embolization is performed by placing several small gelfoam pledgets in the proximal hypogastric artery, in an attempt to stop multiple bleeding sites. Alternatively, a metallic coil can quickly be deposited in the proximal hypogastric artery to facilitate rapid cessation of the bleeding sites. Although rare, the major complications of pelvic embolization include impotence, pelvic ischemia, skin necrosis, and nontarget embolization.

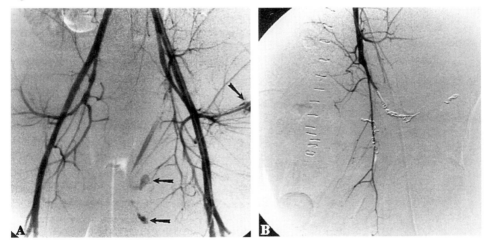

FIGURE 7. Pelvic trauma. *A*, Pelvic angiogram demonstrates bleeding sites off terminal branches of the left hypogastric artery (arrows). *B*, Selective left hypogastric arteriogram after embolization with gelfoam and coils demonstrates cessation of bleeding.

39. What is the role of embolotherapy in gastrointestinal hemorrhage?

Embolotherapy is a mainstay in the treatment of GI hemorrhage. GI hemorrhage can be stopped with embolization or infusion of vasoconstrictors. The tissue distal to the site of vessel occlusion is rendered ischemic. The upper gastrointestinal tract is rich in collateral communications that minimize the impact of ischemia and the incidence of secondary bowel infarction. For upper GI hemorrhage, embolotherapy is preferred over intraarterial infusion of vasoconstrictors. In contrast, embolization of the mesenteric circulation to the lower GI tract is associated with a higher incidence of ischemic complications such as bowel infarction. As a result, intraarterial infusion of vasoconstrictive agents is preferred over embolotherapy for lower GI hemorrhage.

40. What are the indications for transcatheter embolotherapy in gastrointestinal hemorrhage?
Acute arterial hemorrhage from an upper GI source, or failure of intraarterial vasoconstrictors to control bleeding from any gastrointestinal source.

41. What are the embolic agents that are used to treat GI hemorrhage?
Gelatin sponge (Gelfoam; Upjohn, Kalamazoo, MI) and metallic coils.

42. What is the role of embolization for splenic injuries?
Blunt abdominal trauma can cause significant injury to the spleen. The degree of splenic injury is variable, ranging from a superficial laceration to complete fragmentation. Patients who are hemodynamically stable with splenic injury who do not require laparotomy for other reasons can be considered for transcatheter embolization.

43. How is embolization of the spleen performed in this setting?
The main splenic artery is occluded with metallic coils. The goal is to reduce blood flow enough to promote hemostasis at the site of splenic hemorrhage, without inducing splenic infarction. Collateral branches develop and preserve flow to maintain splenic function.

BIBLIOGRAPHY

1. Bakal CW, Cynamon J, Lakritz PS, Sprayregen S: Value of preoperative renal arterial embolization in reducing blood transfusion requirements during nephrectomy for renal cell carcinoma. J Vasc Interv Radiol 4:727–731, 1993.
2. Dick HM, Bigliani LU, Michelsen WJ, et al: Adjuvant arterial embolization in the treatment of benign primary bone tumors in children. Clin Orthop 139:133–144, 1979.
3. Hickman MP, Lucas D, Novak Z, et al: Preoperative embolization of the spleen in children with hypersplenism. J Vasc Interv Radiol 3:647–652, 1992.
4. Hind CRK, Thomas AMK, Pepys MB, Allison DJ: Serum C-reactive protein responsive to therapeutic embolization: Possible role in management. Clin Radiol 36:179–183, 1985.
5. Mucha P, Welch TJ: Hemorrhage in major pelvic fractures. Surg Clin North Am 68:757–773, 1988.
6. Rosen RJ, Riles TS: Arteriovenous malformations. In Strandness DE, van Breda A (eds): Vascular Diseases: Surgical and Interventional Therapy. New York, Churchill Livingstone, 1994, pp 1121–1137.
7. Rowe DM, Becker GJ, Rabe FE, et al: Embolization and surgery for restoration of function. Radiology 150:673–676, 1984.
8. Scalfani SJA, Weisberg A, Scalea TM, Phillips TF, Duncan AO: Blunt splenic injuries: Nonsurgical treatment with CT, arteriography, and transcatheter embolization of the splenic artery. Radiology 181:189–196, 1991.
9. Trastek VF, Pairolero PC, Joyce JW, et al: Splenic artery aneurysms. Surgery 91:694–699, 1982.
10. Yakes WF, Leuthke JM, Parker SH, et al: Ethanol embolization of vascular malformations. RadioGraphics 10:787–796, 1990.

80. THROMBOLYTIC THERAPY

Kenneth D. Murphy, M.D.

1. What is the purpose of thrombolytic therapy?
To rapidly restore blood flow through an occluded artery, vein, or bypass graft. The integrity of the human circulation is maintained by a balance of endogenous fibrinolysis and coagulation to prevent deleterious thrombosis or hemorrhage. Thrombolysis alters physiologic fibrinolysis to remove pathologic clot.

2. What are the clinical applications of thrombolytic therapy?
Thrombolytic therapy can be administered for thrombotic or embolic occlusive disease of the arterial or venous system. Thrombolytic efficacy has been established for occlusion of the peripheral

arteries, peripheral veins, bypass grafts, mesenteric arteries, renal arteries, hemodialysis access sites, pulmonary arteries, and coronary arteries. The use of thrombolytics for treatment of deep venous thrombosis and for stroke is under investigation.

3. What are the indications for thrombolysis?

Acute, subacute, or chronic thrombotic or embolic occlusion of a native artery, vein, or bypass graft (Fig. 1). Peripheral arterial occlusions result in varying degrees of ischemia. Peripheral venous occlusions can result in venous insufficiency or pulmonary embolism. The spectrum of clinical presentations for occlusive disease varies with the chronicity of the obstruction.

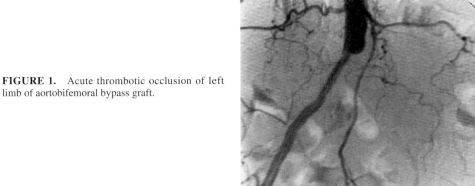

FIGURE 1. Acute thrombotic occlusion of left limb of aortobifemoral bypass graft.

4. What are the absolute contraindications to thrombolysis?

Active internal bleeding, known intracranial pathology, stroke within the last 6 months, craniotomy within the last 2 months, irreversible limb ischemia, and an infected bypass graft.

5. What are the relative contraindications to thrombolysis?

Uncontrolled hypertension, history of GI bleeding, bacterial endocarditis, diabetic retinopathy, coagulopathy, pregnancy, recent major surgery, recent major trauma, and recent CPR. In these patients, it is imperative to carefully analyze the potential risk:benefit ratio in each case.

6. What is the classification of acute limb ischemia?

The Society for Vascular Surgery and the Interventional Society for Cardiovascular Surgery categories for acute ischemia are viable, threatened, and irreversible. Each category is defined by the sensorimotor examination and the status of the arterial and venous Doppler signal. A threatened extremity has mild muscle weakness and sensory loss, with inaudible arterial but audible venous Doppler signals. Irreversible ischemia in an extremity is defined as profound paralysis and sensory loss, with inaudible arterial and venous Doppler signals.

7. How are occlusions classified with respect to the duration of symptoms?

Peripheral occlusive disease is defined by duration of symptoms. In an acute occlusion, the duration of symptoms is less than 24 hours; a subacute occlusion, 1–30 days; a chronic occlusion, more than 30 days.

8. What is the pharmacology of thrombolytic therapy?

Thrombolytic agents accelerate the fibrinolytic system. These agents act as plasminogen activators by hydrolyzing the peptide bond in the plasminogen molecule, converting it to active plasmin. Plasmin promotes degradation of the fibrin within thrombus, to soluble fibrin split products. The result is lysis of clot and restoration of vessel patency.

9. What are the primary thrombolytic agents?

The first-generation thrombolytic agents are streptokinase (SK) and urokinase (UK). The main second-generation agent is tissue plasminogen activator (t-PA). All three activate plasminogen to facilitate clot lysis. The greatest experience in peripheral occlusive disease has been with the first-generation agents. All three agents have been used in the treatment of myocardial infarction.

10. What is streptokinase?

A protein produced by group C beta-hemolytic streptococci. The molecule is not an enzyme but an indirect plasminogen activator. The agent combines with plasminogen to form an intermediate complex that undergoes a conformational change. The intermediate SK-plasminogen complex enzymatically cleaves another plasminogen molecule to form plasmin. Plasmin degrades fibrin clot into fibrin split products. The in vivo half-life of SK is approximately 16 minutes, and it therefore must be infused continuously. Streptokinase is antigenic and capable of inducing allergic reactions. In addition, neutralizing antibodies can develop and limit the thrombolytic effect.

11. What is urokinase?

A protein in human urine that has fibrinolytic activity. It is isolated in tissue culture of human fetal kidney cells. Because urokinase is nonantigenic, antibody neutralization is not a factor when administering UK. UK is a serum protease enzyme that directly cleaves plasminogen to form plasmin. Because the half-life of UK is approximately 16 minutes, continuous infusion is required.

12. What is tissue plasminogen activator?

A fibrinolytic agent produced by recombinant DNA technology from a line of ovarian cells from a hamster. t-PA is nonantigenic and has a half-life of 4 minutes. The agent activates plasminogen bound to fibrin, a theoretical advantage since the agent is targeted for interaction with the fibrin-rich thrombus. As a result, the fibrinolytic activity of t-PA, when complexed with fibrin, is 1,000 times greater than its plasma activity.

13. What are the advantages of urokinase?

In studies comparing the safety and efficacy of UK, SK, and t-PA for thrombolysis of peripheral arterial occlusive disease, urokinase was found to have a higher percent of clot lysis, improved thrombolytic outcome and clinical success, and the lowest complication rate from bleeding. The mean duration of infusion was significantly less for UK compared with SK. For these reasons, UK is the primary thrombolytic agent of choice.

14. How are thrombolytic agents for peripheral occlusive disease delivered, and what is the preferred method of administration?

Thrombolytic agents can be delivered locally into the thrombus or systemically. Despite the simplicity of systemic administration of lytic agents via an intravenous infusion, local administration is preferred. Local thrombolytic therapy is technically more demanding: an infusion catheter must be positioned directly into the pathologic thrombus (Fig. 2).

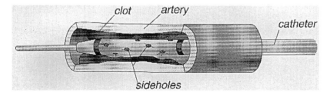

FIGURE 2.   Prototype infusion catheter within arterial thrombus.

15. What are the advantages of local thrombolytic therapy?

Catheter-directed delivery of the lytic agent ensures interaction of the clot with the lytic agent. Intraclot administration also increases the contact area of the drug with thrombus. The agent is effectively contained within the clot, which avoids the deleterious effects of hemodilution and contact with plasmin inhibitors in the plasma. The first-pass clearance of the agent by various filtering organs is eliminated by local infusion. The relative regional "containment" of the agent also reduces the systemic concentration and thereby minimizes hemorrhagic complications. Direct infusion into the thrombus also facilitates administration of higher concentrations of the drug. Higher concentrations promote more rapid thrombolysis.

16. What is continuous infusion thrombolysis?
Regional administration of the lytic agent at a constant rate. The agent "weeps" out of the catheter sideholes into the clot.

17. What is "pulse-spray" pharmacomechanical thrombolysis (PSMT)?
A technique in which the thrombolytic agent is administered into the clot using brief, repeated small-volume (0.2–0.4 ml), high-pressure injections via a multi-sidehole catheter. The theorized advantages of PSMT are clot maceration from the penetrating pulses of the lytic agent, increased contact area of the clot and the drug, and an increased rate of clot dissolution with diminished volume of the lytic agent. The theorized disadvantage is the potential risk of inadvertent embolism from clot maceration. Thrombosed hemodialysis access grafts are treated with this approach without any significant embolic sequelae. The use of PSMT for arterial and venous thrombosis remains under investigation.

18. What are the angiographic features of an embolus?
Peripheral emboli usually lodge at stenoses, vessel branching points, or bifurcations. The emboli appear as occlusive filling defects on angiography, with a characteristic meniscus configuration at the point of luminal cutoff (Fig. 3). Collateral vessels are typically absent. The underlying vessel is usually free of underlying atherosclerotic disease. The most common source of peripheral arterial emboli is a cardiac thrombus.

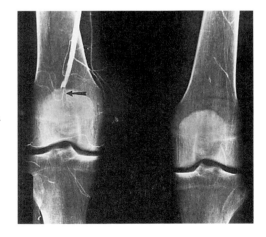

FIGURE 3.   Right popliteal artery embolus (arrow).

19. Can embolic occlusions be treated with thrombolysis?
Arterial emboli can be treated successfully with thrombolytic therapy. The embolus in many cases is lysable. The thrombus that forms proximal and distal to the embolus is also responsive to lytic agents. It is important to exclude cardiac mural thrombus as the source of the emboli because thrombolysis could potentiate further embolization from the heart. Alternative management of peripheral embolic occlusion includes surgical embolectomy. In many instances, a simple surgical embolectomy is preferred because the underlying vessel is usually normal, and no further vascular intervention is required. Surgery also avoids the risk of thrombolytic therapy. Venous emboli to the lung can be treated with systemic or local thrombolytic therapy.

20. What are the angiographic features of thrombotic occlusions?

Thrombotic occlusions typically occur in patients with underlying atherosclerotic disease. The clinical presentation is usually one of long-standing limb ischemia with recent deterioration. The angiographic findings are thrombosis, regional atherosclerosis, and the presence of well-developed collaterals (Fig. 4A). Typically, the thrombosis is secondary to an underlying focal stenosis in the diseased vessel. Conversion of an atherosclerotic occlusion to a focal stenosis is amenable to angioplasty or stent placement and is facilitated by thrombolysis (Figs. 4B and C).

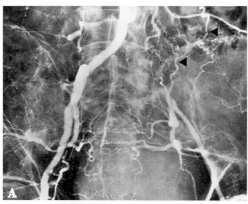
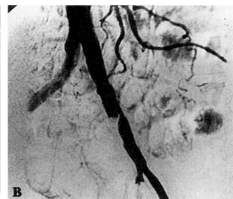
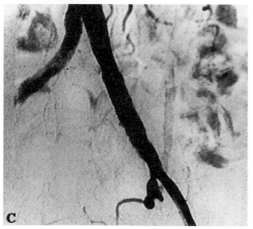

FIGURE 4. Acute ischemia of left lower leg. *A*, Pelvic angiogram demonstrates thrombotic occlusion of the left common iliac artery, with collaterals (arrowheads) reconstituting the external iliac artery. *B*, Pelvic angiogram after catheter-directed thrombolysis demonstrates a patent left common iliac artery with high-grade stenosis. *C*, Pelvic angiogram demonstrates restored patency after placement of a balloon-expandable stent at the stenosis.

21. What is the technique of local intraarterial thrombolysis?

Percutaneous access is established and a sheath is placed in the artery or vein. Thrombolysis can be performed from a femoral, axillary, brachial, or graft approach. The femoral approach is usually favored because the large caliber of the femoral artery decreases the risk of access site complications, especially hematoma. The occlusion is then crossed with a guidewire-catheter technique. The guidewire traversal of thrombus is a favorable prognostic indicator of successful thrombolysis, because it creates a channel for UK to interact with clot. Over the guidewire an infusion delivery system is placed within the thrombus.

22. What are the four major types of catheter delivery systems for thrombolysis?

1. End-hole catheter
2. Coaxial infusion catheter-guidewire system
3. Multi-sidehole infusion catheter
4. Infusion guide wire

23. How do coaxial infusion catheter-guidewire systems work?

An infusion catheter is placed into the proximal portion of the thrombus, and a smaller coaxial infusion guidewire is placed into the distal clot. The coaxial system facilitates infusion of the agent into longer segments of clot. The thrombolytic agents are infused via the delivery system; heparin is administered systemically.

24. Why is heparin administered during thrombolysis?

To prevent pericatheter thrombosis. Heparin also may potentiate the efficacy of the lytic agent. Heparin can be administered via the sheath or intravenously. The standard dose is 600–1200 units per hour. The dose is titrated to maintain the activated thromboplastin time (aPTT) at 1.5 to 2.5 times the control. At the conclusion of thrombolysis, the heparin therapy is discontinued and the percutaneous delivery system removed after the coagulation status normalizes. If further systemic anticoagulation is indicated, heparin can be readministered 6–12 hours after successful groin compression, with close monitoring for puncture site bleeding.

25. What is the transthrombus bolus technique?

Prior to the initiation of continuous infusion therapy, a transthrombus bolus of UK can be administered. The catheter-directed transthrombus bolus is typically 10,000–25,000 IU of concentrated UK per 10 cm of thrombus. There is some evidence that the transthrombus bolus diminishes the duration of lysis, total dose of UK, and the bleeding complication rate.

26. What is the recommended dose of urokinase for peripheral arterial occlusions?

The options include lose dose, high dose, and "higher dose" continuous infusion. Low dose UK therapy is defined as 1,000–2,000 IU/min. High dose UK therapy is 4,000 IU/min. Typically, high dose therapy is instituted for 4 hours, followed by low dose. "Higher" dose is defined as 360,000–500,000 IU/hour. The severity of ischemia determines the dose. In cases of severe ischemia, high dose protocols are used to achieve rapid lysis.

27. What is the guidewire traversal test?

An attempt to negotiate a guidewire across the occluded vessel prior to initiation of lysis. If the wire can be successfully passed across the occlusion, the clot is more likely to lyse. If the guidewire traversal test fails, proximal infusion of lytic agents at the proximal margin of the occlusion via an endhole catheter will typically "soften" the thrombus to facilitate subsequent guidewire passage. The intraclot position of the wire facilitates placement of the infusion catheter within the target thrombus.

28. What factors are predictive of a successful outcome of lytic therapy?

Prosthetic grafts respond more favorably to thrombolytic therapy than venous bypass grafts. In addition, the more proximal a bypass graft, the higher the likelihood of thrombolytic success. Proximal native arterial occlusions are more responsive to thrombolysis than distal occlusions. The age of the occlusion is also a predictor of success. Acute and subacute occlusions respond more favorably than chronic occlusions. Patients with absent circulation distal to the occlusion, absent distal signal on Doppler examination, and a hypercoagulable state respond less favorably to thrombolysis.

29. How are patients managed clinically during thrombolysis?

Patients are carefully monitored in an intensive care or step down unit after transfer from the interventional radiology suite. Vital signs are monitored frequently, and blood pressure is controlled to avoid a hypertensive-induced hemorrhage. Urine, stool, nasogastric aspirate, sputum, and neurologic status are monitored closely for signs of bleeding. Patients are kept on bed rest to minimize the risk of falling and inducing hemorrhage. Intravenous or oral medications are favored over intramuscular and subcutaneous injections to minimize the risk of bleeding. Blood samples are obtained from indwelling lines. All venous lines, arterial lines, and catheter access sites are closely monitored for signs of bleeding. If a hematoma develops at the arterial sheath entry site, the sheath should be upsized. The pulses distal to the infusion catheter should be monitored by palpation or by Doppler for evidence of embolization. The patient's oral intake is withheld in case surgery becomes necessary.

30. What laboratory tests are monitored during thrombolysis?

Specific tests allow the interventionalist to monitor the degree of systemic lysis. A baseline aPTT, prothrombin time (PT), platelet count, fibrinogen level, and hematocrit are obtained. The PT and aPTT are monitored every 6 hours, and the systemic heparin therapy is titrated accordingly. The fibrinogen level is also obtained every 6 hours, and a value of < 100 mg/dl is associated with a systemic lytic state with increased risk of spontaneous hemorrhage. If the fibrinogen is < 100 mg/dl and the patient is not bleeding, the UK dose can be reduced by half. If there is evidence of hemorrhage with a low fibrinogen, UK is discontinued and fresh frozen plasma, cryoprecipitate, E-aminocaproic acid, or aprotinin are administered. The platelet count should be monitored daily for heparin-induced thrombocytopenia. The hematocrit should be checked daily for occult blood loss.

31. What additional medications are given during thrombolysis?

Urokinase is associated with the development of chills after administration. The cause is unknown. Prophylactic administration of acetaminophen (650–1000 mg orally) and diphenhydramine (50 mg orally or IV) can minimize the incidence and severity of UK-induced rigors. Chills can be treated with medperidine and H2-receptor blockers. To minimize bleeding complications, concurrent administration of aspirin and warfarin during thrombolysis is avoided. Pain control is typically managed with intravenous or oral analgesics.

32. What are the endpoints of thrombolysis?

Restoration of antegrade flow (Fig. 5), complete lysis of occlusion—or new thrombus formation, failure to lyse residual thrombus, or a complication of therapy.

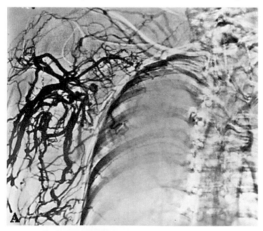

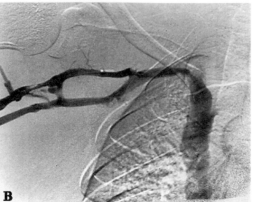

FIGURE 5. Primary axillosubclavian vein thrombosis. *A,* Contrast extremity venogram demonstrates acute thrombosis of right axillary and subclavian veins. *B,* Follow-up venogram after catheter-directed thrombolysis demonstrates restored patency.

33. What are the alternatives to conventional thrombolytic therapy?

In select patients, thrombolytic therapy is contraindicated. Surgical thrombectomy or embolectomy is a widely accepted alternative. The development of percutaneous mechanical thrombectomy catheters continues to expand the therapeutic options for the treatment of thrombotic or embolic occlusive disease.

34. What are the complications of thrombolysis?

The complication rates vary with the thrombolytic agent used. Studies have documented a higher incidence of hemorrhagic complications with t-PA and SK than with UK. Complications include major bleeding (7%), minor bleeding (6%), distal embolization (5%), reperfusion syndrome (< 1%), compartment syndrome (2%), amputation due to preexisting severe ischemia (8%), allergic reactions (< 1%), renal failure (< 1%), a cardiac event (< 1%), and death (< 1%).

35. How can the incidence and severity of complications be minimized?

By early recognition and prompt treatment, proper patient selection, careful patient management, and close monitoring of laboratory data.

BIBLIOGRAPHY

1. Bachmann F: Plasminogen activators. In Colman RW, Hirsch J, Marder VJ, Salzman EW (eds): Hemostasis and Thrombosis: Basic Principles and Clinical Practice, 2nd ed. Philadelphia, J.B. Lippincott, 1987.
2. Bookstein JJ, Valji K: Pulse-spray pharmacomechanical thrombolysis. Cardiovasc Intervent Radiol 15:228–233, 1992.
3. Fears R: Kinetic studies on the effect of heparin and fibrin on plasminogen activators. Biochem J 249:77–81, 1988.
4. Gardiner GA, Sullivan KL: Complications of regional thrombolytic therapy. In Kadir S (ed): Current Practice of Interventional Radiology. Philadelphia, B.C. Decker, 1991, pp 87–91.
5. Korninger C, Stassen JM, Collen D: Turnover of human extrinsic (tissue-type) plasminogen activator in rabbits. Thromb Haemost 46:658–661, 1981.
6. McNamara TO, Fischer JR: Thrombolysis of peripheral arterial and graft occlusions: Improved results using high-dose urokinase. AJR 144:769–775, 1985.
7. McNamara TO, Goodwin SC, Kandarpa K: Complications associated with thrombolysis. Semin Intervent Radiol 2:134–144, 1994.
8. Sullivan KL, Gardiner GA, Shapiro MJ, et al: Acceleration of thrombolysis with a high-dose transthrombus bolus technique. Radiology 173:805–808, 1989.
9. Van Breda A, Katzen BT, Deutsch AF: Urokinase versus streptokinase in local thrombolysis. Radiology 165:109–111, 1987.

81. INFERIOR VENA CAVA FILTERS

Kenneth D. Murphy, M.D.

1. What is the purpose of an inferior vena cava (IVC) filter?

To trap all deep venous emboli, not just clinically significant emboli, while preserving caval patency.

2. What are some characteristics of an ideal inferior vena cava filter?

The filter should be biocompatible, mechanically stable, nonthrombogenic, and relatively inexpensive. The procedure for placing the filter must be simple, safe, and minimally invasive.

3. What are the absolute indications for inferior vena cava filter placement?
- Pulmonary embolism with a contraindication to anticoagulation
- Documented deep venous thrombosis with a contraindication to anticoagulation
- Recurrent pulmonary emboli despite adequate anticoagulation
- A complication of anticoagulant therapy (hemorrhage)

4. **What are the relative indications for IVC filter placement?**
   • Failure of existing filter device
   • Postpulmonary embolectomy
   • Free-floating iliofemoral or IVC thrombus
   • DVT extension despite adequate anticoagulation
   • Pulmonary hypertension with inadequate pulmonary reserve for the patient to survive any additional emboli.

5. **What are the absolute contraindications to inferior vena cava filter placement?**
   • An IVC that cannot be percutaneously accessed
   • Severe coagulopathy that is refractory to corrective therapy

6. **What are relative contraindications to IVC filter placement?**
   Pregnancy and young age.

7. **Where in the IVC should the filter be placed?**
   Above any thrombus. In most circumstances, thrombus is located in the iliac or femoral veins or below, and the filter should be placed in the infrarenal IVC (Fig. 1). The superior margin or "apex" of the device should be positioned at the level of the most caudal renal vein. An infrarenal location is preferred because the potential for retrograde thrombosis of the renal veins from thrombus trapped in the device is minimized. In addition, the flow in the infrarenal IVC is laminar, promoting efficient clot trapping by the filter.

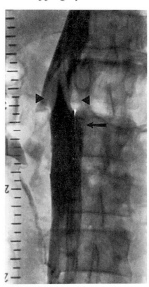

FIGURE 1.   Cavogram demonstrates filter (arrow) positioned just below the renal veins (arrowheads).

8. **When should a caval filter be placed above the renal veins?**
   When there is infrarenal thrombus in the IVC, renal vein thrombosis, or failure of the indwelling infrarenal IVC filter.

9. **Why is an inferior vena caval contrast study performed prior to filter placement?**
   To evaluate IVC patency, the position of the renal veins, the IVC diameter, and to evaluate for any IVC or renal vein anomalies. The renal veins are usually located at the L1–L2 vertebral level. The renal veins appear as negative filling defects due to unopacified blood entering the cava (Fig. 2). If there is uncertainty as to the level or number of renal veins, selective catheterization is warranted.

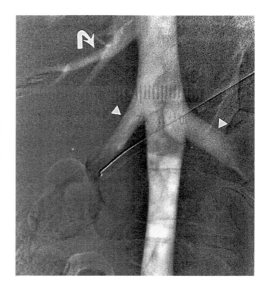

FIGURE 2. Cavogram of a normal inferior vena cava (IVC) demonstrates contrast reflux into hepatic veins (curved arrow) and renal veins (arrowheads). Normally, reflux is not as significant and these veins appear as negative filling defects.

10. What is the technique for performing an inferior vena caval contrast study?

The diagnostic contrast study can be performed from a femoral, jugular, or brachial vein approach. Anticoagulation therapy should be withheld approximately 4 hours prior to the procedure. A pigtail or straight catheter is positioned in the caudal IVC at the iliac venous confluence or in the left iliac vein. Positioning the catheter in the left iliac vein enhances the detection of vena caval anomalies. Images should be obtained using the Valsalva maneuver to facilitate caval distention and accurate assessment of the maximum IVC diameter. A radiopaque grid is placed on the body surface parallel to the IVC axis to localize the filter placement site. After completion of the diagnostic contrast study, the filter is usually deployed via the same access site.

11. What variants of IVC are pertinent to caval filter placement?

1. Caval duplication
2. Left-sided IVC
3. Retroaortic left renal vein
4. Circumaortic renal vein

12. How common is a left-sided or a transposed IVC? What are the implications for filter placement?

A left-sided IVC occurs in 0.2% of the population. A jugular or left femoral approach for filter placement is necessary in such cases.

13. What are the venographic findings of caval duplication?

A duplicated infrarenal IVC occurs in 0.2–3.0% of the population. The venographic findings of caval duplication include opacification of both caval lumens, preferential opacification of the cava on one side, absence of contralateral iliac inflow, and termination of the left IVC into the left renal vein. Catheter placement in the left iliac vein facilitates detection of this anomaly.

14. Where should an IVC filter be placed if a caval duplication is present?

In each IVC, or a single filter can be placed in the suprarenal IVC. In cases of caval duplication with asymmetric size, the smaller cava can be embolized with coils and the larger one interrupted with standard filter placement.

15. What is the anatomy of a circumaortic left renal vein?

A circumaortic left renal vein (Fig. 3), which forms a "ring" around the aorta, is more common than a (single) retroaortic left renal vein. Typically, the more cephalad branch is preaortic and the more caudal branch retroaortic. In cases of circumaortic or retroaortic left renal vein, the retroaortic vein typically inserts lower into the IVC, and deployment of a single short filter into the IVC or dual filters into the iliac veins is recommended.

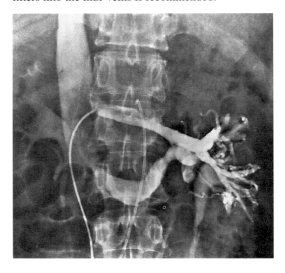

FIGURE 3. Circumaortic left renal vein.

16. What are the four FDA-approved filter devices available in the United States?

1. Greenfield filter (Medi-Tech/Boston Scientific, Watertown, MA)
2. Bird's Nest filter (Cook, Inc., Bloomington, IN)
3. Vena-tech filter (B. Braun Vena-Tech, Evanston, IL)
4. Simon Nitinol (Nitinol Medical Technologies Group, Woburn, MA)

All four filters are permanent devices not intended for temporary use or removal.

17. What are the technical features of a Greenfield filter?

The original filter was a stainless steel device introduced in 1973. It required a large introducer sheath (outer diameter 29.5 French) that limited its acceptance, due to the high incidence of access site (groin) thrombosis. As a result, the titanium Greenfield filter was developed in 1989. The new design featured a smaller introducer sheath (outer diameter 14 French), which diminished access-site complications. Since 1989, the most significant modification has been an "over-the-wire" capability, meaning that it can be deployed over a guidewire. The filter has a conical shape (Fig. 4) that facilitates clot trapping at the apex, with preservation of lateral IVC flow. The filter is designed for IVC diameters not exceeding 28 mm.

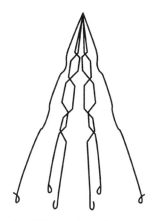

18. Can a patient with a Greenfield filter undergo an MRI examination?

Yes, the device is nonferromagnetic and is MR-compatible.

FIGURE 4. Greenfield filter.

19. What are the technical features of a Bird's Nest filter?

The Bird's Nest filter is a permanent filter composed of four 0.18-mm diameter stainless steel wires that are 25 cm long. The four wires are connected to V struts at each end that secure the smaller wires to the caval wall. When deployed in the IVC, the wire strands form a mesh that traps clot (Fig. 5). The outer diameter of the introducer sheath is 14.5 French. The device is designed for IVC diameters not exceeding 40 mm. The filter is ferromagnetic and therefore creates extensive artifact on MR.

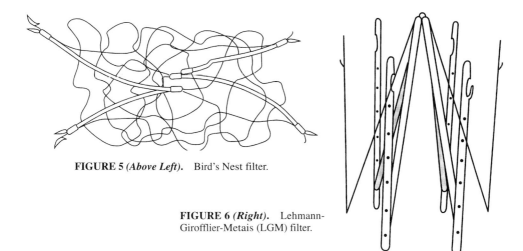

FIGURE 5 *(Above Left)*.   Bird's Nest filter.

FIGURE 6 *(Right)*.   Lehmann-
Girofflier-Metais (LGM) filter.

20. What are the technical features of the Vena-tech filter?

The Vena-tech filter, also known as the Lehmann-Girofflier-Metais (LGM) filter, has a conical shape (Fig. 6) composed of an alloy of eight metals. The LGM filter has flat stabilizing side rails that promote centering of the filter within the IVC. The outer diameter of the introducer sheath is 12.9 French. The LGM filter is MR-compatible and is designed for IVC diameters not exceeding 28 mm.

21. What are the technical features of the Simon Nitinol filter?

Released in 1990, the Simon Nitinol filter is a permanent filter composed of nitinol, a nickel-titanium alloy. The Nitinol has thermal properties that allow the filter to be soft and malleable when the preloaded device is perfused with iced saline via the introducer sheath. After deployment and subsequent exposure to the body's temperature, the filter is instantaneously transformed into a previously imprinted rigid configuration. The filter has a two-level design composed of a dome and legs (Fig. 7). Filtering occurs at each tier (Fig. 8). The introducer sheath has the smallest diameter of any of the approved IVC filters, measuring 9 French in its outer diameter. The device is designed for IVC diameters not exceeding 28 mm.

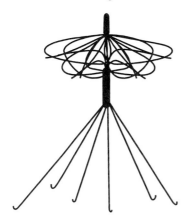

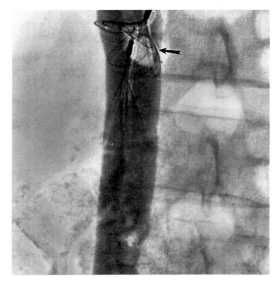

FIGURE 7 *(Above Left)*.   Simon Nitinol filter.
FIGURE 8 *(Right)*.   Filling defect (arrow) represents clot trapped in the dome of a Simon Nitinol filter.

22. Which access routes are available for IVC placement?

All four FDA-approved filters can be placed from a transjugular or a transfemoral venous approach. The right common femoral or right jugular venous approaches are preferred because they allow a more direct course to the IVC, which makes filter deployment easy and accurate. The angulation associated with a left-sided approach may lead to complications including kinking of the introducer sheath and tilting of the filter in the IVC. The Simon Nitinol filter is unique in that it can be placed via a brachial vein approach in addition to the standard femoral and jugular access routes.

23. How can an IVC filter be placed if the cava is significantly enlarged?

A "megacava" is an IVC with a diameter greater than 28 mm. The incidence of megacava is reported to be 3%. If the megacaval diameter is less than 40 mm, a Bird's Nest filter can be deployed in the IVC. If the diameter is greater than 40 mm, a filter should be deployed in each iliac vein.

24. What is the maximum amount of tilt acceptable for the Greenfield filter?

The maximum acceptable tilt with respect to the long axis of the IVC is 15°. A filter with a tilt in excess of 15° has diminished clot trapping efficacy (Fig. 9). Deployment of the Greenfield filter from a left femoral approach promotes tilt and should be avoided unless the new "over-the-wire" device is used.

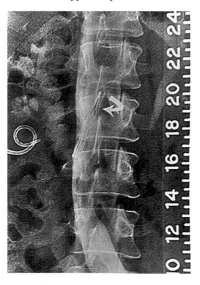

FIGURE 9. Greenfield filter with excessive tilt (curved arrow).

25. Which filter has the shortest length?

The Simon Nitinol filter (38 mm). This feature makes this device ideal for deployment in a short infrarenal IVC, as with a left circumaortic renal vein.

26. What is the recommended timing of filter placement?

A filter should be placed within 24 hours in:
1. Patients with acute pulmonary embolism with contraindication to anticoagulation
2. Patients with acute pulmonary embolism despite therapeutic levels of anticoagulation
3. Patients with free-floating iliofemoral deep venous thrombosis

A filter should be placed within 48 hours in patients with deep venous thrombosis for whom anticoagulation is contraindicated or has failed.

27. What is the incidence of femoral vein thrombosis after transfemoral filter insertion?

The incidence has been reported to be as high as 24–33%. The high incidence of access-site thrombosis was largely attributed to the large introducer sheath size (outer diameter, 29.5 French) required for placement of the stainless steel Greenfield filter. As smaller delivery systems evolved, the incidence of access-site thrombosis diminished. The incidence of femoral vein thrombosis after insertion of the lower profile titanium Greenfield filter is 8.7%.

28. What are the incidence and mechanisms of recurrent pulmonary emboli after filter placement?

The incidence is approximately 3%. Several mechanisms can account for recurrent pulmonary embolism, including caval thrombosis, proximal propagation of clot trapped within the filter, and suboptimal clot trapping efficacy. In addition, pulmonary emboli can originate from the upper extremity or other venous beds not protected by the filter.

29. How are recurrent pulmonary emboli treated in such a situation?

The treatment varies with the source of recurrent pulmonary emboli. In cases of filter failure, anticoagulation or placement of an additional filter above the original device is indicated. If recurrent emboli are from an upper extremity source, filter placement in the superior vena cava should be considered.

30. What is the incidence of caval thrombosis after IVC filter placement?

The incidence is generally below 10%. The mechanism can be primary thrombosis or occlusion following clot trapping. Patients with caval thrombosis are at risk for bilateral leg edema from venous stasis and at risk for recurrent pulmonary emboli. Treatment is variable, ranging from conservative observation to aggressive thrombolysis for the thrombotic occlusion. An additional filter may be necessary if the caval thrombosis is the source of recurrent pulmonary emboli.

BIBLIOGRAPHY

1. Beckmann CF, Abrams HL: Circumaortic venous ring: Incidence and significance. AJR 132:561–565, 1979.
2. Geisinger MA, Zelch MG, Risius B: Recurrent pulmonary embolism after Greenfield filter placement. Radiology 165:383–384, 1987.
3. Greenfield LJ, Cho KJ, Proctor M, et al: Results of a multicenter study of the modified hook-titanium Greenfield filter. Radiology 165:383–384, 1987.
4. Jones TK, Barnes RW, Greenfield LJ: Greenfield vena cava filter: Rationale and current indications. Ann Thorac Surg 42:548–555, 1987.
5. Kellman GM, Alpern MB, Sandler MA, Craig BM: Computed tomography of vena caval anomalies with embryologic correlation. RadioGraphics 8:533–556, 1988.
6. Mayo J, Gray R, St. Louis E, et al; Anomalies of the inferior vena cava. AJR 140:339–345, 1983.
7. Mewissen MW, Erickson SJ, Foley WD, et al: Thrombosis at venous insertion sites after inferior vena caval filter placement. Radiology 173:155–157, 1989.
8. Pais SO, Tobin KD, Austin CB, Queral L: Percutaneous insertion of the Greenfield inferior vena cava filter: Experience with 96 patients. J Vasc Surg 8:460–464, 1988.
9. Prince MR, Novelline RA, Athanasoulis CA, Simon M: The diameter of the inferior vena cava and its implications for the use of vena cava filters. Radiology 149:687–689, 1983.
10. Sardi A, Minken SL: The placement of intracaval filters in an anomalous (left-sided) vena cava. J Vasc Surg 6:84–86, 1987.
11. Wells I: Inferior vena cava filters. In Belli AM (ed): Interventional Radiology of the Peripheral Vascular System. Boston, Little, Brown & Co., 1994, pp 93–117.

82. DEEP VENOUS THROMBOSIS

Kenneth D. Murphy, M.D.

1. What is the incidence of deep venous thrombosis (DVT)?

Approximately 5 million documented cases of DVT and an estimated 600,000 cases of pulmonary embolism occur annually in the United States. The incidence of lower extremity DVT in patients with documented pulmonary embolism (PE) is 70–80%.

2. What are the risk factors for DVT?

• Malignancy	• Pregnancy	• Anesthesia
• Stroke	• Cardiac failure	• Diabetes
• Trauma	• Increasing age	• Smoking
• Surgery	• Bed rest	• Hypercoagulable states

3. What is Virchow's triad?

In 1860, Virchow described a triad of factors necessary for the development of DVT: abnormal venous flow dynamics, an abnormal venous wall, and a hypercoagulable state.

4. What causes abnormal venous flow?

The primary causes that are predisposing factors for DVT include extrinsic venous compression, intraluminal foreign bodies, diminished cardiac function, trauma, and immobilization.

5. What causes an abnormal venous wall?

Prior DVT, indwelling venous lines, and caustic effects of venous infusion.

6. What hypercoagulable states predispose to venous thrombosis?

• Polycythemia vera	• Protein C deficiency
• Malignancy	• Protein S deficiency
• Pregnancy	• Oral estrogens
• Antithrombin III deficiency	

7. What indications should prompt an evaluation for a hypercoagulable disorder as the etiology of DVT?

• Young patients	• Unusual site of thrombosis (e.g., portal vein)
• Positive family history	• Recurrent/multiple thrombosis

8. How does malignancy predispose to the development of DVT?

The mechanism is complex and multifactorial. Specific factors include decreased ambulation, central venous catheters, oncologic surgery, venous invasion or extrinsic compression by tumor, tumor-associated hyperaggregable platelets, and tumor activation of procoagulant blood factors.

9. Does anesthesia predispose to the formation of DVT?

Yes. The associated risk with general anesthesia is greater than with spinal or epidural anesthesia. This is attributed to the muscle relaxation and altered fibrinolytic activity observed with general anesthetic agents.

10. What is the clinical presentation of DVT?

The signs and symptoms of DVT are variable, and the clinical assessment is often unreliable. Studies have documented an unacceptably low sensitivity and specificity of clinical examination alone in detecting DVT. The classic clinical findings include extremity swelling, leg pain, a palpable cord, increased skin temperature, and Homan's sign (pain on dorsiflexion of the foot). Clinical suspicion for DVT warrants further evaluation with imaging.

11. What does the clinical differential diagnosis of DVT include?

Cellulitis, calf hematoma, muscle strain, arthritis, Baker's cyst, and bursitis. These all can mimic the clinical presentation of DVT.

12. What imaging studies are available for detection of DVT?

• Sonography	• Impedance plethysmography
• Contrast venography	• Nuclear medicine phlebography
• Magnetic resonance imaging	

13. What is the most widely used imaging modality for detection of DVT?

Ultrasonography, which incorporates B-mode imaging with pulsed Doppler and color Doppler techniques. B-mode ultrasound is real-time imaging of the deep veins; Doppler ultrasound determines blood flow direction and velocity based on alterations in the sound wave frequency of moving blood. Color Doppler detects blood flow and assigns a color based on the velocity and direction of flow. Pulsed and color Doppler are adjuncts to B-mode ultrasonography in the evaluation for suspected DVT.

14. How is an extremity ultrasound examination for suspected DVT performed?

The exam can be performed in the sonography suite or at the bedside. The deep venous system, from the inguinal ligament to the proximal calf, is evaluated using B-mode (gray-scale) imaging with sequential transverse compression at intervals of 1–2 cm. Pulsed Doppler signal is obtained at various levels with and without augmentation with manual squeezing of the extremity. If the calf is squeezed and the deep venous system is patent, augmentation should increase venous flow.

15. What is the ultrasound appearance of a normal vein?

A normal vein is freely compressible and demonstrates a classic venous Doppler signal (Fig. 1). The vein also demonstrates a change in Doppler signal with the respiratory cycle, called phasicity.

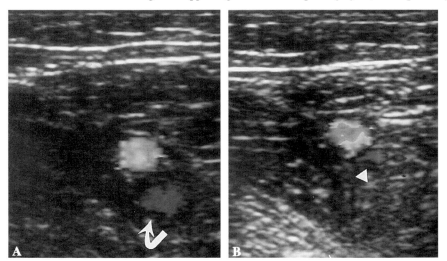

FIGURE 1. Doppler sonogram of normal superficial femoral vein. *A,* Noncompressed image demonstrates Doppler flow in vein (curved arrow). *B,* Image with manual compression demonstrates collapse of the vein (arrowhead) indicating absence of thrombus.

16. What are the ultrasound findings in acute DVT?

The most sensitive and specific finding in DVT is noncompressibility of the vein when gray-scale imaging is performed. Additional findings include absent Doppler signal, isoechoic or hyperechoic intraluminal thrombus, absent phasicity, absent augmentation, and an expanded vein diameter measuring 50% more than the accompanying vein.

17. What are the ultrasound findings of chronic DVT?

1. Thickened venous walls
2. Collateral veins
3. Dampened phasicity
4. Diminished augmentation
5. Patent veins that are noncompressible

18. What are the limitations of extremity ultrasound examination for DVT?

The accuracy for DVT detection is limited by technical factors including extremity edema, overlying arterial calcifications, overlying collateral vessels, large body habitus, unrecognized multiple of duplicated veins, and lack of patient cooperation.

19. What are the complications of extremity ultrasound examination for DVT?

The exam is accurate, noninvasive, and relatively risk free. The only reported complication, inadvertent dislodgment of a femoral DVT and secondary pulmonary embolism during a compression ultrasound, is rare.

20. What is the technique for lower extremity venography?

Lower extremity venography enables evaluation of the deep veins in the pelvis, thigh, and calf. The venogram is performed by placement of a 19- to 23-gauge butterfly needle in a peripheral vein on the dorsum of the foot. The needle should be directed toward the toe to enhance filling of the lateral and medial plantar veins, which empty into the deep venous system. Approximately 50–150 ml of contrast is injected and sequential radiographs in two views are obtained from the foot to the pelvis. Tourniquets are applied around the calf and thigh to direct the contrast into the deep venous system. A study is considered positive if an intraluminal filling defect is detected on more than one view. The sensitivity is 100% for clots greater than 5 mm. The procedure's technical success is limited by extremity edema, poor venous access, preferential filling of the superficial venous system, occasional difficulty in image interpretation, and complications.

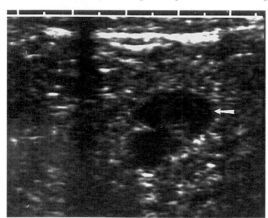

FIGURE 2. Doppler sonogram of deep venous thrombosis (DVT). Echogenic thrombus is noted within the vein lumen (arrow).

21. What are the venographic findings of acute DVT?

The most specific finding is a smooth, intraluminal venous filling defect with contrast outlining the clot, resulting in a "tram-track" appearance (Fig. 3). Additional findings include an abrupt vein cutoff, nonfilling of a venous segment, absence of venous collaterals, and a "capping defect," which refers to the meniscus-like convex superior or inferior margin of the thrombus within the contrast column.

22. What are the venographic findings of subacute and chronic DVT?

Subacute DVT refers to clot that is 1–4 weeks old. A chronic DVT is thrombus more than 4 weeks old. During the subacute and chronic phases, the thrombus undergoes clot retraction. As a result, the once smooth filling defect becomes eccentric, irregular, and adherent to the vein wall. The organized thrombus also can calcify. The incorporation of thrombus into the vein wall results in luminal compromise and narrowing. The thrombus can undergo recanalization, which appears as multiple small thread-like channels within the thrombosed venous segment. The organization, healing, and recanalization of intraluminal thrombus usually damage the underlying valves and render them incompetent. Extensive venous collaterals develop with chronic DVT (Fig. 4).

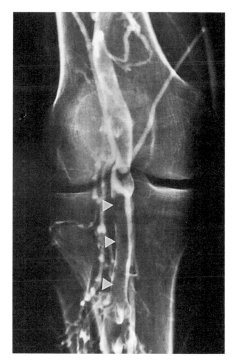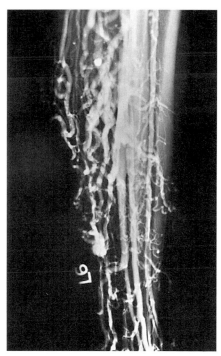

FIGURE 3 *(Left).*   Acute deep venous thrombosis (DVT) of popliteal vein. Note the intraluminal filling defect (arrowheads) and "tram-tracking" of contrast around the thrombus.

FIGURE 4 *(Right).*   Chronic lower-extremity deep venous thrombosis (DVT) with abundant collaterals.

23. What is a free-floating thrombus?

A clot that is nearly completely surrounded by contrast on venography (Fig. 5). There is usually a small attachment to a larger thrombus or the vein wall. These thrombi are at great risk for dislodgment and embolization to the lungs. Free-floating venous thrombus is considered an indication for caval interruption (placement of a inferior vena caval filter) as prophylaxis against pulmonary embolism.

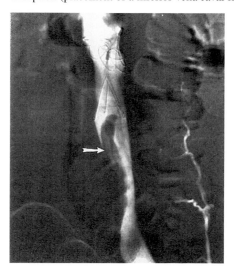

FIGURE 5.   Right common iliac vein deep venous thrombosis (DVT) with extension into the inferior vena cava (arrow).

24. What is the fate of a calf DVT?

About 40% of calf DVTs resolve spontaneously without anticoagulation. An additional 40% retract and become recanalized without extension above the knee. The remaining 20% propagate into the popliteal and femoral veins, a location where there is significant risk of embolization of thrombus into the pulmonary circulation.

25. What venographic artifacts can cause misinterpretations?

Air emboli, contrast layering, pseudothrombus, nonfilling of a venous segment, and venous compression from an extrinsic process. A pseudothrombus is nonopacification of a focal vein segment secondary to inflow from an adjacent nonopacified venous branch. Extrinsic compression of veins from masses, muscle bundles, crossing vessels, or tourniquets can mimic venous occlusion. Recognition of these venographic pitfalls is important to prevent misinterpretation of a study.

26. What are the complications of venography?

Thrombophlebitis, allergic contrast reaction, and extravasation of contrast into the soft tissues. The complication rate varies with the type, volume, and concentration of contrast material. The incidence of postvenography thrombophlebitis is less than 10%. DVT develops as a result of contrast-induced phlebitis. The risk of this complication can be reduced by flushing the limb veins with saline or heparin and by minimizing the contrast volume. Allergic contrast reactions in patients undergoing contrast venography are rare, with minor cases of hives representing most cases. Extravasation of contrast into the soft tissues can result in local skin necrosis, ulceration, or cellulitis. Patients with diabetes or atherosclerotic disease are at greater risk for complications of contrast extravasation.

27. What is the role of magnetic resonance imaging in DVT?

The role of MRI for DVT detection was initially investigational but has found some clinical utility, especially for examination of the deep pelvic veins, which cannot be readily examined with ultrasound. The potential advantages of MRI include its noninvasiveness and the ability to demonstrate extravascular disease. Also, no intravenous contrast is needed. The exact role of MRI in the diagnosis of DVT is unknown; it is usually more expensive than ultrasound.

28. What is the role of impedance plethysmography (IPG) in the diagnosis of DVT?

IPG is a noninvasive exam that is used to detect DVT. The technique is based on the principle that abnormal venous blood flow can produce alterations in impedance (electrical resistance). Impedance is increased in the setting of compromised venous blood flow. The primary limitation of IPG is poor sensitivity and specificity for DVT below the popliteal vessels. False-negative exams occur as IPG detects alterations in venous flow, not the thrombus itself. IPG currently has little role in the workup of suspected DVT.

29. What are the complications of DVT?
- Pulmonary embolism
- Chronic postphlebitic syndrome
- Phlegmasia cerulea dolens
- Phlegmasia alba dolens
- Amputation
- Death

30. What is phlegmasia cerulea dolens?

A rare clinical condition that develops in 1% of patients with DVT. It is characterized by extensive thrombus formation in the deep and superficial venous circulation. The venous thrombosis results in venous hypertension and secondary increased interstitial pressure that limits arterial inflow and causes arterial insufficiency. Clinically, the limb is markedly swollen with a bluish skin discoloration and varying stages of superficial gangrene. This condition is associated with underlying malignancy. Treatment options include anticoagulation, thrombolysis, and surgical thrombectomy. The condition is associated with a high morbidity and mortality. Complications of phlegmasia cerulea dolens include venous gangrene, amputation, pulmonary embolism, and death.

31. What is phlegmasia alba dolens?

A clinical condition associated with iliofemoral DVT. The affected limb is markedly edematous and white. The edema is the result of iliofemoral vein and perivenous lymphatic obstruction. The arterial inflow is preserved. The condition is associated with pelvic surgery and pregnancy. Phlegmasia alba dolens is more common and less severe than phlegmasia cerulea dolens.

32. What is thrombophlebitis migrans?

A rare condition characterized by extremity and mesenteric venous thrombosis. The condition is associated with Buerger's disease, malignancy, and hypercoagulable states.

33. What is the chronic postphlebitic syndrome?

The most common cause of long-term morbidity and disability from DVT. The syndrome is characterized by pain, swelling, chronic venous insufficiency, venous claudication, ulceration, and skin changes. The syndrome is attributed to venous obstruction and to clot organization at the valve level, with secondary valvular dysfunction.

34. What are the treatment options for DVT?

The treatment options for DVT are varied and controversial. The goals of DVT treatment are to prevent postphlebitic syndrome and pulmonary embolism by preserving venous patency and valvular function. The treatment options for DVT are anticoagulation, catheter-directed thrombolysis, and surgical thrombectomy. The treatment should be individualized to the patient's clinical presentation and relative risk-benefit ratio of each therapy considered.

35. What is the conservative treatment for DVT?

A regimen of bedrest, leg elevation, and anticoagulation with heparin followed by conversion to (oral) warfarin. Ambulation is encouraged after resolution of the pain and swelling.

36. How effective is heparin and warfarin treatment for DVT?

The most widely accepted treatment regimen for lower-extremity DVT is anticoagulation with systemic heparin and subsequent conversion to warfarin. Despite acceptance of this protocol, studies have demonstrated the results to be unsatisfactory in terms of vein recanalization and avoidance of postphlebitic syndrome. A published review of 13 studies found that only 18% of patients with acute DVT treated with heparin demonstrated complete or partial clot lysis. The limited efficacy of DVT treatment with heparin and warfarin has led to investigation of alternative treatment strategies.

37. What is the role of systemic thrombolytic therapy for treatment of DVT?

The role is limited. Investigation of DVT treated with intravenous streptokinase found only a 20% clot dissolution rate. The success of streptokinase has been limited by the frequency of incomplete clot lysis, immunity to the agent, and a significant incidence of bleeding complications.

38. What is the role of catheter-directed thrombolysis in treatment of DVT?

Catheter-directed thrombolysis is an alternative treatment for DVT that is under investigation. Given the success of transcatheter thrombolytic therapy for arterial thrombotic disease, the principles and techniques have been applied to venous thrombosis. The rationale of catheter-directed thrombolytic therapy is to deliver the agent to the thrombus in the safest and most efficacious manner.

39. What are the potential advantages or catheter-directed thrombolysis?

- Guaranteed exposure of the lytic agent to clot
- Increased contact area of lytic agent with thrombus
- Containment of lytic agent within a clot to minimize systemic hemodilution and side effects
- Intraclot administration facilitates administration of higher concentrations of the lytic agent
- The first-pass clearance of the lytic agent by the liver is avoided (Fig. 6)

The preliminary results of catheter-directed thrombolysis are encouraging; a 70% complete lysis rate has been reported in one study using urokinase.

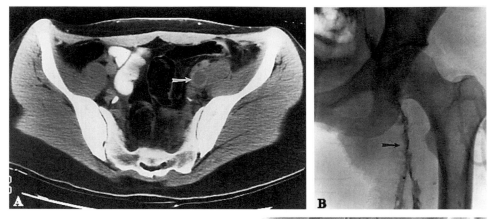

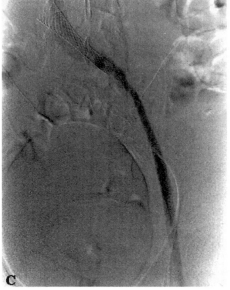

FIGURE 6. Acute iliofemoral deep venous thrombosis (DVT) of left lower-extremity. *A*, CT and *B*, venogram before thrombolysis demonstrates extensive DVT (arrows). *C*, Venogram after catheter-directed thrombolysis demonstrates restored venous patency.

BIBLIOGRAPHY

1. Bettmann MA, Robbins A, Braun SD, et al: Contrast venography of the leg: Diagnostic efficacy, tolerance, and complication rates with ionic and nonionic contrast media. Radiology 165:113–116, 1987.
2. Comerota AJ, Aldridge SC: Appropriate therapy for acute lower-extremity venous thrombosis. In Whittemore AD, Bandyk DF, Cronenwett JL, et al (eds): Advances in Vascular Surgery. St. Louis, Mosby, 1993, pp 213–224.
3. Dale A: Venous gangrene. In Bergan JJ, Yao JST (eds): Vascular Surgical Emergencies. Orlando, FL, Grune & Stratton, 1987, p 443.
4. Dorfman GS, Cronan JJ, Messersmith RN, et al: Occult pulmonary embolism: A common occurrence in deep venous thrombosis. AJR 148:263–266, 1987.
5. Hull RD, Hirsch J, Carter CJ, et al: Pulmonary angiography, ventilation lung scanning, and venography for clinically suspected pulmonary embolism with abnormal perfusion lung scan. Ann Intern Med 98:891–899, 1983.
6. Perlin SJ: Pulmonary embolism during compression US of the lower extremity. Radiology 184:165–166, 1992.
7. Semba CP, Dake MD: Iliofemoral deep venous thrombosis: Aggressive therapy with catheter-directed thrombolysis. Radiology 191:487–494, 1994.
8. Thery C, Bauchart JJ, Lesenne M, et al: Predictive factors of effectiveness of streptokinase in deep venous thrombosis. Am J Cardiol 69:117–122, 1992.

XII. Miscellaneous Topics

---

83. THYROID AND PARATHYROID IMAGING

Zachary D. Grossman, M.D., and Douglas S. Katz, M.D.

---

1. When a nodule is discovered in a patient's thyroid, what is the most accurate diagnostic examination?

If the nodule is believed to be within the thyroid, fine needle aspiration biopsy (FNAB), interpreted by an experienced cytopathologist, is the most accurate diagnostic examination. The biopsy is usually atraumatic and safe.

2. If FNAB is the most accurate and direct diagnostic exam, what is the role of ultrasound?

For additional information prior to potential biopsy. For example, to determine if the nodule is actually in the thyroid, ultrasound is appropriate. Ultrasound also can provide imaging guidance if the nodule is vaguely defined on physical examination.

3. What is the significance of small nodules and what is meant by a "dominant" thyroid nodule on ultrasound examination?

Often, small nodules, usually of no significance, are found incidentally on ultrasound examination. Therefore, ultrasound should be performed only for good reason. Small nodules are so common that patients would be poorly served if all the nodules were biopsied. Some authorities believe that only dominant nodules, 1–2 cm or larger, require tissue diagnosis.

4. Is there anything specific about thyroid cancer on ultrasound?

Unfortunately not. Cancer can have a variety of appearances, none of which are specific.

5. What role does nuclear medicine play in determining the nature of a thyroid nodule?

The most cost-effective approach for diagnosing a palpable nodule is FNAB without imaging. However, if the patient does not want a biopsy initially, or if a nonpalpable dominant abnormality is discovered on ultrasound (and the patient does not want a biopsy), a nuclear scan can be performed. If the nodule has normal or increased activity on a radioiodine scan, cancer is effectively excluded (Fig. 1). "Cold" nodules, or areas of decreased activity on the thyroid scan, are nonspecific and may be due to cancer or benign causes such as adenomas or cysts (Fig. 2).

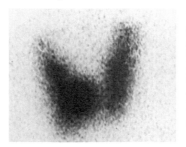 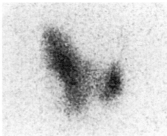

FIGURE 1 *(Left).*   "Hot" nodule at the junction of the right thyroid lobe and the isthmus.

FIGURE 2 *(Right).*   "Cold" nodule in the lateral aspect of the right thyroid lobe.

6. What radiopharmaceutical is usually used instead of radioiodine to scan the thyroid?
Technetium-99m-pertechnetate, a radiopharmaceutical that has a charge and molecular radius similar to that of iodine, is effective. I-123, the isotope of iodine that is used for diagnostic imaging of the thyroid, is expensive and not readily available.

7. Other than for work-up of a nodule, what are the uses for a nuclear scan of the thyroid?
• Evaluating an enlarged thyroid gland
• Evaluating a known or suspected multinodular goiter
• Evaluating a large, tender thyroid

8. On a thyroid nuclear scan, what is the appearance of the thyroid gland in Graves' disease?
The gland is enlarged, there is diffusely increased uptake, and a pyramidal lobe is often visualized.

9. On a thyroid nuclear scan, what is the appearance of the thyroid in toxic multinodular goiter?
There are usually multiple "hot" nodules that suppress the remainder of the gland by producing enough T4 and T3 to suppress TSH by "feedback inhibition."

10. In subacute thyroiditis, what is the appearance of the thyroid on a nuclear scan?
Almost no uptake. The gland is enlarged and tender.

11. In what other noninfectious and noninflammatory condition is there almost no thyroid uptake on a nuclear scan, and yet the patient is hyperthyroid?
Surreptitious intake of thyroid hormone (usually to lose weight).

12. What are the types of thyroid cancer?
Papillary, follicular, medullary, anaplastic, and Hürthle cell.

13. What type of thyroid cancer has the best prognosis?
Papillary cancer, which has an extraordinarily high rate of cure and survival. Even if local lymph node metastases are present, the prognosis is unchanged.

14. To what site does follicular cancer have a tendency to spread?
The lungs.

15. What is the typical appearance of a bony metastasis from thyroid cancer?
A lytic lesion, which may be "bubbly" or have a "blownout" appearance.

16. What is the typical size of a metastasis to the lung from the thyroid?
Thyroid cancer has a tendency to form multiple nodules in the lung, which may create a miliary pattern.

17. What are some other causes of a miliary pattern in the lungs?
Other metastases, tuberculosis, fungal diseases, sarcoidosis, and *Pneumocystis carinii* pneumonia.

18. Thyroid cancer is in the same "family" of metastases as renal cancer and melanoma in that it is quite vascular. How does this manifest on imaging studies?
Vascular metastases tend to be bright (echogenic) on ultrasound (e.g., in the liver). They also have a tendency to bleed (e.g., in the brain).

19. What type of thyroid cancer has a dismal prognosis?
Anaplastic cancer.

20. What type of thyroid cancer is associated with multiple endocrine neoplasia syndromes?
Medullary cancer of the thyroid.

21. Is thyroid cancer common at autopsy?

If one looks carefully at the thyroid histologically, small foci of cancer are common at autopsy. These are almost always incidental findings unrelated to the cause of death. Likewise, in living people, small foci are common, especially in the elderly. This is another reason not to screen the thyroid with ultrasound; subclinical lesions will be discovered that lead to expensive work-ups and therapies.

22. What is the standard treatment for thyroid cancer?

Near-total thyroidectomy with a postoperative ablative dose of radioiodine. Over the next few years, the patient periodically returns to the nuclear medicine department for a thyroid cancer search.

23. How is a thyroid cancer search performed?

The patient is instructed to stop hormone replacement for several weeks so that endogenous thyroid stimulating hormone levels rise, which increases the sensitivity of a thyroid nuclear search scan. The scan is performed after administration of an oral dose of I-131. After 2–3 days, the patient undergoes a whole body scan (the half-life of I-131 is about 8 days) (Fig. 3). If occult abnormal activity is detected, the patient may be treated with a subsequent and larger dose of I-131 in an attempt to ablate the residual disease. If the scan is normal, the patient resumes thyroid hormone replacement. Abnormal uptake in palpable disease, especially in the neck, is sometimes resected (Figs. 4 and 5).

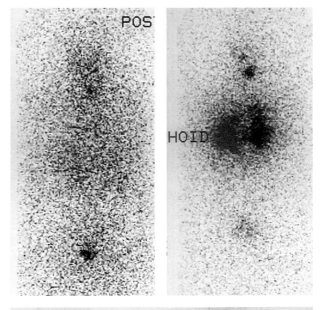

FIGURE 3 *(Left)*. Normal postthyroidectomy I-131 total body thyroid cancer search.

FIGURE 4 *(Right)*. Multiple lung metastases revealed by I-131 total body thyroid cancer search.

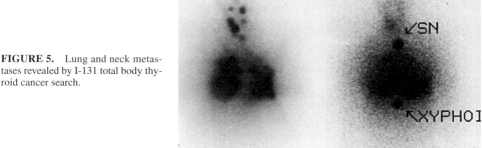

FIGURE 5. Lung and neck metastases revealed by I-131 total body thyroid cancer search.

24. What is the treatment if there is evidence of significant tumor burden such as bony metastases on the thyroid search scan?

Only 29.9 mCi or less of I-131 can be given to an outpatient. Typically, much higher doses are needed to treat metastatic thyroid cancer other than local neck metastases, and the patient must be hospitalized. Specialized procedures are needed to protect the hospital staff from the radiation that is administered to the patient orally. This type of treatment should be performed only by qualified nuclear medicine physicians with the appropriate facilities, training, and nuclear regulatory agency licenses.

25. Is there a role for chemotherapy in the routine treatment of thyroid metastases?

No. No current chemotherapy is as effective as I-131.

26. What is the role of imaging in diagnosing abnormalities of the parathyroid glands?

This is a controversial topic. Many surgeons will operate on the neck of a patient with a suspected parathyroid adenoma without any preoperative imaging, and they will reserve imaging for detecting parathyroid adenomas if the first surgery was unsuccessful. Others want preoperative imaging to localize the suspected site.

27. If imaging is to be performed, what are the options?

Nuclear imaging, ultrasound, MR, CT, and venous sampling.

28. Which imaging test is most frequently used?

Nuclear imaging of the parathyroids. The best nuclear medicine study for the parathyroids is to inject technetium-99m sestamibi intravenously and to image the neck using SPECT (computed tomographic nuclear imaging) soon after injection and with delayed images (1–2 hours later). Parathyroid adenomas have a strong tendency to take up the radiopharmaceutical and hold onto it so that an adenoma is more visible on the delayed images, after the sestamibi washes out of the normal adjacent thyroid (Fig. 6).

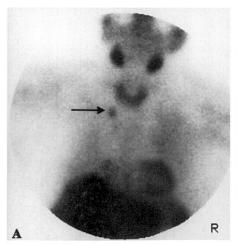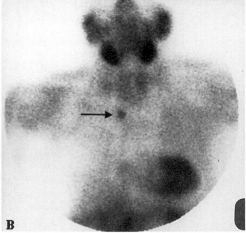

FIGURE 6.   *A*, Early sestamibi parathyroid scan image. Note (from top to bottom) salivary glands, thyroid, parathyroid adenoma (arrow), myocardium, and liver. *B*, Late sestamibi parathyroid image. Thyroid intensity has decreased, but the parathyroid lesion (arrow) remains intense.

29. What are some pitfalls of this exam?

Occasionally a focal thyroid lesion such as an adenoma may take up sestamibi, as will multiple adenomas and hyperplastic glands.

30. Where is an ectopic parathyroid adenoma typically located?
In the thorax, in the region of the tracheoesophageal groove.

31. Is there a role for ultrasound in diagnosing parathyroid adenomas?
Yes. For preoperative localization, ultrasound, in experienced hands using state-of-the-art equipment, is a good examination for finding parathyroid adenomas. They are typically found at the inferior aspect of the thyroid and occasionally may be found within the thyroid itself.

BIBLIOGRAPHY

1. Som PM, Curtin HD: Head and Neck Imaging, 3rd ed. St. Louis, Mosby, 1996.

84. SINUSITIS

Barbara Zeifer, M.D.

1. What are the radiographic features of acute sinusitis?
Acute sinusitis refers to a sinus infection lasting from one day to one month. Acute sinusitis is usually associated with rhinitis. Imaging studies demonstrate thickening of the sinus mucosa—a finding that is not specific for either acute or chronic sinus infection. However, an air-fluid level is indicative of acute sinusitis (Fig. 1).

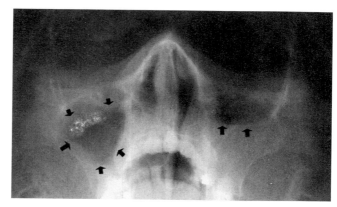

FIGURE 1. Acute sinusitis. Upright Waters' view. There is a sharply defined air-fluid level in the left maxillary antrum (arrows) due to acute sinusitis. Mucosal thickening in the right antrum (arrow) may represent either acute or chronic disease.

2. What are the radiographic features of chronic sinusitis?
Chronic sinusitis refers to a sinus infection that has persisted for longer than three months and is felt to create irreversible mucosal thickening. As mentioned above, this thickening is not radiographically specific and cannot be distinguished from acute mucosal edema. In severe and long-standing sinusitis bony thickening of the sinus walls may occur, particularly in the sphenoid sinus (Fig. 2). This is the only finding that enables the radiologist to make a definitive diagnosis of chronic sinusitis.

3. What is the nasal cycle?
Each individual has a nasal cycle during which the mucosa of the middle and inferior turbinate swells on one side, while the mucosa of the middle and inferior turbinate on the other side constricts. The length of this cycle varies from 30 minutes to 7 hours. The imaging correlate of the nasal cycle is asymmetry of the thickness of the turbinates (on CT). The "swollen" side never occludes the nasal cavity, in contrast to findings in acute rhinitis, and should be recognized as a normal finding.

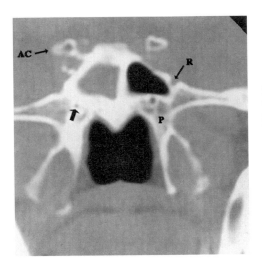

FIGURE 2. Chronic sphenoid sinusitis. Coronal CT. There is marked reactive bony thickening of the right sphenoid sinus walls due to chronic inflammation. The sinus cavity is opacified, which may be due to chronic inflammation or superimposed acute sinusitis. Note the bony encroachment on the Vidian canal (arrow). P = pterygoid process; AC = anterior clinoid process; R = foramen rotundum.

4. What is the role of conventional radiography in the evaluation of suspected sinusitis?

Plain radiography plays a limited role in sinus imaging. The only definite indication for plain films in suspected sinusitis is to determine whether or not an air-fluid level is present in the frontal or maxillary sinus. The plain film otherwise provides inadequate anatomic detail, and cannot precisely define the location and extent of sinus disease.

5. When should computed tomography be performed for acute sinusitis?

To evaluate suspected complications of acute sinusitis, when surgical drainage is planned, and when the diagnosis is uncertain.

Patients with uncomplicated acute sinusitis are managed medically, and CT is not indicated.

6. What are some complications of acute sinusitis?

Orbital cellulitis, orbital abscess, meningitis, cerebritis, epidural abscess, and cerebral abscess.

7. When should a CT be obtained in patients with chronic sinusitis?

Patients with recurrent acute or chronic sinusitis that is incompletely controlled by medical therapy may be candidates for functional endoscopic sinus surgery (FESS). Computed tomography plays a critical role in evaluating these patients, as the exact location and extent of disease is shown. CT also reveals anatomic variations that predispose patients to develop sinusitis; these variations must be identified preoperatively to avoid surgical complications. CT is also indicated if the diagnosis of chronic sinusitis is uncertain.

8. What is the role of MR in the evaluation of sinusitis?

MR plays a limited role. CT reveals the detailed bony anatomy of the sinuses, while cortical bone produces no signal on MR images. MR, however, is the examination of choice for the evaluation of intracranial complications of sinusitis, and to distinguish inflammatory from neoplastic disease within the sinuses.

9. How are secretions normally cleared from the sinuses? How does sinusitis develop?

Normally, mucociliary clearance propels mucus and debris through the narrow channels of the sinus drainage pathways. Any disease process that results in apposition of adjacent mucosal surfaces shuts down mucociliary clearance, producing obstruction of the sinuses and an environment where bacteria can proliferate. Mucosal edema from the common cold is a frequent precipitant of this sequence. Some anatomic variations of sinonasal anatomy distort and further narrow the drainage channels.

10. What is the ostiomeatal unit (OMU)?

The OMU refers to the complex drainage pathway of the maxillary, anterior ethmoid, and frontal sinuses into the middle nasal meatus. The components of the OMU include the uncinate plate, inner maxillary sinus ostium, infundibulum, semilunar hiatus, middle turbinate, middle nasal meatus, and the ethmoidal bulla (Fig. 3).

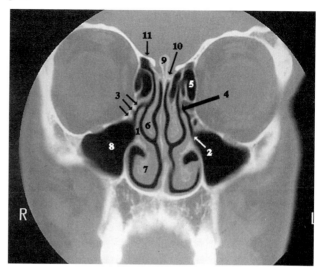

FIGURE 3. Ostiomeatal unit anatomy. Coronal CT: (1) uncinate plate; (2) inner maxillary sinus ostium; (3) infundibulum; (4) semilunar hiatus; (5) ethmoidal bulla; (6) middle turbinate in middle meatus; (7) inferior turbinate in inferior meatus; (8) maxillary antrum; (9) crista galli; (10) cribriform plate; (11) ethmoid roof.

11. What is the uncinate plate (or process)?

The uncinate plate or process is a curvilinear bony projection of the lateral nasal wall which is located behind the nasolacrimal duct. Its central portion has a free superior margin, above which is the slit of the semilunar hiatus. The air space lateral to the uncinate plate is the infundibulum. The infundibulum is continuous below with the inner maxillary sinus ostium and the maxillary antrum. It is continuous above with the semilunar hiatus, which opens directly into the middle nasal meatus.

12. What is the ethmoidal bulla?

The anterior ethmoid air cell that forms the roof of the hiatus semilunaris and at least some of the infundibulum. It may consist of a single large air cell, or 2–4 smaller air cells. The lateral wall of the ethmoidal bulla is the lamina papyracea.

13. How is the OMU optimally evaluated by CT?

The OMU should always be imaged in the direct coronal plane on CT. The anatomic components of the OMU are all clearly seen in this plane. Thin sections (3 mm) are routinely obtained, with the patient's neck extended so that direct coronal images can be acquired. If a patient cannot tolerate neck extension, 1 mm contiguous images can be obtained on a helical CT scanner, and coronal images can be reconstructed from the imaging data set.

14. What is functional endoscopic sinus surgery (FESS)?

A relatively recently developed but now widely accepted surgical technique during which a set of rigid, fiberoptic endoscopes is used to examine the nasal and sinus cavities. The tip of each endoscope is angled, ranging from 30 to 120 degrees, so that any portion of the sinonasal cavity can be visualized. Various specialized instruments (forceps, suction, probes, and small drills) are inserted alongside the viewing endoscope. FESS has essentially replaced external procedures that were used for the surgical treatment of sinusitis.

15. How does FESS alter the course of sinus disease?

The concept of FESS is to treat chronic or recurrent acute sinusitis by restoring normal physiology. The surgery is directed toward the central drainage pathways, especially the OMU, to relieve any obstruction of normal sinus drainage.

16. What is the frontal recess?

The drainage outlet of the frontal sinus. Older texts referred to this area as the nasofrontal duct, a term that is no longer used. The configuration of the frontal recess is determined by the development of the surrounding ethmoid air cells; it is not a discrete anatomic duct. The frontal recess consists of the frontal ostium and the space below it. The frontal recess empties into the middle nasal meatus, the anterior ethmoidal labyrinth, or the infundibulum, depending on the particular individual's anatomy (Fig. 4).

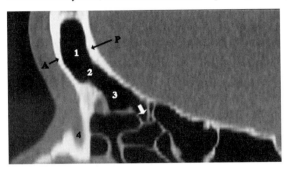

FIGURE 4.   Frontal recess. Sagittal CT reformation: (1) frontal sinus; (2) frontal ostium; (3) frontal recess; (4) nasolacrimal duct; (A) anterior table frontal sinus; (P) posterior table frontal sinus. The frontal recess does not end inferiorly (arrow) but has moved laterally out of the slice, and empties directly into the middle nasal meatus (not seen).

17. What is the sphenoethmoidal recess?

A cleft between the posterior ethmoid and the sphenoid sinus that is directly continuous with the superior nasal meatus below. The sphenoid ostium, located along the anterior wall of the sphenoid sinus, empties directly into the sphenoethmoidal recess. Drainage of the posterior ethmoid is variable and is not demonstrated on imaging studies.

18. What is a Haller cell?

An air cell within the bone of the orbital floor (Fig. 5). It is formed by progressive inferior pneumatization of the anterior ethmoid into the orbital floor. A Haller cell may impinge on the infundibulum.

19. What is a concha bullosa cell?

An air cell that has formed within the middle nasal turbinate (Fig. 5). It will occasionally have a wide and well-delineated superior opening, but usually the ostium is not identified on CT. A concha

FIGURE 5.   Normal variations of sinonasal anatomy. Coronal CT. The anterior ethmoid has pneumatized into the orbital floor, producing a Haller cell (H). Pneumatization of the middle turbinate has produced the concha bullosa cell (CB). In addition, pneumatization of the orbital roof has produced a supraorbital ethmoid air cell (SOE).

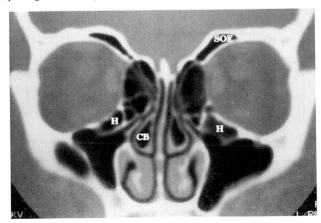

bullosa may interfere with air flow through the middle meatus and may adversely affect OMU drainage.

20. What is an agger nasi cell?

The agger nasi is the most anterior of all the anterior ethmoid air cells. Although it has a separate embryologic origin, it can be thought of as an air cell in the lacrimal bone, occasionally pneumatizing into the orbital plate of the ethmoid (lamina papyracea). A large agger nasi cell may form the floor of the frontal recess.

21. What is an Onodi cell?

A posterior ethmoidal air cell that has extended posteriorly to pneumatize the planum sphenoidale. The importance of this anatomic variation is that it results in a posterior ethmoid air cell bordering the optic canal, instead of the sphenoid sinus. Posterior ethmoid disease in patients with an Onodi cell may therefore affect the optic nerve; the optic nerve can be injured during posterior ethnoidectomy in such patients, as well.

22. What is granulomatous sinusitis?

A group of granuloma-forming inflammatory disorders that have common imaging features. There are many specific etiologies, both infectious and non-infectious. Acutely, granulomatous sinusitis is characterized by smooth as well as nodular soft-tissue swelling of the nasal mucosa. As the disease progresses septal perforation occurs, which is the radiographic hallmark of this disorder. The inflammatory process may eventually spread to the maxillary and ethmoid sinuses. Late in the course of the disease, bony destruction occurs and the mucosal swelling recedes. Endstage disease is characterized by formation of a smooth contiguous cavity that includes the nose and the involved sinuses.

23. What are the etiologies of granulomatous sinusitis?

Actinomycosis, nocardia, tuberculosis, syphilis, blastomycosis, Wegener's granulomatosis, sarcoidosis, and inhalation of beryllium, chromate salts, or cocaine.

24. Is lethal midline granuloma a form of granulomatous sinusitis?

No. This disorder may cause mucosal thickening as well as cartilaginous and bony destruction. However, lethal midline granuloma is now classified as a disorder related to lymphoma.

25. What are the imaging features of sinonasal polyps?

Sinonasal polyps may be single, multiple, or diffuse. All polyps are edematous, and are therefore low in density on CT, low in signal intensity on T1-weighted MR, and hyperintense on T2-weighted MR. Polyps are seen as smooth soft-tissue masses in the nasal cavity, which are most commonly found in the middle meatus. They tend to elongate inferiorly, and "drip" downward. An isolated sinus polyp is less frequent, producing a rounded or pedunculated soft-tissue mass in a sinus cavity.

26. What are the imaging features of diffuse sinonasal polyps?

In diffuse polyposis there are numerous polyps throughout the nose and involved sinus cavities. The pressure of these polyps may affect the surrounding bony structures with widening of the nasal cavity with splaying of the lateral nasal walls and expansion of involved air cells. These changes occur slowly over time so that the bony structures are displaced and possibly thinned, but are never grossly destroyed. There is severe impairment of sinus drainage. Secretions are entrapped and become dessicated, which on CT produces high attenuation material that insinuates between and around the individual low density polyps.

27. What is an antrochoanal polyp?

A specific type of polyp that originates in the maxillary sinus. The antrochoanal polyp initially fills the maxillary sinus, then eventually extrudes medially into the nasal cavity (Fig. 6). As the polyp enlarges, it works its way posteriorly toward the posterior nasal choana, where it may present as a nasopharyngeal mass.

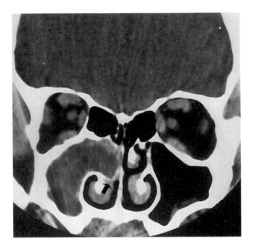

FIGURE 6. Antrochoanal polyp. Coronal CT. There is complete opacification of the right maxillary antrum by low density material. There is localized expansion of the lateral nasal wall. Surrounding the soft tissue material in the nose is a thin rim of bone (arrow), indicating that the polyp is enlarging slowly enough for the bone to remodel around it.

28. What is a retention cyst?

Retention cysts are classified as either mucous or serous cysts. A mucous retention cyst forms when a mucous gland becomes obstructed and expands. A serous retention cyst represents submucosal accumulation of fluid. These two entities are not distinguishable from one another, and both will appear similar to an isolated polyp as well. Retention cysts are most frequently found along the floor of the maxillary antrum, and are incidental findings on plain films in about 10% of the population. On imaging studies, retention cysts are sharply defined, rounded densities that contain fluid. A retention cyst may fill the entire sinus cavity but never alters the thickness or contour of the sinus wall. Clinically, they are of no significance.

29. What is a mucocele?

An obstructed sinus cavity that has expanded due to accumulation of thick secretions. A mucocele is most commonly produced in the frontal sinus (60–65% of all cases), followed by the ethmoid air cells (20–25%), the maxillary sinus (10%), and the sphenoid sinus (1–2%, but may be more common than previously thought).

30. What are the imaging features of a mucocele?

A mucocele produces expansion of a sinus cavity. The sinus walls become extremely thinned or dehiscent. Frontal and ethmoid mucoceles bulge into the orbit and/or the anterior cranial fossa; maxillary mucoceles bulge into the cheek; sphenoid mucoceles may impinge on the optic canal. The wall of a maxillary sinus mucocele may contain areas of both bony thickening and separate areas of bony thinning, due to underlying chronic inflammation and the expansile process, respectively (Fig. 7).

Mucoceles are low in density on CT. Protein content and hydration status affect the signal intensity pattern on MR. Theoretically, any pattern of signal intensity is possible. In practice, mucoceles are hyperintense on T2-weighted MR, and are either hypointense or hyperintense on T1-weighted sequences. The T2-weighted sequence will often demonstrate lower signal intensity mucoid concretions within the high signal fluid.

31. How can chronic fungal sinusitis in the normal host be distinguished from bacterial or viral sinusitis on imaging studies?

Imaging studies cannot reliably distinguish between these two entities, as both produce circumferential mucosal thickening. However, fungal sinusitis in the normal host is usually unilateral, often isolated to a single sinus cavity, and is refractory to standard medical therapy. Fluid collections are uncommon in fungal sinusitis, so that an air-fluid level would direct the diagnosis toward bacterial sinusitis. Chronic fungal sinusitis in the normal host is extremely rare.

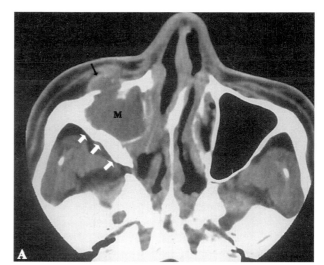

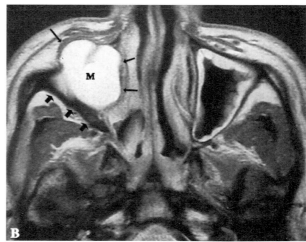

FIGURE 7. Maxillary mucocele. *A*, Axial CT. *B*, Axial T2-weighted MR. The CT scan demonstrates complete opacification of the right maxillary antrum by low density material (M). There is expansion of the entire lateral nasal wall, as well as the anterior maxilla, with marked thinning of bone. There is dehiscence of the anterior bony plate (arrow). There is thickening of the posterior antral wall (arrows), indicating underlying chronic inflammatory disease. On T2-weighted MR, the mucocele (M) is homogeneously high in signal intensity. The bony expansion (thin arrows) and bony thickening (thick arrows) are seen.

32. What organisms cause invasive fungal sinusitis?

Many fungal organisms cause invasive sinusitis. Most commonly, aspergillus is the responsible fungus. Mucormycosis is most often found in poorly controlled diabetics. These organisms invade blood vessels leading to thrombosis, infarction, and necrosis, with frequent intraorbital and intracranial extension.

A subset of diabetic patients with mucormycosis manifest a less aggressive and more chronic course; they recover from intermittent episodes of bony destruction with antifungal medication.

33. What is the radiographic appearance of a mycetoma?

A mycetoma is a collection of fungal hyphae and debris that does not invade the sinus mucosa. A mycetoma is hyperdense on CT. When the sphenoid sinus is involved the sinus walls may be thickened. A mycetoma is isointense to hypointense on T1-weighted MR images and is markedly low in signal on T2-weighted images.

34. What is allergic fungal sinusitis?

Allergic fungal sinusitis is produced by an allergic reaction to fungal antigens without mucosal infection or invasion. It is usually associated with nasal polyps in atopic individuals. Many fungi can produce this syndrome. Allergic fungal sinusitis is characterized by the accumulation of allergic mucin, which is extremely thick. The underlying mucosa is inflamed but not invaded by the fungi. The disease is eradicated by removal of this mucin, which requires endoscopic sinus surgery. Antifungal medication has no effect, but steroids are administered during the active phase of the disease.

35. What are the radiographic features of allergic fungal sinusitis?

A single or several ipsilateral sinus cavities may be involved, or there may be a more diffuse process. There is a thin rim of hypodense tissue, while the predominant sinus content is that of homogeneously dense material, which represents the mucin (Fig. 8). This mucin is denser than any cellular tissue could possibly be without intravenous contrast injection; this entity can therefore be distinguished from tumor. There may be remarkable enlargement of the involved sinus(es), often with bony destruction. The mucin is so hypointense on both T1- and T2-weighted MR images that the sinus erroneously appears aerated.

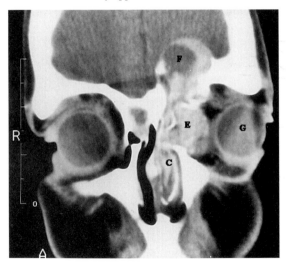

FIGURE 8. Allergic fungal sinusitis. Coronal CT. There is marked lateral expansion of the left anterior ethmoid (agger nasi) into the orbit, with lateral displacement of the globe. There is superior expansion of the left frontal sinus into the anterior cranial fossa; the dura remains intact. The concha bullosa cell is involved as well. Note the high-density contents of the involved sinuses, representing the allergic mucin. The low-density area in the left frontal sinus represents entrapped secretions or polyps. (F) Frontal sinus; (E) ethmoid sinus; (G) globe; (C) concha bullosa.

BIBLIOGRAPHY

1. Blitzer A, Lawson W: Fungal infections of the nose and paranasal sinuses. Otolaryngol Clin North Am 26:1007, 1993.
2. Corey JP, Delsupehe KG, Ferguson BJ: Allergic fungal sinusitis: Allergic, infectious, or both? Otolaryngol Head and Neck Surg 113:110, 1995.
3. Laine FJ, Smoker WR: The ostiomeatal unit and endoscopic surgery: Anatomy, variations, and imaging findings in inflammatory diseases. AJR 159:849, 1992.
4. Som PM, Curtin HD: Head and Neck Imaging, 3rd ed. St. Louis, Mosby, 1996.
5. Stammberger H: Functional Endoscopic Sinus Surgery. Philadelphia, B.C. Decker, 1991.
6. Yousem DM: Imaging of sinonasal inflammatory disease. Radiology 188:303, 1993.

INDEX

Page numbers in **boldface type** indicate complete chapters.